# Endocrine Surgery of the Head and Neck

# Endocrine Surgery of the Head and Neck

## Phillip K. Pellitteri, D.O., F.A.C.S.

Attending, Section of Head and Neck Surgery
Department of Otolaryngology/Head and Neck Surgery
Vice Chief, Division of Surgery
Geisinger Health System
Danville, Pennsylvania
and
Associate Professor of Clinical Surgery
Penn State College of Medicine
Hershey, Pennsylvania

## Thomas V. McCaffrey, M.D.

Department of Otolaryngology, Head and Neck Surgery
University of South Florida
Tampa, Florida

THOMSON

DELMAR LEARNING

Australia Canada Mexico Singapore Spain United Kingdom United States

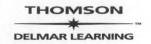

**THOMSON**

**DELMAR LEARNING**

Endocrine Surgery of the Head and Neck
by Phillip K. Pellitteri and Thomas V. McCaffrey

**Health Care Publishing Director:**
William Brottmiller

**Acquisitions Editor:**
Candice Janco

**Editorial Assistant:**
Maria D'Angelico

**Executive Marketing Manager:**
Dawn F. Gerrain

**Executive Editor:**
Cathy L. Esperti

**Project Editor:**
Mary Ellen Cox

**Production Coordinator:**
Anne Sherman

**Art/Design Coordinator:**
Jay Purcell

Library of Congress
Cataloging-in-Publication Data
Endocrine surgery of the head and neck / [edited by] Philip K. Pellitteri, Thomas V. McCaffrey.
    p. ; cm.
Includes bibliographical references and index.
  ISBN 0-7693-0091-X (alk. paper)
1. Thyroid gland—Surgery. 2. Parathyroid glands—Surgery. 3. Endocrine glands—Surgery.
  [DNLM: 1. Parathyroid Glands—surgery. 2. Thyroid Gland—surgery. 3. Endocrine Surgical Procedures. WK 280 E56 2003]
I. Pellitteri, Phillip K. II. McCaffrey, Thomas Vincent.
  RD599.5.T46 E536 2003
  617.5'39—dc21                    2002025605

## NOTICE TO THE READER

# Contents

# Preface

The surgical management of disease of the thyroid and parathyroid glands has evolved substantially over the past 50 years. Influential procedural and technologic developments that aid in diagnosis and therapy have resulted in improved clinical outcomes for patients with these disorders. Advances in the understanding of molecular genetics and oncogenesis, nuclear medicine technology for diagnosis and imaging, immunoradiometrics for hormone assessment, and innovative protocols for minimally invasive surgery are several highlight areas that have underscored the exponential growth of endocrine surgery.

It is with a sense of great pride and accomplishment that we offer this initial edition of *Endocrine Surgery of the Head and Neck*. This text was designed to offer a comprehensive discussion on the surgical management of endocrine disorders of the head and neck, principally those attributed to the thyroid and parathyroid glands. In developing the text, the editors have endeavored to capture the collaborative multidisciplinary philosophy essential to treatment of these disorders by enlisting the contributions of authorities in their focused areas of achievement and expertise so that a comprehensive and broad representation exists across all related disciplines.

The book is divided into two sections composed of thyroid and parathyroid disorders. Each section addresses fundamental pathophysiologic and contemporary management principles for each system. The focus of the text is to present current, state of the art, practical management information that is clinically applicable, pragmatic, and cost-effective. In so doing, the book offers perspectives on embryologic development and anatomy; epidemiology, genetics, and pathophysiology; evaluation and diagnostic protocols; and therapeutics, both medical and surgical, for a comprehensive array of disorders of the thyroid and parathyroid glands. It is our hope that the text will serve as a comprehensive, practical management source and reference standard for physicians and surgeons dedicated to the treatment of patients with endocrine disorders of the head and neck.

Phillip K. Pellitteri D.O., F.A.C.S.

# Contributors

**Mark Aferzon, M.D.**
Otolaryngology Resident
Geisinger Medical Center
Danville, Pennsylvania

**Anil T. Ahuja, M.B.B.S., M.D., F.R.C.R., F.H.K.C.R., K.H.K.A.M.**
Associate Professor
Department of Diagnostic Radiology and Organ Imaging
The Chinese University of Hong Kong
Prince of Wales Hospital
Shatin, NT, Hong Kong

**Peter E. Anderson, M.D.**
Associate Professor
Department of Otlaryngology Head and Neck Surgery
Oregon Health Sciences University
Portland, Oregon

**Zubair W. Baloch, M.D., Ph.D.**
Assistant Professor of Pathology
University of Pennsylvania Medical Center
Philadelphia, Pennsylvania

**Kenneth D. Burman, M.D.**
Washington Hospital Center
Uniformed Services
University of the Health Sciences
Washington, DC

**Fernando Cabanillas, M.D., F.A.C.P.**
Ashbel Smith Professor of Medicine
Chairman, Department of Lymphoma/Myeloma
The University of Texas M.D. Anderson Cancer Center
Houston, Texas

**Joseph Califano, M.D.**
Assistant Professor
Department of Otolaryngology—Head and Neck Surgery
Baltimore, Maryland

**W. Bradford Carter, M.D.**
Associate Professor, Department of Surgery
Director of Endocrine Surgery
University of Maryland Medicine
Baltimore, Maryland

**Bart L. Clarke, M.D.**
Assistant Professor of Medicine
Mayo Medical School
Rochester, Minnesota

**James Cohen, M.D., Ph.D.**
Associate Professor
Department of Otolaryngology Head and Neck Surgery
Oregon Health Sciences University
Portland, Oregon

**Anthony C. De la Cruz, M.D.**
Department of Otolaryngology
Harvard Medical School
Massachusetts Eye and Ear Infirmary
Boston, Massachusetts

**Ann D. Dunn,**
Research Associate Professor of Medicine, Retired
University of Virginia Medical School
Charlottesville, Virginia

**Douglas B. Evans, M.D.**
Professor of Surgery
Department of Surgical Oncology
University of Texas M.D. Anderson Cancer Center
Houston, Texas

**William B. Farrar, M.D.**
Director of Medical Affairs
Chief, Division of Surgical Oncology
The Arthur G. James Cancer Hospital
and
Richard J. Solove Research Institute
Columbus, Ohio

**William C. Faquin, M.D., Ph.D.**
Assistant Professor of Pathology
Harvard Medical School
and
Assistant Pathologist
Department of Pathology
Massachusetts General Hospital
Boston, Massachusetts

**Douglas L. Fraker, M.D.**
Jonathan Rhoads Associate Professor of Surgery, Chief
Division of Surgical Oncology
University of Pennsylvania
Philadelphia, Pennsylvania

**Michael Friedman, M.D.**
Professor and Chairman
Section of Head and Neck Surgery
Department of Otolaryngology and
Bronchoesophagology
Rush Presbyterian-St. Luke's Medical Center
Chicago, Illinois

**Richard M. Gall, F.R.C.S.C.**
Department of Otolaryngology
Mt. Sinai Hospital
Toronto, Ontario, Canada

**Robert F. Gagel, M.D.**
Professor of Medicine, Head (ad interim)
Division of Internal Medicine
The University of Texas M.D. Anderson Cancer Center
Houston, Texas

**Sofia Garcia-Buder, M.D.**

**Brian M. Ginzburg, M.B.B.C.H., F.R.C.P.C.**
Assistant Professor
Department of Medical Imaging
University of Toronto
Toronto, Ontario, Canada

**Ana M. Grau, M.D.**
Surgical Oncology Fellow
Department of Surgical Oncology
The University of Texas M.D. Anderson Cancer Center
Houston, Texas

**Chul S. Ha, M.D.**
Associate Professor of Radiation Oncology
Department of Radiation Oncology
The University of Texas M.D. Anderson Cancer Center
Houston, Texas

**John T. Hansen, Ph.D.**
Professor and Associate Dean
Department of Neurobiology and Anatomy
University of Rochester School of Medicine and Dentistry
Rochester, New York

**Diane Hershock, M.D., Ph.D.**
Assistant Professor of Medicine
Hospital of the University of Pennsylvania
Philadelphia, Pennsylvania

**Ana Olweira Hoff, M.D.**
Albert Einstein Hospital
Centro Paulista de Oncologia
Sao Paulo, Brazil

**Daniel W. Karakla, M.D., F.A.C.S.**
Associate Professor
Department of Otolaryngology/Head and Neck
Surgery
Eastern Virginia Medical School
Norfolk, Virginia

**Thomas Kennedy, M.D., F.A.C.S.**
Associate Professor
Jefferson Medical College
Director, Department of Otolaryngology/Head and
Neck Surgery
Geisinger Medical Center
Danville, Pennsylvania

**Barbara Kinder, M.D.**
Carmalt Professor of Surgery
Department of Surgery
Yale University School of Medicine
New Haven, Connecticut

**Douglas Klotch, M.D.**
Clinical Professor of Surgery
Tampa, Florida

**Dennis H. Kraus, M.D.**
Associate Attending, Head and Neck Service,
Department of Surgery
Director, Speech, Hearing, and Rehabilitation Center
Memorial Sloan-Kettering Cancer Center
New York, New York

**NiNi Ku, M.D.**
Clinical Associate Professor of Pathology
University of South Florida
College of Medicine
Tampa, Florida
and
Director of Cytopathology
Bayfront Medical Center
St. Petersburg, Florida

**Jessica Landsberg, M.D.**
Department of Otolaryngology and Bronoesophagology
Rush Presbyterian-St. Luke's Medical Center
Chicago, Illinois

**Roee Landsberg, M.D.**
Department of Otolaryngology and Bronoesophagology
Rush Presbyterian-St. Luke's Medical Center
Chicago, Illinois

**Jeffrey E. Lee, M.D.**
Associate Professor of Surgery
M.D. Anderson Cancer Center
Houston, Texas

**Roger J. Levin, M.D., F.A.C.S.**
Clinical Associate Professor of Surgery
Section of Otolaryngology Head and Neck Surgery
Penn State University College of Medicine
Milton S. Hershey Medical Center
Hershey, Pennsylvania

**Virginia A. LiVolsi, M.D.**
Professor of Pathology
University of Pennsylvania Medical Center
Philadelphia, Pennsylvania

**Christopher R. McHenry, M.D., F.A.C.E., F.A.C.S.**
Director, Division of General Surgery
MetroHealth Medical Center
Associate Professor of Surgery
Case Western Reserve University School of Medicine
Cleveland, Ohio

**Michael T. McDermott, M.D.**
Professor of Medicine
Division of Endocrinology, Metabolism, and Diabetes
University of Colorado Health Sciences Center
Denver, Colorado

**Steven C. Meschter, M.D.**
Director of Cytopathology
Department of Laboratory Medicine
Geisinger Medical Center
Danville, Pennsylvania

**Elizabeth A. Mittendorf, M.D.**
Chief Resident in General Surgery
MetroHealth Medical Center
Cleveland, Ohio

**Ronald P. Monsaert, M.D., F.A.C.P., F.A.C.E.**
Clinical Professor of Medicine
Jefferson Medical College
Associate Professor
Department of Endocrinology
Penn State Geisinger Health System
Philadelphia, Pennsylvania

**Carlos A. Muro-Cacho, M.D., Ph.D.**
Associate Professor of Oncology, Pathology, and Otolaryngology
H. Lee Moffitt Cancer Center and Research Institute
University of South Florida
Tampa, Florida

**Eugene N. Myers, M.D.**
Professor and Chairman, Department of Otolaryngology
University of Pittsburgh School of Medicine
Pittsburgh, Pennsylvania

**Arnold M. Noyek, M.D., F.R.C.S.C., F.A.C.S.**
Otolaryngologist in Chief, Mount Sinai Hospital
Chairman, Isabel Silverman CISEPO Program
Professor of Otolaryngology
Professor of Medical Imaging
University of Toronto
Toronto, Ontario, Canada

**Yasser H. Ousman, M.D.**
Washington Hospital Center
Uniformed Services
University of the Health Sciences
Washington, DC

**Pranay Patel, M.D., F.A.C.S.**
Associate
The Watson Clinic LLP
Lakeland, Florida
Adjunct Clinical Instructor
Geisinger Medical Center
Danville, Pennsylvania

**Gregory W. Randolph, M.D.**
Director General for Thyroid Surgical Services
Massachusetts Eye & Ear Infirmary
Assistant Professor Otolaryngology—Head and Neck Surgery
Harvard Medical School
Boston, Massachusetts

**Thomas Robbins, M.D.**
University of Florida
Gainesville, Florida

**Sanziana A. Roman, M.D.**
Clinical Instructor
Department of Surgery
Yale University School of Medicine
New Haven, Connecticut

**Sandeep Samant, M.S., F.R.C.S.**
Assistant Professor
Department of Otolaryngology Head and Neck Surgery
University of Tennessee Health Science Center
Memphis, Tennessee

**Ashok R. Shaha, M.D., F.A.C.S.**
Attending Surgeon, Head and Neck Services
Memorial Sloan-Kettering Cancer Center
and

Professor of Surgery
Cornell University Medical Center
New York, New York

**Steven I. Sherman, M.D.**

**Robert A. Sofferman, M.D.**
Fletcher Allen Health Care
UHC Campus
Burlington, Vermont

**John I. Song, M.D.**
Fellow, Advanced Training in Head and Neck
Oncologic Surgery
Department of Otolaryngology
University of Pittsburgh
School of Medicine
Pittsburgh, Pennsylvania

**Bethany B. Tan, M.D.**
Visiting Lecturer
Department of Surgery
Section of Thoracic Surgery
University of Michigan
Ann Arbor, Michigan

**R. Michael Tuttle, M.D.**
Assistant Professor of Medicine
Cornell School of Medicine
Memorial Sloan-Kettering Cancer Center
New York, New York

**Donald P. Vrabec, M.D., F.A.C.S.**
Director Emeritus and Clinical Professor
Department of Otolaryngology Head and Neck Surgery
Geisinger Health System
Danville, Pennsylvania

**Randal S. Weber, M.D.**
Professor and Vice Chair
Department of Otolaryngology
Hospital of the University of Pennsylvania
Philadelphia, Pennsylvania

**Ian J. Witterick, M.D., F.R.C.S.C.**
Staff Otolaryngologist
Mount Sinai Hospital
Head of Otolaryngology
Saint Joseph's Health Centre
Toronto, Ontario, Canada

**W. Edward Wood, M.D.**
Director of Pediatric Otolaryngology
Geisinger Medical Center
Danville, Pennsylvania

# Acknowledgment

Fundamental to the growth of the art and science of surgery is the process of mentoring. The evolution of thyroid and parathyroid surgery has represented a continuum of accomplishments achieved by those who have been mentored by the giants before them. In a much more humble manner, the production of this text is due, in great part, to those who have contributed so much to my career as mentors: Donald Humphrey, Ph.D.; Donald Vrabec, M.D.; Thomas Kennedy, M.D., and K. Thomas Robbins, M.D. I owe you all a great debt of gratitude and am proud to have studied under each of you.

I would like to acknowledge the diligent and often thankless effort of the editorial staff at Delmar Learning: Candice Janco, Maria D'Angelico, and Kristin Banach. I am grateful for their expertise and professionalism.

Finally, special thanks are extended to the expert assistants in the Department of Otolaryngology/Head and Neck Surgery at Geisinger Medical Center who provided valued editorial logistical support throughout the development and production of the text: Rhonda Beaver, Nancy Thompson, and Angela Williams.

Phillip K. Pellitteri, D.O., F.A.C.S.

# Historical Perspectives in Thyroid Surgery

## Donald P. Vrabec, M.D.

*"Only the man who is familiar with the art and science of the past is competent to aid in its progress in the future."*
Albert Christian Theodor Billroth

Nowhere in medical history is there a saga more enthralling, more gripping and more inspiring than that of the history of thyroid surgery. Nowhere were the steps more brilliantly choreographed than in the passage from a problem with nearly 100% surgical mortality to one in which the surgeon can confidently reassure the patient of a surgical risk less than 0.1%.

Undoubtedly there were a substantial number of massive goiters evident, particularly in those endemic goiter areas of Europe and Asia. Undoubtedly there were goiters which had reached massive proportions compressing the airway and esophagus with severe respiratory distress or dysphagia. Undoubtedly there were surgical attempts to decompress these areas; however, in an era prior to the introduction of anesthesia, asepsis and adequate instrumentation, torrential bleeding and sepsis commonly resulted in a fatal outcome. By mid 19th century the mortality rate still persisted at over 50%. Most surgeons were disenchanted and refused to perform thyroidectomy.

In 1848 Diffenbach in Leipzig wrote: *"The operation for goiter is one of the most thankless, most perilous undertakings which, if not altogether prohibited, should at least be restricted . . . . If we review all we know concerning operations upon hard goiters we can only regard with tremendous aversion those fool-hardy performances."*[1]

Later (1866) Professor Samuel D. Gross of Jefferson Medical College wrote in his textbook, *A System of Surgery*, 4th ed.: *"Thus whether we view this operation in relation to the difficulties which must necessarily attend its execution, or with reference to the severity of the subsequent inflammation, it is equally deserving of rebuke and condemnation. No honest and sensible surgeon . . . would ever engage in it."*[2]

It was not until the fourth quarter of the 19th century that there surfaced a determined effort to master the problems of thyroid surgery. During the following 125 years, seven resourceful, creative, brilliant, and skillful surgeons boldly opened the pathway to ultimate success. Each milestone along the way opened new horizons, new problems and new opportunities. These seven pioneer surgeons were Theodor Billroth, Theodor Kocher (the "Father of Thyroid Surgery"), William S. Halsted, Charles H. Mayo, George W. Crile, Frank H. Lahey, and Thomas Peel Dunhill. The contributions of each of these venturesome surgeons will be presented.

## THEODOR BILLROTH (1829–1894)

Theodor Billroth has been widely acclaimed as the most distinguished surgeon of the 19th century. Born in eastern Germany, he was an 1852 medical graduate of the University of Berlin. He served as assistant to Langenbeck, the Chairman of Surgery at the University of Berlin. He was especially interested in the developing science of microscopic pathology and during his three year assistantship to Langenbeck examined and classified the voluminous tumor material in Langenbeck's clinic. He was a dedicated surgeon and research scientist and published numerous articles on operative technique as well as pathologic anatomy. His work was so impressive that he received many offers of academic appointments both in pathology and surgery. In 1860 he assumed the Chair of Surgery at the University of Zurich, a position which he retained for six and one half years. Located in a highly endemic goiter region he began a program of surgery on large suffocating goiters. During his years at Zurich he performed 20 thyroidectomies with a mortality rate of 40%. Discouraged by these results he abandoned thyroid surgery for nearly 10 years.

It should be realized that during this period thyroid surgery was in its infancy. For the most part, it was limited to patients with large goiters compressing the trachea and causing respiratory distress. This was the era before the design of adequate hemostats or artery forceps. Anesthesia was in its infancy and asepsis had not been introduced into surgery. Later, with improvements in anesthesia, antisepsis and artery forceps, Billroth resumed surgery on the thyroid. A subsequent study of 48 thyroidectomies disclosed a mortality rate of 8.3%.[3] By the 1880s Billroth was the most experienced thyroid surgeon in the world; however, his greatest accomplishments were in other areas of surgery. He performed the first laryngectomy, the first total esophagectomy, the first gastrectomy and the first pancreatectomy for cancer. He was one of the most scholarly and prolific medical authors of the 19th century.[4]

In 1867 at the age of 37 he assumed the Chairmanship of Surgery at the University of Vienna, where he remained for 27 years as the Master Surgeon and Surgical Scholar in all Europe.

Greater still than his surgical or literary accomplishments was the inspiration that he conveyed to his many assistants. He was able to arouse in them a spirit of inquisitiveness, thoroughness and surgical perfection that propelled many of them to the surgical chairs of the leading universities of Europe. Their later contributions to medical knowledge were vast. The ones related to the thyroid will be mentioned. Anton Wolfler, a student of Billroth and first assistant for 10 years, was the first to describe in detail post-thyroidectomy tetany and publish a thorough discussion of the danger of operative injury to the recurrent laryngeal nerves. He assumed the Chair of Surgery at the University of Graz and subsequently at the University of Prague. He published two classic monographs on the development and structure of the thyroid gland and of goiter based on Billroth's operative material.[5]

Anton von Eiselsberg succeeded Wolfler as Billroth's first assistant. His experimental work on transplantation of the thyroid and parathyroid attracted world-wide attention. He continued Wolfler's studies of the tetany material in Billroth's clinic. The etiology of postoperative tetany remained unknown until 1891 when Gley reported his finding that post-thyroidectomy tetany was caused either by removal of the parathyroid glands or interference with their blood supply. At age 33 von Eiselsberg accepted the Chair of Surgery at the University of Utrecht, where he remained for three years and then occupied a similar position at the University of Konigsberg. In 1901 he returned to Vienna to succeed Billroth as Professor of Surgery.[3]

Johann von Mikulicz is regarded by many as the most brilliant, productive and prominent pupil of the Billroth school. His contributions to surgery in general and to thyroidectomy in particular almost rival those of Billroth. In 1882 he assumed the Chair of Surgery at Krakaw, Poland which he retained for five years. In 1887 he replaced von Eiselsberg at Konigsberg. Three years later he moved to a similar position at the University of Breslau where he remained until his death in 1905. His important contribution to thyroid surgery was his "new method" of thyroidectomy, which was the single stage subtotal resection of the thyroid leaving a small amount of functioning thyroid tissue and thereby avoiding tetany and myxedema. Although Mikulicz's procedure was either ignored or soon forgotten in favor of Kocher's multi-staged thyroidectomies, his procedure would later resurface to form the basis of modern subtotal thyroidectomy. Thus, it can be seen that the "spirit" of Billroth lived through his students and through the many generations of physicians that followed. Today, at the mention of the name of Billroth, there is immediate recognition and respect. The medical profession has yet to produce his peer.

## THEODOR KOCHER (1841–1917)

Theodor Kocher, the "Father of Thyroid Surgery," a graduate of the University of Berne and a pupil of Billroth, assumed the chairmanship of the department of surgery at the University of Berne at age 31. Following meticulous attention to control of bleeding as well as asepsis, Kocher was able to relentlessly reduce his operative mortality. In an era when the mortality for thyroid surgery approached 40% and even Billroth became discouraged and abandoned thyroid surgery for a period of 10 years, Kocher was able to reduce his mortality rate to 12.8% in 101 thyroid operations during his first 10 years at Berne. By 1889, 250 additional cases were reported with a mortality rate of 2.4%. In 1917, the year of his death, he reviewed his entire surgical experience and reported approximately 5,000 operations with an overall mortality rate of 0.5%.[6]

Early in his career at the University of Berne, Kocher began doing total removal of the thyroid. By careful, meticulous dissection he was able essentially to do a bloodless procedure without disturbing adjacent tissue. One of his first procedures was done on January 8, 1874, on an 11-year-old girl named Marie Richsel. Marie did well postoperatively and was discharged subsequently to the care of her referring physician some distance away. Sometime thereafter Kocher received a report from the referring physician that Marie had undergone marked changes in her personality, becoming listless, mentally dull and lethargic. Kocher, determined to examine Marie, traveled to her village and found her to be as described in the letter with an ugly, almost idiotic appearance. It is important at this point to note that until now no physiologic function had been ascribed to the thyroid itself. However, coincidentally the same year that Kocher performed his total thyroidectomy on Marie Richsel, Gull, in London, described a condition to which he applied the term "cretinoid," characterized by dryness of the skin, coarse features, swelling of the hands and retardation of the mental process.[7] Gull was describing changes he had encountered, not uncommonly, in postmenopausal women. Kocher recognized the similarity of Marie's symptoms to those described in the "cretinoid" state. Kocher pondered the possible relationship between total removal of the thyroid and the altered physical and mental condition. This was a tragic complication, for at this time there was no known treatment for such a condition. Kocher immediately recalled all his prior total thyroidectomy patients for examination. Of the 34 candidates 18 returned and 16 of the 18 were found to have the clinical symptoms similar to those of Marie Richsel. Kocher coined the term "cachexia strumipriva" for the condition. Realizing that such a devastating and potentially fatal condition followed total removal of the thyroid, Kocher stopped doing total thyroidectomies for benign disease, limiting his procedures to unilateral lobectomy. He reserved total thyroidectomy for malignancy or cases of severe airway obstruction secondary to tracheal compression.

In 1878 Ord of London described two similar cases of middle-aged women who developed cretinoid-like symptoms. He thought the swelling in the subcutaneous tissues was caused by the accumulation of mucin and hence introduced the term "myxedema." Ord went on to discover in postmortem examination that the alveoli of the thyroid, instead of being distended with colloid, were replaced by fibrous tissue. This was the first actual demonstration of an association between the thyroid gland and myxedema.[8]

One question that had puzzled Kocher for some time was the high incidence of myxedema in his patients with a relatively rare incidence of tetany, as compared to the experience of Billroth who had a high incidence of tetany with essentially no incidence of myxedema. Halsted explains this by describing the techniques of the two surgeons. Kocher was described as being neat and precise, operating in a bloodless manner, scrupulously removing the entire thyroid gland, doing little damage outside its capsule. Billroth, operating more rapidly and, with less regard for tissue and less concern for hemorrhage, might have easily removed the parathyroids or at least interfered with their blood supply while leaving remnants of the thyroid behind.[9]

In 1883 Kocher presented his classic paper before the 12th German Surgical Congress. In it he described the consequences of total removal of the thyroid, thereby proving that the thyroid gland is essential to normal body function.[10] That same year (1883) Felix Semon described precisely the signs and symptoms of myxedema and suggested that loss of thyroid function was the common cause of cretinism, myxedema, and "cachexia strumipriva."[11]

Unlike most surgeons of his time, Kocher's experience included patients with hyperthyroidism. This was an era when the preoperative preparation of hyperthyroid patients using iodine or propylthiouracil had not yet been discovered. The hazards of surgery in these hypermetabolic, thyrotoxic and thyrocardiac patients were so great that even many of the world's most prominent thyroid surgeons shied away from the hyperthyroid patients. Kocher developed a staged surgical technique for the hyperthyroid patient. The initial stage consisted of ligation of two, three, or sometimes even all four of the major thyroid arteries to reduce blood supply to the gland. At a second procedure a unilateral lobectomy was done. If the patient persisted or recurred with hyperthyroid features, then a third procedure could be done to reduce the size of the opposite lobe, leaving a small remnant behind to avoid the problem of myxedema. By 1911 Kocher had operated on 200 patients with hyperthyroidism with a mortality rate of 4.5%, a remarkable achievement for his time.

Kocher's contributions in the field of thyroid surgery were monumental, including the discovery that total removal of the thyroid led to myxedema, the perfecting of the thyroidectomy operation, the stimulus which he gave to the operative treatment of hyperthyriodism and the realization of the dangers of the indiscriminate use of iodine in patients with goiter.

Kocher made many significant contributions to many areas of general surgery other than the thyroid; however, these are not relevant to the current text.

Kocher received many professional honors including the presidency of the major European surgical societies, as well as the International Surgical Congress. His most prestigious award, however, was the Nobel Prize in Medicine and Physiology which came in 1909 in recognition of "his work in physiology, pathology and surgery on the thyroid gland." He was the first surgeon to receive the Nobel Prize.

By the beginning of the 20th century most of the problems of simple goiter had been solved. The operative mortality had declined to acceptable levels. This is attributed to the introduction of anesthetic agents, antisepsis and the design of new and better instrumentation. A surgeon now could work slower and more cautiously in a bloodless field. The etiology of myxedema following total thyroidectomy had been elicited and methods of management using thyroid extract and iodine were understood and practiced. Tetany had now been demonstrated to be the result of total removal or interference with the blood supply of the parathyroid glands. Although treatment with calcium salts had not yet been recognized, operative techniques were so designed as to protect the parathyroid glands and their blood supply, thus avoiding tetany prophylactically. Finally, vocal paralysis was understood to be secondary to injury to the recurrent laryngeal nerve and/or the external branch of the superior laryngeal nerve. Again careful dissection to identify and preserve these nerves led to a marked decrease in postoperative voice problems. The remaining challenges now were hyperthyroidism and malignancy. It was in the management of these problems that four American surgeons and one Australian surgeon were to play important roles. The Americans include William Stewart Halsted of the Johns Hopkins Hospital, Charles H. Mayo of the Mayo Clinic, George Washington Crile of Cleveland, and Frank H. Lahey of Boston. The Australian surgeon, who is frequently referred to as "the forgotten thyroid surgeon" was the bold pioneer thyroid surgeon, Thomas Peel Dunhill. A comprehensive history of thyroid surgery cannot ignore his contributions.

## W.S. HALSTED (1852–1922)

William Stewart Halsted graduated from Yale and subsequently Columbia University, College of Physicians and Surgeons. Following two years of internship at Bellview and New York Hospitals he continued his studies for two years in Europe visiting the prestigious medical and surgical clinics in Germany and Austria. He developed his interest in thyroid disease working in the laboratory with Wolfler, an assistant of Billroth. He subsequently observed Billroth and other famous surgeons, including Kocher, in their surgery of the thyroid. He returned to New York in 1880 and for six years remained in the New York Hospitals. During those six years only one thyroidectomy was done. Halsted was dismayed by the lack of progress in thyroid surgery by the American surgeons. He researched reports and found only 45 operations for goiter had been recorded in America up to 1883. By that time Billroth and Kocher had been reporting their experience with more than 100 cases each. He attributed the lack of progress in thyroid surgery in the United States to the failure to accept the principles of asepsis and to the lack of proper surgical instruments. The operative mortality was caused primarily by operative hemorrhage or postoperative sepsis, problems which were under relatively good control in Europe using aseptic techniques and proper surgical instruments. Prior to 1890 not a single thyroidectomy in the United States had been performed using aseptic conditions. Furthermore, it was customary to assign only one or two hemostats per operation in the New York Hospitals. Halsted stated that few if any of the New York Hospitals even owned more than five or six hemostats at that time. Halsted remained in New York where his writings, research and his bold surgical approaches earned him widespread recognition. When the Johns Hopkins Hospital opened in 1889, Halsted was recruited as the first chairman of the surgical division, a position he maintained throughout the remainder of his professional career. While still in New York, he made original investigations on regional nerve block using cocaine for this purpose. Working with two other physicians, they apparently used direct injections into the peripheral nerves at their wrists and/or elbows. They repeatedly confirmed cocaine's ability to produce conduction blocks in the nerves into which it was injected. Halsted and his assistants became addicted to cocaine as a result of these experiments. Halsted's work with thyroid surgery, as well as the largest part of his other work came after the addiction was a fact. Whether Halsted was ever completely cured of this addiction is unknown, although some of the notes of Sir William Osler (his medical caregiver) revealed that Halsted wrestled with his problem during his most productive years as Chief of Surgery at Johns Hopkins Hospital. It was remarked that the personality of Halsted was changed markedly by his addiction. He became shy, aloof, obsessed by precision and gentle handling of tissues, and scrupulous in his attention to the most minute surgical detail. Halsted was described as being the most discerning and critical surgical observer that history could ever be expected to provide.[12]

His early work with thyroid surgery was monumental. In 1907 Halsted and Evans (a medical student) reported the results of injection studies that demonstrated the blood supply to the parathyroid glands.[13] His work in developing surgical technique and in laboratory research, particularly with transplant work and the study of parathyroid implants, was classic. He confirmed tetany would be relieved with injections of parathyroid extract. He proved that the small parathyroid transplants would prevent tetany. In 1909 working with McCallum, he was able to control postoperative tetany in a dog with calcium salts introduced by the way of a stomach tube. Halsted was always concerned about the preservation of the parathyroids and would do operations only on one side taking care to identify and preserve the parathyroids on that side. Later if surgery on the opposite lobe was required, there was no danger of tetany. In cases of hyperthyroidism, he did staged arterial ligations and lobectomies as originally described by Kocher. Halsted, however, realized that ligation of all arteries would not cure the patient but made surgery safer by reducing blood loss.

Halsted's contributions to thyroid surgery were many and include the design of artery clamps (which were made in Paris) as well as a number of other retractors, ligature carriers, scalpels, dissectors, etc. which collectively made thyroid surgery safe and orderly. He described a standardized technique of thyroidectomy based on anatomic and physiologic principles. He developed the technique of parathyroid grafts, as well as the recognition that infused calcium salts could reverse postoperative tetany. He introduced fine silk suture material for ligatures. He introduced rubber gloves in the operating room (originally inspired by the desire to protect the hands of the scrub nurse who eventually became Mrs. Halsted). He brought the renowned medical illustrator Max Brödel from Lepzig as the first full time medical illustrator in the United States. Brödel's drawing were used in most of Halsted's monographs and publications adding greatly to their educational value. He was a pioneer in local infiltration anesthesia and finally his classic monograph *The Operative Story of Goiter*[14] remains the principle historical reference in thyroid surgery. Although Halsted had a primary interest in thyroid surgery, he did not amass the large number of thyroidectomies that other pioneers in the field have reported. Halsted's interests were in many areas of surgery to which he made enormous contributions. These contributions go far afield of the current manuscript.

Undoubtedly, Halsted's supreme achievement was the stimulus he created for the concept of a university environment as the proper vehicle for American medical education. According to Becker, American medical education was poorly structured and ill-defined, usually with a two year course in a proprietary school. Halsted's influence, especially his obsession with precision and gentle handling of tissue and his scrupulous attention to surgical detail, was needed to liberate surgery from the bold, rough technology that had emanated from the existing schools.[3] He established a surgical center which was unparalleled, with the possible exception of Billroth's.

## CHARLES H. MAYO (1863–1939)

Dr. Charles H. Mayo was the first to use the term "hyperthyroidism" and has been referred to as the "Father of American Thyroid Surgery." His first introduction to thyroid surgery was the day in 1890 when a Mr. Strain, a brawny Scotsman of 60 years, walked into his office with an enormous goiter. It hung down onto his chest and forced his head up and back as far as it could go—interfering seriously with his respiration. At surgery, the Mayo brothers incised the skin and superficial tissues freely and scooped the tumor out with their hands. Bleeding was torrential, for they could take time only to tie off the largest vessels. The minute the goiter was out, they stuffed sponges soaked with turpentine into the cavity to control the bleeding, and sewed the skin and flesh across it. Several days later they reopened the wound to remove the sponges. The patient did well and in time returned back to his occupation as a farmer.[15] Dr. Charlie Mayo was impressed and enthused about thyroid surgery, whereas Dr. Will Mayo, less impressed, turned his attentions to other areas of the body. Dr. Charlie thus became the thyroid surgeon at the Mayo Clinic. Mortality for his first 16 cases was 25%. At that time, however, the disease was considered medical and the patients were referred for surgery as a last resort. As surgical skills and medical referrals improved so the did the postoperative mortality figures. In 1912, Dr. Charlie did 278 operations for exophthalmic goiter without a death. Dr. Mayo used Kocher's method of staged thyroidectomy initially. Preliminary ligation of the main thyroid arteries on one or both sides was done. Later the patient was returned for removal of one lobe of the thyroid. If symptoms returned or persisted, the other lobe could then be approached surgically leaving behind a small portion to presumably prevent myxedema. The mortality rate for almost 500 cases of exophthalmic goiter decreased to 5%. Much of the later success of Dr. Charlie's surgery for exophthalmic goiter must be credited to Dr. Henry Plummer, his medical counterpart. Dr. Plummer had a profound interest in thyroid disease and surgery and recognized that there were distinct types of hyperthyroidism, including the classic Graves' disease, as well as hyperthyroidism with adenomatous goiter but without exophthalmos. He stressed their significant differences, as well as their therapeutic and prognostic implications. In 1923, Plummer established the value of iodine in the preoperative preparation of patients with Graves' disease.[16] Subsequent statistics show that the introduction of iodine resulted in a decrease of operative mortality from between 3 and 4% to less than 1%, and a decrease in the incidence of multi-staged operations from over 50% down to 2%. The significant contributions credited to Dr. Charlie include the following: 1) He recognized that hyperthyroidism with exophthalmos had the same mortality rate as the adenomatous goiter with hyperthyroidism—presumably caused by myocardial injury. 2) He urged dividing the strap muscles in order to obtain wider surgical exposure. 3) He taught preservation of the parathyroids in order to prevent tetany. 4) He amplified Kocher's multi-staged thyroidectomy procedure, doing preliminary ligations of the thyroid arteries on one or both sides and subsequent lobectomy when the patient's condition had improved.

## GEORGE W. CRILE (1864–1943)

Broad based in investigative as well as clinical sciences, Dr. Crile's interest ranged from the nervous system and anesthesia to areas of transfusion technique and surgery, especially of the head and neck area with special interests in thyroid surgery. Early in his career he was dismayed by the deaths of two young patients with Graves' disease. The procedures had gone well, but both had died from thyroid "storm" a short time postoperatively. He had noticed that both had presented at surgery in a markedly agitated state. Crile felt that the fear of surgery and not surgery itself was the greatest factor in postoperative thyroid "storm.' He developed a technique to eliminate this fear by "stealing" the gland. He named his technique "anoci-association," a name which became almost synonymous with his own. He would essentially condition these patients by having the anesthesiologist visit the patient for several days preoperatively and administer inhalation treatments to familiarize him/her with the techniques of anesthesia. He would actually not tell the patient on which day surgery was to be done. On the appointed day, when the patient was in a suitable frame of relaxation, the anesthesiologist would include preoperative medications in his daily routine intravenous injection and would include nitrous oxide and oxygen in the insufflation treatments. Once the patient was asleep he/she was taken to the operating room where local anesthesia was infiltrated and the thyroid gland slowly and methodically removed under absolutely silent conditions. The technique often worked so well that the patient would not know, often until the time of discharge from the hospital, that the thyroid was ever removed. Dr. Crile and his associates performed more than 22,000 thyroid operations, more than half of which were for hyperthyroidism. The operative mortality rate for the last 5,000 cases had been 1% and his incidence of temporary or persistent hypoparathyroidism was 1%.[17] He emphasized removing enough thyroid to control the hyperthyroid state, while simultaneously preserving enough to avoid myxedema. He left a margin of thyroid behind to protect the recurrent nerve and parathyroid glands. Similarly, the hemostat was directed inside the capsule of the gland to avoid injury to the recurrent nerve and parathyroid glands.

Crile was instrumental in organizing the American College of Surgeons and was one of its original 12 surgeons. He was the second president of the American College of Surgeons and a regent for 28 years. He was Chairman of the Board of Regents for 13 years. During his career he wrote extensively on diseases of the head and neck, including benign thyroid disease as well as malignant thyroid disease. He described the classic technique for radical neck dissection and proposed his ideals for surgical management of cancer of the head and neck, which later were accepted and expanded by Dr. Hayes Martin at the Memorial Hospital in New York.

## FRANK H. LAHEY (1880–1953)

Dr. Lahey, operating in Boston, was perhaps one of the most prolific authors of articles on thyroid diseases. He published more than 150 papers by the mid-20th century. He was the first surgeon in Boston to use the basal metabolic rate (BMR) as a test for hyperthyroidism. Using this study, along with iodine and the use of multi-staged procedures, he was able to decrease mortality to less than 1%.[3] The patients were admitted to the hospital where the metabolic rate was determined. They were allowed to rest for several days to stabilize their metabolic rate after which iodine was administered to bring the metabolic rate down to normal range. Once the metabolic rate reached an irreducible level surgery was performed. Technically he taught the importance of dividing the strap muscles to obtain good exposure and visualizing the recurrent nerve and the parathyroid glands. His philosophy was that the best way to preserve the nerve was to expose it and to keep it in view at all times. He struggled with the internists for degrading surgery and urged earlier referrals in order to have patients in a safer condition for surgery.

By 1941, more than 18,000 thyroid operations had been done at Lahey's Clinic and approximately 5,000 of these were done for Graves' disease. The overall operative mortality had been reduced to 0.7% with tetany in 0.2%. Recurrence of hyperthyroidism in the Graves' disease patient was approximately 3.3%. Lahey continued to operate until two weeks prior to his death in 1953. He personally had done more than 10,000 thyroidectomies while his clinic had done more than 40,000 thyroidectomies during his career. The overall operative mortality on these 40,000 thyroidectomies was 0.1%.

## THOMAS PEEL DUNHILL (1876–1957)

Born in 1876 in the remote sheep raising region of Australia, the family was burdened by poverty caused by the untimely death of his father before Thomas had reached the age of two. Thomas attended local schools and proved to be a brilliant student, eventually graduating as a pharmacist in 1898. Motivated early on to become a physician and surgeon, he worked as a pharmacist and studied at night to fulfill requirements for entrance to the clinical school of medicine at Melbourne Hospital, from which he graduated in 1905. Serving an internship, he proved to be an exceptional physician who, upon completion of his internship, was invited to join the senior medical staff of the newly formed St. Vincent's Hospital. He functioned initially as the outpatient physician and anesthetist, where his introduction to the severe problems of the thyrotoxic patient motivated him to seek relief for these critically ill patients. He entered the arena of thyroid surgery in 1907, during an era which might well be described as the "best of times and the worst of times" for the thyroid surgeon. The golden age of surgery had already arrived. Ether had been introduced as a general anesthetic. Antiseptic surgery had been introduced by Joseph Lister in the 1870s. Von Bergman had described the use of steam sterilization, which laid the foundation for aseptic surgery. Functional hemostats designed by Spencer Wells and William Halsted were efficiently controlling the torrential hemorrhage of thyroid surgery. Local anesthesia had been introduced and was in widespread use. The operative mortality in simple goiter had been reduced to acceptably low levels. The etiology of myxedema was understood, as was the treatment using extracts of thyroid and iodine preparations. The cause of tetany had been elucidated although as of yet there had not been a method for management. Vocal paralysis was understood to be caused by injury to the recurrent laryngeal nerve and/or the external branch of the superior laryngeal nerve. On the other hand, the serious problems of thyrotoxicosis and thyrocardiac disease were formidable for the thyroid surgeon. Until then, Kocher had performed only 200 operations on toxic goiter with a mortality rate of 4.5%. His procedure consisted of unilateral lobectomy, with or without ligation of the contralateral superior thyroid artery. His cure rate reached 70%. Kocher's 1911 *Textbook of Surgery* warned that surgery was contraindicated in the thyrocardiac and in those suffering from auricular fibrillation. Postoperative thyroid crisis with death was not uncommon. Chloroform anesthesia, commonly used in many areas, was cardiotoxic and hepatotoxic and was often the cause for death postoperatively. Recurrence of thyrotoxicosis following lobectomy was not uncommon and undoubtedly was caused by the removal of an in-

sufficient amount of the thyroid gland. Perhaps one of the more serious handicaps to the surgeon was the belief by the internist that thyrotoxicosis was primarily a medical disease and that surgery was contraindicated. Consequently, the patient was subjected to a number of useless drugs and techniques, including the drinking of milk from thyroidectomized goats and the injection of serum from thyroidectomized animals, etc. None of these proved to be of significant value. The patient remained under medical management for years until his condition deteriorated with thyrotoxicosis and thyrocardiac disease, including cardiac myopathy. The patients were grossly emaciated in severe congestive heart failure, blinded from corneal ulcerations and essentially on the verge of death. Only then were the patients referred to surgery, more or less as a last resort. Surgery in these agonal states resulted in an alarmingly high mortality rate, perpetuating the evil reputation of surgery in the thyrocardiac patient. Surgeons in some areas, particularly England, were said to have kept their mortality rates down by refusing to operate on severe cases and not operating at all on the thyrocardiacs. In the United States, even prominent surgeons such as Charles Mayo, who at this time followed Kocher's lobectomy and ligation technique, never attacked the remaining lobe of the thyroid if the patient relapsed. Thus, the vicious cycle of late referral by the medical department, followed by high surgical mortality, perpetuated an even greater disinclination for the medical service to refer the patients to surgery. Thus, it was into this arena of thyroid surgery that Thomas Peel Dunhill entered in 1907. Situated as he was in remote Australia, far from the glamour of the university clinics in Austria, Germany and Switzerland, as well as those famous clinics in the United States, his early work received little worldly recognition. Conversely, the isolation in Australia had a beneficial side for Dr. Dunhill. Thyroid surgery was largely limited to the principal hospitals at the medical centers in Melbourne and Sydney. Word of his surgical success with thyrotoxicosis and thyrocardiac patients quickly spread through the Australian medical community. It was soon recognized by the Australian medical physicians that the role of the internist should be confined to diagnosis and perhaps the presurgical preparation of the patient, and that surgery offered the most likely opportunity for cure. The result was that patients were referred earlier for surgery, allowing even better surgical outcomes.

Early in his career he realized that the secret to successful surgery in the thyrotoxic patient was to remove enough thyroid tissue. He felt removal of a single lobe was insufficient and that subtotal thyroidectomy was required. He operated on the thyrocardiac patient even before Kocher, Halsted, Mayo or Crile attempted these procedures. By 1911 he had amassed 230 cases of thyroidectomy on exophthalmic goiter patients with only four deaths (1.7% mortality).[18] In 1912 his results were presented before the Surgical Section of the Royal Society of Medicine.[19] At that time, England was said to be 20 years behind in thyroid surgery with a current mortality rate of 33% in the thyrotoxic patient. The English surgeons were said to be quite dubious of Dunhill's results, questioning the accuracy of his diagnoses, etc. Dunhill's travels also took him to the United States where he visited surgical clinics in Boston, New York, Washington DC, Cleveland and the Mayo Clinic. He communicated the same data to the renowned thyroid surgeons at these institutions. During this era most of the "giants" of thyroid surgery avoided doing surgery in patients with cardiac failure and auricular fibrillation, considering these findings a contraindication to surgery. Dunhill, on the other hand, considered them indications for surgery and attacked both lobes leaving only small portions of each lobe in the manner originally described by Johann von Mikulicz more than a quarter century earlier, but practically forgotten elsewhere. Following Dunhill's tour of England and the United States in 1911, many reports rapidly flowed from the major thyroid centers describing the abandonment of the classic unilateral lobectomy and arterial ligation procedures in favor of the von Mikulicz procedure. Few of these reports cited Dunhill for his influence, although the timing seems more than coincidental.

Shortly after Dunhill's return to Australia, World War I broke out and he went to war. In France he met Dr. George Gask and impressed him with his surgical talents. Following the war Gask assumed the position of surgeon in charge at St. Bartholomew's Hospital in London. He invited Dunhill to join him and in 1920 Dunhill moved to London. Shortly thereafter, Plummer at the Mayo Clinic reintroduced iodine in the preoperative management of thyrotoxicosis. This was probably the most important therapeutic advance until the introduction of antithyroid drugs some 20–30 years later. Dunhill did introduce iodine therapy into his surgical regimen for the thyrotoxic patient. Dunhill's abilities rapidly acclaimed him the acknowledgement of his English peers. He was recognized as one of the two leading surgeons in England. In 1928 he was appointed Surgeon to the Royal Household and subsequently served four British monarchs (George V, Edward VIII [before his abdication], George VI, Elizabeth II). In 1935 at age 60 he retired from St. Bartholomew's Hospital in London and entered a career in private practice until age 70, at which time he stated that he had only three remaining patients, King George VI, Queen Mary (the queen mother) and Winston Churchill. In 1939 he was awarded honorary Fellowship in the Royal College of Surgeons (FRCS), England, the first time such an award

was bestowed on a surgeon who was still in active surgical practice.

Though often referred to as the "forgotten" pioneer thyroid surgeon, his work in developing safe and effective surgery for the thyrotoxic and the thyrocardiac patient was monumental. Thomas Peel Dunhill truly merits recognition as a peer of the other pioneering giants of thyroid surgery.

As the first half of the 20th century came to a close and the surgical efforts of the seven pioneering thyroid surgeons had concluded, the hesitancy and trepidation that had been an accompaniment of thyroid surgery had now been conquered. But we would be remiss and narrow-minded if we did not recognize and acknowledge the many preceding and concurrent observations and discoveries which contributed to this success. This can best be presented by a brief chronological overview of the non-surgical discoveries that had a significant bearing on the victory over thyroid disease.

Centuries earlier Pliny was aware of the occurrence of goiters in pigs and we now know that in regions of endemic goiter among the human population, the majority of domestic animals are more or less affected. It attacks any species of land or fresh water vertebrate; however, it never occurs in those animals living in the sea.

The first successful thyroidectomy was recorded by Abul Casem Kaalaf Ebn Abbas, commonly referred to today as Abulcasis. The experience was recorded in his medical treaties "Al-Tasrif" in the year 952 A.D. However, progress was at a stand-still and the accomplishments of Abulcasis were forgotten; only to be discovered by scholars 800 years later.

The early writings of Marco Polo in 1271 alluded to people of a certain district he visited as being afflicted with "tumors in the throat occasioned by the nature of the water which they drink."[5]

Toward the end of the 18th century the medical literature contained more articles devoted to the subject of goiter in cretinism. Soon it was observed that there was a more or less definitive geographic distribution of endemic goiter, including the mountainous areas of Europe, and the valleys of Sudan. In the United States the regions surrounding the Great Lakes and the Pacific Northwest were most affected.

For centuries the favorite form of goiter treatment had been the use of ash prepared from the burning of seaweed and sea sponge. In 1812 Courtoir, a French chemist, while heating burnt seaweed in a copper vat with strong sulfuric acid noted a vapor of "a superb violet color." The vapor condensed in the neck of his retort, and when brought to the attention of Gay-Lussac, it was named iodine, for the color of its vapor.

Coindet, a Swiss physician, knowing that for centuries burnt sponges and seaweed were used successfully to treat goiter, was struck by the idea that this new element might be the active principle of this time-honored remedy. He began treating patients with pure iodine either as the tincture or in the form of potassium iodide. He noted startling results. Coindet was thus the first to use iodine per se in the treatment of goiter; although for more than 500 years cures following the administration of burnt sea sponges had depended on this element.

As early as 1830 Prevost of Geneva argued that goiter was an iodine deficiency disease and that the fault would be found in the water supply. Other European scientists went so far as to recommend the official sale of iodine as a prophylactic measure or even suggested that water supplies in goiterous districts be enriched with iodine.

In 1882 Hadden noted that in myxedema there was a decreased secretion of urea which was reversed by the injection or feeding of thyroid extract. In 1895 Magnus-Levy suggested that these alterations in urea indicated an altered metabolism. He investigated the effects of thyroidectomy on the gas exchange and the respiratory metabolism in animals, thus laying the foundation of a knowledge of the chief function of the thyroid gland. Turning his attention from the myxedematous to the hyperthyroid, he noted that in patients with Graves' disease there was a significant increase in oxygen consumption and heat production. This was the first laboratory demonstration that exophthalmic goiter involved abnormal activity of the thyroid gland, and that its essential function was to regulate the body metabolism via an internally secreted hormone.[16]

In 1896 Baumann subjected thyroid tissue to hydrolysis with sulfuric acid in an attempt to produce more highly concentrated preparations from the thyroid gland. He established that the gland contains a high percentage of iodine. He named his preparation iodothyrine. It was found to possess a response similar to, but more powerful than that of dried thyroid gland. It was subsequently found that all the iodine in the gland was found in the protein fraction, which Baumann called iodothyrine. Baumann later made the significant observation that persons living in goiterous regions were deficient in iodine.[20]

Only in recent times has the whole question of iodine distribution in water in relation to the production of goiter been systematically investigated. Principal studies were done in the United States, Switzerland and New Zealand. In 1907 Marine demonstrated that 90% of the dogs in the city of Cleveland, as well as many other domestic animals, showed some degree of enlargement of the thyroid. In 1910 he found that the addition of 1 mg of iodine per liter of water was sufficient to prevent the development of thyroid hyperplasia in brook trout.[21]

Large scale experiments in the prophylaxis of endemic goiter among school children and adults were done in Michigan and Ohio in the 1920s. In Michigan, a striking 70–75% reduction of goiter was observed in the 1928 re-survey, merely four years after the introduction of *iodized* salt. Goiter was practically eliminated among children in three of the four counties with the prevalence being 0.5% or less.[22]

In Ohio the state Department of Health made a rather comprehensive study of goiter throughout the state and planned to support the general use of iodized salt. Approximate 60,000 children were examined for goiter. However, the results of this survey were never published because of strong opposition to the general use of iodized salt by leading goiter surgeons. The surgeons were largely concerned with potential toxicity. However, some smaller studies were conducted on a local level and the introduction of iodized salt was instituted. Thirty-one percent of these school children had goiter in 1924. By 1936 only 7% of those who used iodized salt regularly had goiter. There was no change in goiter prevalence among children who did not use iodized salt. Similar studies in West Virginia and elsewhere confirmed the value of iodized salt in preventing or reducing goiter in endemic areas. Studies in Michigan and Ohio showed no cases of hyperthyroidism developing among children using iodized salt regularly.[21]

The early clinical studies of thyroid established that whatever the physiologically active iodine compound is, it was firmly linked to the thyroid protein which contained all the iodine in the gland. In 1919 Kendall succeeded in obtaining a white crystalline substance containing 65% of the thyroid iodine. It exhibited, qualitatively, the physiologic effects associated with the thyroid gland. He named this substance "thyroxin." Kendall thus provided the final proof of the essential connection of iodine with the activity of the thyroid. Kendall's experiments were not completely efficient since only 65% of the iodine was isolated. This problem was subsequently taken up by Harrington, Professor of Biologic Chemistry at the University of London, who used a slightly different method of hydrolysis to produce a compound which the investigator felt was more active and superior to Kendall's. However, there was still a definite discrepancy between the apparent thyroxin content and the total iodine content of the thyroid. Further research finally resulted in the isolation of diiodotyrosine in 1929. This substance, occurring side by side with thyroxin in the thyroid, accounts for all the remaining glandular iodine. In 1927 thyroxin was synthesized by Harrington and Barger.[23]

It appeared that a disturbance of thyroid function plays an essential part in the production of Graves' disease, although it was uncertain whether the condition represented an intrinsic disorder of the gland. The condition so named was recognized first by Parry of London in 1825, and subsequently described in detail by Graves in 1825 in Dublin and later by Basedow in Germany in 1840. It was suggested that Graves' disease was a condition directly opposite to that of myxedema, cretinism and cachexia strumipriva. Experimentally, it was possible to reproduce the phenomenon of Graves' disease by administering thyroid gland; however, the entire symptom complex could not be so reproduced. It was thus suggested that hyperactivity alone was insufficient to account for the condition but that the syndrome presented by the patient with exophthalmic goiter was caused not only by oversecretion but to abnormal secretion. The available facts seemed to indicate that Graves' disease arose not from an intrinsic abnormality of the thyroid, but rather from the action on the thyroid of an extrinsic stimulus, the true nature of which was yet unknown.

Surgical treatment in the care of goiter still remains the most satisfactory mode of attack. This may be a reflection upon the incompleteness of our knowledge. However, the fact remains that operative removal of part of the gland in Graves' disease and of nodular masses, so called "adenomata," in the other forms of goiter associated with toxic symptoms, produce the most immediate and most satisfactory results.

As mentioned earlier, Coindet in 1820 was the first to use iodine in the treatment of goiter. He reported that iodine benefitted many patients, especially by reducing the size of the thyroid gland. In 1850, Chatin in France demonstrated that small doses of iodine would prevent the development of endemic goiter and cretinism. Following these reports, the use of iodine, usually in the form of potassium iodide, in the treatment of goiter became very common, and as a result it was found that many patients, instead of benefitting, were made much worse. Kocher had emphasized the dangers of indiscriminant administration of iodine to patients with goiter and did not introduce it as a preoperative measure in his surgery practice. Plummer confirmed the opinion of Kocher and others, as he also had repeatedly seen patients with adenomatous goiter without hyperthyroidism "rendered hyperthyroid" by the administration of iodine.

The first extensive studies of the effect of iodine preoperatively in exophthalmic goiter was initiated by Plummer in March 1922. The optimal dose of Lugol's solution was 10 drops well diluted with water. Routine dose in the average moderately severe case was 10 drops daily. With more severe thyrotoxicosis, or impending "storm," the dose was increased to three or four times daily for a few days and then reduced to once a day. Surgery was postponed until it was evident that no further improvement was to be obtained from the Lugol solution. Maximal improvement usually occurred after the drug had been administered eight or ten days but might be delayed two or even three weeks depending on the response. Plummer reported his results in October of 1923. Approximately 600 patients with exophthalmic goiter had been treated with Lugol's solution over a period of 20 months. No patient with unquestioned exophthalmic goiter had been made worse by Lugol's solution. Approximately two-thirds of the patients with exophthalmic goiter benefitted greatly; one fourth benefitted slightly; the remainder or about one patient in 20 (5%) will not benefit. The probability of the iodine doing harm was less than 1 in 600.

When these initially "high-risk" cases were later accepted for surgery (after pre-operative treatment with Lugol's solution), the surgical mortality rate and the frequency of postoperative "storm" resulting in death progressively decreased.

By the end of the first quarter of the 20th century, surgery for hyperthyroidism had become relatively standardized with increased safety and an acceptable mortality rate. These favorable results were primarily caused by the recognition of the importance of careful preoperative preparation. Once the patient was admitted to a private hospital room, careful attention was dedicated to avoiding any anxiety or psychic trauma in the patient. Following an adequate period of time to allow the patient to relax and become accustomed to the hospital surroundings, preoperative iodine was administered in the manner which was described by Dr. Plummer in 1923. Daily treatment was continued until the basal metabolic rate and pulse rate were brought to an irreducible minimum at which time the patient was in the best condition for surgical intervention. Surgery then consisted, for the most part, of a subtotal resection of the thyroid done in the manner originally described by von Mikulicz and later resurrected by Dunhill.

There followed an intensive search to discover chemical compounds which would possess the ability to inhibit the endocrine function of the thyroid gland. Several compounds showed some degree of activity; however, many were accompanied by toxic side effects. In 1943 Astwood found that thiourea and thiouracil did exhibit such properties with fewer side effects.[24] They were used in studies on normal persons and on patients with hyperthyroidism. The patients showed a relief of symptoms and return to normal of the serum cholesterol and basal metabolic rate. The remission was sustained during treatment but the hyperthyroidism returned when therapy was discontinued. Astwood continued his work with various thiouracil compounds and eventually found that propylthiouracil produced the most reliable and predictable results with the fewest side effects.[25] Invariably the patients responded and often felt so well that at times it was said to be difficult to convince them of the importance of proceeding with the operation. Today antithyroid drugs are used in the preoperative preparation of the hyperthyroid patient. In many cases it is also used as the definitive treatment especially since propylthiouracil is available to all practitioners. Most patients with hyperthyroidism can be brought to a state of normal metabolism with propylthiouracil and some can be maintained indefinitely on small maintenance doses. However, recurrence of the symptoms of hyperthyriodism is not uncommon if the drug is stopped. On the other hand, there is the danger of producing myxedema should the treatment be prolonged.

From the surgeon's viewpoint, propylthiouracil should be used primarily in the preoperative preparation of the patient. Thyroidectomy should then be carried out, except perhaps in those patients who are elderly or in patients with severe complicating medical problems.

Although propylthiouracil reliably reverses the hyperthyroid state, it does not affect the blood flow to the gland. The gland usually remains large, soft and highly vascular. It is possible to decrease the gland's vascularity by also administering Lugol's solution for two or three weeks prior to operation. Lugol's solution results in a decrease of the size of the gland. It becomes firmer and the vascularity is decreased, making surgery safer. The mortality rate reliably falls well below 1% with a minimum of complications and with an assurance that permanent cure will result with few exceptions.

Somewhere in the early to mid 1940s ionization with radioactive iodine developed rather serendipitously as a side issue of atomic energy research. In 1949, Solely administered $I^{131}$ to laboratory animals and found that at the end of approximately 30–40 days the thyroid gland had decreased in size by 50% with few normal acini remaining.[26] It followed that a number of researchers and clinicians introduced this new technique in the management of Graves' disease, where it was found that an appropriate dose will destroy subtotally the hyperfunctioning thyroid gland, resulting in remission of the hyperthyriodism. This was first used clinically by Hertz and Roberts.[27] Complicated techniques and equipment were required to handle the radioactive substances, but in those clinics so equipped the use of $I^{131}$ soon became a standard method of treatment. The half-life of $I^{131}$ is eight days, while all the effects disappear by the fifth week. Tissue penetration is but a few millimeters in the form of beta rays. Haines of the Mayo Clinic reported his series in 1948. Forty cases were presented in which 27 produced good results with a single therapeutic dose of $I^{131}$. All symptoms were controlled and the gland was reduced to a "normal size." Myxedema developed in seven patients. No serious side reactions were reported. The $I^{131}$ was effective

both in exophthalmic goiter, as well as hyperthyroidism associated with nodular goiters, although larger doses were required to control the patients with nodular goiter. Early on, no evidence of carcinogenic properties was found with $I^{131}$; however, with the passage of time an incidence of carcinogenic activity similar to that with external irradiation was realized. The use of $I^{131}$ had some distinct advantages over the external beam radiation in that the severe skin reactions were not produced, and quite commonly the hyperthyroidism could be managed with a single dose treatment. A review of the first 600 patients reported in this country showed the major complication to be myxedema occurring in 8.5%. The treatment is especially valuable in severe thyrotoxicosis, in the elderly patient with advanced hyperthyroidism, in some cases of recurrent hyperthyroidism following subtotal thyroid resection, and in patients who are serious surgical risks.

Since its introduction in the early 1940s radioiodine has not only proved beneficial in the preoperative and long term treatment of hyperthyroidism, but also it has helped elucidate a better understanding of thyroid pathophysiology. These advances include a better understanding of radioiodine uptake mechanisms, the basis of its therapeutic effect, complete identification of thyroid hormone synthesis, serum transport mechanisms of thyroid hormones and thyroid imaging.

As we entered the second half of the 20th century, many more problems of thyroid surgery had been solved. Preoperative preparation of the hyperthyroid patient using iodine and antithyroid drugs was now standard and added a large margin of safety to the procedure. The operative techniques themselves were standard since the problems of myxedema and hyperthyroidism, as well as those of voice disturbances and tetany, were now understood and for the most part could be routinely addressed. The technique of subtotal resection of the thyroid was now standardized and essentially used throughout the profession. The principal remaining problem to be understood and managed was that of carcinoma of the thyroid. In 1950 Duffy and Fitzgerald were the first to report the incidence of thyroid carcinoma in patients who had received head and neck radiation therapy during childhood.[28] Often the radiation was low dose and administered for non-malignant conditions, such as lymphoid hyperplasia, acne or thymus enlargement. In 1994 Tezelman et al reported on 373 surgical patients operated on between 1982 and 1993.[29] He found cancer of the thyroid in 7 patients who had previously received radioiodine ($I^{131}$) for an incidence of 1.9%. The average interim between $I^{131}$ treatment and the malignancy was 11.4 years. An even more unusual report was that of Prinz et al who found unexpected parathyroid adenomas and hypertrophy in 8 of 23 patients who had a history of head and neck radiation therapy.[30] His conclusion was that this finding may represent a preclinical form of hyperparathyroidism and therefore was further evidence linking radiation therapy to hyperparathyroidism. In all these cases the preoperative serum calcium levels were normal.

In 1951 Horn described a new variety of thyroid carcinoma, medullary carcinoma.[31] This was clarified by the work of Hazard et al in 1959. In 1962 Cope et al[32] discovered a new hormone, which they named calcitonin, and six years later (1968) Melvin and Tashjian associated carcinoma of the parafollicular C cells (medullary carcinoma) with an excessive production of calcitonin.[33]

Prior to 1961 a uniform system of classification and management of thyroid carcinomas had not been defined. The literature revealed a variety of names applied to the different histologic patterns with equally varied methods of classification. In an attempt to introduce some uniformity in the classification and prognosis of thyroid cancer, Woolner et al reviewed 885 cases of thyroid carcinoma observed over a 30 year period at the Mayo Clinic. In that landmark study, it was revealed that papillary carcinoma represented approximately 60% of the total, and that it was the most readily curable of all types. They noted that regional nodes are involved in approximately 40% but that distant metastasis was uncommon. The characteristics of follicular carcinoma, solid carcinoma and anaplastic carcinoma were similarly documented. This study formed the basis from which the modern classification and treatment of neoplasms of the thyroid gradually evolved.[34]

Thus, the history of thyroid surgery is a dynamic, colorful and exciting one studded with "giants" in surgery, medicine and radiology—thoughtful, dedicated and daring men. Each advance was the result of reasoned deduction, thoughtful research and bold therapeutic strides. Each problem was solved logically as it surfaced—and with each solution the self-confident feeling that mastery of this enigma was finally imminent.

Today after one and one-half centuries of clinical achievements, mortality rates have been reduced from a level of nearly 50% to a level approaching 0.1%. Even today controversy continues regarding the optimal therapeutic approach in individual cases. Surgery, medicine and radioactive isotopes alone or in combination still have their favorable points and their drawbacks—and though many regard them as academic, who can predict what future vistas will unfold. Newer and better scanners are constantly being developed. New and different medicines will be introduced. Technological advances in medicine with faster and smarter computers, implantable computer chips, gene therapy, gamma knives, DNA studies, intrauterine diagnostic and therapeutic maneuvers, etc. may one day make our current therapeutic efforts appear as primitive to future genera-

tions of physicians as do the actions of the Drs. Mayo when they prevented exsanguination of their first thyroidectomy patient by packing the wound with turpentine soaked sponges.

Sir Issac Newton once said—"we can see farther today because we stand on the shoulders of giants." Perhaps one future day others will enjoy an even clearer view as they stand on the shoulders of present day giants. They may smile as their patients log-in to "thyroid.com," pass their mouse over the "computer health chip" implanted into their pectoral muscles and be diagnosed and treated—never leaving the confines of their virtual world. Then again the prophetic words of Professor Samuel D. Gross (1866) may ring true:

*"Can the thyroid gland when in the state of enlargement be removed with a reasonable hope of saving the patient? Experience emphatically answers, NO! . . . no honest and sensible surgeon would ever engage in it."*

## References

1. Diffenbach JF. Die operation des kroppes. *Die Operative Cherurgie, Leipzig.* 1948; 2:331&340. (Quoted by Harrison JS)
2. Gross SD. (1866). *A System of Surgery.* 4th ed. Philadelphia: Lea & Febiger; p. 394. (Quoted by Sedgwick CE and Filtzer HS)
3. Becker WF. Pioneers in thyroid surgery. *Annals of Surgery.* 1977; 185:493–504.
4. Colcock BP. Lest we forget: a story of five surgeons. *Surgery.* 1968; 64:1162–72.
5. Harrison TS. Thyroid surgery in historical perspective. *Leb J Med.* 1970; 23:537–51.
6. Modlin, I.M. Surgical triumvirate of Theodor Kocher, Harvey Cushing, and William Halsted. *World J Surg.* 1998; 22:103–13.
7. Gull W. On a cretinoid state supervening in adult life in women. In: *The Thyroid Gland, Its Chemistry & Physiology.* Harrington. London: Oxford University Press; 1933; pp. 5–6.
8. Ord WM. Quoted by Foss HL. In: The thyroid gland, its chemistry and physiology. *Transactions of the American Association for the Study of Goiter.* 1934.
9. Rutkow IM. William Halsted and Theodor Kocher: "an exquisite friendship." *Ann Surg.* 1978; 188:630–7.
10. Kocher TE. Uber kropfextripation und ihre Folgen. *Arch. für Klinische Chirurgie.* 1883; 29:254. Quoted by Becker WF. Pioneers in thyroid surgery. *Ann Surg.* 1977; 185:493:503.
11. Semon F. (1883). Discussion on a case of myxedema. Quoted by Foss HL. Reprinted from the *Transactions of the American Association for the Study of Goiter.* 1934.
12. Harwick RD. Our legacy of thyroid surgery. *Am J Surg.* 1988; 56:230–4.
13. Halsted WS, Evans HM. The parathyroid glandules, their blood supply and their preservation in operation upon the thyroid gland. *Ann Surg.* 1907; 46:489–506.
14. Halsted WS. The operative story of goitre: the author's operation. *Johns Hopkins Hospital Report.* 1920; 19:71–257.
15. Nelson CW. Thyroid surgical procedures of the Mayo brothers. *Mayo Clinic Proceedings.* 1994; 69:1130.
16. Plummer HS, Boothby WM. The value of iodine in exophthalmic goiter. *Collected Papers of the Mayo Clinic and the Mayo Foundation.* 1923; 15:565–76.

17. Foss HL. Surgical treatment of hyperthyroidism. *Penn Med J.* 1949; 52:822–24.
18. Vellar ID. Thomas Peel Dunhill: pioneer thyroid surgeon. *Aust NZ J Surg.* 1999; 69:375–87.
19. Dunhill TP. Partial thyroidectomy under local anesthesia with special reference to exophthalmic goiter. *Proc Royal Soc Med.* 1912; 1:61–84.
20. Marine D. The pathogenesis and prevention of simple or endemic goiter. *JAMA.* 1935; 104:2234–2241.
21. Marine D, Kimball OP. Prevention of simple goiter in man. *Arch Int Med.* 1920; 25:661–72.
22. Park YK. Historical evidence of benefits of iodized salt in the United States. *Publication of U.S. Food & Drug Administration.* January 31, 1997.
23. Foss HL. The evaluation of our knowledge of the thyroid gland. *Reprinted from 1934 Transaction of the American Association for the Study of Goiter.* 1934
24. Astwood EB. Treatment of hyperthyroidism with thiourea and thiouracil. *JAMA.* 1943; 122:78–81.
25. Astwood EB. The use of antithyroid drugs in the treatment of hyperthyroidism. *Transactions of the American Goiter Association.* Springfield IL Charles C. Thomas, Publishers; 1950; 210–212.
26. Soley MH, Miller ER, Foreman N. Graves' disease: treatment with radioiodine (I[131]). *Transactions of the American Goiter Association.* Springfield, IL: Charles C. Thomas, publisher; 1949; 113–119.
27. Hertz S, Roberts A. Application of radioactive iodine in therapy of Graves' disease (abstract). *J Clin Invest.* 1942; 21:624.
28. Duffy BJ, Fitzgerald PJ. Thyroid cancer in childhood and adolescence: report on 28 cases. *J Clin Endocrinol.* 1950; 10:1296–1308.
29. Tezelman S, Grossman RF, Siperstein AE, Clark OH. Radioiodine associated thyroid cancers. *World J Surg.* 1994; 18:522–28.
30. Prinz RA, Lawrence AM, Barbato AL, Braithwaite SS, Brooks, MH. (1981). Unexpected parathyroid disease discovered at thyroidectomy in irradiated patients. *Am J Surg.* 1981; 142:355–7.
31. Horn RC. Carcinoma of the thyroid: description of distinctive morphological variant and report of 7 cases. *Cancer.* 1951; 4:697–707.
32. Cope DH., Cameron EC, Cheney BA et al. Evidence for calcitonin—a new hormone from the parathyroid that lowers blood calcium. *Endocrinology.* 1962; 70:638–49.
33. Melvin KE, Tashjian AH. The syndrome of excessive thyrocalcitonin produced by medullary carcinoma of the thyroid. *Proc Natl Acad Sci.* 1968; 59:1216–22.
34. Woolner LB, Beahrs OH, Black BM, McConahey WM, Keating, FR. Classification and prognosis of thyroid carcinoma. *Am J Surg.* 1961; 102:354–387.

# 2

# Embryology and Anatomy of the Thyroid Glands

## John T. Hansen, Ph.D.

## EMBRYOLOGY

The thyroid gland begins its development around the 24th day after fertilization and is the first endocrine gland to appear in the embryo. The thyroid anlage begins as a thickened median endodermal derivative in the floor of the primitive pharynx. The thickening forms a small herniation or pouch, called the thyroid diverticulum, which appears just caudal to the future site of the median tongue bud. During differentiation and elongation of the embryo, the thyroid diverticulum descends subcutaneously anterior and inferior to the hyoid bone and laryngeal cartilages to assume its definitive position in the neck.

A lateral anlage, derived from the fourth–fifth pharyngeal pouch complex, also contributes to the thyroid gland.[1] This contribution is called the ultimobranchial (postbranchial) body and becomes incorporated into the gland as the parafollicular or C cells. Recent evidence suggests that the ultimobranchial body is not a pure pharyngeal endodermal derivative, but that the C cells are of neural crest origin.[2] Parafollicular, or C cells, produce the polypeptide hormone calcitonin, which reduces the blood concentration of calcium. Most C cells are concentrated in the superior and mediolateral region of the adult human thyroid gland.

For a brief period of time following its descent, the primitive thyroid gland is connected to the tongue by a narrow tube called the thyroglossal duct. By the end of the fifth week of development, the thyroglossal duct normally breaks down and the thyroid diverticulum, which is initially hollow, now becomes a solid mass of tissue and divides into right and left lobes connected by an isthmus. At this time, the definitive thyroid gland lies anterior to the second and third tracheal rings just below the cricoid cartilage, and by the seventh week of embryonic development, assumes its adult position. Often a small amount of thyroid tissue extends superiorly from the isthmus and is known as the pyramidal lobe. A pyramidal lobe is present in about 50% of humans and more commonly is associated with the left side of the isthmus.[3] Occasionally, the pyramidal lobe may be attached to the hyoid bone by fibrous tissue or smooth muscle (levator glandulae thyroideae). The pyramidal lobe and its associated smooth muscle represent a persistent portion of the distal thyroglossal duct. Aberrant thyroid tissue may be found anywhere along its embryonic migratory pathway, but most commonly appears just posterior to the foramen cecum of the tongue (lingual thyroids).

Although the thyroglossal duct normally atrophies and disappears, cysts may form anywhere along the course of the duct. Cysts most commonly appear at the base of the tongue or in the anterior part of the neck, usually just below the hyoid bone. When thyroglossal duct cysts are present, about 63% contain normal thyroid tissue.[4] Accessory thyroid gland tissue that originates from remnants of the thyroglossal duct also may appear in the thymus superior to the thyroid gland or in the neck lateral to the thyroid cartilage. When located in the lateral neck, the accessory thyroid gland usually lies on the thyrohyoid muscle.

## HISTOLOGY

The thyroid gland is enveloped by a thin, dense connective tissue capsule derived from the pretracheal fascia, which splits to envelop the gland. From this connective tissue capsule, septa penetrate the gland and subdivide it into lobules. The thyroid parenchyma is composed of spherical follicles whose walls are lined by squamous to low columnar epithelial cells that encircle a central lumen (Figure 2–1). The lumen contains colloid, a gelatinous substance composed of a glycoprotein (thyroglobulin) with a molecular weight of 660,000 daltons. The hormones $T_4$ (thyroxin) and $T_3$ (triiodothyronine) are stored in the colloid bound to the thyroglobulin. When the hormones are to be released, the hormone bound thyroglobulin is endocytosed by the follicular epithelial cells, and the $T_3$ and the $T_4$ liberated into the cell cytoplasm where they cross the cell memberane to gain access to the capillaries. $T_4$ is the more abundant of the compounds released by the follicular cells, accounting for approximately 90% of the circulating thyroid hormone, although $T_3$ acts more rapidly and is more potent.[5,6] When there is a great demand for thyroid hormone, the follicular cells will extend pseudopods into the follicle lumen to envelop the colloid, which then is absorbed. As demand declines, additional colloid accumulates. The lumen of the follicles range in size from 0.2 to 0.9 mm in diameter and may store sufficient hormone to supply the organism for up to three months. Consequently, the thyroid is the only endocrine gland whose secretory product is stored to any significant degree.

Pale-staining parafollicular cells are found individually or in clusters between the follicle cells but their apex does not reach the lumen of the follicle. These cells generally are two to three times larger than the thyroid follicle cells, but account for only 0.1% of the thyroid parenchyma. The parafollicular cells contain numerous small cytoplasmic granules that contain the hormone calcitonin, which is involved in lowering blood calcium by inhibiting bone resorption. Secretion of calcitonin is stimulated by an elevation in blood calcium concentration.

The septa which penetrate into the parenchyma of the thyroid gland also provide a conduit for the neurovascular elements and lymphatic vessels to enter or leave the gland. The endothelial cells of the thyroid capillaries are fenestrated, similar to endothelial cells of other endocrine glands. The innervation of the thyroid gland is provided by both sympathetic and parasympathetic divisions of the autonomic nervous system, and their function is essentially vasomotor. Adrenergic fibers of the sympathetic system do terminate near the basal lamina of the follicular cells and their stimulation influences thyroid iodine metabolism, suggesting that neurogenic stimuli may directly influence thyroid function.[5] However, the major regulator of the thyroid gland is thyroid-stimulating hormone (TSH or thyrotropin) that is secreted by the basophils of the anterior pituitary gland and binds to receptors on the basal membrane of the follicle cells.

In summary, the synthesis and secretion of thyroid hormone from the gland is a regulated process stimulated largely by TSH. $T_4$ is the major product of the follicular cells and serves as a precursor to the active form of the thyroid hormone, $T_3$. In general, the physiologic actions of thyroid hormone are related to their effects on basal metabolic rates. These hormones increase the

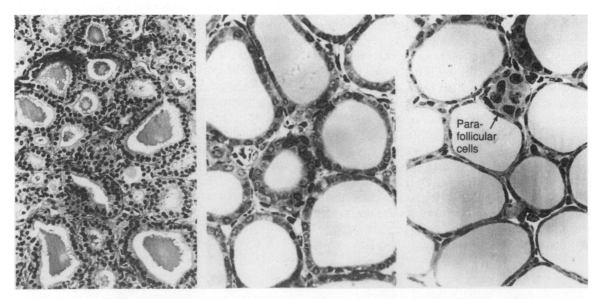

**Figure 2–1.** Histological sections that show the parenchyma of the thyroid gland at three different stages of activity. Note that the size of the follicular cells is proportional to activity of the gland. Parafollicular, or C cells, which produce calcitonin are shown in the photomicrograph on the right. (Reproduced, with permission, from Junqueira et al, 1998. *Basic Histology*, Appleton & Lange, and with the permission of The McGraw-Hill Companion.)

absorption of carbohydrates from the intestine, regulate lipid metabolism, influence growth and development, and feed back to suppress TSH release. Thyroid hormone also plays a role in body growth and differentiation during fetal life.[5,6]

## ANATOMY

The thyroid gland consists of two lateral lobes, a right and left lobe, connected in the middle by a narrow isthmus. About 50% of the time, a small pyramidal lobe is present and extends as high as the hyoid bone. This pyramidal lobe demarcates the mid-line migratory route of the embryonic thyroid gland. Although the human thyroid gland is variable in size, it normally weighs 20 to 30 grams, is somewhat larger in women, and may become enlarged during pregnancy.[7]

Normally, the lateral lobes of the thyroid gland appear as conical lobes with the apex of the lobe extending cranially. Each lobe is about five centimeters in length and extends inferiorly as far as the fifth or sixth tracheal rings. The posterior extensions of the lateral lobes, which lie at the level of Berry's ligament, are termed the tubercles of Zuckerkandl and have an important relationship to the recurrent laryngeal nerves. The isthmus of the gland connects the caudal portions of the two lateral lobes and measures about 1.25 centimeters in width. The isthmus lies anterior to the second and third tracheal rings. The thyroid gland is encased within a thin fibrous capsule derived from the pretracheal layer of the deep cervical fascia. The origin of the thyroid gland's capsule is controversial and has been referred to as the pretracheal fascia, the perithyroid shealth, the thyroid fascia, and the false thyroid capsule.[3] The true connective tissue capsule of the gland is derived from the pretracheal fascia and this is the true capsule of the gland which sends connective tissue septa into the gland parenchyma. Using this terminology, Hollinshead[3] refers to the capsule as an integral part of the gland, inseparable from the parenchyma except by sharp dissection. Above the gland, pretracheal fascia extends cranial to the isthmus and invests the pyramidal lobe if one is present.

Variations associated with the thyroid gland often are related to its embryology. Variations include small "ectopic accessory glands" associated with the migratory route of the gland from the foramen cecum at the base of the tongue, or consist of cysts or fistulae that form as remnants of the thyroglossal duct.[8,9] Suprahyoid, infrahyoid, and prethyroid accessory glands may lie anywhere along the normal migratory route of the thyroid gland from the tongue to the neck.

## Blood Supply

The thyroid gland possesses an extremely rich blood supply. The thyroid gland is supplied by four primary arteries, the paired superior and inferior thyroid arteries. The superior thyroid arteries originate from the most superior portion of the common carotid artery or, more commonly, as the first branch of the external carotid artery. The superior thyroid artery often courses alongside the external branch of the superior laryngeal nerve as they both descend into the neck. This close association should be noted by surgeons as clamping of the superior thyroid artery may damage the external branch of the superior laryngeal nerve when they run together. Consistent branches of the superior thyroid artery include a small infrahyoid branch, a branch to the sternocleidomastoid muscle, a superior laryngeal artery that travels with the internal branch of the superior laryngeal nerve through the thyrohyoid membrane, and a small cricothyroid branch to the muscle of the same name. When the superior thyroid artery reaches the gland it divides into anterior and posterior branches. These branches then ramify into numerous small arteries to the gland and often anastomose with their counterparts from the contralateral side.

The anatomy of the inferior thyroid arteries is more variable. These paired arteries may even be absent on one side in about 0.2 to 6% of cases.[10,11] When absent, it occurs more frequently on the left side. Normally, the paired inferior thyroid arteries arise from the thyrocervical trunk (variable) and ascend into the neck just medial to the anterior scalene muscles, beneath the prevertebral fascia. These arteries then loop medially and inferiorly to the anterior surface of the longus colli muscles, pierce the prevertebral fascia, and cross the vertically ascending recurrent laryngeal nerves (Figure 2–2). Usually the inferior thyroid arteries divide into two branches, a superior branch to the posterior aspect of the gland and an inferior branch to the lower pole of the gland. As with the superior thyroid artery, anastomoses between the inferior thyroid arteries are common across the midline, and they also anastomose with the superior thyroid arteries. Additional blood supply to the gland may occur from smaller arteries, including the ascending cervical artery, tracheal, pharyngeal, and esophageal branches. Blood supply also may come from the inferior laryngeal artery that accompanies the recurrent laryngeal nerve on its course posterior to the gland.[3]

In about 1.5 to 12.2% of cases, a thyroid ima artery may be present.[10] This artery usually arises on the right side and ascends anterior to the trachea. While the origin of the thyroid ima artery is variable, it commonly arises either from the brachiocephalic, right common carotid, or directly from the aorta arch. Very rarely, the artery may arise from the internal thoracic (mammary) artery.[3]

Usually, three large pairs of veins drain the thyroid gland. These veins anastomose freely within the parenchyma of the gland. The superior thyroid vein

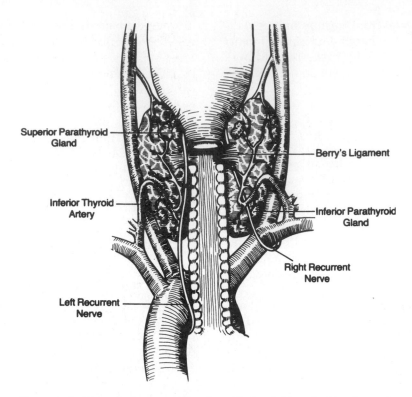

**Figure 2–2.** Posterior aspect of the thyroid gland. Note the blood supply to the gland and the course of the recurrent laryngeal nerves. On the right side, the nerve passes anterior to the inferior thyroid artery and Berry's ligament. On the left side, the nerve passes posterior (deep) to both structures. This variable pattern is discussed in the text. (Reproduced, with permission, from Falk, SA ed., *Thyroid Disease*, Lippincott Williams & Wilkins, 1997.)

drains the upper pole of the gland and accompanies the superior thyroid artery, ultimately emptying into the internal jugular vein or common facial vein near the carotid bifurcation. The middle pair of thyroid veins is variable in size and occurrence. Middle thyroid veins are present in slightly more than 50% of the bodies examined, emerge from the lateral side of the gland, cross the common carotid artery anteriorly, and then drain into the internal jugular veins.[12] The inferior thyroid veins form two trunks that drain the lower aspect of the gland. The right inferior thyroid vein passes just anterior to the brachiocephalic artery and drains into the right brachiocephalic vein while the left inferior thyroid vein descends in front of the trachea and drains into the left brachiocephalic vein. Frequently, the right and left inferior thyroid veins join and drain by a common branch (thyroid ima vein) into the left brachiocephalic vein. Anastomoses between the inferior thyroid veins are common. When present, these veins form a plexus anterior to the trachea known as the plexus thyroideus impar.[3]

## Lymphatics

The lymphatic vessels of the thyroid gland run on the penetrating septa of the thyroid gland connective tissue capsule and communicate with the capsular network of lymphatic vessels on the surface of the gland. Lymph then drains to prelaryngeal, pretracheal and paratracheal lymph nodes, ultimately collecting in deep cervical lymph nodes by coursing in small lymphatic vessels associated with the thyroid veins.[13] Some lymphatic vessels may drain directly into the large veins in the root of the neck or into the thoracic duct.[7]

## Innervation

Autonomic sympathetic nerves to the thyroid gland are derived from the cervical sympathetic chain ganglia. Periarterial nerve plexuses accompany the thyroid arteries to the gland and most of these fibers are vasomotor in function (vasoconstrictive) (see Histology section).[13] The majority of these fine nerves apparently arise from the middle cervical ganglion and course with the inferior thyroid artery to the gland.[7] The vagus supplies parasympathetic fibers to the thyroid gland.

## Recurrent Laryngeal Nerve

The recurrent, or inferior, laryngeal nerves are of great importance because of their anatomical relationship to the thyroid gland. On the right side, the recurrent laryngeal nerve arises from the vagus nerve as the latter passes anterior to the right subclavian artery (Figure 2–2). The right recurrent nerve loops inferior and around the right subclavian artery and ascends superiorly toward the larynx in close association with the tracheoesophageal groove. On the left side, the left recurrent nerve arises from the vagus nerve as the latter crosses the aortic arch anteriorly in the superior mediastinum. The left recurrent branch loops under the aortic arch in close association with the ligamentum arteriosum, and then ascends superiorly toward the larynx in the tracheoesophageal groove. Several small cardiac parasympathetic branches may arise from the left recurrent nerve as it loops under the aortic arch, and small fibers also may arise from these recurrent branches to supply the trachea (sensory and parasympathetic) and esophagus (motor).[3,13]

As the recurrent laryngeal nerves ascend superiorly, they come into direct anatomical relationship with the pair of inferior thyroid arteries. Unfortunately, this relationship is variable. The nerve may pass anterior or posterior to the artery, or between the first subdivision of the artery (Figure 2–2). Hollinshead[3] has concluded that on the right side, the recurrent nerve passes between either the main or minor branches of the inferior thyroid artery about 50% of the time. About 25% of the time, the nerve passes posterior to the artery. On the left side, the nerve passes posterior to the artery about 50% of the time, and rarely passes anterior to the artery or its other branches (about 10–12% of cases).

The recurrent nerves also display a variable relationship to the tracheoesophageal groove. Berlin[14] found that the right recurrent nerve may lie as much as 1 cm lateral to the trachea and lie in the groove only about 59% of the time. The position of the left recurrent is more consistent, lying in the groove about 70% of the time.

At the level of the thyroid gland, the recurrent nerves are in direct relationship to the gland and its attachment to the trachea. The lateral lobes of the gland are fixed to the upper two or three tracheal rings by a thickened portion of pretracheal fascia called Berry's ligament (suspensory or lateral ligament, but sometimes incorrectly called the posterior suspensory ligament) (Figure 2–2).[15] The recurrent nerves may pass posterior (deep) to Berry's ligament (75% of the time), through the ligament (25% of the time), or even course through the substance of the thyroid gland for a brief distance (7–10% of the time).[14] Regardless of its course, the recurrent nerve usually may be identified at the level of this important landmark. Once the nerves enter the larynx, they divide into anterior and posterior branches to supply the muscles and mucosa of the larynx. The recurrent nerves innervate all the intrinsic muscles of the larynx except the cricothyroid muscle, which is innervated by the small external branch of the superior laryngeal nerve. These nerves also supply sensory innervation to the mucosa lining the larynx below the level of the vocal folds. Most important, the recurrent nerves innervate the posterior cricoarytenoid muscles which are the primary abductors of the vocal folds. Denervation of these muscles because of trauma to the recurrent nerves will compromise the action of the abductors, and the vocal folds will tend to approximate one another in the adducted position. Under normal conditions and without significant laryngeal edema, the airway may remain open but inspiratory stridor and dyspnea may occur. The ability to speak will be compromised as well, producing hoarseness of the voice.[16]

Rarely, the recurrent nerve on either side may arise from the vagus nerve at about the anatomical level of the thyroid gland. If this occurs on the right side (more common), the nerve does not loop around the right subclavian artery but courses directly to the larynx posterior to the common carotid artery.[3] Often, this variation is associated with an anomalous retroesophageal right subclavian artery.

## References

1. Sugiyama S. The embryology of the human thyroid gland including ultimobranchial body and others related. *Adv Anat Embryol Cell Biol.* 1970; 44(H2): 6–110.
2. Carlson BM. *Human Embryology and Developmental Biology.* 2nd ed. St. Louis: Mosby; 1999.
3. Hollinshead WH. *Anatomy for Surgeons, Vol 1. The Head and Neck.* 2nd ed. New York: Harper & Row; 1968.
4. LiVolsi VA, Perzin KH, Savetsky L. Carcinoma arising in median ectopic thyroid (including thyroglossal duct tissue). *Cancer.* 1974; 34: 1301–1315.
5. Junqueira LC, Carneiro J, Kelly RO. *Basic Histology.* 9th ed. Stamford, CT: Appleton & Lange; 1998.
6. LoPresti JS, Singer PA. Physiology of thyroid hormone synthesis, secretion, and transport. In: Falk SA, ed. *Thyroid Disease: Endocrinology, Surgery, Nuclear Medicine, and Radiotherapy.* 2nd ed. Philadelphia: Lippincott-Raven; 1997.
7. Clemente CD. *Gray's Anatomy.* 30th ed. Philadelphia: Lea & Febiger; 1985.
8. LiVolsi VA. Pathology of thyroid disease. In: Falk SA, ed. *Thyroid Disease: Endocrinology, Surgery, Nuclear Medicine, and Radiotherapy.* 2nd ed. Philadelphia: Lippincott-Raven; 1997.

9. Hansen JT. Embryology and surgical anatomy of the lower neck and superior mediastinum. In: Falk SA, ed. *Thyroid Disease: Endocrinology, Surgery, Nuclear Medicine, and Radiotherapy*. 2nd ed. Philadelphia: Lippincott-Raven; 1997.

10. Faller A, Scharer O. Uber die variabilitat der arteriaw thyreoidcac. *Acta Anat (Basel)*. 1947; 4: 119–122.

11. Hunt PS. A reappraisal of the surgical anatomy of the thyroid and parathyroid glands. *Br J Surg*. 1968; 55: 63–66.

12. Bachhuber CA. Complications of thyroid surgery: anatomy of recurrent laryngeal nerve, middle thyroid vein, and inferior thyroid artery. *Am J Surg*. 1943; 60: 96–100.

13. Moore KL, Dalley AF. *Clinically Oriented Anatomy*. 4th ed. Baltimore: Lippincott Williams & Wilkins; 1999.

14. Berlin DD. The recurrent laryngeal nerves in total ablation of the normal thyroid gland. *Surg Gynecol Obstet*. 1935; 60: 19–26.

15. Lore JM. Surgery of the thyroid gland. In: Tenta LT, Keyes GR, eds. *Symposium on Surgery of the Thyroid and Parathyroid Glands*, Vol 13. Philadelphia: WB Saunders; 1980. 69–83.

16. Kaplan EL. Thyroid and parathyroid. In: Schwartz SI, ed. *Principles of Surgery*, Vol 2. New York: McGraw-Hill; 1989. 1613–1685.

# 3

# Tumors and Tumor-like Lesions of the Thyroid Gland

Carlos A. Muro-Cacho, M.D., Ph.D.
NiNi Ku, M.D.

## INTRODUCTION

Every year, 18,000 new thyroid cancer cases and 1,200 deaths are reported in the USA. This accounts for 1.2 % of the total number of new cancer cases of all sites and 0.2 % of the total number of deaths related to cancer, respectively.[1-4] The annual incidence of thyroid malignancies in different parts of the world varies from 0.5 to 10 per 100,000 individuals.[2,4] Despite its infrequency, it is important to remember that thyroid carcinoma is as prevalent as multiple myeloma, twice as common as Hodgkin's disease, and as frequent as cancers of the esophagus, larynx, mouth, and uterine cervix.[2,4] Furthermore, thyroid cancer is the most common malignant endocrine tumor, responsible for 64% of deaths attributable to malignant endocrine neoplasms, more than all other endocrine cancers combined. Nevertheless, treatment of thyroid cancer is very successful, and in the United States alone, approximately 500,000 patients have survived it.[2,4] Here, we review the histologic and cytologic features of benign and malignant tumors of the thyroid gland and the most recent scientific progress in thyroid pathogenesis.

## NORMAL THYROID GLAND

The thyroid gland is formed by two lobes joined by an isthmus and, in a significant percentage of individuals, the "pyramidal lobe," a vestige of the thyroglossal duct extending upward from the isthmus.[4] The adult gland weighs approximately 15 to 25 g, and on average each lobe measures 4.0 x 2.0 x 4.0 cm and the isthmus 2.0 x 2.0 x 0.6 cm.[2,5] A fibrous capsule surrounds the gland and connects with intrathyroidal fibrous septa forming "lobules" that become grossly evident in pathologic conditions. Each lobule is supplied by a single artery and contains 20 to 40 "follicles" that average 200 nm in size (Figure 3–1A) and contain "colloid."[2,4-8] Follicles are lined by a monolayer of low-cuboidal *follicular* cells surrounded by a basement membrane. In fine needle aspiration biopsy (FNAB) specimens, normal follicular cells are typically arranged in follicles, and monolayered sheets arranged in a honeycomb pattern with well-defined borders and nuclei which maintain polarity. Minute tissue fragments and naked nuclei resembling lymphocytes are not uncommon, and colloid may be seen in various amounts.[9-13]

The other epithelial cell type in the thyroid gland is the "C" or *parafollicular* cell, which contains calcitonin in secretory granules (Figure 3–1B). In normal adults, C cells are found along the central axis of the lobes, predominantly in the middle to upper third regions, often in clusters of 50 or more.[14-16]

## THYROID TISSUE IN ABNORMAL LOCATIONS

The bilobate thyroid anlage descends from the foramen cecum of the tongue to the anterior neck along the thyroglossal duct.[8,17,18] Follicular cells appear at the ninth

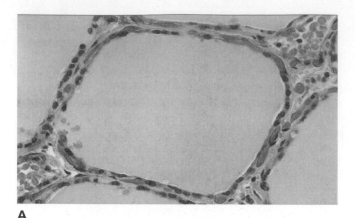

A

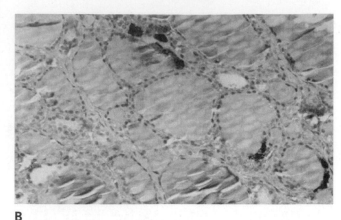

B

**Figure 3–1.** **A.** Normal thyroid follicles. **B.** Parafollicular cells. Calcitonin immunostain.

week, lumina at the tenth week, and colloid secretion at the twelfth week. Neural crest-derived C cells migrate to the ultimobranchial bodies before their incorporation into the thyroid.[17,18]

Abnormalities in migration result in ectopic thyroid tissue anywhere between the base of the tongue (lingual and sublingual thyroid) and the mediastinum.[17-24] Other sites where ectopic thyroid tissue has been reported include larynx, trachea, aortic arch, heart, pericardium, esophagus, diaphragm, gallbladder, common bile duct, retroperitoneum, vagina, sella turcica, inguinal region and ovarian teratomas (struma ovarii).[23-27] Occasionally, thyroid "parasitic" nodules disconnect from the gland and acquire their own vascular supply,[2] and in the context of chronic thyroiditis may be confused with lymph node metastasis.[2,4] Some authors consider the presence of thyroid tissue within lymph nodes (inclusions) a metastasis,[2,4] particularly if the thyroid tissue replaces one third or more of the node, if several nodes are affected, if psammoma bodies are present, or if the thyroid tissue shows cytoarchitectural features of papillary carcinoma.[2,4,19,21,22] Ectopic thyroid tissue may undergo malignant transformation.[22]

## CLASSIFICATION OF THYROID TUMORS

Table 3–1 shows a simplified classification of thyroid tumors based on the WHO classification,[28-32] and modified according to widely accepted criteria established by Rosai, Carcangiu and DeLellis in *Fascicle 5 of the Atlas of Tumor Pathology* (Third Series).[2]

### Epithelial Tumors

The thyroid gland contains only two major types of epithelial cells, the *follicular* cell and the *parafollicular* or C cell. Epithelial tumors are, therefore, divided into those that exhibit follicular cell differentiation and those that

**Table 3–1.** Classification of tumors of the thyroid gland[2,4,28,29]

I.   Epithelial
   A. Derived from follicular cells
      1. Benign: Adenoma
         a. Conventional
         b. Variants
      2. Malignant: Carcinoma
         a. Differentiated
           • Follicular carcinoma
              Minimally invasive
              Widely invasive
           • Papillary carcinoma
              Conventional
              Variants
         b. Poorly differentiated
           • Insular carcinoma
           • Other
         c. Undifferentiated (anaplastic)
   B. Derived from parafollicular (C) cells
      1. Medullary carcinoma
      2. Other
   C. Mixed tumors with follicular and parafollicular differentiation
   D. Tumors with oncocytic differentiation
      1. Adenoma
      2. Carcinoma
   E. Tumors with clear cell features
   F. Tumors with squamous differentiation
   G. Mucin-producing tumors
II.  Sarcomas
III. Lymphoma
IV.  Plasmacytoma
V.   Secondary and metastatic tumors

exhibit C cell differentiation (see Table 3–1) although rare tumors showing differentiation along both cell lines have also been reported. "Medullary carcinoma" (and its variants) is the only major type of neoplasm showing C cell differentiation.[2,4]

Neoplasms with follicular cell differentiation are divided into benign and malignant. Benign tumors are designated as "follicular adenomas" and their malignant counterparts are divided into two major categories, "follicular" and "papillary." Tumors that show no obvious differentiation are classified as "undifferentiated" or "anaplastic." The recognition of a tumor as poorly differentiated is more important, from a prognostic point of view, than its recognition as follicular or papillary. A variety of histopathological appearances (ie oncocytic, clear cell, squamous, mucinous) can be seen in tumors of both follicular and parafollicular origin.

## Tumors with Follicular Differentiation

### Follicular Adenoma

Adenomas are benign, encapsulated follicular tumors found in approximately 3% of otherwise normal glands at autopsy and rarely in association with thyroiditis, nodular hyperplasia or other lesions.[33,34] They are nearly always solitary, although two or more adenomas (that satisfy diagnostic criteria) can rarely occur in the same gland. A clonal origin has been supported by several studies.[35-37] They occur most frequently in euthyroid, middle-aged women, and present as painless lumps that may compress the trachea and produce pain caused by hemorrhage and other complication.[2,38-48] They usually measure between 1 and 3 cm and are round or oval with a homogeneous surface showing no internal lobulation, and surrounded by a fibrous capsule of variable thickness (Figure 3–2B). Their color depends on the degree of vascularity and colloid content. Hemorrhage, fibrosis, calcification and ossification are less common than in hyperplastic nodules (Figure 3–2A) and necrosis is rare, although it may complicate FNAB. The tumor cells are polygonal with minimal pleomorphism and round-to-oval normochromatic nuclei and several architectural patterns can be recognized: *Trabecular/solid (embryonal)* tumors are very cellular with diffuse trabecular or solid architecture and few or no follicles. They resemble the prefollicular stage of thyroid development. *Microfollicular (fetal)* adenomas have smaller follicles than the surrounding gland and contain little colloid. In *Normofollicular (simple)* tumors,

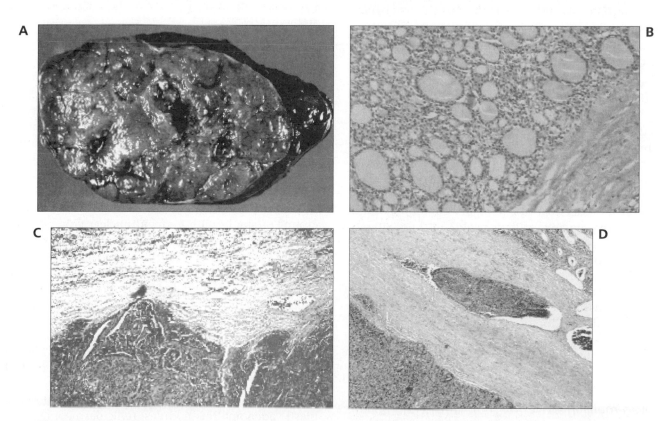

**Figure 3–2. A.** Follicular adenoma. Variegated gross appearance. **B.** Follicular adenoma. The periphery of the tumor is surrounded by a fibrous capsule. **C.** Follicular adenoma. Indentation of the inner aspect of the tumor capsule. **D.** Follicular carcinoma. Vascular invasion with tumor attachment to the endothelium.

follicles are of similar size than those of the non-neoplastic gland. In *macrofollicular (colloid)* tumors, follicles are larger than the normal adjacent gland and are difficult to distinguish from hyperplastic nodules.[2,4,47] Some adenomas have histologic features that distinguish them from the conventional type: oncocytic or Hürthle cell adenoma, adenoma with clear cells, adenoma with bizarre nuclei, hyalinizing trabecular adenoma, adenolipoma, adenochondroma. Most of these variants do not differ from conventional ones with regard to clinical behavior, but their recognition is important in order to avoid confusion with other lesions.

The differential diagnosis of conventional follicular adenoma includes dominant hyperplastic nodule, minimally invasive follicular carcinoma, and encapsulated follicular variant of papillary carcinoma. The typical uncomplicated adenoma lacks the internal lobulation of nodular hyperplasia. The diagnosis of adenoma should be favored over that of dominant hyperplastic nodule if the lesion is single and completely encapsulated (Figure 3–2C), compresses the surrounding gland, and has a microscopic, uniform appearance that is substantially different from that of the rest of the gland. On the other hand, the presence of inflammation, papillary projections within dilated follicles (Sanderson's polsters), and smaller nodules of similar appearance in the rest of the gland should suggest the diagnosis of hyperplastic nodule.[2,4,48]

## Follicular Carcinoma

Follicular carcinoma (FC) is a malignant follicular tumor that lacks features typical of other specific types of thyroid malignancy.[2,47,48] This definition excludes the follicular variant of papillary carcinoma (papillary carcinoma with predominant or exclusive follicular architecture), the follicular oncocytic carcinoma, and the poorly differentiated "insular" carcinoma.

FC is more prevalent in women at an age on average 10 years older than for papillary carcinoma[43] and typically presents as a solitary "cold" nodule without detectable cervical adenopathy or signs of hyperthyroidism. In contrast to papillary carcinoma, it is unusual for FC to be clinically occult although distant metastases, particularly to the bone, are often the first manifestations of the disease.[40,42] From a morphologic and prognostic standpoint, follicular carcinomas are divided into two major categories on the basis of their pattern of local invasion: minimally invasive and widely invasive.[2]

### Minimally invasive follicular carcinoma (MIFC)

The gross appearance of MIFC is similar to that of follicular adenoma, but the peritumoral capsule tends to be thicker and more irregular. MIFC is typically larger than 1 cm and is light-tan to brown with a solid bulging cut surface, microfollicular architectural growth pattern, and frequent secondary hemorrhagic, cystic or fibrotic changes.[19] The differential diagnosis of MIFC includes follicular adenoma, the dominant nodule often found in nodular hyperplasia, follicular variant of papillary carcinoma, and tubular-follicular variant of medullary carcinoma. The diagnosis of malignancy requires the demonstration of unequivocal capsular and/or vascular invasion. To be regarded as unequivocal capsular invasion, the tumor must penetrate the entire thickness of the capsule. Vascular invasion is a much more reliable sign of malignancy than capsular invasion (Figure 3–2B). To qualify as vascular invasion, the neoplastic cells should attach to the wall of a large caliber extracapsular vessel obliterating its lumen either partially or totally (Figure 3–2D).[50-58]

### Widely invasive follicular carcinoma (WIFC)

In WIFC, gross examination reveals extensive invasion of gland and surrounding tissues. Microscopically, most tumors exhibit solid areas, trabecular pattern, high mitotic activity, marked nuclear anaplasia and necrosis, features that overlap with those of poorly differentiated carcinomas (see below). WIFC metastasize in 80% of cases, usually to the lung, bone, brain and liver.[50-53,58,59]

## Cytopathology of Follicular Neoplasms

FNAB is generally considered unreliable in the differential diagnosis of follicular lesions of the thyroid gland. The diagnostic cytological criteria of follicular adenoma overlap with those of well-differentiated follicular carcinoma and, therefore, the non-committed terminology of "follicular neoplasm" is often used as a diagnostic term. Follicular neoplasms are typically hypercellular showing little or no colloid (Figure 3–3A). The cells are predominantly arranged in microfollicles, syncytial groups or singly with frequent nuclear crowding and overlapping. Rarely, macrofollicles can also be noted (Figure 3–3B and 3–3C). The cells have scant cytoplasm, slightly enlarged nuclei and fine chromatin. Aspirates from poorly differentiated follicular carcinomas are usually cellular and show architectural features similar to those seen in better differentiated follicular neoplasms, but the cells display typical features of malignancy, such as enlarged nuclei, irregular nuclear membrane, nuclear hyperchromasia and prominent nucleoli (Figure 3–3D). The cytological appearance of well-differentiated tumors can be confused with that of hyperplastic adenomatous nodules, follicular neoplasms of Hürthle cell (oncocytic) type, and the follicular variant of papillary carcinoma. Differentiation from nodular hyperplasia is, however, quite accurate with only 1 to

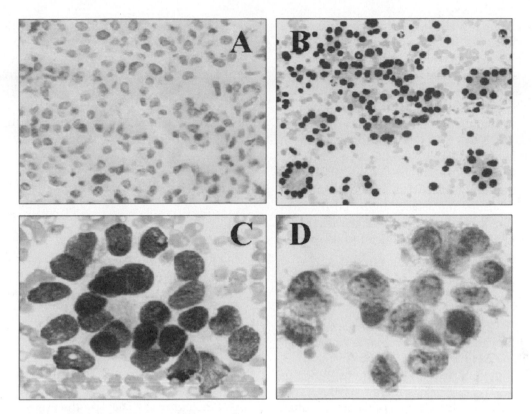

**Figure 3–3.** Cytologic patterns of follicular neoplasms of thyroid by FNA biopsy. **A.** Microfollicular adenoma, cell block preparation (Hematoxylin-Eosin stain, X400). **B.** Cellular adenoma with microfollicular pattern and syncytial-type tissue fragments exhibiting uniformly enlarged and crowded nuclei (Diff-Quik stain, X400). **C.** Follicular carcinoma with much larger and crowded nuclei of variable sizes and shapes in follicular pattern (Diff-Quik stain, X630). **D.** Follicular carcinoma with enlarged and hyperchromatic nuclei in syncytial-type tissue fragments (Papanicolaou stain, X630).

2% of false negatives. In general, the diagnosis of follicular carcinoma is correctly made in approximately 75% of cases, while the cytopathological diagnosis of follicular variant of papillary carcinoma is usually done accurately in more than 95% of cases.[60-62]

## Pathogenesis of Follicular Carcinoma

Follicular carcinoma frequently exhibits loss of heterozygosity on chromosomes 10q and 3p, with most of the abnormalities involving 3p21-25 and 17p13.1-13.3, the sites for the VHL (3p25-26) and p53 (17p13.1) tumor suppressor genes. Mutation studies of these chromosomal regions indicate, however, that neither p53 nor VHL genes play a significant role, implicating possible novel tumor suppressor genes on chromosomes 3p and 17p.[63-68] Recently, abnormalities of transforming growth factor β (TGF-β) signaling pathway have been reported.[65] TGF-β interacts with specific surface receptors (TβR) to elicit a series of intracellular phosphorylation events that culminate in growth arrest at the G1 phase of the cell cycle. Although in the vast majority of conventional adenomas all components of the TGF-β pathway are normally expressed, in minimally invasive follicular carcinomas TGF-β type II receptors (TβR-II) and activating Smad proteins, intracellular mediators, are downregulated. As a consecuence, TGF-β-mediated growth inhibitory signals cannot reach the nucleus, and cell cycle progresses to cell division leading to tumor formation.

## Papillary Carcinoma

Papillary carcinoma (PC) is a malignant follicular tumor characterized by distinctive nuclear features.[2] It is the most common type of thyroid cancer (65 to 80 % in USA) and it constitutes approximately 90% of childhood thyroid cancers.[1,2] PC typically presents in the third to fifth decades, with a ratio of women to men of 2–3:1 in Caucasian populations and 10:1 in Japanese populations.[69-75] In about 6% of cases there is a history of previous irradiation to the neck with an average interval of approximately 20 years.[71] Graves' disease, hyperplastic nodules, adenomas and Hashimoto's disease are found in glands with PC but a definitive association has not been established.[76-79] PC has also been reported in a familial form.[2,4,72]

The typical PC is whitish, firm and granular and has ill-defined margins. It is often multi-centric and in one third of the cases there is extrathyroid extension into the soft tissues of the neck and direct extension into larynx, trachea, esophagus or skin can also be seen.[78] Half of the patients have clinically evident lymphadenopathy at the time of presentation. Nodal metastases of papillary carcinoma tend to grow with a papillary pattern even when these features are not well developed in the primary tumor.[2,4,78] Blood-borne metastases also occur, although less commonly than with most other thyroid malignant tumors. Lung metastases are by far the most common and can occur in the absence of cervical nodal involvement. Other sites include skeletal system, liver, and central nervous system.

## Conventional

Conventional PC (Figure 3–4A) has complex papillae with a central fibrovascular stalk of variable thickness interspersed with neoplastic follicles that have similar nuclear features although in various proportions. A fibrous stroma with wide hyaline bands traversing the tumor and dividing it into irregular lobules is a common feature[76,77] (Figure 3–4B). Associated with papillae (Figure 3–4C) there may be psammoma bodies or other calcific concretions. The diagnosis, however, requires the presence of distinct nuclear features (Figure 3–4D): empty nuclear appearance known as "Orphan Annie's eyes" and overlapping nuclei that are larger than normal, round or slightly oval and have indentations, folds, pseudo-inclusions and grooves (Figure 3–5).[80-91] Mitotic figures are rare and, when significantly increased, they may indicate poor differentiation and aggressive behavior.

## Variants

### Papillary microcarcinoma

This tumor usually measures 1.0 cm or less and is found incidentally in approximately 10% of population-based autopsy studies and in 6% of surgical series (Figure 3–6A). It typically has a scar-like configuration with neoplastic cells in the periphery of the fibrotic area. It is also known as "occult sclerosing carcinoma" or "non-encapsulated sclerosing tumor."[92]

### Encapsulated variant

Approximately 10% of PC are totally surrounded by a fibrous capsule that may be intact or focally infiltrated by tumor growth. They produce nodal metastases in 25% of cases but blood-borne metastases are rare and the survival rate is nearly 100%.[2,4,77]

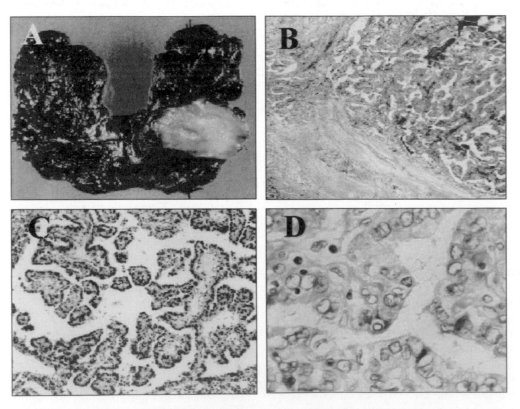

**Figure 3–4.** Papillary carcinoma. **A.** Gross appearance of a single focus invading the thyroid capsule. **B.** Fibrotic bands. **C.** Papillae. **D.** Nuclear clearing and nuclear grooves.

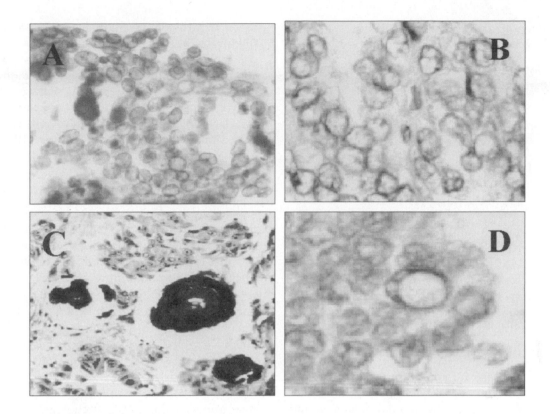

**Figure 3–5.** Papillary carcinoma. **A.** Nuclear clearing. **B.** Higher magnification of clear and early psammoma body. **C.** Psammoma bodies. **D.** Intranuclear pseudoinclusion.

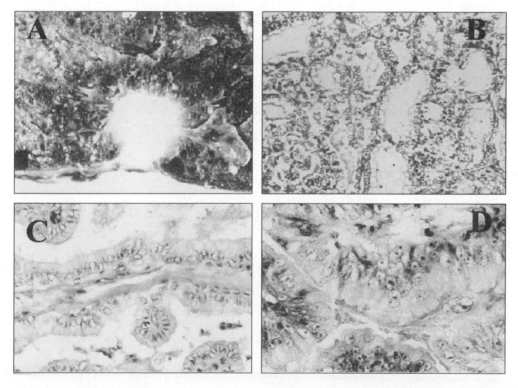

**Figure 3–6.** Papillary carcinoma. **A.** Papillary microcarcinoma (occult papillary carcinoma). Gross appearance. **B.** Follicular variant. Typical nuclear features of papillary carcinoma with follicular growth pattern. **C.** Tall cell variant. Follicular cells are twice as tall as they are wide. **D.** Columnar cell variant. Pseudostratification and marked atypia of tumor nuclei.

### Follicular variant

They have an exclusively or almost exclusively follicular pattern of growth but the tumor cells have the typical nuclear features of PC (Figure 3–6B).[93]

### Solid/trabecular variant

This is a rare tumor with solid and/or trabecular appearance and typical nuclear features of PC.[2,4,77]

### Diffuse sclerosing variant

In this tumor, one or (more commonly) both lobes are diffusely replaced by numerous small papillary formations located within intrathyroidal cleft-like spaces (probably representing lymph vessels), extensive squamous metaplasia, numerous psammoma bodies, and prominent lymphocytic infiltration and fibrosis.[2,4,71,77]

### Tall and columnar cell variants

The incidence of these tumors is approximately 10% and they tend to occur in older patients. They are usually larger than 5 cm and extrathyroidal extension and vascular invasion are frequent. In the tall cell variant (Figures 3–6C and 3–6D), papillae are well formed and covered by cells that are twice as tall as they are wide and have abundant acidophilic cytoplasm similar to oncocytes. Mitoses are frequent. In contrast with both the conventional and the tall cell forms of papillary carcinoma, in columnar cell carcinomas there is prominent nuclear stratification and nuclei may lack the typical features of PC.[94-97]

## Cytopathology of Papillary Carcinoma

Cytological specimens obtained by FNAB are typically hypercellular with cells organized in monolayered sheets, papillary fragments with branching fronds, and syncitial-type tissue fragments with or without follicles. The amount of colloid is minimal and appears as thick, ropy or stringy (Figure 3–7A). The cells are low-columnar or cuboidal showing enlarged, irregular, crowded nuclei with loss of polarity and pale "powdery" or "dusty" chromatin, occasional chromocenters (Figures 3–7B and 3–7C), frequent nuclear grooves and intranuclear pseudo-inclusions (cytoplasmic invaginations) (Figure 3–7D). The cytoplasm is variable in size and may appear pale, foamy, vacuolated, dense or finely

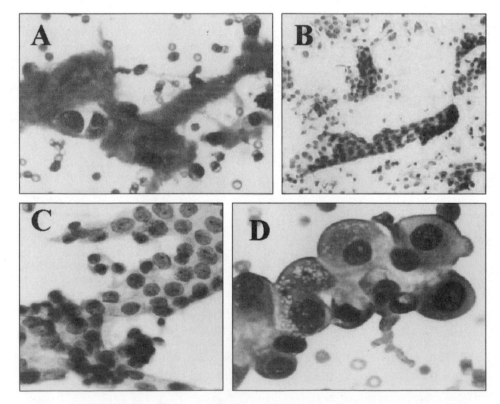

**Figure 3–7.** Cytologic patterns of papillary carcinoma by FNA biopsy. **A.** Colloid. **B.** Sheet of cells in tubular pattern. **C.** Sheet of cells with minimal atypia. **D.** Higer magnification showing intracytoplasmic vacuolation (Papanicolau, X630).

granular, mimicking that of Hürthle cells. Psammoma bodies and multinucleated giant cells may also be identified. Difficult diagnoses are cystic papillary carcinoma, cystic degeneration, and follicular variant of papillary carcinoma. In the former, numerous lymphocytes, foamy macrophages and inflammatory debris with insufficient representative cells may lead to a false negative diagnosis. Despite focal nuclear features typical of conventional PC, the presence of prominent microfollicles in follicular variant of papillary carcinoma may lead to the diagnosis of follicular neoplasm. Other diagnostic pitfalls include nodular hyperplasia, papillary hyperplasia, oncocytic tumors and medullary carcinoma. Tall cell and columnar cell types have not been extensively studied cytologically.[98-115]

## Pathogenesis of Papillary Carcinoma

A wide variety of molecular abnormalities in signal transduction pathways (ie TNF-α, TGF-β, gsp, ret, trk, ras, met, ret,and p53)[116-127] have been found in papillary carcinoma in association with different tumor phenotypes of variable biological and clinical behavior. In fact, recent cytogenetic and molecular analyses strongly suggest that thyroid cancer is an excellent model for the study of epithelial carcinogenesis.[121] This recent interest in pathogenesis research in thyroid cancer is also in part because of the discovery that well-differentiated PC are characterized by the activation of the receptor tyrosine kinases RET and NTRK1 proto-oncogenes, caused, in the majority of cases, by intrachromosomal inversions of chromosome 10 and chromosome 1, respectively.[128,129] The RET proto-oncogene, located on chromosome subband 10q11.2, encodes a receptor tyrosine kinase expressed in tissues and tumors derived from neural crest. RET germline mutations lead to multiple endocrine neoplasia type 2 (MEN 2) and to some sporadic medullary carcinomas.[130] In some PC, the RET gene fuses with the D10S170 locus resulting in the generation of the RET/PTC1 oncogene; in others with the gene encoding the regulatory subunit RI alpha of PKA forming the RET/PTC2 oncogene; and finally, in others, a newly discovered gene, localized on chromosome 10 and called ELE1 leads to the formation of the RET/PTC3 oncogene.[131-140] A novel gene, ELKS, has also been described in PC.[131] The ELKS gene encodes a novel 948 amino acid peptide expressed ubiquitously in human tissues. In this gene, the 5' portion is fused to the RET caused by the translocation t(10;12)(q11;p13).[131,135-143] Loss of heterozygosity for chromosome 1 (D1S243) and the p53 gene (TP53) have been reported in the tall cell variant but not in the columnar cell variant.[144] As in follicular carcinoma, it has become evident that cell cycle abnormalities are also responsible for tumor progression and tumor growth in PC. TβR-II are markedly decreased in PC and this down-regulation is responsi-

ble, at least in part, for the overexpression of cyclin D1 and cell cycle progression. In fact, the amount of cyclin D1 has been shown to correlate with disease stage in PC.[145,146] Also, a high prevalence of TPS3 point mutations has been detected in undifferentiated or anaplastic carcinomas.[132]

## Poorly Differentiated Carcinoma

Some carcinomas that arise from follicular cells do not fit easily into any category, and occupy both morphologically and behaviorally an intermediate place between the well-differentiated and undifferentiated (anaplastic) carcinomas. It is arguable whether they represent independent tumor entities or a higher grade of existing ones.[148]

One characteristic morphological variant of poorly differentiated follicular carcinoma is insular carcinoma (IC).[2,4] The incidence of IC varies with geographic location. Thus, in Paraguay IC is not an uncommon tumor while in the United States it is extremely rare.[2,4] IC is solid and often necrotic measuring over 5 cm at the time of diagnosis. It has an invasive pattern of growth and metastases to regional lymph nodes and distant sites, particularly lung and bone, are common. It is composed of small cells with round nuclei and scant cytoplasm (Figures 3–8A and 3–8B).[148-156] A variable number of mitosis is always present and blood vessel invasion is common. Foci of necrosis are frequently in the center of the insulae and around blood vessels. It can be confused with medullary carcinoma and other neuroendocrine neoplasms because of its carcinoid-like insular configuration, and it may be misdiagnosed as undifferentiated (anaplastic) carcinoma when the predominant pattern of growth is solid. The tumor cells are positive for keratin and thyroglobulin, and negative for calcitonin.

The rest of poorly differentiated thyroid carcinomas is a heterogeneous group in which some tumors may have nuclear features similar to those of papillary carcinoma, architectural configuration consistent with a follicular carcinoma, or oncocytic features.[2,4,150]

## Cytopathology of Poorly Differentiated Carcinoma

FNAB specimens from poorly differentiated carcinomas are highly cellular and often have a necrotic background. Trabeculae and/or cell clusters are sometimes associated with microfollicles. Cells have poorly defined, vacuolated cytoplasm and mild to moderate nuclear atypia with occasional intranuclear pseudo-inclusions and grooves.[157-159]

## Undifferentiated (Anaplastic) Carcinoma

Anaplastic carcinoma (AC) is a highly malignant tumor that appears partially or totally undifferentiated by routine histopathological assessment. Evidence of epithe-

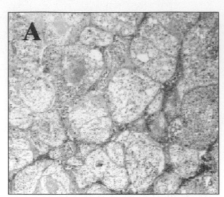 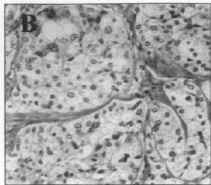

**Figure 3–8.** Poorly differentiated carcinoma. **A.** Insular carcinoma. Islands of tumor cells separated by bands of fibrotic stroma. **B.** Insular carcinoma. Higher magnification.

lial differentiation can be found, at least focally, by immunohistochemistry or electron microscopy.[152,160-165] AC is also known as pleomorphic carcinoma, sarcomatoid carcinoma, metaplastic carcinoma, and carcinosarcoma (Figures 3–9A and 3–9B). AC is characteristically a tumor of elderly individuals and below 50 years of age, the diagnosis of AC should be made with caution.[158-165] The tumor presents as a rapidly enlarging and invasive neck mass of few weeks to few months duration with frequent compression signs such as dyspnea, dysphagia and hoarseness. Occasionally, patients first present with symptoms or signs related to distant metastatic involvement (skin, bowel, bone, adrenal glands, lung, and digestive tract), but usually a thyroid mass will be readily detected. AC is fatal in most cases with the longest survival time being 2.5 years.[160-165] The tumor usually replaces most of the thyroid gland and, in many cases, metaplastic cartilage or bone can be seen at the gross level. The microscopic appearance shows considerable variation with three distinct morphologic patterns, and transitions and intermediate forms among them often occur. These patterns are "squamoid," "spindle cell" and "giant cell" types. The spindle cell pattern is indistinguishable from a true sarcoma (fibrosarcoma or a malignant fibrous histiocytoma). The giant cell pattern shows marked pleomorphism and numerous tumor giant cells with bizarre (sometimes multiple) hyperchromatic nuclei. The immunohistochemical profile of undifferentiated carcinoma is somewhat related to the pattern of growth. In the squamoid type there is strong expression of both high and low molecular weight keratins. Spindle and giant cell foci generally lack high molecular weight keratins but may show variable reactivity for low molecular weight cytokeratin.[166]

## Oncocytic (Hürthle Cell) Tumors

Oncocytic tumors are composed exclusively or predominantly (over 75 %) of follicular cells exhibiting on-cocytic features (Figures 3–10A through C). The oncocyte has an abundant granular acidophilic cytoplasm containing a large number of mitochondria (Figure 3–10D). Most authors consider that oncocytic tumors have gross, microscopic, behavioral, cytogenetic and perhaps etiopathogenetic features that justify their separation from other neoplasms.[167-173]

## Oncocytic (Hürthle Cell) Adenoma

Oncocytic adenoma is a benign, encapsulated, round-to-oval, solitary thyroid neoplasm with a homogeneous brown color caused by mitochondrial cytochrome content.[167,168] Sometimes the entire tumor undergoes a massive infarct-type necrosis, either spontaneously or after FNAB. The pattern of growth is usually follicular but it can also be trabecular or solid. Ultrastructurally, some mitochondria have a normal appearance and others have marked abnormalities of size, shape and content. Immunoreactivity for cytokeratin and thyroglobulin is less intense than in conventional follicular cells.[174,175]

## Oncocytic (Hürthle Cell) Carcinoma

Oncocytic carcinoma is a malignant thyroid neoplasm composed exclusively or predominantly (over 75 %) of oncocytes.[2] It accounts for 2–3 % of all thyroid carcinomas and 20 % of follicular carcinomas. On average, oncocytic carcinomas are larger than oncocytic adenomas, but they are also brown color and solid. Degenerative changes are more common than in the adenoma. Minimally invasive oncocytic carcinomas possess a complete capsule (encapsulated form) while widely invasive carcinomas invade the capsule often as sharply outlined nodules that connect with each other and with the main tumor mass, but that may appear as separate tumors.[169,173] The differential diagnosis includes parathyroid oncocytoma (benign or malignant) and the oncocytic variant of medullary carcinoma. Laboratory data, ultrastructural evaluation and immunohistochemistry may be necessary for diagnosis.

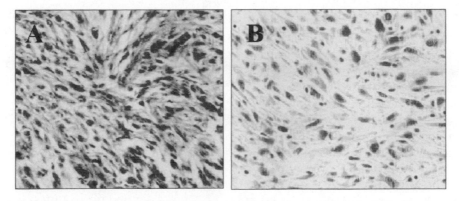

**Figure 3–9.** Undifferentiated (anaplastic) carcinoma. **A.** Spindle cells with storiform growth pattern. **B.** Prominent hyperchromatism and atypia of tumor cells.

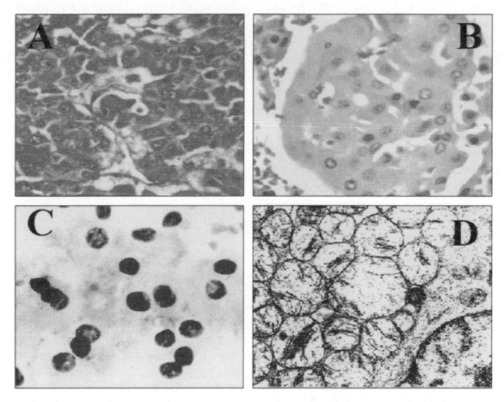

**Figure 3–10.** Oncocytic tumor. **A** and **B.** Oncocytic cells. Eosinophylic cytoplasm. **C.** Cytological features of oncocytic cells. Oncocytic cells in large polygonal cellular clusters, abundant granular cytoplasm and uniform nuclei with macronucleoli (Diff-Quik stain, X630). **D.** Abnormal mitochondriae within oncocytic cells (electron micrograph).

## Cytopathology of Oncocytic Tumors

As in conventional follicular neoplasms, Hürthle cell adenoma and well-differentiated carcinoma cannot be reliably distinguished on cytological grounds. Generally, Hürthle cells are discohesive, large, polygonal and with granular cytoplasm (Figures 3–10B and 3–10C). The nucleus is large, round to oval with fine chromatin and prominent nucleoli and binucleation and marked nuclear atypia are not uncommon. Aspirates are hypercellular with cells either singly or in loose aggregates, minimal or no colloid and no lymphocytes or conventional follicular cells in the background. In Hürthle cell carcinoma, pleomorphism may be prominent. Occasional intranuclear pseudo-inclusions and small oncocytic cells with high nucleus:cytoplasm ratio may be seen. The differential diagnosis includes non-neoplastic lesions containing Hürthle cells (ie, nodular hyperplasia with oncocytic metaplasia, chronic lymphocytic Hashimoto's thyroiditis and the oncocytic variant of papillary carcinoma).[177]

## Pathogenesis of Oncocytic Tumors

Oncocytic tumors share many of the abnormalities found in other neoplasms of follicular origin. However, there are also clear differences that may justify the worse clinical behavior often attributed to oncocytic lesions. Thus, *ras* gene point mutations in codons 12, 13 and 61 are found in more than 50% of Hürthle cell carcinomas,[177] and the presence of these mutations seem to correlate with poor prognosis.[178,179] Microsatellite polymorphisms are also found in Hürthle cell neoplasms with more frequency than in other neoplasms derived from follicular cells.[180,181] In addition, the majority of Hurthle cell adenomas show loss of heterozygosity on either chromosome 3q or 18q, in contrast to other tumor types.[182] Furthermore, hypermethylation of the E-cadherin 5' CpG followed by mutational inactivation is observed in 40% of Hürthle's cell carcinoma, suggesting a mechanism for invasion and metastasis.[183]

## Tumors with Special Features

### Clear cell tumors

These are primary thyroid neoplasms in which 75% or more of the tumor cells show marked cytoplasmic clearing caused by the presence of cytoplasmic vesicles (dilated mitochondriae, endoplasmic reticulum or Golgi apparatus), glycogen, lipid (lipid-rich adenoma), mucin (signet-ring cell carcinoma) or thyroglobulin. Clear cells can be seen in oncocytic and non-oncocytic tumors and in benign conditions.[184,185]

### Mucinous tumors

Both extracellular hyaluronic acid and intracytoplasmic acid glycoproteins can be detected in a variety of thyroid neoplasms: signet-ring follicular adenoma, follicular carcinoma with signet-ring features, mucoepidermoid carcinoma, sclerosing mucoepidermoid carcinoma with eosinophilia, mucinous carcinoma, papillary carcinoma, medullary carcinoma and undifferentiated carcinoma.[2,4] In rare tumors, transitions between areas of typical thyroid carcinoma and mucinous adenocarcinoma are seen.

### Squamous differentiation

Focal or extensive squamous differentiation can be found in many thyroid tumors. Squamous metaplasia is rare in follicular and medullary carcinomas but is found in approximately 30% of papillary carcinomas. The term *"squamous cell carcinoma"* is reserved for those tumors with obvious squamous differentiation and prominent cytologic atypia sometimes mixed with undifferentiated areas. Some tumors may produce mucin (adenosquamous carcinoma). Secondary involvement by a non-thyroidal squamous cell carcinoma should be ruled out.[2]

## Tumors with Parafollicular Differentiation

### C Cell Hyperplasia

C cell hyperplasia (CCH) is an uncommon multifocal proliferation of C cells within the follicles of the thyroid gland [186-193] that has been recognized as a pre-neoplastic condition in MEN IIA and IIB and is used histologically to distinguish sporadic and familial forms of medullary carcinoma.[193-198] It was initially reported in patients having a history of familial medullary thyroid carcinoma and abnormal calcitonin secretory reserves but it can be found in a variety of situations.[189-192, 196]

The diagnosis of *diffuse (non-nodular) C cell hyperplasia* should be made when the process involves both thyroid lobes with at least 50 C cells per low-power field.[194-198] C cells should completely obliterate the follicular space in a diffuse, bilateral and multifocal manner occupying an intrafollicular position separated from the interstitium by the follicular basal lamina and from the colloid by extensions of the follicular cell cytoplasm.[197,199-202]

### Medullary Carcinoma

Medullary carcinoma (MC) is a rare neoplasm that arises from C or parafollicular cells and accounts for 5–10% of all thyroid malignancies.[2] Approximately 70% of the cases occur sporadically and are associated with Hashimoto's disease or chronic hypercalcemia but they seem to be unrelated to irradiation.[204-206] The rest of the cases are familial and inherited in an autosomal dominant form [207-210] and occur in association with tumors of the adrenal medulla and parathyroid gland, in the context of multiple endocrine neoplasia (see below).[203-205]

Sporadic MC is a tumor of middle-aged adults [210-215] with an indolent course and 5-year survival rates of 60–70 % after surgery. Patients with MEN IIA are usually in the second decade and often have slow-growing, multicentric bilateral tumors. Patients with MEN IIB (III) are slightly younger (average 15 years) and harbor aggressive neoplasms that metastasize early and have poor prognosis.[212-215]

The typical MC is solid with a lobular, trabecular, insular or sheet-like architecture and composed of a mixture of round, polygonal or spindle-shaped cells (Figure 3–11). Necrosis, hemorrhage, and mitotic activity are uncommon and lymphatic and vascular invasion may be seen at the periphery of the tumor and in advanced cases in the contralateral lobe. The stroma contains collagen and, in most cases, amyloid deposits that

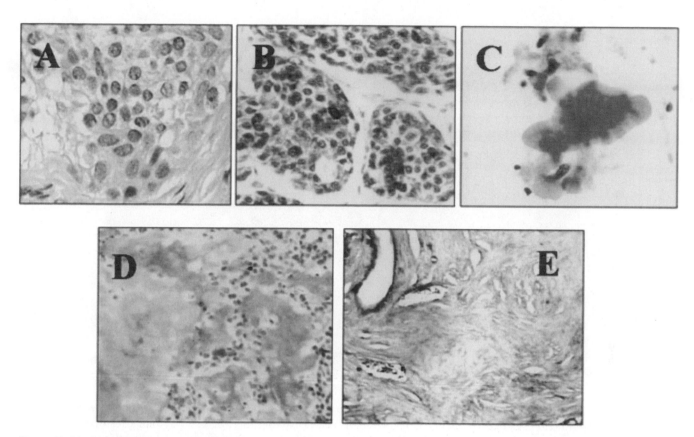

**Figure 3–11.** Medullary carcinoma. **A.** Homogeneous cellularity with minimal atypia and solid growth pattern. **B.** Calcitonin immunostain **C.** Amyloid (FNAB specimen). **D.** Amyloid (Hematoxylin-Eosin stain). **E.** Amyloid (Congo red stain).

are Congo red-positive and show green birefringence with polarized light (Figure 3–12E). In familial MC foci of C cell hyperplasia are present sometimes away from the main tumor. By immunohistochemistry, MCs are typically positive for low molecular weight cytokeratin, CEA, calcitonin (Figure 3–12B), neuron-specific enolase, synaptophysin, and chromogranin. Chromogranin may, in fact, be a more specific marker than calcitonin.[216,217] Ultrastructurally, calcitonin and other hormonal products are stored in two types of membrane-bound secretory granules. Type I granules (280 nm) are moderately electron-dense with finely granular contents closely applied to the membrane. Type II granules (130 nm) are more electron-dense and their contents are separated from the membrane by a narrow electron-lucent space.[2]

The probability of nodal metastases increases with the size of the primary tumor. Nodal metastases have been reported in 20 % of patients with tumors less than 0.7 cm, 30 % of patients with tumors between 0.7 and 1.5 cm, and 80 % of patients with tumors greater than 1.5 cm.[207-209] Sites of metastasis are central and lateral cervical nodes, lung, liver, bone, and adrenal glands. Survival correlates with age and sex of the patient and stage of the disease. Patients less than 40 years old at the time of diagnosis have a significantly better progno-

sis than older patients, even when individuals with the familial form of the disease are excluded from analysis. In addition, women have a better prognosis than men.

Many variants of MC have been described and, therefore, MC may mimic a wide variety of benign and malignant primary thyroid neoplasms.[207-209]

## Multiple Endocrine Neoplasia Syndrome

Multiple endocrine neoplasia syndromes (MEN) are autosomal dominantly inherited diseases characterized by the syn- or metachronous development of neoplastic and hyperplastic neuroendocrine lesions in several glands of an affected patient.[212-227] MEN appears in two major forms referred to as type 1 (MEN-1) and type 2 (MEN-2). MEN-1 is characterized by neuroendocrine lesions in parathyroid, pancreas, duodenum and pituitary, and occasionally adrenocortical, lipomatous and neuroendocrine tumors in other locations. The genetic defect of MEN-1 involves a new form of tumor suppressor gene called MU located on chromosome 11q13. MU codes for a protein called "menin" which is expressed in a variety of human tissues and organs.[224] MEN-1 gene carriers have inactivating germline frameshift, nonsense, missense and in-frame deletion mutations scattered throughout the 10 coding exons. The MEN-2 syndrome is divided into three clinical vari-

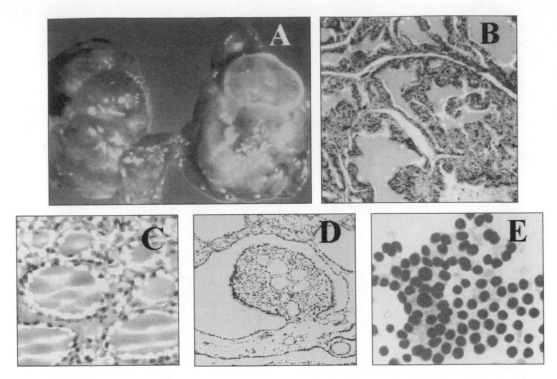

**Figure 3–12.** Nodular hyperplasia. **A.** Gross appearance of multinodular gland. **B.** Hyperplastic thyroid epithelium. **C.** Resorption of colloid in hyperplasia. **D.** Sanderson's polster. **E.** Cytologic features. Follicular epithelial cells with uniform, small nuclei in a monolayer-honeycomb and follicular patterns (Diff-Quik stain, X400).

ants referred to as MEN-2A, MEN-2B and familial medullary thyroid carcinoma (FMTC). In MEN-2A, pheochromocytomas and parathyroid hyperplasia, and in MEN-2B, additional skeletal abnormalities and ganglioneuromatosis can also be found. All three MEN-2 phenotypes are associated with oncogenic point mutations of the RET proto-oncogene on chromosome 10q11.2. Direct mutational analysis of germline DNA allows for the unambiguous identification of gene carriers and, therefore, the discrimination of MEN-associated and sporadically occurring neuroendocrine tumors.[216,218] The detection of these abnormalities can be used in early diagnosis and should lead to preventive total thyroidectomy, especially in affected families, to prevent the fatal outcome of delayed diagnosis.[227]

## Cytopathology of Medullary Carcinoma

FNAB are variably cellular depending on the amount of fibrosis. Amyloid appears as amorphous clumps of pale pink to violet Congo Red positive material (see Figure 3–12C). Tumor cells are seen singly or in loosely cohesive groups with poorly defined cell borders. The cells are of variable morphology and appear as small, round, oval, cuboidal, polygonal or spindle-shaped. The nuclei are round or elongated and eccentrically located (plasmacytoid appearance) and the coarsely granular chro-

matin is described as "salt and pepper." Nuclear molding (neuroendocrine-like features), inconspicuous nucleoli, bi- and multinucleation, indistinct delicate cytoplasmic borders with occasional fine and granular cytoplasm, and dendritic cell processes are common. The main diagnostic pitfalls are lymphoma, papillary carcinoma and Hürthle cell carcinoma.[229-235]

## Non-Epithelial Tumors

### Lymphoma

Primary lymphoma constitutes 8% of all thyroid malignancies.[235-255] The term is reserved for those cases where the thyroid gland is the predominant and often exclusive site of involvement, and therefore it should not be used for secondary involvement by systemic lymphoma or leukemia, which are found in 10% of autopsies.[240-242] In approximately 80% of thyroid lymphomas, the residual non-neoplastic gland exhibits features of Hashimoto's or lymphocytic thyroiditis[249,250] but only a very small percentage of patients with thyroiditis develop lymphoma.

Most primary thyroid lymphomas occur in middle-aged or elderly patients with a ratio of women to men ranging from 2:1 to 8:1.[251,254] They present as a relatively rapid thyroid enlargement accompanied by hoarseness, dysphagia and/or dyspnea in about 25% of the cases and cord paralysis in about 17%.[251-254] In most cases, the tumor is an ill-defined, solid mass with homogeneous, bulging white surface lacking encapsulation.

Most tumors are diffuse large B cell or immunoblastic non-Hodgkin lymphomas and, less frequently, poorly differentiated lymphocytic (small-cleaved) and intermediate types. T cell lymphomas are exceptionally rare.[251] Like lymphomas of mucosal sites, thyroid lymphoma appears to derive from parafollicular ("centrocyte-like") B-cells, and the high grade thyroid lymphomas appear to be derived from low grade tumors. There are histologic, immunohistologic, and clinical similarities between low and high grade non-Hodgkin's lymphomas of the thyroid and those of other mucosal sites, and some authors consider them neoplasms of mucosa-associated lymphoid tissue (MALT).[251]

Histopathologic evaluation requires adequate tissue sampling and proper pathologic interpretation, but surgical resection of the thyroid mass is not routinely part of the management strategy,[238] although some authors favor a more aggressive surgical approach since the amount of residual disease after debulking procedures has been shown to correlate with local and distant recurrences. Routine use of immunocytochemical analysis has led to the recognition that many thyroid neoplasms previously diagnosed as anaplastic or small cell carcinomas are actually lymphomas of the thyroid.[239-240,243,252-255]

## Hodgkin's Disease

It is exceptional for Hodgkin's disease to involve primarily the thyroid gland. As in many other extranodal sites, most cases so diagnosed in the past would be classified otherwise today. However, indisputable cases of Hodgkin disease of the thyroid exist.[256] Most are of the nodular sclerosis type and some have involved the regional lymph nodes.

## Cytopathology of Lymphoma

Cytologic specimens from malignant lymphomas are characterized by a monotonous population of non-cohesive atypical cells with large irregular vesicular nuclei, prominent nucleoli and scant cytoplasm. Although it is possible to diagnose primary high grade thyroid lymphoma in material obtained by FNAB, the distinction of low grade B cell lymphoma from lymphocytic thyroiditis is sometimes problematic. The most important differential diagnosis is from Hashimoto's thyroiditis where the lymphoid population is polymorphic and accompanied by plasma cells, macrophages and oncocytic cells. It should be remembered that Hashimoto's thyroiditis and malignant lymphoma often coexist. Ancillary techniques such as immunohistochemistry, flow cytometry and gene rearrangement studies can help to establish the definitive diagnosis.[255] Definitive diagnosis of lymphoma on cytologic specimens may be facilitated by the documentation of a clonal lymphoid proliferation within the specimen by flow cytometric immunophenotyping or immunocytochemistry. Recently, molecular techniques have also been developed to detect clonal lymphoid proliferation based on immunoglobulin (Ig) or T cell receptor gene rearrangement.[257]

## Plasmacytoma

Involvement of the thyroid gland by a plasma cell malignancy can be seen as an expression of widespread myeloma or as the only manifestation of the disease (plasmacytoma). Plasmacytoma should be distinguished from lymphoma exhibiting plasmacytoid features (ie immunoblastic lymphoma), some forms of small lymphocytic lymphoma, and "pleomorphic immunocytoma." In true plasmacytoma, all tumor cells have the appearance of plasma cells exhibiting various degrees of immaturity or atypia, whereas in lymphomas, the plasmacytoid elements alternate with cells of lymphoid type. The disease, even if localized, may be accompanied by detectable immunoglobulin abnormalities in the serum, and immunoglobulin light-chain restriction can be demonstrated immunohistochemically. Plasmacytoma may be associated with amyloid deposits and foreign-body reaction, features that may simulate a medullary carcinoma. Primary plasmacytoma of the thyroid is often accompanied by evidence of autoimmune thyroiditis in the remainder of the gland.[258-269]

## Sarcoma

Sarcomas are malignant tumors of mesenchymal derivation arising within the thyroid gland. Often, undifferentiated (anaplastic) carcinoma can be impossible to distinguish from sarcoma. Sarcoma-like tumors of the thyroid should be regarded as undifferentiated thyroid carcinomas until proven otherwise, although the issue is of no great practical significance since sarcoma's natural history and response to therapy do not differ significantly from those of undifferentiated carcinoma.[270-272]

The exception is thyroid angiosarcoma, a malignant tumor exhibiting endothelial cell differentiation (malignant hemangioendothelioma)[273-275] described in European, iodine-deficient mountainous areas, in elderly patients with a history of long-standing goiter and sudden painful enlargement of the gland and, in some instances, pleuropulmonary spread producing chest pain and hemothorax. The tumor is typically large with extensive areas of necrosis and hemorrhage and may resemble a hematoma. Although almost always invasive, it may exhibit a nodular well-circumscribed appearance on the cut surface. Histologically, freely anastomosing channels lined by atypical endothelial cells are often associated with a papillary configuration resulting from a predominantly intraluminal pattern of growth. The nuclei of the epithelioid endothelial cells are often large, vesicular, of regular outlines, and endowed with a large basophilic or amphophilic nucleolus connected by chromatin strands to the nuclear membrane. Mitoses, typical and atypical, are invariably found, often in large numbers. The pattern of growth is nearly always highly invasive and tumor necrosis is prominent. The tumor cells express vascular markers such as Factor VIII, CD31, CD34, and Ulex Europeus.

## Secondary/Metastatic Tumors

The thyroid gland may be invaded by carcinomas of pharynx, larynx, trachea, and esophagus, and by metastatic lesions in adjacent cervical lymph nodes. In view of the rarity of primary squamous cell carcinoma of the thyroid, the possibility of a metastasis should be considered whenever such a tumor type is present in a thyroid biopsy, particularly if the tumor is well to moderately well-differentiated. The discovery at autopsy of metastases to the thyroid from melanoma and carcinomas (lung, gastrointestinal tract, head and neck region, breast, and kidney) occurs in 9.5% of patients.[276,277]

## Cytopathology of Secondary/Metastatic Tumors

### Metastatic melanoma

Aspirates are hypercellular with single, discohesive cells with enlarged eccentrically placed nuclei with frequent bi- or multinucleation, prominent nucleoli, intranuclear pseudo-inclusions and moderately abundant cytoplasm with or without intracytoplasmic melanin pigment. Unusual cytologic features and previous history of melanoma do not help in reaching the diagnosis.

### Metastatic sarcoma

Aspirates may be hypocellular to cellular and the cytologic features reflect the histology of sarcomas ranging from malignant spindle cells in syncytial arrangements (malignant fibrous histiocytoma, fibrosarcoma, leiomyosarcoma) to lipoblasts of varying maturation in liposarcoma. The background may contain metachromatic myxoid or chondroid matrix material.

### Metastatic squamous cell carcinoma

Aspirates are cellular with malignant squamous cells singly or in syncytial arrangements with enlarged nuclei, prominent nucleoli and cytoplasm with squamoid or keratinizing features.

## Tumor-like Conditions

### Nodular Hyperplasia

Nodular hyperplasia (uninodular, multinodular or adenomatoid goiter, adenomatous hyperplasia) is a common thyroid disease (Figure 3–12). The endemic form, because of low iodine content of the water and soil, is the result of an increase in thyroid-stimulating hormone secretion. Initially the gland responds with hyperplastic (tall) follicular epithelium and scanty colloid production (parenchymatous goiter). Later, however, the gland becomes atrophic and stores abundant colloid (colloid goiter). The sporadic form is by far the most common in the United States, with an incidence in the general adult population of 3–5% and in autopsy series of 50%.[278] Some cases are considered the nodular forms of lymphocytic or Hashimoto's thyroiditis. Clinically, most patients are euthyroid and present with a multinodular gland that may cause tracheal obstruction. Hyperfunctional cases are called "*toxic nodular hyperplasia.*" The thyroid capsule is intact and on cross section multiple partially encapsulated nodules are seen, some composed of dilated follicles lined by flattened epithelium, others extremely cellular, and still others with oncocytes or clear cells. Some of the dilated follicles have small active follicles at one pole called "Sanderson polsters" (Figure 3–12D). Rupture of follicles may provoke a granulomatous reaction to the colloid and fresh and old hemorrhage, fibrosis, calcification, and osseous metaplasia are not uncommon. Nodular hyperplasia can simulate malignancy caused by the presence of hypercellularity, vesicular (ground-glass-like) nuclei, papillae, and parasitic nodules.

*Cytological features.* Aspirates are hypocellular and cytologic features reflect the stages of histological evolution. Often there is a mixture of colloid and follicular cells arranged in macro- or microfollicles or sheets with small round to oval nuclei with regular nuclear outline and finely granular chromatin. Also present are naked nuclei of follicular cells and histiocytes with and without hemosiderin. Squamous metaplasia and hemosiderin-laden macrophages can be seen and the amount and quality of colloid varies with some nodules being very cellular and containing minimal colloid. Oncocytic change can be confused with oncocytic tumors. The main diagnostic pitfalls are follicular neoplasms and colloid cyst or goiter. Cells with small nuclei and abundant cytoplasm are arranged in sheets with a honeycomb pattern.

## Diffuse Hyperplasia (Graves' Disease)

The diffusely hyperplastic gland may simulate malignancy because of the presence of well-developed papillary formations, large vesicular nuclei in the follicular epithelium and occasional extension of the hyperplastic process into the skeletal muscle of the neck. Cytological appearance varies with degree of activation.

## Dyshormonogenetic Goiter

This is a genetic hyperplasia resulting from enzymatic defects in the synthesis of thyroid hormones and secondary hypersecretion of thyroid-stimulating hormone. The gland is hypercellular and nuclear atypia can be prominent.

## Hashimoto's Thyroiditis

Hashimoto's disease presents with a combination of epithelial damage and proliferation, prominent interstitial polymorphous inflammatory infiltrate with germinal center formation (Figure 3–13), fibrotic bands and frequent "oxyphylic" change in follicular cells. Active phases are associated with multinodularity and enlargement of the gland and later phases with atrophy and fibrosis. Diffuse (Hashitoxicosis), nodular (nodular

Hashimoto's thyroiditis), and fibrous variants should be distinguished from primary and metastatic squamous cell carcinoma and from sclerosing mucoepidermoid carcinoma with eosinophilia.

*Cytological features.* Aspirates are usually cellular with numerous Hürthle cells singly or in discohesive clusters, forming micro- or macrofollicles in a background rich in lymphocytes, plasma cells and scant colloid. A background of atypical lymphocytes often justify the collection of non-fixed material for flow cytometric studies. The main diagnostic pitfalls are malignant lymphoma, Hürthle cell neoplasms and nodular hyperplasia with Hürthle cell metaplasia.

### Granulomatous (DeQuervain) thyroiditis

It can simulate a malignancy clinically and grossly due to ill-defined nature of the margins (Figure 3–14).

### Fibrosing (Riedel) thyroiditis

The fibrous process extends outside the thyroid into the surrounding soft tissues mimicking malignancy. Microscopically, the abundant collagen and prominent lymphoplasmacytic infiltrate and the lack of atypia

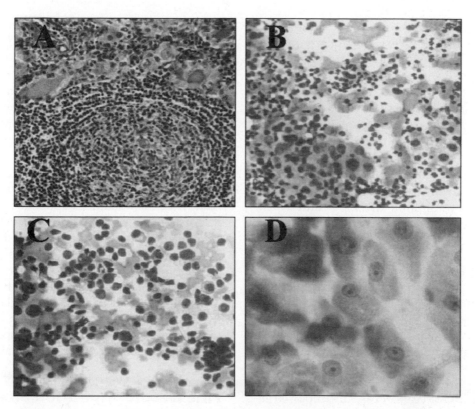

**Figure 3–13.** Hashimoto's thyroiditis. **A.** Germinal center. **B, C** and **D.** Cytologic features. **B.** Oncocytic follicular cells. **C.** Inflammatory cells (lymphocytes and monocytes. **D.** Higher magnification of sheets of follicular cells with oncocytic features.

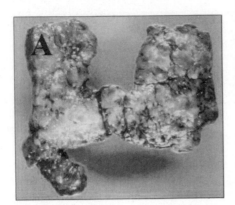
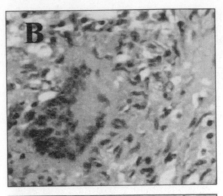
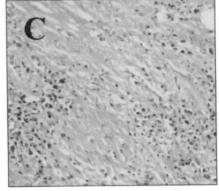

**Figure 3–14.** Granulomatous thyroiditis. **A.** Gross appearance with multinodularity and fibrosis. **B.** Multinucleated giant cell. **C.** Fibrosis and necrosis.

should facilitate the distinction from spindle cell anaplastic carcinoma, desmoplasia in papillary carcinoma, and lymphoma with sclerosis.

### Amyloid goiter

In most cases, the disease is accompanied by amyloid deposition in other organs. The amyloid deposits may be unilateral or bilateral and are often associated with a foreign body type giant cell reaction and adipose tissue. The differential diagnosis includes medullary carcinoma, the amyloidosis of multiple myeloma, and hyalinizing trabecular adenoma.

## THE THYROID NODULE

Thyroid nodules are extremely common. It has been estimated that there is a 5 to 10% lifetime risk of developing a palpable thyroid nodule. Approximately 4% of Americans between the ages of 30 and 60 years have one or more palpable thyroid nodules (one in 12 to 15 women and one in 40 to 50 men).[279] Since only approximately 18,000 new thyroid cancer cases are reported annually, most of these nodules are benign, and clinicians should be as selective as possible in recommending surgical removal.

The evaluation of a nodule should include the following considerations: *Age.* The incidence of malignancy is higher in children and the elderly. *Sex.* The incidence of malignancy is higher in males. *Geographic location* (iodine-deficiency). *Family history.* A strong family history (unrelated to dietary iodine deficiency) suggests the diagnosis of either dyshormonogenetic goiter or medullary carcinoma. *Rate of growth.* Most adenomas and well-differentiated follicular or papillary carcinomas are slow growing. Rapid enlargement of a pre-existing nodule may be related to the emergence of an undifferentiated malignant component or to spontaneous hemorrhage. *Characteristics of the nodule.* Solitary nodules are more likely to be malignant than multiple ones. One third of clinically solitary nodules are however multiple on scan or after pathologic examination. A malignancy should be suspected if the nodule is hard or if there are irregular nodules in a multinodular gland, if the gland is fixed when swallowing, or if there is vocal cord paralysis. *Ipsilateral adenopathy.* In the absence of infection, this is the strongest clinical indicator of malignancy.

## Fine Needle Aspiration Biopsy (FNAB)

This technique is quick, inexpensive and diagnostically accurate in experienced hands.[279-291] Its accuracy can be further improved by ultrasound guidance and is considered the test of choice in the initial evaluation of any thyroid nodule.[279-282] The most important aspect of FNAB interpretation is obtaining a high quality sample since most mistakes are made when interpretation is attempted in a poor-quality sample. Patients are placed in supine position with their head slightly elevated. Generally, a 22½ to 25-gauge needle is used. Minimal or no suction is applied to avoid aspirating excessive blood that may complicate interpretation. Tumor seeding or implantation has not been reported with thyroid tumors. For optimal results, 2–3 needle passes are recommended and both Papanicolaou and Diff-Quik stained smears should be prepared.[289] In addition, the cytopathologist must be familiar with potential limitations and pitfalls, and must use strict criteria for specimen adequacy. For proper smear interpretation of solid lesions, a minimum of six well-preserved cellular clusters with at least 10 cells in each cluster is needed. For cystic lesions, clinical judgment must be made before rendering a benign diagnosis. FNAB may result in transient elevation of thyroglobulin serum levels, partial or complete infarct of the tumor (particularly in oncocytic lesions), papillary hyperplastic changes, hemorrhage and thrombosis. These changes can be misinterpreted as papillary carcinoma or angiosarcoma.

The diagnostic accuracy of thyroid FNAB is generally reported in the range of 70% to 90% but it is highly aspirator and interpreter dependent. Generally accepted false negative rates and false positive rates are 1–8% and 1–2%, respectively.[279-289] Although FNAB is sufficiently sensitive in the diagnosis of thyroiditis and carcinomas, such as papillary, medullary, poorly differentiated and anaplastic, it has a limited value in the distinction of benign from malignant follicular lesions because of overlapping cytologic criteria.[290,291] Ancillary techniques such as quantitative image analysis, DNA ploidy, immunohistochemistry for several markers and quantitation of nucleolar organizing regions have shown variable results.

## Frozen-Section Examination

The role of frozen section (FS) in the management of thyroid nodules has greatly diminished after the widespread use of FNA. Its use, however, remains a subject of debate and indications have to be established for each institution. Lesions that are usually identifiable by FS include: conventional type of papillary carcinoma, widely invasive follicular carcinoma, poorly differentiated (insular) carcinoma, undifferentiated (anaplastic) carcinoma, medullary carcinoma, thyroiditis, and nodular hyperplasia (adenomatoid goiter).[292-306]

The most common diagnostic problem is the differential diagnosis of a single encapsulated nodule with follicular pattern. In this case, the differential diagnosis includes: dominant hyperplastic nodule, follicular adenoma, minimally invasive follicular carcinoma and encapsulated follicular variant of papillary carcinoma. The difficulty is caused by the very focal nature of capsular and vascular invasion in minimally invasive follicular carcinoma, and the absence of recognizable ground-glass nuclei on frozen tissue. In these circumstances, it is justified to "defer" diagnosis until permanent sections are examined.

Several authors have reported similar sensitivity and specificity for FNA and FS when used independently.[307-338] It is generally agreed that FS adds little to the intraoperative decision process if a definitive diagnosis of malignancy has been issued by preoperative FNA. Less definitive interpretations, however, decrease the sensitivity, specificity and accuracy of the FNA diagnosis. On the other hand, an FNAB diagnosis of "follicular neoplasm" is unlikely to be changed at the time of FS when follicular tumors are often "deferred to permanent." For these reasons, some authors have concluded that routine use of FS is unnecessary and that adequate preoperative FNAB diagnosis and sound clinical judgment at the time of surgery can adequately guide the extent of surgical resection. In fact, FS influences clinical management in a low number of cases (between 3% and 5%) and, in some cases, it can actually mislead the surgeon. On the other hand, FS should be strongly considered whenever the FNAB diagnosis is "suspicious." In 54% of these cases, a cancer is finally demonstrated by histological evaluation and, although FNAB is a reliable first diagnostic step, a negative FNAB should never be considered an exclusion of malignancy if there is strong clinical suspicion.[329-334] In general, when strict histologic and cytologic criteria are applied, the combined use of both methods decreases the false positive and false negative values of each of the methods used individually. Also, intraoperative evaluation of the tissue allows gross examination and intraoperative cytopathological assessment by touch preps, smears or scrapings. This cytological analysis at the time of frozen section together with recent modifications of the technique enhances overall diagnostic accuracy and, in particular, the recognition of papillary carcinomas. If by combining these methodologies malignancy is strongly suspected, definitive surgery can be confidently planned because in 90% of these cases final histological analysis will reveal malignancy. In contrast, if intraoperative evaluation is not diagnostic of malignancy, a conservative lobectomy-isthmusectomy is recommended, because in 71 % of these cases final histological evaluation will reveal a benign lesion.

## References

1. Landis SH, Murray T, Bolden S, Wingo P. Cancer statistics, 1998. CA. *A Cancer Journal for Physicians.* 1998;48(1):6–29.

2. AACE Clinical Practice Guidelines for the Diagnosis and Management of Thyroid Nodules. *Endocr Pract.* 1996;2:78–84.

3. Rosai J, Carcangiu ML, DeLellis RA. *Tumors of the Thyroid Gland. Atlas of Tumor Pathology.* Vol. 5. Washington, DC: Armed Forces Institute of Pathology; 1992.

4. LiVolsi VA. Surgical pathology of the thyroid. In: Bennington JL ed. *Major Problems in Pathology;* Vol 22. Philadelphia: WB Saunders; 1990.

5. Hoyes AD, Kershaw DR. Anatomy and development of the thyroid gland. *Ear Nose Throat J.* 1985;64:318–33.

6. Messina G, Viceconti, N, Trinti, B. Variations in the anatomy and physiology of the thyroid gland in old age. *Recenti Prog Med.* 1997;88(6): 281–6.

7. Licata, A, Bonanno G, Naso P et al. Surgical anatomy of the thyroid gland. Morphofunctional peculiarities and surgical pictures. *Minerva Chir* 1989;44(1-2): 83–86.

8. Hoyes, AD, Kershaw DR. Anatomy and development of the thyroid gland. *Ear Nose Throat J.* 1985;64(7): 318–33.

9. Frable WJ, Frable MA. Fine-needle aspiration biopsy of the thyroid. histopathologic and clinical correlations. In: Fenoglio CM, Wolff M, eds. *Progress in Surgical Pathology, Vol I.* New York: Masson; 1980:105–18.

10. Kline TS. *Handbook of Fine Needle Aspiration Biopsy Cytology.* St. Louis: CV Mosby; 1981.

11. Nunez C, Mendelsohn G. Fine-needle aspiration and needle biopsy of the thyroid gland. *Pathol Annu.* 1989; 24:161–98.

12. Oertel YC, Oertel JE. Diagnosis of benign thyroid lesions: fine-needle aspiration and histopathologic correlation. *Annals Diagn Pathol.* 1998;2(4):250–263.

13. Oertel YC, Oertel JE. Diagnosis of malignant thyroid lesions: fine-needle aspiration and histopathologic correlation. *Annals Diagn Pathol.* 1998;2(6):377–400.

14. Braunstein H, Stephens CL. Parafollicular cells of the human thyroid. *Arch Pathol.* 1968;86:659–66.

15. Gibson WC, Peng T-C, Croker BP. C-cell nodules in adult human thyroid. a common autopsy finding. *Am J Clin Pathol.* 1981;75: 347–50.

16. McMillan PJ, Hooker WM, Deftos LJ. Distribution of calcitonin-containing cells in the human thyroid. *Am J Anat.* 1974;140:73–80.

17. Baughman RA. Lingual thyroid and lingual thyroglossal tract remnants. a clinical and histopathologic study with a review of the literature. *Oral Surg.* 1972;34:781–99.

18. Williams ED, Toyn CE, Harach HR. The ultimobranchial gland and congenital thyroid abnormalities in man. *J Pathol.* 1989;159: 135–41.

19. Block MA, Wylie JH, Patton RB et al. Does benign thyroid tissue occur in the lateral part of the neck? *Am J Surg.* 1966;112:476–81.

20. Ward R. Relation of tumors of lateral aberrant thyroid tissue to malignant disease of the thyroid gland. *Arch Surg.* 1940;40:606–15.

21. Okstad S, Mair IW, Sundsfjord TA et al. Ectopic thyroid tissue in the head and neck. *J Otolaryngol.* 1986;15(1):52–5.

22. Kaplan M, Kauli R. Ectopic thyroid gland. a clinical study of 30 children and review. *J Pediatr.* 1978;92(2):205–9.

23. Larochelle D, Arcand P, Belzille M et al. Ectopic thyroid tissue. a review of the literature. *J Otolaryngol.* 1979;8(6):523–30.

24. Lewis M, Holleran WM. Ectopic thyroid gland in children. *Am J Surg.* 1968;115(5):688–90.

25. Eyuboglu E, Kapan M, Ipek T et al. Ectopic thyroid in the abdomen: report of a case. *Surg Today.* 1999;29(5):472–4.

26. Shiraishi, T, Imai H, Fukutome K et al. Ectopic thyroid in the adrenal gland. *Hum Pathol.* 1999;30(1):105–8.

27. Richmond I, Whittaker JS, Peiraniya AK et al. Intracardiac ectopic thyroid: a case report and review of published cases. *Thorax.* 1990;5(4):293–4.

28. Hedinger CE, Williams ED, Sobin LH. Histological typing of thyroid tumours. In: Hediger CE, ed. *International Histological Classification of Tumours, Vol 11.* 2nd ed. Berlin: Springer-Verlag; 1988.

29. Hedinger C, Williams ED, Sobin LH. The WHO histological classification of thyroid tumors: a commentary on the second edition. *Cancer.* 1989;63(5):908–11.

30. Veronesi U, Cascinelli N, Pilotti, S. Epidemiology, etiological factors and histological classification of malignant tumors of the thyroid. *Minerva Med.* 1971;62(6):272–4.

31. Pansa E, Maggi G. Classification and morphology of malignant tumors of the thyroid. *Minerva Med.* 1967;58(1):10–23.

32. Klein M, Aubert V, Weryha G et al. Classification and epidemiology of thyroid tumors. *Rev Prat.* 1996;46(19):2288–95.

33. Hamburger JI. Solitary autonomously functioning thyroid lesions. Diagnosis, clinical features and pathogenetic considerations. *Am J Med.* 1975;58:740–8.

34. Festen C, Otten BJ, van de Kaa CA. Follicular adenoma of the thyroid gland in children. *Eur J Pediatr Surg.* 1995;5(5):262–4.

35. Namba H, Matsuo K, Fagin JA. Clonal composition of benign and malignant human thyroid tumors. *J Clin Invest.* 1990;86:120–5.

36. Thomas GA, Williams D, Williams ED. The clonal origin of thyroid nodules and adenomas. *Am J Pathol.* 1989;134:141–7.

37. Hicks DG, LiVolsi VA, Neidich JA, Puck JM, Kant JA. Clonal analysis of solitary follicular nodules in the thyroid. *Am J Pathol.* 1990;137:553–62.

38. Bisi H, Fernandes VS, Asato de Camargo RY, Koch L, Abdo AH, de Brito T. The prevalence of unsuspected thyroid pathology in 300 sequential autopsies, with special reference to the incidental carcinoma. *Cancer.* 1989;64:1888–93.

39. Johannessen JV, Sobrinho-Simoes M. Well differentiated thyroid tumors. problems in diagnosis and understanding. *Pathol Annu.* 1983;18(Pt. 1):255–85.

40. Cuello C, Correa P, Eisenberg H. Geographic pathology of thyroid carcinoma. *Cancer.* 1969;23:230–9.

41. Russell WO, Ibanez ML, Albores-Saavedra JT et al. Thyroid carcinoma. Classification, intraglandular dissemination and clinico-pathological study based upon whole organ sections of 80 glands. *Cancer.* 1963;16:1425–60.

42. Lang W, Choritz H, Hundeshagen H. Risk factors in follicular thyroid carcinomas. a retrospective follow-up study covering a 14-year period with emphasis on morphological findings. *Am J Surg Pathol.* 1986;10:246–55.

43. Harness JK, Thompson NW, Mcleod MR et al. Follicular carcinoma of the thyroid gland: trends and treatment. *Surgery.* 1984;96:972–80.

44. Crile G, Hazard JB. Relationship of the age of the patient to the natural history and prognosis of carcinoma of the thyroid. *Ann Surg.* 1953;138:33–8.

45. Brennan MD, Bergstralh EJ, van Heerden JA et al. Follicular thyroid cancer treated at the Mayo Clinic, 1946 through 1970: initial manifestations, pathologic findings, therapy, and outcome. *Mayo Clin Proc.* 1991;66:11–22.

46. Emerick, G, Duh QY, Siperstein AE et al. Diagnosis, treatment, and outcome of follicular thyroid carcinoma. *Cancer.* 1993;72(11): 3287–95.

47. Franssila KO, Ackerman LV, Brown CL, Hedinger CE. Follicular carcinoma. *Semin Diagn Pathol.* 1985;2:101–22.

48. Kahn NF, Perzin KH. Follicular carcinoma of the thyroid: an evaluation of the histology criteria used for diagnosis. *Pathol Annu.* 1983;18:221–53.

49. Schmid K, Totsch WM, Ofner D et al. Minimally invasive follicular thyroid carcinoma: a clinico-pathological study. *Curr Top Pathol.* 1997;91:37–43.

50. Schmidt RJ, Wang CA. Encapsulated follicular carcinoma of the thyroid: diagnosis, treatment, and results. *Surgery.* 1986;100(6): 1068–77.

51. De Micco, C. Anatomo-pathology and histological prognosis of follicular thyroid carcinoma. *Ann Endocrinol.* 1992;58(3):172–82.

52. Woolner LB. Thyroid carcinoma: pathologic classification with data on prognosis. *Semin Nucl Med.* 1971;1(1):101–502.

53. Yamashina M. Follicular neoplasms of the thyroid. Total circumferential evaluation of the fibrous capsule. *Am J Surg Pathol* 1992; 16(4):392–400.

54. Iida F. Surgical significance of capsule invasion of adenoma of the thyroid. *Surg Gynecol Obstet.* 1977;144:710–2.

55. Warren S. Invasion of blood vessels in thyroid cancer. *Am J Clin Pathol.* 1956;26:64–5.

56. Galera-Davidson H, Bibbo M, Baotels PH et al. Differential diagnosis between follicular adenoma and follicular carcinoma of the thyroid by marker features. *Anal Quant Cytol Histol.* 1986;8(3): 195–200.

57. Montironi, R, Alberti R, Sisti S et al. Discrimination between follicular adenoma and follicular carcinoma of the thyroid: preoperative validity of cytometry on aspiration smears. *Appl Pathol.* 1989;7(6):367–74.

58. Sprenger E, Lowhagen T, Vogt-Schaden M et al. Differential diagnosis between follicular adenoma and follicular carcinoma of the thyroid by nuclear DNA determination. *Acta Cytol.* 1977;21(4): 528–30.

59. Galera-Davidson H, Bartels PH, Fernandez-Rodriquez A et al. Karyometric marker features in fine needle aspirates of invasive follicular carcinoma of the thyroid. *Anal Quant Cytol Histol.* 1990; 12(1):35–41.

60. Harach HR, Virgili E, Soler G et al. Cytopathology of follicular tumours of the thyroid with clear cell change. *Cytopathology.* 1991;2(3):125–35.

61. Kini SR, Miller JM, Hamburger TI et al. Cytopathology of follicular lesions of the thyroid gland. *Diagn Cytopathol.* 1985;1(2): 123–32.

62. Miller JM, Kini SR, Hamburger JI. The diagnosis of malignant follicular neoplasms of the thyroid by needle biopsy. *Cancer.* 1985; 55:2812–7.

63. Dal Cin P, Sneyers W, Aly MS et al. Involvement of 19q13 in follicular thyroid adenoma. *Cancer Genet Cytogenet.* 1992;60(1): 99–101.

64. Roque L, Castedo S et al. Translocation t(5;19): a recurrent change in thyroid follicular adenoma. *Genes Chromosomes Cancer.* 1992; 4(4):346–7.

65. West J, Munoz-Antonia TA, Johnson JG, Klotch D, Muro-Cacho CA. TGF-β Type II receptors and Smad proteins in follicular thyroid tumors. *Laryngoscope.* (in press).

66. Pilotti S, Manenti G, DeGregorio L et al. Identification of the same HRAS1 mutation in a primary minimally invasive follicular carcinoma of the thyroid gland and its bone metastasis developed 15 years later. *Diagn Mol Pathol.* 1995;4(1):73–4.

67. Grebe SK, McIver B, Hay ID et al. Frequent loss of heterozygosity on chromosomes 3p and 17p without VHL or p53 mutations suggests involvement of unidentified tumor suppressor genes in follicular thyroid carcinoma. *J Clin Endocrinol Metab.* 1997;82(11): 3684–91.

68. Jenkins RB, Hay ID, Herath TF et al. Frequent occurrence of cytogenetic abnormalities in sporadic nonmedullary thyroid carcinoma. *Cancer.* 1990;66:1213–20.

69. Carcangiu ML, Zampi G, Pupi A et al. Papillary carcinoma of the thyroid. A clinicopathologic study of 241 cases treated at the University of Florence, Italy. *Cancer.* 1985;55:805–28.

70. Hawk WA, Hazard JB. The many appearances of papillary carcinoma of the thyroid. *Cleve Clin Q.* 1976; 43:207–16.

71. LiVolsi V. Papillary neoplasms of the thyroid. Pathologic and prognostic features. *Am J Clin Pathol.* 1992;97:426–34.

72. Hay ID. Papillary thyroid carcinoma. *Endocrinol Metab Clin North Am.* 1990;19:545–76.

73. Mazzaferri EL. Papillary thyroid carcinoma: factors influencing prognosis and current therapy. *Semin Oncol.* 1987;14:315–32.

74. Vickery AL Jr. Thyroid papillary carcinoma. Pathological and philosophical controversies. *Am J Surg Pathol.* 1983;7:797–807.

75. Carcangiu ML, Zampi G, Rosai J. Papillary thyroid carcinoma: a study of its many morphologic expressions and clinical correlates. *Pathol Annu.* 1985;20(Pt.1):1–44.

76. Kulacoglu S, Ashton-Key M, Buley I. Pitfalls in the diagnosis of papillary carcinoma of the thyroid. *Cytopathology.* 1998;9(3): 193–200.

77. Rigaud, C. Papillary carcinoma of the thyroid: development of the histological criteria for diagnosis. Study of 29 cases and review of the literature. *Ann Pathol.* 1998;8(3):211–9.

78. Frazell EL, Foote FW Jr. Papillary thyroid carcinoma. Pathological findings in cases with and without clinical evidence of cervical node involvement. *Cancer.* 1955;8:1165–6.

79. Rosai J, Carcangiu ML. Pitfalls in the diagnosis of thyroid neoplasms. *Pathol Res Pract.* 1987;182:169–79.

80. Christ ML, Haja J. Intranuclear cytoplasmic inclusions (invaginations) in thyroid aspirations. Frequency and specificity. *Acta Cytol.* 1979;23:327–31.

81. Yang GC, Greenebaum E. Clear nuclei of papillary thyroid carcinoma conspicuous in fine-needle aspiration and intraoperative smears processed by ultrafast papanicolaou stain. *Mod Pathol.* 1997;10(6):552–5.

82. Chetty R,. Learmonth GM, Kalan MR. The significance of nuclear grooves and phagocytosis in the diagnosis of metastatic papillary carcinoma of the thyroid. *Cytopathology.* 1991;2(1):43–5.

83. Dominguez-Malagon HR, Szymanski-Somez TT, Gaytan-Sasier SR. Optically clear and vacuolated nuclei. Two useful signs for the transoperative diagnosis of papillary carcinoma of the thyroid. *Cancer.* 1988;62(1):105–8.

84. Shurbaji MS, Gupta PK et al. Nuclear grooves: a useful criterion in the cytopathologic diagnosis of papillary thyroid carcinoma. *Diagn Cytopathol.* 1988;4(2):91–4.

85. Ellison E, Lapuerta P, Martin S. Psammoma bodies in fine needle aspirates of the thyroid. *Cancer Cytopathol.* 1988;84:169–75.

86. Crile G Jr, Sobrinho-Simoes M. The origin and significance of thyroid psammoma bodies. *Lab Invest.* 1980;43:287–96.

87. Klinck GH, Winship T. Psammoma bodies and thyroid cancer. *Cancer.* 1959;12:656–62.

88. Deligeorgi-Politi H. Nuclear crease as a cytodiagnostic feature of papillary thyroid carcinoma in fine-needle aspiration biopsies. *Diagn Cytopathol.* 1987;3:307–10.

89. Gray A, Doniach I. Morphology of the nuclei of papillary carcinoma of the thyroid. *Br J Cancer.* 1969;23.49–51.

90. Chan JK, Saw D. The grooved nucleus. A useful diagnostic criterion of papillary carcinoma of the thyroid. *Am J Surg Pathol.* 1986; 10:672–9.

91. Satoh Y, Sakamoto A, Yamada K, Kasai N. Psammoma bodies in metastatic carcinoma to the thyroid. *Mod Pathol.* 1990;3:267–70.

92. Lang W, Borrusch H, Bauer L. Occult carcinomas of the thyroid. Evaluation of 1,020 sequential autopsies. *Am J Clin Pathol.* 1988;90: 72–76.

93. Albores-Saavedra J, Gould E, Vardaman C et al. The macrofollicular variant of papillary thyroid carcinoma. A study of 17 cases. *Human Pathol.* 1991;22:1195–205.

94. Akslen LA, Varhaug JE. Thyroid carcinoma with mixed tall-cell and columnar-cell features. *Am J Clin Pathol.* 1990;94:442–5.

95. Flint A, Davenport RD, Lloyd RV. The tall cell variant of papillary carcinoma of the thyroid gland. Comparison with the common form of papillary carcinoma by DNA and morphometricanalysis. *Arch Pathol Lab Med.* 1991;115:169–71.

96. Evans HL. Columnar-cell carcinoma of the thyroid. A report of two cases of an aggressive variant of thyroid carcinoma. *Am J Clin Pathol.* 1986;85:77–80.

97. Sobrinho-Simoes M, Nesland JM, Johannessen JV. Columnar-cell carcinoma. Another variant of poorly differentiated carcinoma of the thyroid. *Am J Clin Pathol.* 1988;89:264–67.

98. Harach HR, Virgili E, Soler G, Zusman SB, Saravia-Day E. Cytopathology of follicular tumours of the thyroid with clear cell change. *Cytopath.* 1991;2:125–35.

99. Ohori NP, Schoedel KE. Cytopathology of high-grade papillary thyroid carcinomas: tall-cell variant, diffuse sclerosing variant, and poorly differentiated papillary carcinoma. *Diagn Cytopathol.* 1999;20(1):19–23.

100. Zacks JF, de las Morenas A et al. Fine-needle aspiration cytology diagnosis of colloid nodule versus follicular variant of papillary carcinoma of the thyroid. *Diagn Cytopathol.* 1998;18(2):87–90.

101. Akhtar M, Ali MA, Hug M et al. Fine-needle aspiration biopsy of papillary thyroid carcinoma: cytologic, histologic, and ultrastructural correlations. *Diagn Cytopathol.* 1991;7(4):373–9.

102. Francis, IM, Das DK, Sheikh ZA et al. Role of nuclear grooves in the diagnosis of papillary thyroid carcinoma. A quantitative assessment on fine needle aspiration smears. *Acta Cytol.* 1995;39(3):409–15.

103. Vinette, DS, MacDonald LL, Yazdi HM. Papillary carcinoma of the thyroid with anaplastic transformation: diagnostic pitfalls in fine-needle aspiration biopsy. *Diagn Cytopathol.* 1991;7(1):75–8.

104. Kupp M, H Ehya. Nuclear grooves in the aspiration cytology of papillary carcinoma of the thyroid. *Acta Cytol.* 1989;33(1):21–6.

105. Schmid KW, Lucciarini P, Jadurner D et al. Papillary carcinoma of the thyroid gland. Analysis of 94 cases with preoperative fine needle aspiration cytologic examination. *Acta Cytol.* 1987;31(5):591–4.

106. Kini SR, Miller JM, Hamburger TI et al. Cytopathology of papillary carcinoma of the thyroid by fine needle aspiration. *Acta Cytol.* 1980;24(6):511–21.

107. Deligeorgi-Politi, H. Nuclear crease as a cytodiagnostic feature of papillary thyroid carcinoma in fine-needle aspiration biopsies. *Diagn Cytopathol.* 1987;3(4):307–10.

108. Hugh JC, Duggan MA, Chang-Poon V et al. The fine-needle aspiration appearance of the follicular variant of thyroid papillary carcinoma: a report of three cases. *Diagn Cytopathol.* 1988;4(3):196–201.

109. Mesonero CE, Jugle JE, Wilbur DC et al. Fine-needle aspiration of the macrofollicular and microfollicular subtypes of the follicular variant of papillary carcinoma of the thyroid. *Cancer.* 1988;84(4):235–44.

110. Doria MI, Jr, H Attal, Wang HH et al. Fine needle aspiration cytology of the oxyphil variant of papillary carcinoma of the thyroid. A report of three cases. *Acta Cytol.* 1996;40(5):1007–11.

111. Martinez-Parra D, Campos Fernandez J, Hierro-Guilmain CC et al. Follicular variant of papillary carcinoma of the thyroid: to what extent is fine-needle aspiration reliable? *Diagn Cytopathol.* 1996;15(1):12–6.

112. Harach HR, Zusman SB. Cytopathology of the tall cell variant of thyroid papillary carcinoma. *Acta Cytol.* 1992;36(6):895–9.

113. Filie AC, Chiesa A, Bryant BR et al: The tall cell variant of papillary carcinoma of the thyroid. Cytologic features and LOH of metastatic and/or recurrent neoplasms and primary neoplasms. *Cancer.* 1999;87:238–42.

114. Putti TC, Bhuiya TA, Wasserman PG. Fine needle aspiration cytology of mixed tall and columnar cell papillary carcinoma of the thyroid. A case report. *Acta Cytol.* 1998;42(2):387–90.

115. Kaw YT. Fine needle aspiration cytology of the tall cell variant of papillary carcinoma of the thyroid. *Acta Cytol.* 1994;38(2):282.

116. Pang XP, Ross NS, Hershman TM. Alterations in TNF-alpha signal transduction in resistant human papillary thyroid carcinoma cells. *Thyroid.* 1996;6(4):313–7.

117. Gagel RF. An overview of molecular abnormalities leading to thyroid carcinogenesis: a 1993 perspective. *Stem Cells.* 1999;15 (Suppl 2):7–13.

118. Pierotti, MA, Bongarzone I, Borello MG et al. Cytogenetics and molecular genetics of carcinomas arising from thyroid epithelial follicular cells. *Genes Chromosomes Cancer.* 1996;16(1):1–14.

119. Farid NR. Molecular pathogenesis of thyroid cancer: the significance of oncogenes, tumor suppressor genes, and genomic instability. *Exp Clin Endocrinol Diabetes.* 1996;104(Suppl 4):1–12.

120. Ito T, Seyama T, Mizuno T et al. Genetic alterations in thyroid tumor progression: association with p53 gene mutations. *Jpn J Cancer Res.* 1993;84(5):526–31.

121. Wynford-Thomas, D. Molecular basis of epithelial tumorigenesis: the thyroid model. *Crit Rev Oncog.* 1993;4(1):1–23.

122. Sozzi G, Bongarzone I, Miozzo M et al. Cytogenetic and molecular genetic characterization of papillary thyroid carcinomas. *Genes Chromosomes Cancer.* 1992;5(3):212–8.

123. Namba HS, Rubin A, Fagin TA et al. Point mutations of ras oncogenes are an early event in thyroid tumorigenesis. *Mol Endocrinol.* 1990;4(10):1474–9.

124. Jenkins RB, Hay ID, Herath TF et al. Frequent occurrence of cytogenetic abnormalities in sporadic nonmedullary thyroid carcinoma. *Cancer.* 1990;66(6):1213–20.

125. Namba H, Gutman RA, Matsuo K et al. H-ras protooncogene mutations in human thyroid neoplasms. *J Clin Endocrinol Metab.* 1990;71(1):223–9.

126. Gire V, Wynford-Thomas D. Origin and progression of thyroid epithelial tumors: molecular and cellular mechanisms. *Arch Anat Cytol Pathol.* 1998;46(1-2):11–8.

127. Nakayama T, Ito M, Ohtsuru A et al. Expression of the ets-1 proto-oncogene in human thyroid tumor. *Mod Pathol.* 1999;12(1):61–8

128. Saji M, Westra WH, Chen H et al. Telomerase activity in the differential diagnosis of papillary carcinoma of the thyroid. *Surgery.* 1997;122(6):1137–40.

129. Weiss M, Baruch A, Keydas I et al. Preoperative diagnosis of thyroid papillary carcinoma by reverse transcriptase polymerase chain reaction of the MUC1 gene. *Int J Cancer.* 1996;66(1):55–9.

130. Eng C. RET proto-oncogene in the development of human cancer. *J Clin Oncol.* 1999;17(1):380–93.

131. Nakata T, Kitamura Y, Shimizu K et al. Fusion of a novel gene, ELKS, to RET due to translocation t(10;12)(q11;p13) in a papillary thyroid carcinoma. *Genes Chromosomes Cancer.* 1999;25(2):97–103.

132. Pierotti MA, Vigneri P, Bougarzone I. Rearrangements of RET and NTRK1 tyrosine kinase receptors in papillary thyroid carcinomas. *Recent Results Cancer Res.* 1998;154:237–47.

133. Durick K, Gill GN, Taylor SS. Shc and Enigma are both required for mitogenic signaling by Ret/ptc2. *Mol Cell Biol.* 1998;18(4):2298–308.

134. Komminoth P. The RET proto-oncogene in medullary and papillary thyroid carcinoma. Molecular features, pathophysiology and clinical implications. *Virchows Arch.* 1997;431(1):1–9.

135. Santoro M, Chiappetta G, Cerrato A et al. Development of thyroid papillary carcinomas secondary to tissue-specific expression of the RET/PTC1 oncogene in transgenic mice. *Oncogene.* 1996;12(8):1821–6.

136. Viglietto G, Chiappetta G, Martinez-Tello FJ et al. RET/PTC oncogene activation is an early event in thyroid carcinogenesis. *Oncogene.* 1995;11(6):1207–10.

137. Minoletti F, Butti MG, Coronelli S et al. The two genes generating RET/PTC3 are localized in chromosomal band 10q11.2. *Genes Chromosomes Cancer.* 1994;11(1):51–7.

138. Bongarzone I, Butti MG, Coronelli S et al. Frequent activation of ret protooncogene by fusion with a new activating gene in papillary thyroid carcinomas. *Cancer Res.* 1994;54(11):2979–85.

139. Santoro M, Sabino N, Ishizaka Y et al. Involvement of RET oncogene in human tumours: specificity of RET activation to thyroid tumours. *Br J Cancer.* 1993;68(3):460–4.

140. Santoro M, Carlomagno F, Hay ID et al. Ret oncogene activation in human thyroid neoplasms is restricted to the papillary cancer subtype. *J Clin Invest.* 1992;89(5):1517–22.

141. Herrmann MA, Hay ID, Bartelt DH et al. Cytogenetic and molecular genetic studies of follicular and papillary thyroid cancers. *J Clin Invest.* 1991;88(5):1596–604.

142. Grieco M, Santoro M, Berlingieri MT et al. PTC is a novel rearranged form of the ret proto-oncogene and is frequently detected in vivo in human thyroid papillary carcinomas. *Cell.* 1990;60(4):557–63.

143. Grieco M, Santoro M, Berlingieri MT et al. Molecular cloning of PTC, a new oncogene found activated in human thyroid papillary carcinomas and their lymph node metastases. *Ann N Y Acad Sci.* 1988;551:380–1.

144. Filie AC, Chiesa A, Bryant BR et al. The tall cell variant of papillary carcinoma of the thyroid: cytologic features and loss of heterozygosity of metastatic and/or recurrent neoplasms and primary neoplasms. *Cancer.* 1999;87(4):38–42.

145. Muro-Cacho CA, Holt T, Klotch D et al. Cyclin D1 expression as a prognostic parameter in Papillary Carcinoma of the thyroid. *Otolaryngol Head Neck Surg.* 1999;120(2):200–207.

146. Muro-Cacho CA, Munoz-Antonia T, Livingston S et al. Transforming growth factor receptors and p27kip in thyroid carcinoma. *Arch Otolaryngol Head Neck Surg.* 1999;125(1):76–81

147. Nishida, T, Katayama S, Tsujimoto M et al. Clinicopathological significance of poorly differentiated thyroid carcinoma. *Am J Surg Pathol.* 1999;23(2):205–11.

148. Sakamoto A. Poorly differentiated carcinoma of the thyroid: an aggressive type of tumour arising from thyroid follicular epithelium. *Curr Top Pathol.* 1997;91:45–50.

149. Sakamoto A, Kasai N, Sugano H et al. Poorly differentiated carcinoma of the thyroid. A clinicopathologic entity for a high-risk group of papillary and follicular carcinomas. *Cancer.* 1983;52(10):1849–55.

150. Pilotti S, Collini P, Manzari A et al. Poorly differentiated forms of papillary thyroid carcinoma: distinctive entities or morphological patterns? *Semin Diagn Pathol.* 1995;12(3):249–55.

151. Killeen RM, Barnes L, Watson CG et al. Poorly differentiated ("insular") thyroid carcinoma. Report of two cases and review of the literature. *Arch Otolaryngol Head Neck Surg.* 1990;116(9):1082–6.

152. Begin LR, Allaire GS. Insular (poorly differentiated) carcinoma of the thyroid: an ultrastructural and immunocytochemical study of two cases. *J Submicrosc Cytol Pathol.* 1997;28(1):121–31.

153. Mizukami Y, Nonomura A, Michigishi T et al. Poorly differentiated (insular) carcinoma of the thyroid. *Pathol Int.* 1995;45(9):663–8.

154. Carcangiu ML, Zampi G, Rosai J. Poorly differentiated (insular) thyroid carcinoma. A reinterpretation of Langhans' "wuchernde Struma." *Am J Surg Pathol.* 1984;8:655–68.

155. Flynn SD, Forman BH, Stewart AF, Kinder BK. Poorly differentiated (insular) carcinoma of the thyroid gland: an aggressive subset of differentiated thyroid neoplasms. *Surgery.* 1988;104:963–70.

156. Kuhel WI, Kutler DI, Santos Buck CA. Poorly differentiated insular thyroid carcinoma. A case report with identification of intact insulae with fine needle aspiration biopsy. *Acta Cytol.* 1998;42(4):991–7.

157. Pereira EM, Maeda SA, Alves F et al. Poorly differentiated carcinoma (insular carcinoma) of the thyroid diagnosed by fine needle aspiration (FNA). *Cytopathology.* 1996;7(1):61–5.

158. Zakowski MF, Schlesinger K, Mizrachi HH. Cytologic features of poorly differentiated "insular" carcinoma of the thyroid. A case report. *Acta Cytol.* 1992;36(4):523–6.

159. Pietribiasi F, Sapino A, Papotti M et al. Cytologic features of poorly differentiated 'insular' carcinoma of the thyroid, as revealed by fine-needle aspiration biopsy. *Am J Clin Pathol.* 1990;94(6):687–92

160. Rosai J, Saxen EA, Woolner L. Undifferentiated and poorly differentiated carcinoma. *Semin Diagn Pathol.* 1985;2:123–36.

161. Bronner MP, LiVolsi VA. Spindle cell squamous carcinoma of the thyroid: an unusual anaplastic tumor associated with tall cell papillary cancer. *Mod Pathol.* 1991;4:637–43.

162. Casterline PF, Jaques DA, Blom H, Wartofsky L. Anaplastic giant cell and spindle-cell carcinoma of the thyroid: a different therapeutic approach. *Cancer.* 1980;45:1689–92.

163. Berry B, MacFarlane J, Chan N. Osteoclastomalike anaplastic carcinoma of the thyroid. Diagnosis by fine needle aspiration cytology. *Acta Cytol.* 1990;34(2):248–50.

164. Aldinger KA, Samaan NA, Ibanez M et al. Anaplastic carcinoma of the thyroid: a review of 84 cases of spindle and giant cell carcinoma of the thyroid. *Cancer.* 1978;41:2267–75.

165. Carcangiu ML, Steeper T, Zampi G, Rosai J. Anaplastic thyroid carcinoma. A study of 70 cases. *Am J Clin Pathol.* 1985;83:135–58.

166. Pilotti S, Collini P, Del Bo R et al. A novel panel of antibodies that segregates immunocytochemically poorly differentiated carcinoma from undifferentiated carcinoma of the thyroid gland. *Am J Surg Pathol.* 1994;18(10):1054–64.

167. Hamperl H. Benign and malignant oncocytoma. *Cancer.* 1962;15:1019–27.

168. Bondeson L, Bondeson A-G, Ljunberg O et al. Oxyphil tumors of the thyroid: follow-up of 42 surgical cases. *Ann Surg.* 1981;194:677–80.

169. Tallini G, Carcangiu ML, Rosai J. Oncocytic neoplasms of the thyroid gland. *Acta Pathol Jpn.* 1992;42:305–15.

170. Caplan RH, Abellera RM, Kisken WA. Hürthle cell tumors of the thyroid gland. A clinicopathologic review and long-term follow-up. *JAMA.* 1984;251:3114–7.

171. McLeod MK, Thompson NW. Hürthle cell neoplasms of the thyroid. *Otolaryngol Clin North Am.* 1990;23:441–52.

172. Lazzi S, Spina D, Als C, et al. Oncocytic (Hurthle cell) tumors of the thyroid: distinct growth patterns comparedwith clinicopathological features. *Thyroid.* 1999;9(2):97–103.

173. Berho M, Suster S. The oncocytic variant of papillary carcinoma of the thyroid: a clinicopathologic study of 15 cases. *Hum Pathol.* 1997;28(1):47–53.

174. Tallini G, Ladanyi M, Rosai L. Analysis of nuclear and mitochondrial DNA alterations in thyroid and renal oncocytic tumors. *Cytogenet Cell Genet.* 1994;66(4):253–9.

175. Matias C, Moura Nunes JF, Sobrinho LG et al. Giant mitochondria and intramitochondrial inclusions in benign thyroid lesions. *Ultrastruct Pathol.* 1991;15:221–9.

176. Kini SR, Miller JM, Hamburger JI. Cytopathology of Hurthle cell lesions of the thyroid gland by fine needle aspiration. *Acta Cytol.* 1981;25:647–52.

177. Bouras M, Bertholon J, Dutrieux-Berger N et al. Variability of Ha-ras (codon 12) proto-oncogene mutations in diverse thyroid cancers. *Eur J Endocrinol.* 1998;139(2):209–16.

178. Schark C, Fulton N, Yashiro T et al. The value of measurement of ras oncogenes and nuclear DNA analysis in the diagnosis of Hurthle cell tumors of the thyroid. *World J Surg.* 1999;16(4):745–51

179. Schark C, Fulton N, Jacobi JF et al. N-ras 61 oncogene mutations in Hurthle cell tumors. *Surgery.* 1990;108(6):994–9

180. Takiyama Y, Saji M, Clark DP et al. Polymerase chain reaction-based microsatellite analysis of fine-needle aspirations from Hurthle cell neoplasms. *Thyroid.* 1997;7(6):853–7.

181. Segev DL, Saji M, Phillips GS et al. Polymerase chain reaction-based microsatellite polymorphism analysis of follicular and Hurthle cell neoplasms of the thyroid. *J Clin Endocrinol Metab.* 1998;83(6):2036–42.

182. Zedenius J, Wallin G, Svensson A et al. Allelotyping of follicular thyroid tumors. *Hum Genet.* 1995;96(1):27–32.

183. Graff JR, Greenberg VE, Hermann JG et al. Distinct patterns of E-cadherin CpG island methylation in papillary, follicular, Hurthle's cell, and poorly differentiated human thyroid carcinoma. *Cancer Res.* 1998;58(10):2063–6.

184. Carcangiu ML, Sibley RK, Rosai J. Clear cell change in primary thyroid tumors. A study of 38 cases. *Am J Surg Pathol.* 1985;9:705–22.

185. Civantos F, Albores-Saavedra J, Madji M et al. Clear cell variant of thyroid carcinoma. *Am J Surg Pathol.* 1984;196:361–370

186. Braunstein H, Stephens CL. Parafollicular cells of the human thyroid. *Arch Pathol.* 1968;86:659–66.

187. Pearse AG, Polak JM. Cytochemical evidence for the neural crest origin of mammalian ultimobranchial C cells. *Histochemie.* 1976;27:96–102.

188. DeLellis RA, Wolfe HJ. The pathobiology of the human calcitonin (C)-cell: a review. *Pathol Annu.* 1981;16(2):25–52.

189. McMillan PJ, Hooker WM, Deftos LJ. Distribution of calcitonin-containing cells in the human thyroid. *Am J Anat.* 1974;140: 73–80.

190. Teitelbaum SL, Moore KE, Shieber W. Parafollicular cells in the normal human thyroid. *Nature.* 1971;230:334–45.

191. DeLellis RA, Nunnemacher G, Wolfe HJ. C-cell hyperplasia: an ultrastructural analysis. *Lab Invest.* 1977;36:237–48.

192. Kaserer K, Scheuba C, Neuhold N et al. C-cell hyperplasia and medullary thyroid carcinoma in patients routinely screened for serum calcitonin. *Am J Surg Pathol.* 1998;22(6):722–8.

193. Black WC, Haff RC. The surgical pathology of parathyroid chief cell hyperplasia. *Am J Clin Pathol.* 1970;53(5): 565–79.

194. Perry A, Molberg K, Albui-Seranedra J. Physiologic versus neoplastic C-cell hyperplasia of the thyroid: separation of distinct histologic and biologic entities. *Cancer.* 1996;77(4):750–6.

195. Matias-Guiu X, Peiro G, Eggvius J et al. Proliferative activity in C-cell hyperplasia and medullary thyroid carcinoma. Evaluation by PCNA immunohistochemistry and AgNORs staining. *Pathol Res Pract.* 1995;191(1):42–7.

196. Scopsi L, Di Palma S, Ferrari C et al. C-cell hyperplasia accompanying thyroid diseases other than medullary carcinoma: an immunocytochemical study by means of antibodies to calcitonin and somatostatin. *Mod Pathol.* 1991;4(3):297–304.

197. Albores-Saavedra J, Monforte H, Madji M et al. C-cell hyperplasia in thyroid tissue adjacent to follicular cell tumors. *Hum Pathol.* 1988;19(7):795–9.

198. Gibson WG, Peng TC, Croker BP et al. Age-associated C-cell hyperplasia in the human thyroid. *Am J Pathol.* 1982;106(3): 388–93.

199. Asaadi AA. Ultrastructure in C cell hyperplasia in asymptomatic patients with hypercalcitoninemia and a family history of medullary thyroid carcinoma. *Hum Pathol.* 1981;12(7):617–22.

200. Deftos LJ, d. Bone HG, Parthermore JG. Immunohistological studies of medullary thyroid carcinoma and C cell hyperplasia. *J Clin Endocrinol Metab.* 1980;51(4):857–62.

201. Wolfe HJ, Melvin KE, Cerri-Skinner SJ et al. C-cell hyperplasia preceding medullary thyroid carcinoma. *N Engl J Med.* 1973; 289(9):437–41.

202. Black WC, Haff RC. The surgical pathology of parathyroid chief cell hyperplasia. *Am J Clin Pathol.* 1970;53(5):565–79.

203. Giuffrida D, Gharib H. Current diagnosis and management of medullary thyroid carcinoma. *Ann Oncol.* 1998;9(7):695–701.

204. Heshmati HM, Gharib H, Van Heerden JA et al. Advances and controversies in the diagnosis and management of medullary thyroid carcinoma. *Am J Med.* 1997;103(1):60–9.

205. DeLellis RA.The pathology of medullary thyroid carcinoma and its precursors. *Monogr Pathol.* 1993;35:72–102.

206. Wolfe HJ, Delellis RA. Familial medullary thyroid carcinoma and C cell hyperplasia. *Clin Endocrinol Metab.* 1981;10(2):351–65.

207. Lairmore TC, Wells SA, Jr. Medullary carcinoma of the thyroid: current diagnosis and management. *Semin Surg Oncol.* 191;7(2): 92–9.

208. Bindewald H, Raue F, Merkle MP. The diagnosis and therapy of medullary thyroid carcinoma in childhood. *Prog Pediatr Surg.* 1983;16:43–6.

209. Graze K, Spiler IJ, Taskjian AH et al. Natural history of familial medullary thyroid carcinoma: effect of a program for early diagnosis. *N Engl J Med.* 1978;299(18):980–5.

210. Wells SA, Jr, Baylin SB, Gann DS et al. Medullary thyroid carcinoma: relationship of method of diagnosis to pathologic staging. *Ann Surg.* 1978;188(3):377–83.

211. Skogseid B. Multiple endocrine neoplasia type I. Clinical genetics and diagnosis. *Cancer Treat Res.* 1997;89:383–406.

212. Heshmati HM, Hofbauer LC. Multiple endocrine neoplasia type 2: recent progress in diagnosis and management. *Eur J Endocrinol.* 1997;137(6):572–8.

213. Komminoth P. Multiple endocrine neoplasia type 1 and 2: from morphology to molecular pathology 1997. *Verh Dtsch Ges Pathol.* 1997;81:125–38.

214. Komminoth P. Multiple endocrine neoplasia type 1 and 2. 1997 diagnostic guidelines and molecular pathology. *Pathologe.* 1997;18(4): 286–300.

215. Kambouris M, Jackson CE, Teldman GL. Diagnosis of multiple endocrine neoplasia [MEN] 2A, 2B and familial medullary thyroid cancer [FMTC] by multiplex PCR and heteroduplex analyses of RET proto-oncogene mutations. *Hum Mutat.* 1996;8(1): 64–70.

216. Harach HR, Wilander E, Srimehus L et al. Chromogranin A immunoreactivity compared with argyrophilia, calcitonin immunoreactivity, and amyloid as tumour markers in the histopathological diagnosis of medullary (C-cell) thyroid carcinoma. *Pathol Res Pract.* 1992;188(1-2):123–30.

217. Hayashida, C. Y., V. A. Alves, Kanamura CT et al. Immunohistochemistry of medullary thyroid carcinoma and C-cell hyperplasia by an affinity-purified anti-human calcitonin antiserum. *Cancer.* 1993;72(4):1356-63.

218. Takano T, Miyauchi A, Yokorana T et al. Preoperative diagnosis of medullary thyroid carcinoma by RT-PCR using RNA extracted from leftover cells within a needle used for fine needle aspiration biopsy. *J Clin Endocrinol Metab.* 1999;84(3):951–5.

219. Lagercrantz J, Larsson C, Grimmond S et al. Candidate genes for multiple endocrine neoplasia type 1. *J Intern Med.* 1995;238(3): 245–8.

220. Hofstra RM, Stelwagen T, Stulp RP et al. Extensive mutation scanning of RET in sporadic medullary thyroid carcinoma and of RET and VHL in sporadic pheochromocytoma reveals involvement of these genes in only a minority of cases. *J Clin Endocrinol Metab.* 1996;81(8):2881–4.

221. Cohen R, Giscard-Darteville S, Braeg S et al. Calcitonin genes (I and II) expression in human nervous and medullary thyroid carcinoma tissues. *Neuropeptides.* 1994;26(3):215–9.

222. Takai S, Tateishi H, Nishisho I et al. Loss of genes on chromosome 22 in medullary thyroid carcinoma and pheochromocytoma. *Jpn J Cancer Res.* 1987;78(9): 94–8.

223. Biarnes J, Miranda M, Corral J et al. The molecular pathology of RET protooncogene in families with multiple endocrine neoplasia type 2A. *Med Clin (Barc).* 1996;107(9):321–5.

224. Ledger GA, Khosla S, Lindon NM et al. Genetic testing in the diagnosis and management of multiple endocrine neoplasia type II. *Ann Intern Med.* 1995;122(2):118–24.

225. Matias-Guiu X. RET protooncogene analysis in the diagnosis of medullary thyroid carcinoma and multiple endocrine neoplasia type II. *Adv Anat Pathol.* 1998;5(3):196–201.

226. Lips CJ, Leo JR, Berends MJ et al. Thyroid C-cell hyperplasia and micronodules in close relatives of MEN-2A patients: pitfalls in early diagnosis and reevaluation of criteria for surgery. *Henry Ford Hosp Med J.* 1987;35:133–8.

227. Melvin KE, Miller HH, Tashjian AH Jr. Early diagnosis of medullary carcinoma of the thyroid gland by means of calcitonin assay. *N Engl J Med.* 1971;285:1115–20.

228. Forrest CH, Frost FA, De Boer WB et al. Medullary carcinoma of the thyroid: accuracy of diagnosis of fine-needle aspiration cytology. *Cancer.* 1998;84(5):295–302.

229. Zeppa P, Vetrani A, Marin M et al. Fine needle aspiration cytology of medullary thyroid carcinoma: a review of 18 cases. *Cytopathology.* 1990;1(1):35–44.

230. Bauman A, Strawbridge HT, Bauman WA. The clinical value of fine needle aspiration biopsy in a patient with medullary thyroid carcinoma and pseudofollicular carcinoma. *N Y State J Med.* 1989;89(9):527–9.

231. Soderstrom N, Telenius-Berg M, Akerman M. Diagnosis of medullary carcinoma of the thyroid by fine needle aspiration biopsy. *Acta Med Scand.* 1975;197(1-2):71–6.

232. Green I, Ali S, Allen E, Zakowski M. A spectrum of cytomorphologic variations of medullary thyroid carcinoma, Fine needle aspiration findings in 19 cases. *Cancer Cytopathol.* 1997;81:40–4

233. Miller JM, Kini SR, Hamburger JI. *Needle Biopsy of the Thyroid.* New York: Praeger; 1983.

234. Suen KC, Quenville NF. Fine needle aspiration biopsy of the thyroid gland: a study of 304 cases. *J Clin Pathol.* 1983;36:1036–45.

235. Anscombe AM, Wright DH. Primary malignant lymphoma of the thyroid—a tumour of mucosa-associated lymphoid tissue: review of seventy-six cases. *Histopathology.* 1985;9:81–97.

236. Uzasa K, Inoue A, Tajima K, Miyauchi A, Matsuzuka F, Kuma K. Malignant lymphomas of the thyroid gland. Analysis of 79 patients with emphasis on histologic prognostic factors. *Cancer.* 1986;58:100–4.

237. Burke JS, Butler JJ, Fuller LM. Malignant lymphomas of the thyroid: a clinical pathologic study of 35 patients including ultrastructural observations. *Cancer.* 1977;39:1587–602.

238. Ansell SM, Grant CS, Haberman TM. Primary thyroid lymphoma. *Semin Oncol.* 1999;26(3):316–23.

239. Coltrera MD. Primary T-cell lymphoma of the thyroid. *Head Neck.* 1999;21(2):160–3.

240. Singer JA. Primary lymphoma of the thyroid. *Am Surg.* 1998; 64(4):334–7.

241. Pedersen RK, Pedersen NT. Primary non-Hodgkin's lymphoma of the thyroid gland: a population based study. *Histopathology.* 1996;28(1): 25–32.

242. Junor EJ, Paul J, Reed NS. Primary non-Hodgkin's lymphoma of the thyroid. *Eur J Surg Oncol.* 1992;18(4):313–21.

243. Tupchong L, Hughes F, Harmer CL. Primary lymphoma of the thyroid: clinical features, prognostic factors, and results of treatment. *Int J Radiat Oncol Biol Phys.* 1986;12(10):1813–21

244. Mizukami Y, Matsubara F, Hashimoto T et al. Primary T-cell lymphoma of the thyroid. *Acta Pathol Jpn.* 1987;37(12):1987–95.

245. Aozasa K, Inoue A, Ueda T et al. Immunologic and immunohistologic analysis of 27 cases with thyroid lymphomas. *Cancer.* 1987;60:969–73.

246. Tennvall J, Cavallin-Stahl E, Arerman M. Primary localized non-Hodgkin's lymphoma of the thyroid: a retrospective clinico-pathological review. *Eur J Surg Oncol.* 1987;13(4):297–302

247. Anscombe AM, Wright DH. Primary malignant lymphoma of the thyroid—a tumour of mucosa- associated lymphoid tissue: review of seventy-six cases. *Histopathology.* 1985;9(1):81–97.

248. Woolner LB, McConahey WM, Beahrs OH et al. Primary malignant lymphoma of the thyroid. Review of forty-six cases. *Am J Surg.* 1996;111(4):502–23.

249. Scholefield JH, Quayle AR, Harris SC et al. Primary lymphoma of the thyroid, the association with Hashimoto's thyroiditis. *Eur J Surg Oncol.* 1992;18(2):89–92.

250. Hyjek E, Isaacson PG. Primary B cell lymphoma of the thyroid and its relationship to Hashimoto's thyroiditis. *Hum Pathol.* 1998;19(11):1315–26.

251. Mizukami Y, Matsubara F, Hashimoto T et al. Primary T-cell lymphoma of the thyroid. *Acta Pathol Jpn.* 1987;37:1987–95.

252. Skarsgard ED, Connors JM, Robius RE. A current analysis of primary lymphoma of the thyroid. *Arch Surg.* 1991;126(10): 1199–203.

253. Tennvall J, Cavallin-Stahl E, Akerman A. Primary localized non-Hodgkin's lymphoma of the thyroid: a retrospective clinico-pathological review. *Eur J Surg Oncol.* 1987;13(4):297–302

254. Chak LY, Hoppe RT, Burke JS, Kaplan HS. Non-Hodgkin's lymphoma presenting as thyroid enlargement. *Cancer.* 1981;48: 2712–6.

255. Mizukami Y, Michigishi T, Nonomura D et al. Primary lymphoma of the thyroid: a clinical, histological and immunohistochemical study of 20 cases. *Histopathology.* 1990;17(3):201–9.

256. Feigin GA, Buss DH, Paschal B, Woodruff RD, Myers RT. Hodgkin's disease manifested as a thyroid nodule. *Hum Pathol.* 1982;13:774–6.

257. Lovchik J, Lane MA, Clark DP. Polymerase chain reaction-based detection of B-cell clonality in the fine needle aspiration biopsy of a thyroid mucosa-associated lymphoid tissue (MALT) lymphoma. *Hum Pathol.* 1997;28(8):989–92.

258. Ohshima M, Momiyama T, Souda S et al. Primary plasmacytoma of the thyroid: a case report and comparative literature study between Western nations and Japan. *Pathol Int.* 1994; 44(8):645–51.

259. Kovacs CS, Mant MJ, Nguyen GK et al. Plasma cell lesions of the thyroid: report of a case of solitary plasmacytoma and a review of the literature. *Thyroid.* 1994;4(1):65–71.

260. Rubin J, Johnson JT, Killeen R. Extramedullary plasmacytoma of the thyroid associated with a serum monoclonal gammopathy. *Arch Otolaryngol Head Neck Surg.* 1994;116(7):855–9.

261. Beguin Y, Boniver J, Bury F et al. Plasmacytoma of the thyroid: a case report, a study with use of the immunoperoxidase technique, and a review of the literature. *Surgery.* 1987;101(4): 496–500.

262. Gruber B, Goldman M, Pecant W. Plasmacytoma of the thyroid. *Otolaryngol Head Neck Surg.* 1987;97(6):567–71.

263. Chen KT, Bauer V, Bauer F et al. Localized thyroid plasmacytoma. *J Surg Oncol.* 1986;32(4):220–2.

264. Aozasa K, Inoue A, Yoshimura H et al. Plasmacytoma of the thyroid gland. *Cancer.* 1986;58(1):105–10.

265. Matsubayashi S, Tamai H, Svzuki T et al. Extramedullary plasmacytoma of the thyroid gland producing gamma heavy chain. *Endocrinol Jpn.* 1985;32(3): 427–33.

266. Lopez M, Di Lauro L, Marolla P et al. Plasmacytoma of the thyroid gland. *Clin Oncol.* 1993;9(1):61–6.

267. Macpherson TA, Dekker A, Kappadia SB, Thyroid-gland plasma cell neoplasm (plasmacytoma). *Arch Pathol Lab Med.* 1981;105(11): 570–2.

268. Buss DH, Marshall RB, Holleman IL Jr et al. Malignant lymphoma of the thyroid gland with plasma cell differentiation (plasmacytoma). *Cancer.* 1980;46(12):2671–5.

269. More JR, Dawson DW, Ralston AJ et al. Plasmacytoma of the thyroid. *J Clin Pathol.* 1968;21(5):661–7.

270. Hedinger CE. Sarcomas of the thyroid gland. In: Hedinger CE, ed. *Thyroid cancer.* Berlin: Springer-Verlag, 1969:47–52. (UICC monograph series; Vol 12.)

271. Griem KL, Robb PK, Caldaselli DD et al. Radiation-induced sarcoma of the thyroid. *Arch Otolaryngol Head Neck Surg.* 1989; 115(8):991–3.

272. Chesky VE, Hellwig CA, Welch JW. Fibrosarcoma of the thyroid gland. *Surg Gynecol Obstet.* 1960;111:767–70.

273. Chan YF, Ma L, Boey JH, Yeung HY. Angiosarcoma of the thyroid. An immunohistochemical and ultrastructural study of a case in a Chinese patient. *Cancer.* 1986;57:2381–8.

274. Krauth PH, Katz JF. Kaposi's sarcoma involving the thyroid in a patient with AIDS. *Clin Nucl Med.* 1989;12(11):848–9.

275. Egloff B. The hemangioendothelioma of the thyroid. *Virchows Arch [A].* 1983;400:119–42.

276. McCabe DP, Farrar WB, Petkov TM, Finkelmeier W, O'Dwyer P, James A. Clinical and pathologic correlations in disease metastatic to the thyroid gland. *Am J Surg.* 1985;150:519–23.

277. Wychulis AR, Beahrs OH, Woolner LB. Metastases of carcinoma to the thyroid gland. *Ann Surg.* 1964;160:169–77.

278. Sidawy M, Del Vecchio D, Knoll S. Kennedy JS. The pathology of dyshormonogenetic goiter. *J Pathol.* 1969;99:251–64.

279. Holleman F, Hoekstra JB, Ruitenberg HM. Evaluation of fine needle aspiration (FNA) cytology in the diagnosis of thyroid nodules. *Cytopathology.* 1995 Jun;6(3):168–75.

280. Taneri F, Poyraz A, Tekin E et al. Accuracy and Significance of Fine-Needle Aspiration Cytology and Frozen Section in Thyroid Surgery. *Endocr Regul.* 1998;32(4):187–191.

281. Vojvodich, Ballagh RH, Cramer H et al. The fine needle aspiration in the pre-operative diagnosis of thyroid neoplasia. *J Otolaryngol.* 1994;23(5):360–5

282. Gharib H. Fine-needle aspiration biopsy of thyroid nodules: advantages, limitations, and effect. *Mayo Clin Proc.* 1994;69(1):44–9

283. Dwarakanathan AA, Staren ED, D'Amore MJ, Kluskens LF, Martirano M, Economou SG. Importance of repeat fine-needle biopsy in the management of thyroid nodules. *Am J Surg.* 1993;166(4):350–2

284. Griffies WS, Donegan E, Abel ME. The role of fine needle aspiration in the management of the thyroid nodule. *Laryngoscope.* 1985;95(9 Pt 1):1103–6

285. Leonard N, Melcher DH. To operate or not to operate? The value of fine needle aspiration cytology in the assessment of thyroid swellings. *J Clin Pathol.* 1997;50(11):941–3

286. Shemen LJ, Chess Q. Fine-needle aspiration biopsy diagnosis of follicular variant of papillary thyroid cancer: therapeutic implications. *Otolaryngol Head Neck Surg.* 1998;119(6):600–2

287. Silverman JF, West RL, Larkin EW et al. The role of fine-needle aspiration biopsy in the rapid diagnosis and management of thyroid neoplasm. *Cancer.* 1986;57: 1164–70.

288. Bouvet M, Feldman JI, Gill GN et al. Surgical management of the thyroid nodule: patient selection based on the results of fine-needle aspiration cytology. *Laryngoscope.* 1992;102(12 Pt 1):1353–6

289. Basolo F, Baloch ZW, Baldanzi A, Miccoli P, LiVolsi VA Usefulness of ultrafast Papanicolaou-stained scrape preparations in intraoperative management of thyroid lesions. *Mod Pathol.* 1999;12(6):653–7

290. Chen H, Zeiger MA, Clark DP, Westra WH, Udelsman R. Papillary carcinoma of the thyroid: can operative management be based solely on fine-needle aspiration?. *J Am Coll Surg.* 1997;184(6):605–10

291. Mesonero C, Jugle J, Wilbur D, Nayar R. Fine needle aspiration of the macrofollicular and microfollicular subtypes of the follicular variant of papillary carcinoma of the thyroid. *Cancer.* 1998;84:235–44.

292. Lin, HS, Komisar A, Opher E et al. Surgical management of thyroid masses: assessing the need for frozen section evaluation. *Laryngoscope.* 1999;109(6):868–73.

293. Guyetant S, Saint-Andre JP. Frozen section examination in thyroid pathology. Technique and effective indications. *Arch Anat Cytol Pathol.* 1998;46(1-2):121–7.

294. McHenry CR, Raeburn C, Strickland T et al. The utility of routine frozen section examination for intraoperative diagnosis of thyroid cancer. *Am J Surg.* 1996;172(6):658–61.

295. DeMay RM. Frozen section of thyroid? Just say no. *Am J Clin Pathol.* 1990;110(4):423–4.

296. Chen H, Nicol TL, Udelsman R. Follicular lesions of the thyroid. Does frozen section evaluation alter operative management?. *Ann Surg.* 1995;222(1): 101–6.

297. Andrew AC, Williamson JM. Frozen section simulation of trabecular adenoma and medullary cancer by papillary thyroid carcinoma. *J Clin Pathol.* 1993;46(8):776–7.

298. Kingston GW, Bugis SP, Davis N. Role of frozen section and clinical parameters in distinguishing benign from malignant follicular neoplasms of the thyroid. *Am J Surg.* 1992;164(6):603–5.

299. Hamburger JI, Hamburger SW. Declining role of frozen section in surgical planning for thyroid nodules. *Surgery.* 1985;98: 307–12.

300. Hamburger JI, Husain M. Contribution of intraoperative pathology evaluation to surgical management of thyroid nodules. *Endocrinol Metab Clin North Am.* 1990;19:509–22.

301. Kraemer BB. Frozen section diagnosis and the thyroid. *Semin Diagn Pathol.* 1987;4(2):169–89.

302. Hamburger, JI, Hamburger SW. Declining role of frozen section in surgical planning for thyroid nodules. *Surgery.* 1985;98(2): 307–12.

303. Rosen Y, Rosenblatt P, Saltzman E. Intraoperative pathologic diagnosis of thyroid neoplasms. Report on experience with 504 specimens. *Cancer.* 1990;66:2001–6.

304. Lin HS, Komisar A, Opher E, Blaugrund SM. Surgical management of thyroid masses: assessing the need for frozen section evaluation. *Laryngoscope.* 1999 ;109(6):868–73.

305. Shaha A, Gleich L, DiMaio T et al. Accuracy and pitfalls of frozen section during thyroid surgery. *J Surg Oncol.* 1990;44(2):84–92.

306. Paphavasit A, Thompson GB, Hay ID et al. Follicular and Hurthle cell thyroid neoplasms. Is frozen-section evaluation worthwhile? *Arch Surg.* 1997 Jun;132(6):674–8

307. Tworek JA, Giordano TJ, Michael. Comparison of intraoperative cytology with frozen sections in the diagnosis of thyroid lesions. *Am J Clin Pathol.* 1998 Oct;110(4):456–61

308. McHenry CR, Raeburn C, Strickland T, Marty JJ. The utility of routine frozen section examination for intraoperative diagnosis of thyroid cancer. *Am J Surg.* 1996 Dec;172(6):658–61

309. Multanen M, Haapiainen R et al. The value of ultrasound-guided fine-needle aspiration biopsy (FNAB) and frozen section examination (FS) in the diagnosis of thyroid cancer. *Ann Chir Gynaecol.* 1999;88(2):132–5.

310. Ersoy E, Taneri F, Tekia E et al. Preoperative fine-needle aspiration cytology versus frozen section in thyroid surgery. *Endocr Regul.* 1999;33(3):141–144.

311. Boyd LA, Earnhardt RC, Dunn JT et al. Preoperative evaluation and predictive value of fine-needle aspiration and frozen section of thyroid nodules. *J Am Coll Surg.* 1998;187(5):494–502.

312. Galimberti A, Vitri P, DePasquale L et al. Utility of fine needle aspiration and frozen section in the diagnosis of uncommon thyroid malignancies. *J Exp Clin Cancer Res.* 1997;16(4):425–6.

313. Sabel MS, Staren ED, Siankakisan et al. User of fine-needle aspiration biopsy and frozen section in the management of the solitary thyroid nodule. *Surgery.* 1997;122(6):1021–6.

314. Chang HY, Lin JD, Chen TF et al. Correlation of fine needle aspiration cytology and frozen section biopsies in the diagnosis of thyroid nodules. *J Clin Pathol.* 1997;50(12):1005–9.

315. Aguilar-Diosdado M, Contreras A et al. Thyroid nodules. Role of fine needle aspiration and intraoperative frozen section examination. *Acta Cytol.* 1997;41(3):677–82.

316. Rodriguez JM, Parrilla P et al. Comparison between preoperative cytology and intraoperative frozen- section biopsy in the diagnosis of thyroid nodules. *Br J Surg.* 1994;81(8):1151–4.

317. McHenry CR, Rosen IB, Sola T et al. Influence of fine-needle aspiration biopsy and frozen section examination on the management of thyroid cancer. *Am J Surg.* 1993;166(4):353–6.

318. Aguilar M. Use of aspiration cytology and frozen section examination for management of benign and malignant thyroid nodules. *Cancer.* 1992;70(4): 903–4.

319. Layfield LJ, Mohrmann RL, Kopald Ktl et al. Use of aspiration cytology and frozen section examination for management of benign and malignant thyroid nodules. *Cancer.* 1991;68(1):130–4.

320. Shaha AR, DiMaio T, Webber C et al. Intraoperative decision making during thyroid surgery based on the results of preoper-

ative needle biopsy and frozen section. *Surgery.* 1990;108(6): 964–7

321. Kopald KH, Layfield LJ, Mohrmann R et al. Clarifying the role of fine-needle aspiration cytologic evaluation and frozen section examination in the operative management of thyroid cancer. *Arch Surg.* 1989;124(10):1201–4.

322. Schmid KW, Ladurner D, Zehmann W et al. Clinicopathologic management of tumors of the thyroid gland in an endemic goiter area. Combined use of preoperative fine needle aspiration biopsy and intraoperative frozen section. *Acta Cytol.* 1989;33(1): 27–30.

323. Keller MP, Crabbe MM, Norwood SH et al. Accuracy and significance of fine-needle aspiration and frozen section in determining the extent of thyroid resection. *Surgery.* 1987;101(5):632–5.

324. Bugis SP, Young JE, Archibald SD, Chen VS. Diagnostic accuracy of fine-needle aspiration biopsy versus frozen section in solitary thyroid nodules. *Am J Surg.* 1986;152:411–6.

325. Keller MP, Crabbe MM, Norwood SH. Accuracy and significance of fine-needle aspiration and frozen section in determining the extent of thyroid resection. *Surgery.* 1987;101:632–5.

326. Kopald LH, Layfield LJ, Mohrmann R, Foshag LJ, Giuliano AE. Clarifying the role of fine-needle aspiration, cytologic evaluation and frozen section examination in the operative management of thyroid cancer. *Arch Surg.* 1989;124:1201–5.

327. Layfield LJ, Mohrmann RL, Kopald KH, Giuliano AE. Use of aspiration cytology and frozen section examination for management of enign and malignant thyroid nodules. *Cancer.* 1991;68(1): 130–4.

328. Bugis SP, Young JE, Archibald SD, Chen VS. Diagnostic accuracy of fine-needle aspiration biopsy versus frozen section in solitary thyroid nodules. *Am J Surg.* 1986;152(4):411–6.

329. Boyd LA, Farnhardt RC, Dunn JT, Frierson HF, Hanks JB. Preoperative evaluation and predictive value of fine-needle aspiration and frozen section of thyroid nodules. *J Am Coll Surg.* 1998;187(5):494–502.

330. Multanen M, Haapiainen R, Leppaniemi A, Voutilainen P, Sivula A. The value of ultrasound-guided fine-needle aspiration biopsy (FNAB) and frozen section examination (FS) in the diagnosis of thyroid cancer. *Ann Chir Gynaecol.* 1999;88(2):132–5.

331. Taneri F, Poyraz A, Tekin E, Ersoy E, Dursun A. Accuracy and significance of fine-needle aspiration cytology and frozen section in thyroid surgery. *Endocr Regul.* 1998;32(4):187–191.

332. Sabel MS, Staren ED, Gianakakis LM, Dwarakanathan S, Prinz RA. Use of fine-needle aspiration biopsy and frozen section in the management of the solitary thyroid nodule. *Surgery.* 1997; 122(6):1021–6.

333. Boyd LA, Earnhardt RC, Dunn JT, Frierson HF, Hanks JB. Preoperative evaluation and predictive value of fine-needle aspiration and frozen section of thyroid nodules. *J Am Coll Surg.* 1998;187(5):494–502.

334. Hamming JF, Vriens MR, Goslings BM, Songun I, Fleuren GJ, van de Velde CJ. Role of fine-needle aspiration biopsy and frozen section examination in determining the extent of thyroidectomy. *World J Surg.* 1998;22(6):575–9.

335. Mulcahy MM, Cohen JI, Anderson PE, Ditamasso J, Schmidt W. Relative accuracy of fine-needle aspiration and frozen section in the diagnosis of well-differentiated thyroid cancer. *Laryngoscope.* 1998;108(4 Pt 1):494–6.

336. Davoudi MM, Yeh KA, Wei JP. Utility of fine-needle aspiration cytology and frozen-section examination in the operative management of thyroid nodules. *Am Surg.* 1997;63(12):1084–9.

337. Chen H, Nicol TL, Udelsman R. Follicular lesions of the thyroid. Does frozen section evaluation alter operative management? Adequate FNAB, routine frozen section is not cost effective. *Ann Surg.* 1995;222(1):101–6

338. Rimm D, Stastny J, Rimm E, Ayer S, Frable W. Comparison of the costs of fine needle aspiration and open surgical biopsy as methods for obtaining a pathologic diagnosis. *Cancer Cytopathol.* 1997; 81:51–6.

# 4

# Thyroid Physiology

**Ann D. Dunn, Ph.D.**

The thyroid gland produces two hormones, 3,5,3'-triiodothyronine ($T_3$) and 3,5,3',5'-tetraiodothyronine or thyroxine ($T_4$). Both are iodinated derivatives of tyrosine. The structural formulas of the hormones and their iodinated precursors are shown in Figure 4–1. Hormone production is dependent on an external iodine supply and on intrathyroidal mechanisms for concentrating ingested iodide and then incorporating it into the tissue specific protein, thyroglobulin (Tg). The thyroid gland is unique within the endocrine system in having a large extracellular space, the follicular lumen, which is used for storage of the hormones and their precursors. As hormone is needed by the organism, Tg is retrieved by the cell where the biologically active hor-

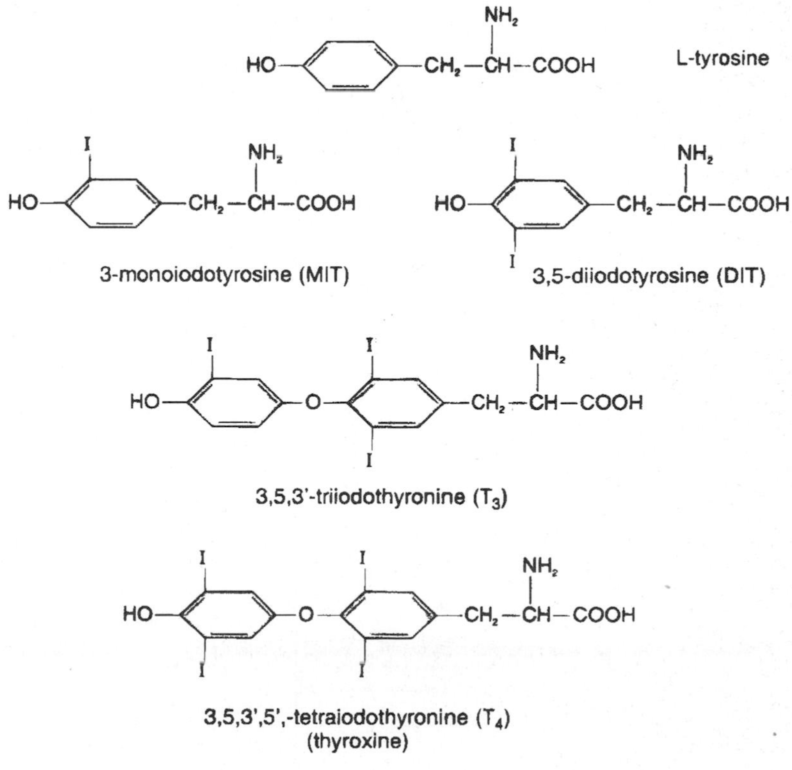

**Figure 4–1.** Structures of the thyroid hormones and their precursors.

mones are released from Tg before being passed into the circulation.

## THYROID HORMONE SYNTHESIS AND RELEASE (see Figure 4–2)

### Iodide Transport

A daily dietary intake take of at least 100μg of iodine per day is required in man to ensure adequate production of thyroid hormone. In North America the average daily intake is somewhat higher than this largely because of the use of iodine as a food additive.[1] In many parts of the world, however, consumption is significantly below the minimum level and iodine-deficiency is the leading cause of thyroid related disorders.

The thyroid normally concentrates iodide some 20–40 fold over the extracellular space and against an electrical gradient of ~40 mV. Key to this trapping action is a protein located in the basal membrane of the thyroid cell known as the sodium/iodide symporter (NIS).[2] NIS couples the influx of $Na^+$ down its electrochemical gradient with the simultaneous influx of $I^-$ up its electrochemical gradient. A $Na^+/K^+$ ATPase acts to maintain the $Na^+$ gradient. Iodide then travels down its electrochemical gradient to the apical surface of the thyrocyte where it is incorporated into Tg. Recent evidence suggests an apical membrane protein, pendrin, aids in releasing iodide into the follicular lumen.[3] Mutations in the gene encoding for this protein are responsible for the common hereditary disorder known as Pendred's syndrome, which is associated with mild hypothyroidism, goiter and hearing loss.[3] Mutations in the gene coding for NIS have been identified in patients with iodide trapping defects, a relatively rare cause of congenital hypothyroidism.[2]

### Thyroglobulin

Thyroglobulin is central to thyroid physiology. It is a tissue specific protein which serves both as matrix for the synthesis of hormone and as vehicle for its storage.[4] The human Tg gene has been cloned and is located on

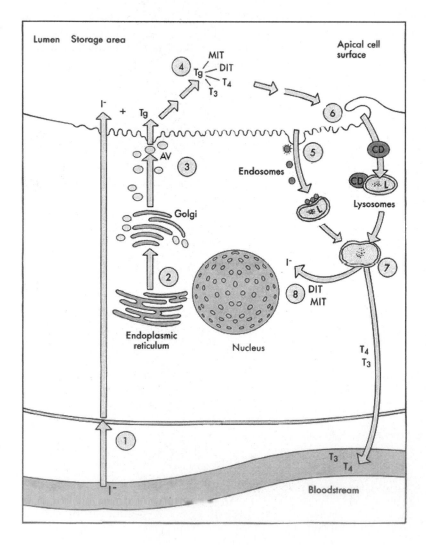

**Figure 4–2.** Synthesis and release of thyroid hormone. 1) Iodide, transported into the thyrocyte at the basal cell membrane by the symporter (NIS) travels down its electrochemical gradient to the apical surface. 2) Tg's polypeptide chain is synthesized on the surface of the endoplasmic reticulum (ER) then translocated into its lumen. Here synthesis of carbohydrate units begins and conformational changes transform the polypeptide chains into stable dimers. Tg enters the Golgi where carbohydrate units are completed. 3) Uniodinated Tg travels to the apical surface in small vesicles (AV). 4) Here, Tg is iodinated and iodotyrosyls coupled to form $T_4$ and $T_3$ by thyroperoxidase in the presence of $H_2O_2$. 5) Tg, retrieved by micropinocytosis enters the endosome-lysosomal pathway where proteolysis and hormone release occurs. 6) Alternatively Tg, retrieved by macropinocytosis travels to lysosomes in colloid droplets (CD). 7) Thyroid hormones and precursors leave the lysosomes, $T_4$ and $T_3$ enter the bloodstream. 8) MIT and DIT are deiodinated and released iodide is recirculated. (From Dunn JT, Dunn AD in *The Thyroid.* Braverman LE, Utiger RD eds. Philadelphia: Lippincott Williams & Wilkins, 2000).

the long arm of chromosome 8Q24. Tg is a large dimeric glycoprotein of ~660 kDa consisting in man of two identical polypeptide chains each of 2,750 amino acids. About 10% of its weight is as carbohydrate and about 0.1–1.0% is as iodine. Tg does not have a high tyrosine content, despite the biological importance of its iodinated residues. Synthesis and maturation of Tg follows a pathway typical of proteins destined for secretion. The polypeptide chain is synthesized on the surface of the rough endoplasmic reticulum. It then passes through a series of intracellular compartments where it undergoes important post-translational modifications prior to reaching the follicular lumen.[5] Carbohydrate units are added to the polypeptide chain as it is translocated into the lumen of the rough endoplasmic reticulum. Folding and dimerization of the polypeptide chain occurs within this compartment, aided by folding enzymes and a group of proteins known as molecular chaperones. Any perturbations of this process result in block of protein transport beyond this point and can cause congenital hypothyroidism.[5] Under normal circumstances, the properly folded Tg dimers migrate to the Golgi complex where processing of the carbohydrate units are completed. Mature but as yet uniodinated Tg is transferred from the Golgi to the apical cell surface in small vesicles.

## Iodination and Thyroperoxidase

Newly formed Tg and iodide meet at the apical cell surface where hormone synthesis occurs. This process includes 1) the oxidation of iodide; 2) its subsequent transfer to tyrosyl residues on Tg, producing monoiodotyrosine (MIT) and diiodotyrosine (DIT); and 3) coupling of two iodotyrosine molecules, either one each of MIT and DIT to form $T_3$ or two of DIT to form $T_4$. Thyroperoxidase (TPO), an enzyme present in the apical cell membrane, is responsible for each of these steps.[6] Hydrogen peroxide, required in the iodinating and coupling reactions, is generated at the apical membrane by an NADPH oxidase.[7] Mutations in the TPO gene have been found in patients with congenital hypothyroidism caused by defective organification. Abnormalities in $H_2O_2$ generation appear to be more rare.

Under normal circumstances, iodide, once trapped, is rapidly incorporated into Tg so that little free iodide exists within the thyroid gland at any given time. The extent to which Tg is iodinated depends on the thyroid's iodide supply. At a level of 0.5% iodine (26 atoms iodine per molecule of 660 kDa) the Tg dimer in man contains on average 5 residues of MIT, 5 of DIT, 2.5 of $T_4$ and 0.7 of $T_3$ out of a total of 132 residues of tyrosine.[4] Questions are frequently raised as to the apparent inefficiency of a system that utilizes only five or six of the

more than 5,000 amino acid residues in Tg to produce hormone. A partial answer to this may lie in Tg's function as a storage vehicle, where hormone and iodine in the form of MIT and DIT may remain for a long time.

Hormone formation involves the coupling of two residues of iodotyrosine within the Tg polypeptide chain. At the hormonogenic site the "acceptor" diiodotyrosyl receives the iodinated phenol ring of the "donor" iodotyrosyl (MIT or DIT) located at some distal site on the polypeptide chain. In the process, the alanine side chain of the donor remains behind, now presumably in the form of dehydroalanine. Iodination *in vitro* of low iodine human Tg indicates that certain tyrosyl sites are favored for early iodination and that three or four major sites exist for hormone formation.[4] The most important hormonogenic site is located five residues from the amino terminal of Tg, while a second major site is located three residues from the carboxy terminal. The locations of donor tyrosyls is incomplete. To date only one has been identified in human Tg and this resides in the amino terminal region of the molecule.[4]

## Storage and Release of Hormone

Most mature iodinated Tg is stored in the colloid as soluble dimers, although some (~10%) highly iodinated molecules associate as tetramers. The colloidal nature of the follicular lumen is caused by its high concentration of protein (~100mg/ml). This extracellular space thus contains a large supply of both iodine and hormone available to the organism, which protects it against times of iodine privation.

Hormone release is initiated by the retrieval of Tg from the follicular lumen. Under stimulatory conditions in some species, this process may occur by macropinocytosis. Pseudopods form at the thyrocyte's apical surface and engulf Tg as large colloid droplets. However, under physiological conditions in most species, including man, Tg is retrieved by micropinocytosis into small vesicles. It is then passed through the endosome-lysosomal system, where the combined action of several acid proteases including cathepsins, B, D, and L and lysosomal dipeptidase I release the hormones and their iodotyrosine precursors from the polypeptide backbone.[4] Evidence suggests the iodoamino acids may be preferentially cleaved first, but ultimately Tg is broken down into amino acids or small peptides within the lysosomes.

Once released from Tg, the thyroid hormones and their precursors enter the cytosol. There MIT and DIT are deiodinated by an iodotyrosine-specific deiodinase and the released iodide reenters the iodide pool. Some $T_4$ is deiodinated to $T_3$ before its release into the circulation by a 5'-iodothyronine deiodinase similar to that found in peripheral tissue.[8] The mechanism by which

$T_4$ and $T_3$ are released from the thyrocyte is not known, but recent evidence suggests a carrier protein may be involved.[9]

## CIRCULATING THYROID HORMONES

Less than 1 % of circulating thyroid hormones exist as free iodoamino acids. The remainder is bound in reversible, non-covalent linkage to one of several plasma proteins.[10] In man the most important of these is thyroxine binding protein (TBG), accounting for about 70% of circulating hormone. The TBG molecule has one hormone binding site with a very high affinity for $T_4$ and a somewhat lower affinity for $T_3$. A second plasma protein, transthyretin, accounts for about 10% of circulating $T_4$ and $T_3$. Each transthyretin molecule has two hormone binding sites but the affinity of the first is somewhat lower than that of TBG, and that of the second site is very low for both hormones. Albumin also serves as a thyroid hormone transport protein. Although it has a low affinity, its abundance allows it to account for 10–20% of bound circulating hormone.

The plasma binding proteins aid in a rapid and uniform distribution of hormone to peripheral tissues, protecting the small hydrophobic hormone molecules from uptake by the first cells they encounter. The bound hormones are in equilibrium with the minute fraction of free circulating hormone that is available for use in peripheral tissue. Under euthyroid conditions about 0.02% of $T_4$ and about 0.3% of $T_3$ in circulation is unbound. The larger free to bound ratio of $T_3$ relative to $T_4$ is caused by the lower affinity of TBG for $T_3$.[10] To date, no change in thyroid state has been attributed to abnormalities in these hormone binding proteins despite their apparent role in thyroid economy.

## METABOLISM OF THYROID HORMONES

Thyroxine must first be deiodinated to $T_3$ in order to exert most of its biological actions. Since relatively little $T_3$ is directly synthesized on thyroglobulin, this transformation becomes an important step in hormonogenesis. Three iodothyronine deiodinases are present in mammals.[8] These are membrane bound enzymes that are closely related structurally and are distinguished by the presence of selenocysteine at their active sites. Each has distinctive substrate preferences, activity characteristics, inhibitor sensitivities and relative tissue specificity. Types I and II deiodinases are activating enzymes that remove iodide from the 5' position of the outer ring of $T_4$ to form $T_3$. Their combined actions are responsible for generating about 80% of the total $T_3$ production. Type I deiodinase is the primary source of circulating $T_3$

and is found in liver, kidney, thyroid (where it is activated by TSH), and to a lesser extent, in other tissues. This enzyme also catalyses the 5' deiodination of 3,3',5' triiodothyronine, known as reverse $T_3$ ($rT_3$), a major metabolite of $T_4$. Type I deiodinase is positively regulated by thyroid hormones and is greatly reduced under pathophysiological states such as starvation and nonthyroidal illnesses. It is inhibited by the antithyroid drug propylthiouracil. Type II deiodinase is present primarily in the central nervous system, the pituitary, the placenta, the skin, brown adipose tissue (in rodents) and has recently been found also in the thyroid.[11] Its major role is thought to be in the local production of $T_3$ but it may also contribute to circulating $T_3$. In contrast to type I deiodinase, the type II enzyme is negatively regulated by thyroid hormone and is unaffected by propylthiouracil. Type III deiodinase inactivates $T_4$ and $T_3$ by inner ring deiodination in the 5 position, forming respectively $rT_3$ or 3,3'diiodothyronine. The enzyme is present in the adult brain, skin and placenta and is also present in high levels in fetal tissues where it is thought to be important in protecting developing tissue from excess levels of thyroid hormone.[12]

## CONTROL OF THYROID FUNCTION

The anterior pituitary is the primary internal regulator of thyroid function, influencing virtually all phases of thyroid metabolism.[13] It secretes thyroid stimulating hormone (TSH), also known as thyrotropin, which is a 28–30 kilodalton glycoprotein consisting of two subunits, α and β. The α subunit is common to the pituitary hormones FSH and LH and to chorionic gonadotropin. The β subunit, however, is unique to TSH, and is responsible for the binding of the hormone to its receptor in the basal membrane of the thyroid cell. On interaction with TSH, the receptor, a member of a family of G protein coupled receptors, undergoes conformational changes that activate one or two regulatory pathways. Most TSH effects are mediated by activation of the cAMP pathway; others involve the $Ca^{+2}$/phosphatidylinositol cascade. The pathway used to elicit a given effect may vary among species. Some of the major effects of TSH on hormone synthesis and release in human thyrocytes are shown in Table 4–1. TSH stimulates both the efflux of $I^-$ into the follicle and the resorption of colloid into the cell within minutes. Later effects include increased expression of the NIS, Tg and TPO genes, stimulation of $H_2O_2$ production, promotion of glycosylation, and increased production of $T_3$ relative to $T_4$.

Circulating levels of TSH are controlled by the opposing influences of thyroid hormone and of thyrotropin releasing hormone (TRH) from the hypothala-

**Table 4–1.** TSH effects on hormone synthesis and release in human thyroid gland

| Event | Mechanism | Regulatory Pathway |
| --- | --- | --- |
| $I^-$ Trapping | Increased expression of Na/I symporter | cAMP |
| $I^-$ efflux | Unknown | $Ca^{+2}$/phosphatidylinositol |
| $H_2O_2$ production | Unknown | $Ca^{+2}$/phosphatidylinositol |
| Iodination & coupling | Increased expression of TPO gene | cAMP |
| Thyroglobulin | | |
|   Synthesis | Increased expression of Tg gene | cAMP |
|   $T_3$:$T_4$ ratio | Increased $T_3$ synthesis relative to $T_4$ | unknown |
| $T_4$ to $T_3$ deiodination | Increased expression of type I deiodinase | cAMP |
| Hormone secretion | | |
|   Tg endocytosis | Unknown | cAMP |
|   Tg proteolysis | Increased activities of cathepsins B, L | unknown |

mus.[14] The latter is a modified tripeptide secreted to the anterior pituitary via the hypothalamo-hypophysial portal system. TRH binds to the plasma membrane of the thyrotrope and stimulates both the release of TSH and the expression of its gene. Levels of circulating TSH are under strict control by the thyroid in a classic negative feedback system. As levels of thyroid hormone rise in response to TSH stimulation, $T_4$ and $T_3$ block the TRH stimulated release of TSH in the thyrotrope. The thyroid hormones also act indirectly by inhibiting TRH gene expression in the hypothamus.

Other internal factors that influence TSH secretion include somatostatin (inhibitory), neurotransmitters, such as dopamine (inhibitory) or adrenergic activators (stimulatory), and cytokines eg interleukin 1b and tumor necrosis factor a (both inhibitory).[14]

Iodine supply is the major external factor influencing thyroid state. Autoregulatory mechanisms present in the thyroid help to compensate for variations in iodide intake. In response to increasing doses of iodine, the thyroid initially increases hormone synthesis but then reverses this process as intrathyroidal levels of iodide reach a critical level and further organification is inhibited. This phenomenon, known as the Wolff-Chaikoff effect is believed to be caused by the inhibition of $H_2O_2$ generation by iodinated lipids.[15] The effect itself, however, is transitory, as the thyroid adapts after a 48 hour exposure to high levels of iodide by altering its trapping mechanism, probably through reduced expression of the NIS gene.[16]

Withdrawal of iodide from the diet leads to a rapid decrease in serum $T_4$ and an increase in serum TSH. Serum $T_3$ levels initially are unaffected but eventually fall with prolonged withdrawal. In response to TSH stimulation, the thyroid increases iodide uptake and organification, alters the distribution of iodoamino acids

within Tg by increasing the ratios of MIT:DIT and $T_3$:$T_4$[4] and increases the intrathyroidal conversion of $T_4$ to $T_3$ by types I and II deiodinases,[8] all of which contribute to a more efficient use of the limited iodine supply. With prolonged iodine deficiency, TSH-stimulated cell proliferation eventually leads to goiter.

## ANTITHYROID COMPOUNDS

Antithyroid drugs can inhibit thyroid hormone synthesis, secretion or metabolism.[17] Common agents and their major actions are summarized in Table 4–2. Although the monovalent ions are no longer used to suppress iodide transport because of their toxicity, the perchlorate discharge test remains a useful diagnostic tool in the evaluation of impaired iodide organification. Thiocyanate is a metabolic product of vegetables such as broccoli, cabbage, and cassava, and if ingested in high enough quantities can interfere with both iodide trapping and Tg iodination. All the thionamide drugs are potent inhibitors of thyroperoxidase, but of those listed, only propylthiouracil also inhibits thyroid hormone deiodination. Carbimazole, not available in the United States, is a potent antithyroid agent *in vitro* but probably exerts most of its effects *in vivo* after its conversion to methimazole. In addition to its effects on Tg endocytosis, excess iodide may also have an inhibitory effect on Tg proteolysis.[4] The β-adrenergic blocking agent, propranolol, has an inhibitory effect on thyroid hormone deiodination but its primary action appears to be in reducing the response to thyroid hormone at the tissue level.[18]

A number of agents utilized in the treatment of nonthryoidal illnesses may have profound effects on thyroid hormone production. Notable among these are

**Table 4–2.** Antithyroid agents and their effect on thyroid hormone synthesis and action

| Step | Drug | Action |
|---|---|---|
| Iodide transport | Monovalent anions: $ClO_4^-$, thiocyanate | Inhibit NIS |
| Tg iodination | Thiocyanate Thionamide drugs: Propylthiouracil, Methimazole, Carbimazole | Inhibit TPO |
| Thyroid hormone release | Iodide | Unknown mechanism, requires organification of $I^-$ |
| Iodotyrosine deiodination | Nitrotyrosines | Inhibit thyroidal deiodination of MIT, DIT. |
| Iodothyronine deiodination | Propylthiouracil | Inhibits type I deiodinase |
| Thyroid hormone action | Propranolol | Blocks β adrenergic receptors |

the iodinated radiocontrast agents which are potent inhibitors of thyroid hormone deiodination and can also interfere with hepatic uptake of $T_4$[19] and binding of $T_3$ to nuclear receptors.[20] The antiarrhythmic agent amiodarone, which is also heavily iodinated, elicits similar alterations in thyroid hormone metabolism and action. Lithium, used in the treatment of bipolar illness, is a potent inhibitor of thyroid hormone release and acts by blocking Tg endocytosis.[21]

## ACTION OF THYROID HORMONES

The thyroid has multiple effects on development, growth and metabolism. The first named are widespread phylogenetically and can be dramatically observed during the course of amphibian metamorphosis. The appropriate levels of thyroid hormone during fetal and neonatal stages in man are critical for the normal maturation of the central nervous system as well as for muscle, bone and lung. In severe cases of thyroid hormone deficiency during this period, the syndrome of cretinism results with its associated mental retardation, deaf mutism and stunted growth.[22] Similarly, an excess of thyroid hormone during these critical developmental periods can also result in neurological abnormalities. The metabolic effects of thyroid hormone appear to be confined to birds and mammals, presumably evolving in response to the increased metabolic pressures of thermogenesis. $O_2$ consumption as well as the metabolism of proteins, carbohydrates and fats are all under thyroid hormone control.

Most effects of thyroid hormone are now believed to be exerted by interactions with specific nuclear thyroid hormone receptors resulting in the altered expression of specific genes.[23] Thyroxine has little affinity for the nuclear receptors and must first be converted to $T_3$ to be effective. The receptors themselves belong to a large superfamily of nuclear receptors, which includes the steroid hormones, retinoic acid and vitamin D. The thyroid hormone receptors are closely related isoforms, despite being encoded by two different genes (α and β). Alternate processing of both gene transcripts produces a total of four isoforms α1, α2, β1 and β2. All have a central DNA-binding domain that binds to specific sequences within the targeted gene, called hormone response elements, and three of the four have carboxy terminal domains that bind $T_3$. Because of amino acid substitutions in this region the α2 isoform is unable to bind $T_3$ and hence does not function as a hormone dependent modulator of gene expression, but instead may inhibit the action of the thyroid hormone dependent isoforms. The thyroid hormone receptors may bind to DNA as homodimers, but probably do so more commonly as heterodimers by associating with any of several other nuclear proteins, usually with members of the same receptor superfamily. The receptor dimer, on association with $T_3$ may have either a positive or negative influence on gene expression, depending on the specific gene involved. Stimulatory actions have been determined for a number of genes, including those encoding for growth hormone, malic enzyme, myelin basic protein, myosin heavy chain alpha, and type I deiodinase, while inhibitory actions have been documented on the expression of genes for myosin heavy chain beta, TSH (α and β subunits), TRH and type II deiodinase. Abnormalities in the receptor-β gene result in reduced $T_3$ binding and are associated with the thyroid hormone resistance syndrome.

The thyroid hormones may have some nongenomic actions, including plasma and mitochondrial membrane transport, polymerization of actin in astrocytes, and modulation of the activities of several enzymes including type II deiodinase.[24] Such nongenomic effects tend to occur rapidly, and unlike nuclear events, $T_4$ may be as effective or more so than $T_3$. Further work is needed to understand the mechanisms by which these events occur.

# References

1. Dunn JT. Sources of dietary iodine in industrialized countries. In: Delange F, Dunn JT, Glinoer D, eds. *Iodine Deficiency in Europe: A Continuing Concern*. New York, NY: Plenum Press; 1993:17–21.

2. Levy O, De la Vieja A, Carrasco N. The Na$^+$/I$^-$ symporter (NIS): recent advances. *J Bioenergetics Biomembranes*. 1998; 30:195–206.

3. Royaux IE, Suzuki K, Mori A et al. Pendrin, the protein encoded by the Pendred syndrome gene (PDS), is an apical porter of iodide in the thyroid and is regulated by thyroglobulin in FRTL-5 cells. *Endocrinology*. 2000;141:839–845.

4. Dunn JT, Dunn AD. Thyroglobulin:chemistry, biosynthesis, and proteolysis. In: Braverman LE, Utiger RD, eds. *The Thyroid*. 8th ed. Philadelphia,PA: Lippincott Williams & Wilkins; 2000:91–104.

5. Kim PS, Arvan P. Endocrinopathies in the family of endoplasmic reticulum (ER) storage diseases: disorders of protein trafficking and the role of ER molecular chaperones. *Endocrine Rev*. 1998;19: 173–202.

6. Ohtaki S, Nakagawa H, Nakamura M, Kotani T. Thyroid peroxidase: experimental and clinical integration. *Endocrine J*. 1996;43: 1–14.

7. Michot JL, Deme D, Virion A, Pommier J. Relationship between thyroid peroxidase, H$_2$O$_2$ generating system and NADPH-dependent reductase activities in thyroid particulate fractions. *Mol Cell Endocrinol*. 1985; 41:211–221.

8. Köhrle J. Local activation and inactivation of thyroid hormones: the deiodinase family. *Mol Cell Endocrinol*. 1999;151:103–119.

9. Cavalieri RR, Simeoni LA, Park SW et al. Thyroid hormone export in rat FRTL-5 thyroid cells and mouse NIH-3T3 cells is carrier-mediated, verapamil-sensitive, and stereospecific. *Endocrinology*. 1999; 140:4948–4954.

10. Schussler GC. The thyroxine-binding proteins. *Thyroid*. 2000; 10:141–149.

11. Salvatore D, Tu H, Harney JW, Larsen PR. Type 2 iodothyronine deiodinase is highly expressed in human thyroid. *J Clin Invest*. 1996; 98:962–968.

12. Bates JM, St. Germain DL, Galton VA. Expression profiles of the three iodothyronine deiodinases, D1, D2, and D3, in the developing rat. *Endocrinology*. 1999;140:844–851.

13. Vassart G, Dumont JE. The thyrotropin receptor and the regulation of thyrocyte function and growth. *Endocr Rev*. 1992;13: 596–611.

14. Scanlon MF, Toft AD. Regulation of thyrotropin secretion. In: Braverman LE, Utiger RD eds. *The Thyroid*. 8th ed. Philadelphia PA: Lippincott Williams & Wilkins; 2000:234–253.

15. Corvilain B, Van Sande J, Dumont JE. Inhibition by iodide of iodide binding to proteins: the "Wolff-Chaikoff" effect is caused by inhibition of H$_2$O$_2$ generation. *Biochem Biophys Res Comm*. 1988; 154:1287–1292.

16. Uyttersprot N, Pelrims N, Carrasco N et al. Moderate doses of iodide in vivo inhibit cell proliferation and the expression of thyroperoxidase and Na$^+$/I$^-$ symporter mRNAs in dog thyroid. *Mol Cell Endocrinol*. 1997;131:195–203.

17. Cooper DS. Antithyroid drugs for the treatment of hyperthyroidism caused by Graves' disease. *Endocrinol Metab Clin North Am*. 1998;27:225–247.

18. Wiersinga WM. Propranolol and thyroid hormone metabolism. *Thyroid*. 1991; 1:273–277.

19. Felicetta JV, Green WL, Nelp WB. Inhibition of hepatic binding of thyronine by cholecystographic agents. *J Clin Invest*. 1980;65: 1032–1040.

20. DeGroot LJ, Rue PA. Roentgenographic contrast agents inhibit triiodothyronine binding to nuclear receptors in vitro. *J Clin Endocrinol Metab*. 1979;49:538–542.

21. Lazarus JH. The effects of lithium therapy on thyroid and thyrotropin-releasing hormone. *Thyroid*. 1998;8:909–913.

22. Boyages SC, Halpern JP. Endemic cretinism: toward a unifying hypothesis. *Thyroid*. 1993;3:59–69.

23. Brent GA. The molecular basis of thyroid hormone action. *N Engl J Med*. 1994;331:847–853.

24. Davis PJ, Davis FB. Nongenomic actions of thyroid hormone. *Thyroid*. 1996;6:497–504.

# 5

# Physical Examination and Diagnosis in Thyroid Disease

Donald P. Vrabec, M.D., F.A.C.S.
Ronald P. Monsaert, M.D.

The scope of problems relating to thyroid disease can be so complex and encompassing as to create a major challenge to the diagnostic capabilities of the clinician. The patient may present with such a variety of seemingly unrelated signs and symptoms as to lull the practitioner into a suspicion of hypochondriasis. This is especially true in our current "cost-effective" frame of mind where screening batteries of diagnostic tests are no longer en vogue and time is of the essence. The patient's symptoms can be confusing and bizarre leading the physician at times to nonspecific diagnoses, such as psychological problems of depression or anxiety, chronic fatigue syndromes, cardiac failure, fibromyalgia and a host of other nonspecific entities. The dilemma is more than simply one of hyperfunction versus hypofunction or nodular versus diffuse or benign versus malignant. Nor should the examination be merely one of placing the thumb on the lower neck while the patient swallows a few sips of water and answers a couple of quick questions about heat intolerance, weight changes and gastrointestinal function.

In actuality the thyroid gland controls body metabolism and has a profound effect on all bodily functions. Additionally, the peculiarities of development and the strategic location of the thyroid gland may produce symptom complexes which divert the physician's attention away from the thyroid gland and toward the symptom itself. To be proficient in the management of thyroid disease, the physician must be knowledgeable about all phases of the embryology, anatomy, endocrine function, genetic implications and environmental issues which may affect the thyroid, and he must be keenly suspicious of all the patient's signs and symptoms.

The patient's history and review of systems should be comprehensive. Postmenopausal women are most commonly affected by hypothyroidism in a ratio of female to male of 10:1. Generalized symptoms include weakness and fatigue with cold intolerance, weight gain, hair loss, edema of the hands and face, thick dry skin and hair, as well as a decreased tendency to sweating. Otolaryngologic symptoms may include hearing loss, dizziness, tinnitus, voice aberrations, middle ear effusion and a slurred speech with an enlarged tongue. The gastrointestinal symptoms include constipation, anorexia, intermittent nausea and vomiting, as well as dysphagia and bloating. Dysphagia is especially common if there is external compression on the esophagus by a circumferential or enlarged thyroid. Genitourinary symptoms include menstrual disorders and a tendency toward polyuria. Cardiovascular symptoms include bradycardia, some elevation of the blood pressure, intermittent angina, at times pericardial effusion and peripheral ischemia. Central nervous system symptoms may include daytime somnolence but insomnia at night, headaches and dizziness, mental and physical slowness, delayed reflexes and psychological symptoms suggestive of depression or anxiety may be present. Pulmonary symptoms may include shortness of breath if there is tracheal compression or pleural effusion. Finally, musculoskeletal symptoms include arthritis and stiffness of the joints with muscle cramps and weakness.

The symptoms of hyperthyroidism commonly include a rapid heartbeat or perceptible palpitations, irritability, anxiety, easy fatigue, increased number of bowel movements with weight loss, and heat intolerance. Again, the incidence is approximately ten times more common in the female than the male with a mean age in the upper 40s. Physical findings may include tachycardia with or without arrhythmia, moist warm skin, a fine tremor of the fingers, and the thyroid is usually enlarged. Eye signs may be present including a lid lag, eyelid retraction and exophthalmos.

Other patient complaints may include the presence of a mass or nodule in the lower neck in the region of the thyroid or in other areas of the neck. These may or may not be associated with the above described signs of hyper- or hypothyroidism. Other symptoms directly related to the thyroid may include acute pain over the thyroid which may suggest a thyroiditis.

The thyroid gland is strategically located in the lower anterior neck in close relationship to the larynx, the trachea, the esophagus, the carotid sheath structures, the sympathetic chain, the recurrent laryngeal nerve and the mediastinal structures. Diffuse or nodular enlargement whether benign or malignant may cause compression or invasion of these adjacent structures. Resulting symptomatology may include dysphagia, dyspnea, voice aberrations, vocal cord paralysis, Horner's syndrome, superior vena caval syndrome and at times pericardial or pleural effusions.

Past medical history may disclose a history of thyroid agenesis, prior thyroidectomy surgery, therapeutic irradiation using either I[131] or external radiation therapy, Hashimoto's thyroiditis, past history of laryngeal cancer or laryngectomy surgery, a history of cancer elsewhere with possible metastasis to the thyroid and a history of other recent head and neck infections, which may have resulted in an abscess within the thyroid.[1]

History of family members with elevated serum calcitonin levels or a medullary carcinoma of the thyroid should arouse suspicion of a similar lesion in the patient, since medullary carcinoma may be transmitted in an autosomal dominant inheritance pattern and is bilateral in most cases, involving the parafollicular or C cells of neural crest origin.[2] Serum calcitonin levels also are of value to determine the presence of metastatic disease or residual tumor in patients treated surgically for medullary carcinoma of the thyroid.

## PHYSICAL EXAMINATION

Facility with the examination of the thyroid and surrounding structures is essential for accurate diagnosis and appropriate management of malignant as well as benign thyroid disease. The patient is initially observed anteriorly. Some findings may be obvious. Others may be more subtle. The hypothyroid patient will usually appear more lethargic, perhaps somewhat overweight and slower in responses. The skin may appear dry and coarse as does the hair.

On the other hand, the hyperthyroid patient may appear more anxious, thinner, somewhat more apprehensive with moist, warm skin and perhaps a visible tremor may be noted in his/her fingers. Eye signs may or may not be present. These may include exophthalmos, lid lag or lid retraction.

In either the hypothyroid or the hyperthyroid patient a diffuse or nodular goiter may not uncommonly be visible in the neck on simple inspection. The patients may have some aberrations of their voice. The hypothyroid patient with myxedematous infiltration of the vocal folds will have a husky, raspy type of voice. On the other hand, the patient whose recurrent laryngeal nerve is compromised by pressure or tumor infiltration will elicit the voice of a paralyzed vocal cord, which will be breathy, barely audible and inefficient as far as air usage is concerned. In other circumstances, the voice may have a gutteral quality signifying obstruction of the aerodigestive passageway usually at the level of the tongue base. This, of course, would suggest a lingual thyroid which has failed to descend along normal developmental pathways. Horner's syndrome may be present with either benign or malignant thyroid disease. The patient may appear to have a hearing deficit in normal conversational situations. This may be the result of middle ear effusions which can be drained and reversed. On the other hand, inner ear myxedematous changes involving the cochlear and vestibular structures may contribute to a sensorineural type of hearing loss accompanied by tinnitus and vertigo.

Facial swelling or plethora and distention of the jugular veins may signify obstruction of the superior vena cava from benign or malignant substernal thyroid disease. Pemberton's sign should be elicited in patients with large goiters. Pemberton's sign is elicited by having the patient extend both arms above the head and watching for facial erythema, swelling and/or distention of the jugular veins.

Following careful observation of the patient's general appearance, the neck is examined. The thyroid may be examined either from the front or from behind the patient depending on the preference of the examiner. The thyroid is palpated initially for gross pathology. The patient is then asked to swallow several sips of water. This will move the thyroid cephalad and make the lower portion of the thyroid more easily approached. If the patient extends the neck less fully the more inferior aspects of the thyroid (especially in patients with substernal goiters or kyphosis) may be easily and accurately examined. Moderate pressure in the tracheal groove on one side will facilitate more accurate palpation of the contralateral thyroid lobe. The examiner will note the size relative to a normal thyroid gland. Similarly, the size and locations of nodules should be accurately recorded. A pyramidal lobe of the thyroid can sometimes be palpated in patients, especially those with Graves' or Hashimoto's disease. A thyroid nodule with recent hemorrhage may be moderately tender, while an acute suppurative or subacute viral thyroiditis is usually exquisitely tender to palpation. Not uncommonly, the pain from the thyroid will radiate to the ipsilateral ear.

The texture of the thyroid may suggest the etiology of the disease. Autoimmune thyroid disease often presents as a firm, bosselated (cobblestone-like) gland. This, in conjunction with a low or elevated serum TSH, should strongly suggest Graves' disease or Hashimoto's thyroiditis, respectively. Smooth nodularity of the thyroid usually represents colloid goiter. Although firm nodules may represent thyroid cancer, this clinical characteristic is not diagnostic. Most if not all thyroid nodules should be biopsied to determine etiology.

Attention is next turned to the areas of lymphatic drainage of the thyroid. The superior pole and the lateral lobes drain superiorly and laterally toward the jugular lymph nodes, while the isthmus and the lower poles of the thyroid drain inferiorly along the tracheoesophageal groove and into the mediastinum. Each side of the neck should be examined methodically from the mandible to the supraclavicular notch. One author's preference is to palpate deep to the sternomastoid muscle by placing the thumb in the groove between the trachea and the sternomastoid and the index and middle fingers lateral to the sternomastoid muscle grasping it and elevating it while feeling down into the depths of the carotid sheath. In this manner it is quite easy to feel the carotid artery as well as the lymph node structures deep to the carotid sheath. This examination is then repeated on the opposite side. Every attempt is made to palpate as deeply into the supraclavicular space as possible without causing the patient undue discomfort.

Finally, examination of the upper neck above the larynx is performed. Nodules just below the hyoid bone in the midline are frequently thyroglossal duct cysts or remnants. Examination of these can be done by having the patient swallow or protrude his tongue which will then cause retraction of the nodule cephalad.

Once the observation of the external surfaces as well as examination of the external neck is accomplished attention is turned to the internal examination of the aerodigestive system. Intraorally, the tongue in the myxedematous patient may be enlarged and thickened. Careful examination of the base of the tongue should be done in order to rule out a lingual thyroid

gland. This would indicate a developmental anomaly. The lingual thyroid can enlarge during periods of increased hormonal demands such as puberty and pregnancy. When this occurs the gutteral qualities of the voice may be even more profound. Additionally, bleeding may occur from the lingual thyroid and finally enlargement of the lingual thyroid may continue to the point of dysphagia and airway obstruction which may precipitate a semiemergent condition. Most commonly hormonal treatment will reduce the size of the mass on the back of the tongue. Occasionally surgical intervention is required to ensure a safe airway. This area of the oropharynx and tongue base is usually readily examined with the aid of a tongue blade and a laryngeal mirror. However, in patients with an extremely active gag reflex a better examination is usually obtained using the fiberoptic nasopharyngolaryngoscope.

Assessment of the etiology of the patient's hoarseness is determined using the fiberoptic nasopharyngolaryngoscope to obtain a dynamic examination of the hypopharynx and larynx. In the hypothyroid patient, the vocal cords are mobile. However, they may exhibit myxedematous changes causing them to be thickened and at times even polypoid along the edges of the vocal cords. The voice in these instances is quite harsh and raspy. The airway may become partially compromised by the thickened myxedematous polypoid tissue and at times it is necessary to surgically trim this back in order to ensure an adequate airway.

When one vocal cord is paralyzed, the airway initially becomes incompetent. The patient may cough or choke on liquids or his own secretions unless he is careful as he swallows. The larynx is inefficient and will produce only two or three words per each breath of air. The voice is of an exaggerated, forced, whispered quality. As time passes, the larynx will compensate somewhat by having the mobile vocal cord cross the midline to partially close the deficit in the airway. This will improve speech and swallowing almost to normal levels. It is important that preoperative laryngeal examinations be done prior to thyroid surgery to establish the mobility of the vocal cords. Since it is possible to have a nearly normal sounding voice with one cord paralyzed, it is important for the operating surgeon to know that there is a paralyzed cord, as injury to the opposite cord would then precipitate the more emergent situation of bilateral vocal cord paralysis and the probable need for subsequent tracheostomy and/or thyroplasty. Paralysis of the vocal cords usually implies compromise of the recurrent laryngeal nerve on the ipsilateral side. This may be secondary to pressure on the nerve but more likely is caused by infiltration of the nerve by malignancy.

It is not uncommon for a laryngeal carcinoma to extend through the anterior commissure region into the thyroid gland. Needle biopsies of these glands then will show squamous carcinoma. The vocal cord may be paralyzed but, in these instances, it will be paralyzed secondary to the squamous carcinoma within the larynx rather than from recurrent nerve involvement. It is also important to know that the etiology is within the larynx rather than within the thyroid. Surgical approach including simultaneous laryngectomy and thyroidectomy can then be accomplished.

External compression on the trachea and/or esophagus by thyroid masses can lead to severe dyspnea and/or dysphagia.[3] It is important to know if the airway and esophageal involvement are secondary to external compression alone or whether there is an element of tumor infiltration within these organs. Therefore, internal examination with bronchoscope and esophagoscopes are necessary in order to determine the status of these organs. At times, radiographic studies are necessary to complement the examinations and to aid in planning of surgery. Under such circumstances, barium swallow of the esophagus may outline the areas of obstruction. CT scans of the trachea and mediastinum can depict areas of involvement by tumor. Appropriate surgical approaches can then be designed and performed.

In summary, elucidating the various etiologies of thyroid disease is often accomplished by considering the aggregate data available from the patient's history, clinical examination, thyroid function studies and the presence or absence of various thyroid autoantibodies. Imaging studies and radioiodine uptake may help clarify the diagnosis. For example, a patient with hyperthyroid symptoms, elevated thyroid function studies, a low TSH, a diffuse goiter and the presence of thyroid stimulating immunoglobulin will easily be diagnosed with Graves' disease. Similarly, a patient with a diffuse goiter, hypothyroid indices and antithyroid antibodies should initially suggest Hashimoto's thyroiditis, and tissue examination of the thyroid may not be necessary for the definitive diagnosis and management.[4]

## THYROID NEEDLE BIOPSY

While obtaining thyroid tissue by percutaneous or surgical biopsy is only occasionally needed in the diagnosis and management of diffuse goiters, biopsy is usually necessary in elucidating the etiology of nodular disease of the thyroid.[5] Thyroid nodules are common (3–7% of adult population) and fortunately thyroid cancers are relatively uncommon (6–8% of all nodules). Thus, a safe, reliable, cost-effective, diagnostic test is important in determining the etiology of disease in patients with nodular disease of the thyroid. Thyroid needle biopsy fulfills these criteria and is indispensable in

the diagnosis and management of these patients.[6] The procedure is essentially painless. The principal reported morbidity is an occasional small hematoma. Sensitivity and specificity have been reported to be greater than 90% and 70%, respectively. The incidence of finding benign thyroid disease at surgery has dropped from 80% before the initiation of this procedure to about 10–20% after biopsy screening. An additional benefit is that the patient and surgeon can better prepare for the type of surgical procedure or other intervention that may be required in the event of a positive or suspicious biopsy. While a thyroid scan or ultrasound may provide useful information, using these techniques alone or together does not approach the usefulness of biopsy alone. Thus, fine needle aspiration biopsy has emerged as the preferred diagnostic procedure in the management of patients with thyroid nodules. Several studies have confirmed the cost-effectiveness of a paradigm using biopsy as the initial procedure.[6,7]

Thyroid biopsy is easily performed in the office with the patient supine. A pillow is placed beneath the shoulders to extend the neck and make the nodule more readily accessible. Antiseptic solution is applied over the nodule and the superficial tissues are infiltrated with 1% lidocaine solution. The nodule is then punctured and gently aspirated. The biopsy contents are then applied to glass slides or fixative solutions for subsequent cytological evaluation. Three to six specimens are obtained trying to sample all areas of the tumor. Small gauge needles without suction may avoid obscuring the specimen with blood. This is especially helpful when biopsying very vascular colloid nodules. Most clinicians use a 22–26 gauge needle although in some cases larger bore needles (14–18 gauge) may ultimately be helpful if the initial biopsy was not diagnostic. The use of larger needles, however, may not be associated with greater accuracy and may be associated with more morbidity. Only larger, well-positioned nodules are suitable for biopsy with larger needles. Finally, the clinician should be aware that cases of cancer seeding along the needle track have been reported when using large bore needles.[8]

While 70% of biopsies are clearly benign or malignant, the remainder may require a more global assessment of the clinical aspects of the case in order to use the biopsy results proficiently. Discussion of these aspects with a cytologist is often helpful.

Pitfalls with thyroid biopsy include the fact that adequate cellularity must be present in the biopsy material. Most cytologists will comment as to whether they consider the cellularity adequate. Inadequate biopsies must be repeated. With larger nodules (greater than 4 cm) the biopsy should be representative with sampling obtained from all four quadrants of the nodule with some consideration given to surgical biopsy if uncertainty persists. Obtaining sufficient cellularity is sometimes a challenge in colloid nodules and in most cystic nodules. In the former case, these nodules are quite vascular often obscuring the specimen with blood. Puncturing the nodule with small gauge needles (26 gauge) without aspiration is often helpful in this situation. While cystic nodules are infrequently malignant, most cysts have a solid component. Since cyst fluid is largely acellular or contains only degenerative cells, it is frequently nondiagnostic. Any nodular components that are apparent after cyst evacuation should be sampled. Small cysts often do not recur following aspiration, but the larger ones (greater than 3 cm) usually do. Thus, concern about a malignancy may arise, especially if the cystic fluid is hemorrhagic. In this instance, surgical biopsy should be considered. Cyst fluid is often yellow or chocolate brown, but occasionally one encounters water-clear fluid. These commonly are parathyroid cysts which usually do not recur following aspiration. It is rare that they are accompanied by the syndrome of hyperparathyroidism.

Perhaps 10–15% of biopsies will be classified as suspicious because they contain Hürthle cells, microfollicular architecture or otherwise suggest a follicular neoplasm. It is not common that a follicular cancer will be so differentiated that the diagnosis can be made by needle biopsy alone. Definitive diagnosis may rest on the demonstration that there is capsular or vascular invasion and this degree of detail can only be seen in a surgical biopsy. Thus, some patients will require surgery for definitive diagnosis. At this point the thyroid scan may be helpful as sometimes these follicular lesions will be "hot" (remainder of thyroid tissue suppressed) and one can then be reassured that this is a benign lesion. Hürthle cells may be prominent in patients with Hashimoto's thyroiditis. If there is other clinical evidence (increased TSH, positive antithyroid antibodies) for Hashimoto's thyroiditis, a more conservative approach may be offered by administering thyroid hormone.[9] Often the nodule will then regress over four to six months. Hashimoto's disease may present with a thyroid nodule and lymphocytes may be the principle finding on biopsy. The cytopathologist may then wish to rule out lymphoma. In this situation repeating the biopsy and sending the specimen for flow cytometry usually resolves the issue.[10] Patients with Hashimoto's disease will have polyclonal lymphocyte populations, whereas patients with lymphoma will have monoclonal populations of lymphocytes. Sometimes a larger bore needle biopsy will be helpful in differentiating these two entities.

Occasionally, the cytologist may have difficulty differentiating anaplastic carcinoma from lymphoma. Again flow cytometry may be helpful; or providing a larger biopsy specimen may resolve the issue. There may be uncertainty about whether a lesion is a medullary carcinoma. In this setting, staining the biopsy for amyloid or calcitonin will usually be positive in the presence of medullary carcinoma. Additionally, the serum calcitonin will usually be elevated in patients with this disease. While most patients with medullary carcinoma of the thyroid have calcitonin elevation, an occasional patient may have this finding as part of the multiple endocrine neoplasia (MEN) syndrome type II or type III. Patients with these syndromes may have pheochromocytoma and this diagnosis should be ruled out before considering surgery for medullary carcinoma of the thyroid. Hyperparathyroidism is often seen in patients with MEN type II. Patients with MEN II, III or familial medullary carcinoma of the thyroid can also be screened by obtaining genetic testing for the RET proto-oncogene; a thorough disscussion of their entities may be found elsewhere in this text.

## SUMMARY

In summary an understanding of thyroid embryology, anatomy and physiology is a necessary prerequisite for interpreting physical examination findings and diagnostic test results and for determining a management scheme for thyroid disorders.

## References

1. Vrabec DP, Heffron TJ. Hypothyroidism following treatment for head and neck cancer. *Ann Otol, Rhinol Laryngol.* 1981;444-453.
2. O'Riordain DS, O'Brien T, Weaver AL, et al. Medullary thyroid carcinoma in multiple endocrine neoplasia types 2A and 2B. *Surgery.* 1994;116(6):1017–23.
3. Alfonso A, Christoudias G, Amaruddin Q, Herbsman H, Gardner B. Tracheal or esophageal compression due to benign thyroid disease. *Am J Surg.* 1981;143(3):350–4
4. Slatosky J, Shipton B, Wahba H. Thyroiditis: differential diagnosis and management. *Am Fam Physician.* 2000;61(4):1047–52, 1054.
5. Shaha AR. (2000 Feb.). Controversies in the management of thyroid nodule. *Laryngoscope.* 2000;110(2 Pt 1):183–93.
6. Woeber KA. Cost-effective evaluation of the patient with a thyroid nodule. *Surg Clin North Am.* 1995;75(3):357-63.
7. Bi J, Lu B. Advances in the diagnosis and management of thyroid neoplasms. *Curr Opin Oncol.* 2000;12(1):54–9.
8. Moosa M, Mazzaferri EL. Disorders of the thyroid gland In: Cummings, CW et al, eds. *Otolaryngol—Head Neck Surg.* 3rd ed. Mosby; 1998; pp. 2450–79.
9. Tollin SR, Fallon EF, Mikhail M, Goldstein H, Yung E. The utility of thyroid nuclear imaging and other studies in the detection and treatment of underlying thyroid abnormalities in patients with endogenous subclinical thyrotoxicosis. *Clin Nucl Med.* 2000;25(5):341–7.
10. Kossev P, Livolsi V. Lymphoid lesions of the thyroid: review in light of the revised European-American lymphoma classification and upcoming World Health Organization classification. *Thyroid.* 1999;9(12):1273–80.

# 6

# Diagnostic Imaging of the Thyroid

Richard M. Gall, M.D., F.R.C.S.C., Ian J. Witterick, M.D., F.R.C.S.C.
Brian Ginzburg, F.R.C.P.C., Arnold M. Noyek, M.D., F.R.C.S.C.,
F.A.C.S

Thyroid nodules are a common finding in the general population. Many of these nodules are detected by the patient or clinician during routine physical examination. This is caused in part by the superficial location of the thyroid gland in the anterior neck. It has been estimated that 4% to 15% of adult Americans have a palpable thyroid lesion,[1,2] with an even higher number having subclinical non-palpable thyroid nodules. When a suspicious lesion is suggested on clinical examination, the use of ancillary diagnostic tests are often required for further work-up of the patient. This includes a wide and ever increasing battery of diagnostic imaging techniques to help in the diagnosis and treatment of thyroid disease. The rapid development of newer diagnostic imaging techniques, with differing strengths and weaknesses, makes it difficult for the clinician/surgeon to properly select which test is most appropriate and cost-effective for any given scenario. This chapter focuses primarily on imaging of the thyroid gland as it relates to surgical thyroid disease and relies largely on illustrative examples of the various imaging techniques.

Imaging can give us the most basic information, such as whether a lesion is present or not, the size of the lesion, the consistency of a lesion—solid, cystic, or both, as well as suggest whether a lesion is benign or malignant. Imaging can also provide us with information regarding function of the gland. It is in this area that much of the newer diagnostic tests have a role to play. Often with the aid of the Department of Diagnostic Imaging the most appropriate test or tests can be selected that will tell us the extent of the thyroid disease, the functional status of the gland, or the involvement of surrounding structures. The challenge is to provide the patient with the most appropriate care without any unnecessary risk or expense. It should be remembered that the use of the various tests available should not be considered as "routine investigations," but rather as tools to be used to appropriately answer a specific clinical question.

No single test is ever going to be 100% sensitive or specific, nor will any of the tests discussed below ever make the need for a tissue sample obsolete. It is the role of the clinician/surgeon to collate the information obtained from the tests performed and put them within the framework of the clinical setting. It is believed that fine needle aspiration (FNA), despite the abundance of new tests available, should still be the initial investigation for the majority of thyroid lesions. It has even been suggested that with the improvements in diagnostic techniques using FNA, thyroid imaging no longer has a role to play.[3] However, while FNA of suspected lesions of the thyroid gland is the most reliable diagnostic test that can currently be performed,[4] development of a non-invasive test that could work as well as FNA would be beneficial. Technologic advances arise faster than literature to support them and make diagnostic imaging of the thyroid gland a challenging and exciting field of study.

## CONVENTIONAL IMAGING

Conventional radiography of the thyroid gland, while inexpensive and widely available, is almost never performed today when investigating thyroid disease. On the other hand, indirect information about the thyroid gland is occasionally detected incidentally on chest X-ray, such as displacement of the trachea or the presence of calcification of the thyroid gland (Figure 6–1). These abnormalities will direct one to other thyroid imaging tests that will be more beneficial. Conventional radiography does not provide any information regarding thyroid function.

## DIAGNOSTIC ULTRASOUND

Diagnostic ultrasound, which relies on the reflection of high frequency sound waves on tissue planes, has over the last 10 years become the initial imaging investigation of choice for clinicians wishing to assess the thyroid gland. It provides consistent images of the thyroid gland that are safe, inexpensive, non-invasive and comfortable for the patient (Figure 6–2).

State of the art "small parts" or high resolution (5–10 MHz) transducers allow for improved resolution of nodules as small as 3.0 mm.[5,6] This is obviously much more sensitive than clinical palpation. However, ultrasound does not differentiate well between various tissue types and, thus, has limitations when trying to differentiate between benign and malignant disease.[7-9] Calcifications large enough to be seen on ultrasound can be seen in both benign and malignant lesions.[10] Ultrasound also does not differentiate lymphadenopathy located deeper in the head and neck as well as CT or MRI, but may be better suited than CT or MRI for detecting enlarged lymph nodes that are more superficially located. Ultrasound can also be extremely dependent on the experience of the radiologist interpreting the study.[11] Some of the more common indications for use of diagnostic ultrasound are listed below.

### Thyroid Nodules

Confirming the presence of a mass is the most common indication for ultrasonography of the thyroid gland. Thyroid ultrasound is much more sensitive in detecting

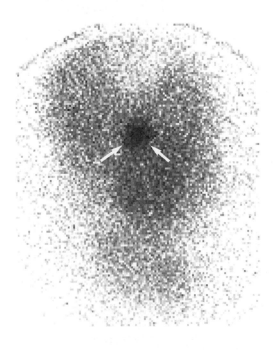
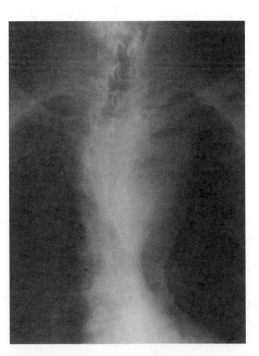

**Figure 6–1.** Chest X-ray showing deviation of the intra-thoracic trachea toward the right. On conventional imaging the cause for the displacement is non-specific. An I$^{123}$ scintigram with a marker in the suprasternal notch (arrows) confirms that the deviation is caused by a retrosternal thyroid.

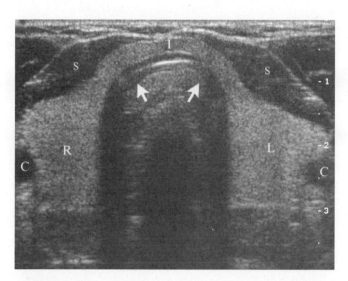

**Figure 6–2.** Transverse ultrasound image with a 12 MHz high frequency transducer provides excellent resolution of the normal thyroid anatomy. (C = common carotid arteries; I = isthmus; L = left lobe of thyroid; R = right lobe of thyroid; S = strap muscles; arrows = trachea).

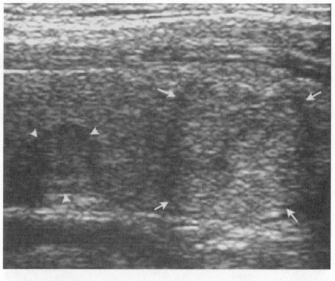

**Figure 6–3.** Two solid nodules: one small and deep in the thyroid parenchyma and, therefore, non-palpable (arrow heads); the other larger, more superficial and, therefore, palpable (arrows).

thyroid masses than physical examination alone.[12] There has been an increase in the number of non-palpable thyroid masses detected thanks to the use of high resolution ultrasound (Figure 6–3).[13-15] These subclinical nodules have been reported to have a malignancy rate of 0.45% to 13%.[17]

Thyroid ultrasound can be used to assess the remainder of a gland after a thyroid nodule has already been detected via manual palpation. It may reveal other nodules that are present or may indicate that the nodule is part of a multinodular goiter (Figure 6–4).[1,16,17,18]

Once a mass has already been identified, thyroid ultrasound can accurately determine whether it is solid or cystic (Figure 6–5). Currently, there is debate regarding the significance of this. Some authors feel that small cystic thyroid lesions have a very low incidence of malignancy, while solid lesions much more frequently prove to be malignant.[19] Others feel that the incidence of malignancy in cystic lesions is much more common than previously reported.[5]

Thyroid ultrasonography has also been used in the detection of cancerous metastases to the thyroid gland. Though relatively uncommon, they are more frequently seen after malignancies that disseminate hematogenously, such as seen in lung cancer, renal cancer, breast cancer and melanoma. Suspicious nodules from these types of cancer should be biopsied as they may be amenable to surgical treatment.[20]

Thyroid ultrasound can also be used in the detection of neck metastases in patients diagnosed with thy-

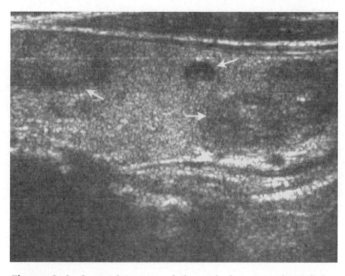

**Figure 6–4.** Sagittal image of thyroid shows multinodular goiter with several nodules (arrows) of different sizes and consistencies.

roid cancer, as well as in patients previously treated for thyroid carcinoma to determine recurrence or spread post-thyroidectomy.

It must be stressed that the high sensitivity of ultrasound to pick up small nodules does have its drawbacks. As mentioned earlier, a significant proportion of the general population will have small asymptomatic thyroid nodules that are found incidentally after thyroid ultrasound, of which the majority will be benign.[13]

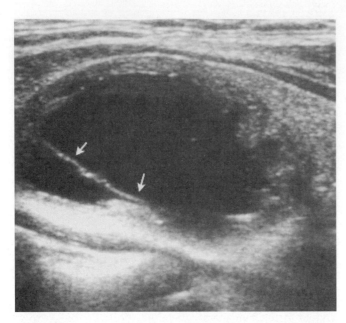

**Figure 6–5.** Predominantly cystic nodule with a septation (arrows).

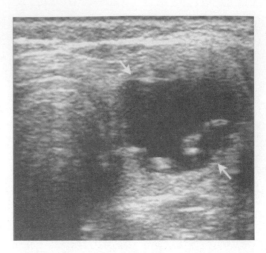

**Figure 6–6.** Cystic nodule with internal debris.

One must take this fact into account and consider the patient's age, past history, possible past radiation exposure, family history and any other related factors before proceeding with a wide range of tests to further work up the patient. Confounding the issue further is the importance of detecting, for example, a small occult papillary carcinoma, as the clinical significance of this is unknown. Using characteristic ultrasound findings as a guide to detect whether a lesion is benign or malignant is also unreliable. Findings typically associated with benign lesions, such as a cystic nodule or a hypoechoic band surrounding the nodule, or those commonly associated with malignancy, such as a solid nodule, one with fine calcifications, and an irregular or indistinct margin are to be used as a guide only, and not to be relied upon (Figures 6–6 through 6–9).[21]

## Ultrasound Guided Biopsy

Ultrasound has been an effective tool for obtaining thyroid gland biopsies. The use of ultrasound guided biopsies are especially useful in deep lesions, difficult to feel masses, and lesions less than 2 cms.[22] The use of ultrasound coupled with fine needle aspiration has been shown to yield better results than aspiration alone, which has resulted in a reduction in the number of unnecessary surgical procedures (Figures 6–10 and 6–11).[22] Ultrasound has also been used to direct the percutaneous injection of ethanol as a treatment for both functioning and non-functioning nodules.[23]

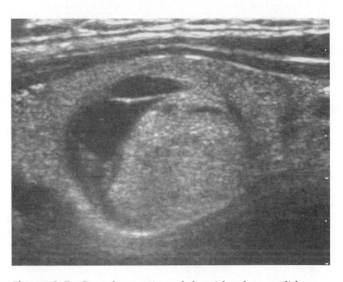

**Figure 6–7.** Complex cystic nodule with a large solid component and a septation.

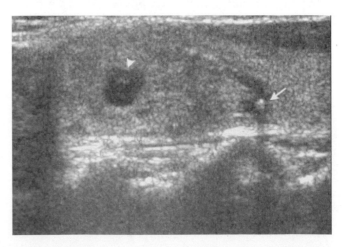

**Figure 6–8.** Predominantly solid nodule with a small cystic component (arrow head) and a small peripheral calcification (arrow).

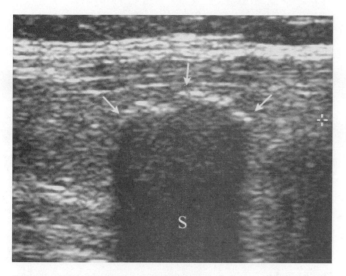

**Figure 6–9.** Nodule with peripheral rim calcifications (arrows). The calcification produces distal loss of ultrasound signal or acoustic shadowing (S).

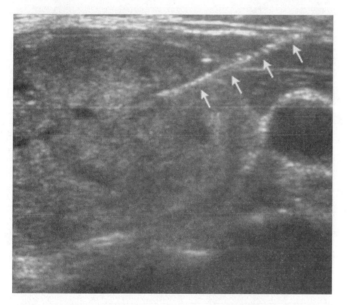

**Figure 6–10.** Ultrasound-guided biopsy of a solid thyroid nodule. The needle (arrows) can be seen traversing the subcutaneous tissues and sampling the nodule.

## Thyroid Volume

Aside from its other uses, ultrasound can be used to assess thyroid gland volume. This can have implications with regard to treatment of various thyroid disorders. It can be used to follow patients with Graves' disease and may be used in determining the appropriate dose of radio-iodine for therapy.[24] Serial thyroid volume measurements are also useful in following patients with diffuse non-toxic goiter on thyroid suppression.[25] PET

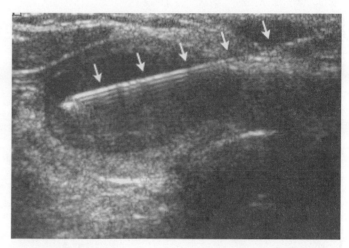

**Figure 6–11.** Ultrasound-guided needle (arrows) aspiration of a cystic thyroid lesion.

scanning has recently become the modality of choice for determining thyroid gland volume (see below).

## Other Uses

Color and power Doppler are used to assess changes in the local vascularity of a thyroid lesion that may indicate eradication of thyroid disease.[26] Color and power Doppler are also used to study functioning thyroid adenomas after injection of percutaneous ethanol.[26] The use of this modality in differentiating benign from malignant disease has been disappointing.[27,28]

## COMPUTED TOMOGRAPHY

Although not considered a first line investigation for thyroid disease, computed tomography (CT) scanning, which relies on attenuation of X-ray photons by tissue density, provides valuable information in a number of disease processes related to the thyroid gland. The CT appearance of the thyroid gland is more dense than the surrounding soft tissue structures,[17] falling between 80–100 Hounsfield units. This is secondary to its high iodine concentration.[29] After the administration of intravenous contrast, the thyroid gland density further increases. Predictably, patients suffering from hypothyroidism may have a lower density on CT scan.[17]

Like ultrasonography, computed tomography is able to provide information regarding the size, consistency, location and shape of a thyroid mass (Figure 6–12). CT is able to discern both extracapsular extension of thyroid disease as well as invasion of adjacent structures and obliteration of fascial planes (Figure 6–13).[17,30,31] It

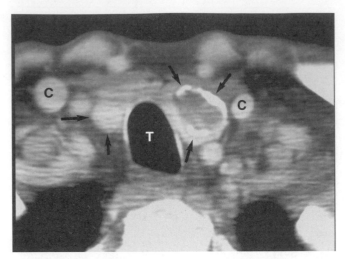

**Figure 6–12.** Transverse CT scan of the thyroid. Arrows outline a left lobe nodule with circumferential ring calcification. Note the normal high density in the normal right lobe (arrowheads). C = common carotid arteries; T = trachea.

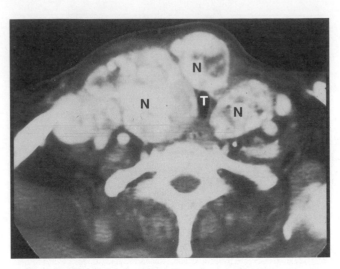

**Figure 6–14.** Multi-nodular goiter with multiple enhancing nodules bilaterally (N). Note compression and narrowing of trachea (T).

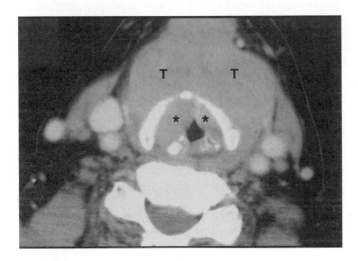

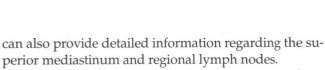

**Figure 6–13.** Thyroid lymphoma with marked enlargement of the thyroid (T) and extension into larynx (asterisks).

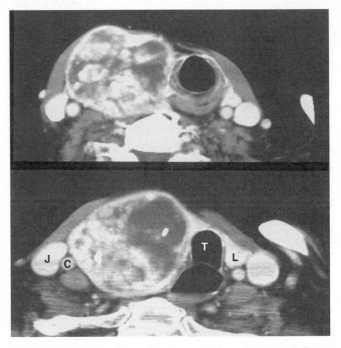

**Figure 6–15.** Very large heterogeneous thyroid nodule in right lobe causing marked displacement of trachea and superior mediastinum to the left. Note the normal high density, uniformly enhancing left thyroid lobe (L). C = common carotid artery; J = internal jugular vein.

can also provide detailed information regarding the superior mediastinum and regional lymph nodes.

CT scanning has a particularly important role to play in the management of thyroid carcinoma and large goiters. It provides excellent resolution of surrounding structures, such as the trachea, esophagus, and adjacent vessels (Figures 6–14 and 6–15). This allows the thyroid surgeon to better plan a surgical approach and decreases the risk of any intra-operative surprises.

As in ultrasonography, CT scanning does not provide any information with regard to histologic tissue type or the benign versus malignant nature of any thyroid disease. As mentioned earlier, certain characteristics of a lesion may point toward a benign or malignant

lesion, but this is certainly not foolproof, and tissue sampling is required to confirm any diagnosis.

CT scanning also can provide important information in the assessment of benign disease processes. For example, when assessing thyroglossal duct cysts, the relationship of the cyst to the hyoid bone or tongue base can be accurately determined. CT can also be used to assess patients suspected of having a lingual thyroid gland (Figures 6–16A & B). This, again, has obvious benefits when doing presurgical planning.[30] Spiral CT imaging has also been used to reliably assess volume of enlarged thyroid glands.[32]

## MAGNETIC RESONANCE IMAGING

Like computed tomography, magnetic resonance imaging (MRI) is not a first line imaging modality when investigating thyroid disease. It has essentially the same uses and applications as CT for investigation of thyroid disease but provides more anatomic detail (Figure 6–17).[33] It has similar limitations as well. CT and MRI have been shown to be less sensitive than ultrasound in detecting intra-thyroidal lesions,[34,35] but better than ultrasound in assessing mediastinal extension of thyroid lesions.[36] One advantage that MRI has over CT is that contrast (gadolinium) does not interfere with iodide uptake or organification by the thyroid gland. A second advantage is that MRI is able to detect blood vessels which appear as a signal void; on CT these may be confused with lymph nodes.[11]

The normal thyroid gland is more intense than the overlying strap muscles but less intense than fat on T1 weighted images. It is more intense than the strap muscles on T2 weighted images. Gadolinium administration results in diffuse enhancement of the gland.

To date, MRI has been unable to differentiate various thyroid gland disease states based on T1 and T2 weighted characteristics (Figure 6–18). High intensity lesions on T1 weighted images have been found to be indicative of hemorrhage into, or colloid degeneration of, a nodule.[37]

MRI has recently been investigated with regard to MRI guided biopsies of the thyroid gland, in cases where ultrasound guided biopsies are not possible because of an intra-thoracic component of the thyroid gland. While feasible and safe, it does not provide any additional benefits as compared to ultrasound guided

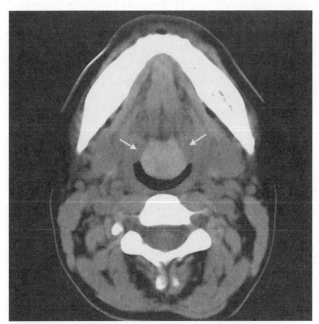

**A**

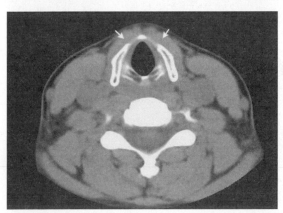

**B**

**Figure 6–16.** Lingual thyroid. **A.** CT showing high density thyroid tissue (arrows) base of tongue; **B.** CT showing absence of thyroid tissue at expected location of thyroid gland (arrows).

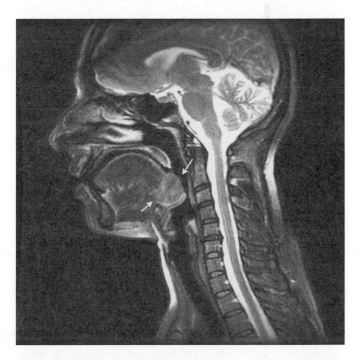

**Figure 6–17.** Lingual thyroid (arrows) seen at base of tongue on mid-sagittal MRI.

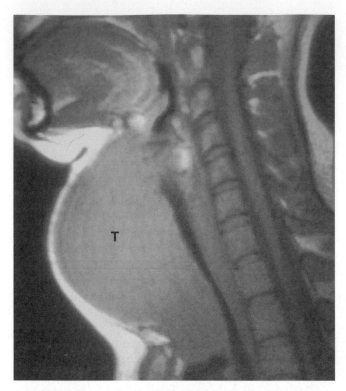

**Figure 6–18.** T1-weighted mid-sagittal MRI showing non-specific massive enlargement of thyroid (T). Pathology was lymphoma.

biopsy technique, providing the lesion can be seen by ultrasound.[38]

## RADIONUCLIDE IMAGING

Until the development of ultrasonography as an imaging modality for the thyroid gland, radionuclide scanning had been the first line investigation of choice for thyroid disease. It owes its popularity to its ability to provide information related to both anatomy and function.

Convention has dictated that thyroid nodules be classified at imaging with respect to the amount of activity that is present. This has been broken down into four categories: hot/hyperfunctioning nodules—when the thyroid nodule concentrates more radionuclide than other parts of the normal gland; warm/functioning/non-delineated nodules—when the nodule concentrates radionuclide equally as well as the normal portions of the gland; cool/hypofunctioning nodules—when the nodule concentrates some radionuclide but less than normal portions of the gland; and cold/nonfunctioning—when the nodule does not concentrate radionuclides at all.[39] Hot nodules have been found to carry less than a 5% risk of malignancy, whereas cold nodules carry approximately a 20% risk of malignancy, with warm and cool somewhere in between these two figures.[40]

While this type of investigation has been available for decades, recent advances in technology, as well as the many newer types of radionuclide agents that are becoming available, make this area of thyroid imaging challenging to keep abreast of. We will now review some of the more commonly used agents as well as some of the newer ones currently being used.

## I¹²³ SCINTIGRAPHY

An I¹²³ scan provides an accurate physiologic picture of the thyroid gland, giving good resolution with a rapid scanning time.[6,31] It also delivers a relatively low radiation dose to the patient. Disadvantages include high (though decreasing) cost and a short half-life.[41] Another disadvantage of radioiodine scintigraphy is that patients on thyroid hormone replacement must have it stopped prior to performing the scan. This hypothyroid state may induce tumor growth[42] and result in significant discomfort to the patient. Imaging is performed from 4 to 24 hours after ingestion of I¹²³.

Iodine radionuclide scans have been used effectively in cases of hyperthyroidism. In Graves' disease, the stimulatory immunoglobulins induce hormonogenesis, thus increasing trapping and organification of iodine. This results in a diffuse increased uptake on imaging (Figure 6–19).[41,43] I¹²³ imaging is often able to differentiate between Graves' disease and acute thy-

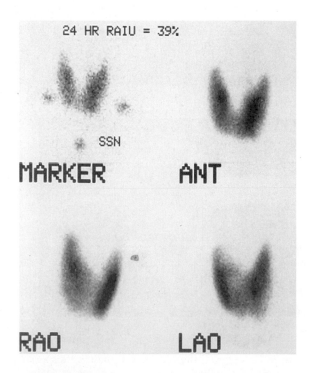

**Figure 6–19.** I¹²³ scintigram showing diffusely increased uptake in the thyroid in a patient with Graves' disease.

roiditis, despite both often presenting with hyperthyroidism. There is usually less uptake of I[123] by the gland in acute thyroiditis, as compared to that seen in Graves' disease (Figure 6–20). This is important to differentiate, as the treatment of the two diseases may be different.

Toxic multi-nodular goiter, on the other hand, presents as focal increased areas of uptake, with the intervening tissue being non-functioning secondary to feedback suppression (Figure 6–21).[43]

## I[131] SCINTIGRAPHY

Though less expensive than I[123], I[131] is not the imaging agent of choice because of its poor resolution. Despite

this, it still has an important role to play in routine quantitative assessment of radioactive iodine uptake. Imaging is performed from 24 to 72 hours after administration of I[131].

I[131] is commonly used in the detection and treatment of well-differentiated thyroid carcinoma. This is based on the ability of papillary and follicular carcinomas to concentrate iodine. I[131] imaging can be used after a total thyroidectomy for well-differentiated thyroid carcinoma to detect local, regional or distant metastases or residual thyroid tissue (Figure 6–22).[44] The incidence of I[131] uptake in thyroid cancer metastases has been reported to be between 60–70%.[45] A positive result after radioiodine scanning is a relatively good indicator of recurrent or persistent disease. This study is often undertaken after an elevated thyroglobulin level has been

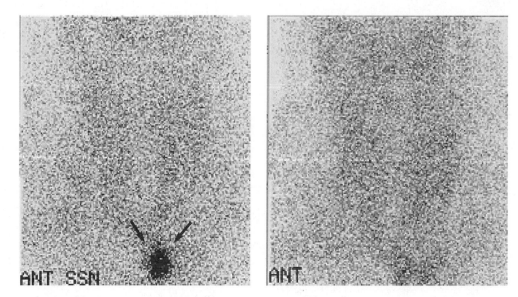

**Figure 6–20.** I[123] scintigram showing diffusely decreased uptake in the thyroid in a patient with thyroiditis. The thyroid uptake is difficult to discern from background. The 2-hour uptake was 4% and the 24-hour uptake was 1%. (Arrows indicate a marker at the suprasternal notch.)

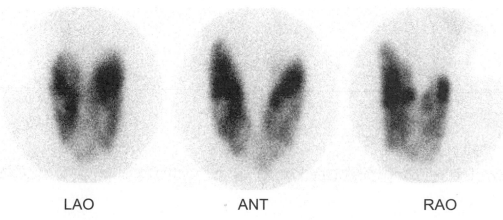

LAO       ANT       RAO

**Figure 6–21.** Multi-nodular goiter.

detected. Prior to radio-iodine imaging, patients should be off all thyroid hormone replacement therapy. This results in an elevated thyroid stimulating hormone level that will increase the uptake of $I^{131}$ into any residual or recurrent thyroid tissue. A negative $I^{131}$ (or $I^{123}$) scan does not rule out a malignancy.[42] If clinical suspicion of primary or recurrent thyroid carcinoma exists despite the negative radio-iodine, then imaging using other radio-pharmaceuticals, such as Thallium-201, Tc-99m-sestamibi or Tc-99m-tetrofosmin may be used.[46] These oth-

er pharmaceuticals may detect up to 80%–90% of thyroid carcinomas measuring greater than 1.5 cm.[47]

The advent of recombinant human thyrotropin (rTSH) allows the thyroid tissue to be stimulated without requiring the withdrawal of thyroid hormone therapy. This has had a significant improvement in the quality of life of these patients, as it makes the necessity of coming off their thyroid hormone therapy, which results in hypothyroidism, unnecessary.[47,48]

As in $I^{123}$ discussed above, diffuse increased uptake is noted in patients with Graves' disease.[41,43] There are also focal areas of increased uptake in patients with toxic multi-nodular goiter.[43] $I^{131}$ is still used in the treatment of Graves' disease and toxic adenoma in order to reduce thyroid function.

Radionuclide imaging with iodine has been used, and is now the investigation of choice, to assess suspected congenital abnormalities such as thyroid agenesis, dysgenesis, ectopic thyroid tissue, lingual thyroid gland or thyroglossal duct cysts (Figures 6–23 and 6–24).

## TC-99M-PERTECHNETATE

This is the most widely used biologic tracer in thyroid imaging. It is inexpensive, easy to obtain, and delivers a low dose of radiation to the patient.[6,31,49] For these reasons, many centers consider this to be the initial agent to be used. Imaging is performed approximately 20 minutes after administration of pertechnetate (Figure 6–25). Despite radio-iodine and Tc-99m-pertechnetate having

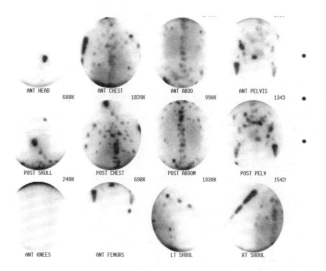

**Figure 6–22.** $I^{131}$ total body scan post-thyroidectomy and ablation showing multiple bony metastases in spine, pelvis, femur, humerus and ribs.

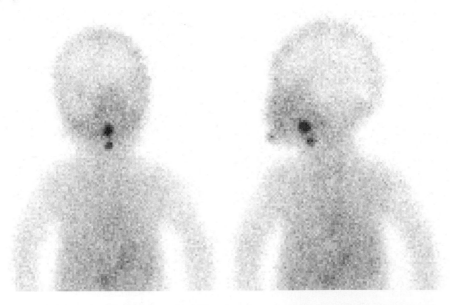

**Figure 6–23.** Lingual (superior focus) and ectopic (inferior focus) thyroid tissue in a 12 day old girl with congenital hypothyroidism. No activity is seen in expected location of thyroid.

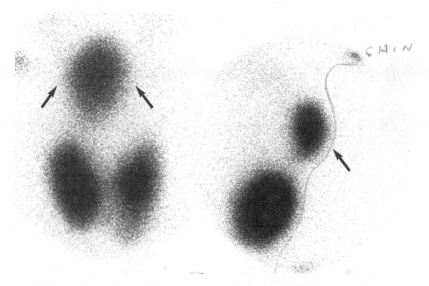

**Figure 6–24.** Anterior and lateral views of the neck show functioning thyroid tissue in a thyroglossal duct cyst (arrows) superior to the normal functioning thyroid gland in a 50-year-old man with an anterior neck mass.

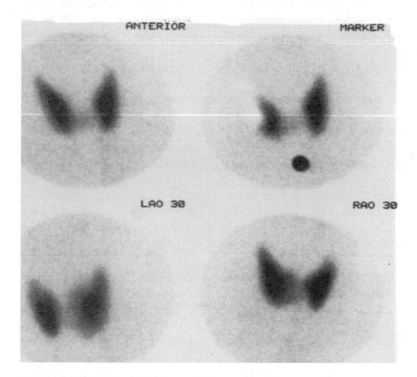

**Figure 6–25.** Normal Tc-99m-pertechnetate scan.

the same mechanism of cellular uptake, pertechnetate is not organified by the thyroid gland, but only trapped by it. This can at times limit its use because the actual physiologic status of the gland cannot be demonstrated and can result in differing results between this test and radioiodide scans.

As is the case with I[123] and I[131] studies, use of this radionuclide agent results in diffuse increased uptake in patients with Graves' disease.[41,43] Patients with toxic multi-nodular goiter also show increased uptake, but scintigraphy is believed to be able to differentiate between these two disease processes.[50]

When this type of scan reveals no abnormality or a cold nodule, no further imaging work-up is usually needed. Cold nodules usually indicate a non-functional thyroid cyst or a malignancy (Figure 6–26). The risk of a cold nodule being malignant has been discussed previously and should be managed appropriately.

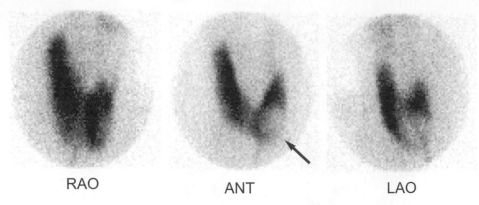

RAO                    ANT                    LAO

**Figure 6–26.** Cold nodule in lower pole left lobe of thyroid gland (arrow). Pathology was papillary carcinoma.

Warm or hot nodules found with Tc-99m-pertechnetate imaging should have I[123] imaging performed to assess the physiologic state of the nodule.[51,52] Some well-differentiated thyroid malignancies are able to trap pertechnetate, thus giving the appearance of a warm or hot nodule.[53] These usually prove to be cold on I[123] imaging and should therefore be classified as a cold nodule (Figure 6–27). Hot nodules on Tc-99m-pertechnetate and iodine imaging usually represent either an adenoma or a toxic solitary nodule (Figure 6–28).[41]

Reduced Tc-99m-pertechnetate uptake may be seen in cases of subacute thyroiditis or other inflammatory thyroid disorders.[54] In cases of diffusely reduced Tc-99m-pertechnetate uptake, Tc-99m-methoxyisobutyl isonitrile scintigraphy (Tc-99m-MIBI) may aid in the diagnosis of thyroid disease.[55] It provides a better image quality than radio-iodine or thallium-201 (Tl-201), which accounts for the increasing popularity of this agent.[45] In fact, Alam et al. have proposed that Tc-99m-MIBI be the first line scintigraphy agent of choice for evaluation of patients with metastatic thyroid disease.[45]

## OTHER RADIONUCLIDES

There are currently a number of newer radionuclides available that may in the future prove to be extremely important in the diagnosis and management of well-differentiated thyroid cancer. Many of these agents are now used when thyroglobulin levels are elevated in the face of a negative radio-iodine scan. Both Tc-99m-sestamibi as well as Tl-201 may prove useful in differentiating benign from malignant disease and may also aid in the detection of thyroid carcinoma metastases.[31,46,56-58] Evidence suggests that Tc-99m-sestamibi and Tl-201 may be better than radio-iodine imaging in detecting lymph node and bone metastases (Figure 6–29), while I[131] may be superior at detecting pulmonary metastases (Figure 6–30).[59] One of the benefits of Tl-201 and Tc-99m-sestamibi is that, unlike I[131], patients need not go off thyroid hormone replacement during the time period of the scan. In patients with a positive Tl-201 scan suspicious for recurrent well-differentiated thyroid carcinoma without a prior radio-iodine scan, a whole-body radio-iodine scan should be performed.[42] Tc-99m-tetrofosmin has also been shown to accurately identify recurrent or metastatic well-differentiated thyroid carcinoma in patients with negative radio-iodine scans without the need to withdraw thyroid hormone replacement.[60-62] Indium-111-pentreotide has also been shown effective in detecting distant metastases in patients with elevated thyroglobulin levels.[63]

Other imaging agents are also being investigated for their use in detecting primary or metastatic medullary thyroid carcinoma.[64] These agents include Tl-201[65], Tc-99m pentavalent dimercaptosuccinic acid (Tc-99m (V) DMSA),[66,67] 131-Indium-meta-iodobenzyl guanidine (I[131]-M MIBG),[68] Tc-99m-sestamibi,[69] somatostatin receptors,[70-72] and indium-111-labelled monoclonal antibodies to carcinoembryonic antigen.[73-76] Gallium-67 has shown promise in detecting poorly differentiated thyroid malignancies, such as anaplastic thyroid carcinoma and thyroid lymphoma.[77]

## POSITRON EMISSION TOMOGRAPHY

Positron emission tomography (PET) has been in use to some extent since the early sixties. It allows for imaging of biologic activity in vivo. PET has now gained widespread acceptance and its use has become increasingly popular. This coincides with an increase in the number of intravenously administered radiotracers that are similar to endogenous compounds that are currently being developed.

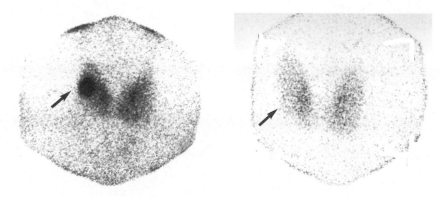

**Figure 6–27.** Discrepancy between Tc-99m-pertechnetate (on left) and I[123] (on right). Note right lobe nodule (arrows) hot on Tc99m and cold on I[123]. This should be considered a cold nodule.

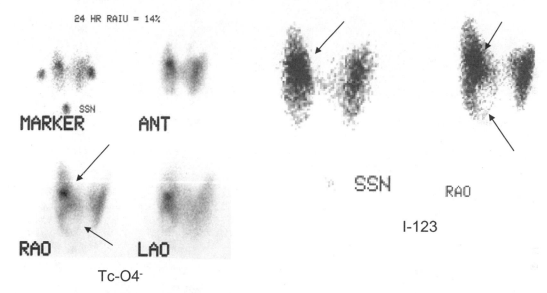

**Figure 6–28.** Concordant nodules with a hot nodule (upper arrow) and a cold nodule (lower arrow) seen on both Tc-99m (left) and on I[123] (right) imaging.

The most common positron emitting radiotracer currently in use is the glucose analogue 2-[fluorine-18] fluoro-2-deoxy-D-glucose (FDG), which is excreted in the urinary tract. FDG has been shown to have an increased uptake in various malignancies including thyroid carcinoma (Figure 6–31).[78-81] This is secondary to intracellular trapping of FDG (as FDG-6-phosphate) by neoplastic cells. FDG-PET may be most important in assessing tumor recurrence in patients with well-differentiated thyroid carcinoma who have negative radio-iodine scans but elevated thyroglobulin levels.[82] It has been shown that high FDG uptake in a thyroid mass suggests that a malignancy is present.[83-86] Low levels of FDG uptake, however, do not rule out the presence of a malignancy as FDG-negative thyroid tumors have also been identified.[81,87,88] There is concern that FDG-PET may miss small lung metastases and, therefore, spiral CT should be considered in those cases where it may be suspected.[89] Diffuse thyroid uptake of FDG has also been demonstrated in patients with chronic thyroiditis.[90]

PET can also be used to assess the functional thyroid gland volume, not an anatomic volume as obtained with ultrasound. This has important implications when determining the appropriate dose for patients scheduled to undergo radio-iodine therapy. Crawford et al have suggested that the ratio of PET (functional volume) to ultrasound (anatomic volume) was, on average, 0.68 in a select group of patients.[91] The presence of thyroid nodules, as well as non-uniform distribution of radio-iodine is the reason for this difference. PET scanning allows a much more precise calculation of appropriate radio-iodine dose.

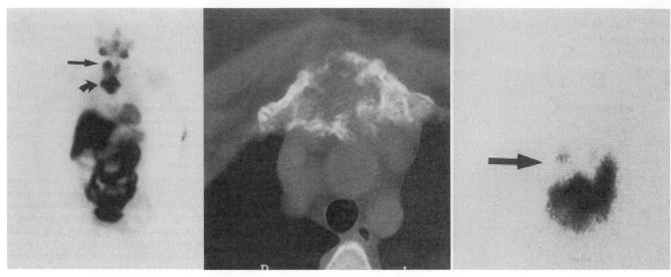

## Tc-Sestamibi                                              I-123

**Figure 6–29.** Tc-Sestamibi (left) showing greater conspicuity for sternal and neck node metastases than I[123] (right). CT (center) shows large destructive follicular thyroid metastatic mass in sternum.

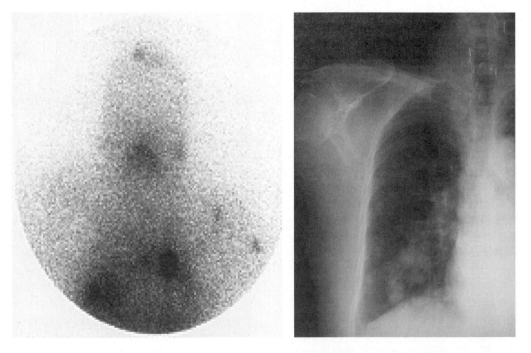

**Figure 6–30.** Iodine radioisotope scan showing pulmonary metastases with correlative chest X-ray.

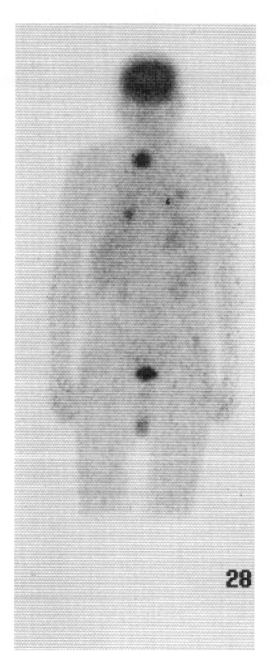

**Figure 6–31.** FDG total body scan. Note thyroid carcinoma metastases in superior mediastinum and both lungs.

## ANGIOGRAPHY

The majority of angiographic investigations performed for thyroid disease involve identification of the surrounding vascular structures and their relationship to the thyroid gland. However, recent studies have indicated that it may be possible to differentiate malignant versus benign nodules by examining the characteristics of the feeding vessel, the margin of the tumor blush, and the density of the tumor blush with contrast.[92] Further investigations in this field are required.

**Acknowledgment.** This work is supported by the Saul A. Silverman Family Foundation as an Isabel Silverman Canada International Scientific Exchange Program (CISEPO) project, the R.S. McGlauglin Foundation, and the Freeman Centre for Endocrine Oncology, Mount Sinai Hospital, Toronto, Canada.

## References

1. Vander JB, Gaston EA, Dawber TR. The significance of non-toxic thyroid nodules. Final report of a 15-year study of the incidence of thyroid malignancy. *Ann Intern Med.* 1968;69:537–540 .
2. Tunbridge WMG, Evered DC, Hall R, et al. The spectrum of thyroid disease in a community: The Wickham Survey. *Clin Endocrinol.* 1977;7:481–493.
3. Goellner JR, Gharhib H, Grant CS, Johnson DA. Fine needle aspiration cytology of the thyroid, 1980-86. *Acta Cytologica.* 1987;31: 587–590.
4. Mazzaferri EL. Management of a solitary thyroid nodule. *N Engl J Med.* 1993;328:553–559.
5. Al-Sayer HM, Bayliss AP, Krukowski ZH, Matheson NA. The limitation of ultrasound in thyroid swelling. *J R Coll Surg Edinb.* 1986;31:27–31.
6. Smith O, Noyek AM. Advances in imaging, scanning and intervention. In: Gray RF, Rutka JA, eds. *Recent Advances in Otolaryngology (6).* New York: Churchill Livingstone; 1988:49–71.
7. Lu C, Chang TC, Hsiao YL, Kuo MS. Ultrasonographic findings of papillary thyroid carcinoma and their relation to pathologic changes. *J Formosan Med Assoc.* 1994;93:933–938.
8. Garretti L, Cassinis MC, Cesarani F, et al. The reliability of echotomographic diagnosis in assessing thyroid lesions. A comparison with cytology and histology. *Radiologia Medica.* 1994;88:598–605.
9. Tramalloni J, Leehardt L. Echography of the thyroid nodules. What the clinician is waiting for. *J Radiol.* 1994;75:187–190.
10. Solbiati L, Ballarati E, Cioffi V, et al. Microcalcifications: a clue in the diagnosis of thyroid malignancies. *Radiology.* 1990;177 (Suppl): 140.
11. Loevner LA. Imaging of the thyroid gland. *Semin US CT MR.* 1996;17:539–562.
12. Schneider AB, Bekerman C, Leland J, et al. Thyroid nodules in the follow-up of irradiated individuals: comparison of thyroid ultrasound with scanning and palpation. *J Clin Endocrinol Metab.* 1997;82:4020-4027.
13. Brander A, Viikinkoski P, Nickels J, et al. Thyroid gland: US screening in a random adult population. *Radiology.* 1991;181: 683–687 .
14. Bruneton JN, Balu-Maestro C, Marcy PY, et al. Very high frequency (13MHz) ultrasonographic examination of the normal neck: detection of normal lymph nodes and thyroid nodules. *J Ultrasound Med.* 1994;13:87–90.
15. Ezzat S, Sarti DA, Cain DR, et al. Thyroid incidentalomas. Prevalence by palpation and ultrasonography. *Arch Intern Med.* 1994;154:1838–1840.
16. Tan GH, Gharib H. Thyroid incidentalomas: management approaches to non-palpable nodules discovered incidentally on thyroid imaging. *Ann Intern Med.* 1997;126:226–231.
17. McShane DP, Freeman JL, Noyek AM, Steinhardt MI. A review of conventional and CT imaging in the evaluation of thyroid malignancies. *J Otolaryngol.* 1987;16:1–9.
18. Brander A, Viikinkoski P, Tuuhea J, et al. Clinical versus ultrasound examination of the thyroid gland in common clinical practice. *J Clin Ultrasound.* 1992;20:37–42.
19. Noyek AM, Finkelstein DM, Witterick IJ, Kirsh JC. Diagnostic imaging of the thyroid gland. In: Falk SA, ed. *Thyroid Disease:*

*Endocrinology, Surgery, Nuclear Medicine and Radiotherapy (2).* New York: Lippincott-Raven; 1997:135–182.

20. Ferrozzi F, Bova D, Campodonico F, et al. US and CT findings of secondary neoplasms of the thyroid gland—a pictorial essay. *Clin Imaging.* 1998;22:157–161.

21. Mann WJ. *Ultraschall im kopf-hals-Bereich.* Berlin: Springer-Verlag; 1984.

22. Hatada T, Okada K, Ishii S, Utsunomiya J. Evaluation of ultrasound-guided fine-needle aspiration biopsy for thyroid nodules. *Am J Surg.* 1998;175:133–136.

23. Goletti O, Monzani F, Lenziardi M, et al. Cold thyroid nodules: a new application of percutaneous ethanol injection treatment. *J Clin Ultrasound.* 1994;22:175–178.

24. Yokoyama N, Nagayama Y, Kakezono F, et al. Determination of the volume of the thyroid gland by a high resolution ultrasonic scanner. *J Nucl Med.* 1986;9:1475–1479.

25. Perrild H, Hansen JM, Hegedii L, et al. Triiodothyronine and thyroxine treatment of diffuse non-toxic goiter evaluated by ultrasonic scanning. *Acta Endocrinol (Copenh).* 1982;100:382–387.

26. Lagalla R, Caruso G, Finazzo M. Monitoring treatment response with color and power Doppler. *Eur J Radiol.* 1998;27 (Suppl 2):S149–S156.

27. Clark KJ, Cronan JJ, Scola FH. Color Doppler sonography: anatomic and physiologic assessment of the thyroid gland. *J Clin Ultrasound.* 1995;23:215–223.

28. Hubsch P, Niederle B, Barton P, et al. Color-coded Doppler sonography of the thyroid: an advance in carcinoma diagnosis? *ROFO.* 1992;156:125–129.

29. Wolf BS, Nakagawa H, Yeh HC. Visualization of the thyroid gland with computed tomography. *Radiology.* 1977;123:368.

30. Syenave P. Surgical pathology of the thyroid gland—diagnostic contribution of computed tomography. *Acta Otorhinolaryngol Belg.* 1987;41:677–684.

31. Friedman M, Toriumi DM, Mafee MF. Diagnostic imaging techniques in thyroid cancer. *Am J Surg.* 1988;155:215–223.

32. Hermans R, Bouillon R, Laga K, et al. Estimation of thyroid gland volume by spiral computed tomography. *Eur Radiol.* 1997;7:214–216.

33. Glazer HS, Niemeyer JH, Balfe DM, et al. Neck neoplasms: MR imaging. 1. Initial evaluation. *Radiology.* 1986;160:343–348.

34. Funari M, Campos Z, Gooding GAW, et al. MRI and ultrasound detection of asymptomatic thyroid nodules in hyperparathyroidism. *J Comput Assist Tomogr.* 1992;16:1615–1619.

35. Stark DD, Clark OH, Gooding GAW, et al. High resolution ultrasound and computerized tomography of thyroid lesions in patients with hyperparathyroidism. *Surgery.* 1983;94:863–868.

36. Brown LR, Aughenbaugh GL. Masses of the anterior mediastinum: CT and MR imaging. *Am J Radiol.* 1991;157:1171–1180.

37. Higgins CB, McNamara MT, Fisher MR, Clark OH. MR imaging of the thyroid. *Am J Radiol.* 1986;145:1255–1261.

38. Kacl GM, Bicik I, Schonenberger AW, et al. Interactive MR-guided biopsies of the thyroid gland: validation of a new method. *Eur Radiol.* 1998;8:1173–1178.

39. Noyek AM, Witterick IJ, Kirsh JC. Radionuclide imaging in otolaryngology—head and neck surgery. *Arch Otolaryngol Head Neck.* 1991;117:372–378.

40. Ashcraft MW, Van Herle AJ. Management of thyroid nodules. II: Scanning techniques, thyroid suppressive therapy, and fine needle aspiration. *Head Neck Surg.* 1981;3:297–322.

41. Chevigne-Brancart M, Baudoux A, Salamon E. Thyroid imaging using 99m-TC, [123]I and [131]I. *Acta Otorhinolaryngol Belg.* 1987;41:637–648.

42. Unal S, Menda Y, Adalet I, et al. Thallium-201, technetium-99m-tetrofosmin and iodine-131 in detecting differentiated thyroid carcinoma metastases. *J Nucl Med.* 1998;39:1897–1902.

43. Fogelman I, Cooke SG, Maisey MN. The role of thyroid scanning in hyperthyroidism. *Eur J Nucl Med.* 1986;11:397–440.

44. Pacini F, Lippi F, Formica N, et al. Therapeutic doses of Iodine-131 reveal undiagnosed metastases in thyroid cancer patients with detectable serum thyroglobulin levels. *J Nucl Med .*1987;28:1888–1891.

45. Alam MS, Kasagi K, Misaki T, et al. Diagnostic value of technetium-99m methoxyisobutyl isonitrile ([99m]Tc-MIBI) scintigraphy in detecting thyroid cancer metastases: a critical evaluation. *Thyroid.* 1998;8:1091–1100.

46. Jadvar H, McDougall IR, Segall GM. Evaluation of suspected recurrent papillary thyroid carcinoma with [18F] fluorodeoxyglucose positron emission tomography. *Nucl Med Commun.* 1998;19:547–554.

47. Maxon HR. Detection of residual and recurrent thyroid cancer by radionuclide imaging. *Thyroid.* 1999;9:443–446.

48. Ladenson PW, Braverman LE, Mazzaferri EL, et al. Comparison of administration of recombinant human thyrotropin with withdrawal of hormone for radioactive iodine scanning in patients with thyroid carcinoma. *N Engl J Med.* 1997;337:888–896.

49. Beckers C. Trends in thyroid imaging. *Horm Res.* 1987;26:28–32.

50. Naik KS, Bury RF. Imaging the thyroid. *Clin Radiol.* 1998;53:630-639.

51. Frank K, Raue F, Lorenz D, et al. Importance of ultrasound examination for the follow-up of medullary thyroid carcinoma: comparison with other localization methods. *Henry Ford Hosp Med J.* 1987;35:122–123.

52. Miskin M, Rosen IB, Walfish PG. Ultrasonography of the thyroid gland. *Radiol Clin North Am.* 1975;13:475–492.

53. Clarke SEM. Radionuclide imaging in thyroid cancer. *Nucl Med Commun.* 1988;9:79–84.

54. Shigemasa C, Teshima S, Taniguchi S, et al. Pertechnetate thyroid uptake is not always suppressed in patients with subacute thyroiditis. *Clin Nucl Med.* 1997;22:109–114.

55. Alonso O, Mut F, Lago G, et al. 99Tc(m)-MIBI scanning of the thyroid gland in patients with markedly decreased pertechnetate uptake. *Nucl Med Commun.* 1998;19:257–261.

56. Corstens H, Huysmans D, Kloppenborg P. Thallium-201 scintigraphy of the suppressed thyroid: an alternative for Iodine-123 scanning after TSH stimulation. *J Nucl Med.* 1988;29:1360-1363.

57. el-Desouki M. Tl-201 thyroid imaging in differentiating benign from malignant thyroid nodules. *Clin Nucl Med.* 1991;16:425–430.

58. Hoefnagel CA, Delprat CC, Marcuse HR, et al. Role of thallium-201 total-body scintigraphy in follow-up of thyroid carcinoma. *J Nucl Med.* 1986;27:1854–1857.

59. Miyamoto S, Kasagi K, Misaki T, et al. Evaluation of technetium-99m-MIBI scintigraphy in metastatic differentiated thyroid carcinoma. *J Nucl Med.* 1997;38:352–356.

60. Lind P, Gallowitsch HJ, Langsteger W, et al. Technetium-99m-tetrofosmin whole-body scintigraphy in the follow-up of differentiated thyroid carcinoma. *J Nucl Med.* 1997;38:348–352.

61. Akcay G, Uslu H, Varoglu E, et al. Assessment of thyroid nodules by technetium-99m-tetrofosmin scintigraphy. *Br J Clin Prac.* 1997;51:5–7.

62. Erdem S, Bashekim C, Kizilkaya E, et al. Clinical application of Tc-99m tetrofosmin scintigraphy in patients with cold thyroid nodules. Comparison with color Doppler sonography. *Clin Nucl Med.* 1997;22:76–79.

63. Boni G, Ferdeghini M, Grosso M, et al. Indium-111 pentreotide, Technetium-99m sestamibi and Iodine-131 scan in metastases of differentiated thyroid carcinoma (abstract). *J Nucl Med.* 1997;38(suppl 5):236P.

64. Hoefnagel CA, Delprat CC, Zanin D, et al. New radionuclide tracers for the diagnosis and therapy of medullary thyroid carcinoma. *Clin Nucl Med.* 1988;13:159–165.

65. Bigsby RJ, Lepp EK, Litwin DE, et al. Technetium 99m pentavalent dimercaptosuccinic acid and thallium 201 in detecting recurrent medullary carcinoma of the thyroid. *Can J Surg.* 1992;35:388–392.

66. Clarke SEM, Lazarus C, Mistry R, et al. The role of technetium-99m pentavalent DMSA in the management of patients with medullary carcinoma of the thyroid. *Br J Radiol.* 1987;60:1089–1092.

67. Udelsman R, Ball D, Baylin SB, et al. Preoperative localization of occult medullary carcinoma of the thyroid gland with single-photon emission tomography dimercaptosuccinic acid. *Surgery.* 1993;114:1083–1089.

68. Itoh H, Sugie K, Toyooka S, et al. Detection of metastatic medullary thyroid cancer with 131-I-M MIBG scans in Sipple's syndrome. *Eur J Nucl Med.* 1986;11:502–504.

69. Lebouthillier G, Morais J, Picard M, et al. Tc-99m sestamibi and other agents in the detection of metastatic medullary carcinoma of the thyroid. *Clin Nucl Med.* 1993;18:657–661.

70. Biersack HG, Briele B, Hotze AL, et al. The role of nuclear medicine in oncology. *Ann Nucl Med.* 1992;6:131–136.

71. Dorr U, Wurstlin S, Frank-Raue K, et al. Somatostatin receptor scintigraphy and magnetic resonance imaging in recurrent medullary thyroid carcinoma: a comparative study. *Horm Metabol Res.* 1993;27(Suppl):48–55.

72. Dorr U, Sautter-Bihl ML, Bihl H. The contribution of somatostatin receptor scintigraphy to the diagnosis of recurrent medullary carcinoma of the thyroid. *Semin Oncol.* 1994;21:42–45.

73. Edington HD, Watson CG, Levine G, et al. Radioimmunoimaging of metastatic medullary carcinoma of the thyroid gland using an indium-111-labeled monoclonal antibody to CEA. *Surgery.* 1988;104;1004–1010.

74. Vuillez JP, Peltier P, Caravel JP, et al. Immunoscintigraphy using 111-In-labeled F(ab')2 fragments of anticarcinoembryonic antigen monoclonal antibody for detecting recurrences of medullary thyroid carcinoma. *J Clin Endocrinol Metab.* 1992;74:157–163.

75. O'Byrne KJ, Hamilton D, Robinson I, et al. Imaging of medullary carcinoma of the thyroid using 111-In-labeled anti-CEA monoclonal antibody fragments. *Nucl Med Commun.* 1992;13:142–148.

76. Peltier P, Curtet C, Chatal JF, et al. Radioimmunodetection of medullary thyroid cancer using a bispecific anti-CEA/anti-indium-DTPA antibody and an indium-111-labeled DTPA dimer. *J Nucl Med.* 1993;34:1267–1273.

77. Higashi T, Ito K, Nishikawa Y, et al. Gallium-67 imaging in the evaluation of the thyroid malignancy. *Clin Nucl Med.* 1988;792–799.

78. Di Chiro G. Positron emission tomography using [$^{18}$F]fluorodeoxyglucose in brain tumors: a powerful diagnostic and prognostic tool. *Invest Radiol.* 1986;22:360–371.

79. Nolop KB, Rhodes CG, Bruden LH, et al. Glucose utilization in vivo by human pulmonary neoplasms. *Cancer.* 1987;60:2682–2689.

80. Okada J, Yoshikawa K, Imaseki K, et al. The use of FDG-PET in the detection and management of malignant lymphoma: correlation of uptake with prognosis. *J Nucl Med.* 1991;32:686–691.

81. Feine U, Lietzenmayer R, Hanke JP, et al. Fluorine-18–FDG and iodine-131 Iodine uptake in thyroid cancer. *J Nucl Med.* 1996;37:1468–1472.

82. Altenvoerde G, Lerch H, Kuwert T, et al. Positron emission tomography with F-18–deoxyglucose in patients with differentiated thyroid carcinoma, elevated thyroglobulin levels, and negative iodine scans. *Langenbecks Arch Surg.* 1998;383:160–163.

83. Adler LP, Bloom AD. Positron emission tomography of thyroid masses. *Thyroid.* 1993;3:195–200.

84. Bloom AD, Adler LP, Shuck JM. Determination of malignancy of thyroid nodules with positron emission tomography. *Surgery.* 1993;114:728–735.

85. Sisson JC, Ackermann RJ, Meyer MA, et al. Uptake of 18-fluoro-2-deoxy-D-glucose by thyroid cancer: implications for diagnosis and therapy. *J Clin Endocrinol Metab.* 1993;77:1090–1094.

86. Scott GC, Meier DA, Dickinson CZ. Cervical lymph node metastasis of thyroid papillary carcinoma imaged with fluorine-18-FDG, technetium-99m-pertechnetate and iodine-131-sodium iodide. *J Nucl Med.* 1995;36:1843–1845.

87. Grunwald F, Schomburg A, Bender H, et al. Fluorine-18-fluorodeoxyglucose positron emission tomography in the follow-up of differentiated thyroid cancer. *Eur J Nucl Med.* 1996;23:312–319.

88. Fridrich L, Messa C, Landoni C, et al. Whole-body scintigraphy with Tc-$^{99}$m-IBI, $^{18}$F-FDG and $^{131}$I in patients with metastatic thyroid carcinoma. *Nucl Med Commun.* 1997;18:3–9.

89. Dietlein M, Scheidhauer K, Voth E, et al. Fluorine-18 fluorodeoxyglucose positron emission tomography and iodine-131 whole-body scintigraphy in the follow-up of differentiated thyroid cancer. *Eur J Nucl Med.*1997;24:1342–1348.

90. Yasuda S, Shohtsu A, Ide M, et al. Chronic thyroiditis: diffuse uptake of FDG at PET. *Radiology.* 1998;207:775–778.

91. Crawford DC, Flower MA, Pratt BE, et al. Thyroid volume measurement in thyrotoxic patients: comparison between ultrasonography and iodine-124 positron emission tomography. *Eur J Nucl Med.* 1997;24:1470–1478.

92. Morita Y. Selective thyroid angiography: techniques, diagnosis and indications. *Hokkaido J Med Sci.* 1993;68:251–264.

# 7

# Evaluation of the Nodular Thyroid Gland

Yasser Ousman, M.D.
Kenneth D. Burman, M.D.

Determining the appropriate approach to a patient with a thyroid nodule is a common problem in endocrinology practice. Thyroid nodules are often discovered by the patient or the practitioner during a routine physical examination. The widespread use of imaging techniques such as ultrasonography, computerized tomography and magnetic resonance imaging to evaluate neck or chest structures other than the thyroid gland has resulted in the increasing discovery of "incidental thyroid nodules". The physician is faced with the task of assessing the significance and determining the best approach to evaluate both palpable and incidentally discovered nodules. For our purposes, an incidental thyroid nodule is one that does not cause associated signs or symptoms, such as hoarseness, discomfort, or dysphagia, and is typically diagnosed during a radiologic examination performed to evaluate a different organ system or structure.

A substantial body of literature has been devoted to delineating an appropriate approach to patients with thyroid nodules and multiple management algorithms have been suggested. The application of fine-needle aspiration biopsy of the thyroid has fundamentally changed the diagnostic approach and improved our ability to distinguish benign from malignant thyroid disease. Indeed, we believe that in most circumstances all euthyroid patients with thyroid nodules larger than about 8–10 mm should have a fine needle aspiration. This chapter will review the prevalence, differential diagnosis and diagnostic evaluation of thyroid nodules.

In this era of increased health cost and managed care, it is important for the physician to understand the significance of the clinical finding and be familiar with the indications of the various diagnostic tools that are available so that an expeditious, cost-effective and logical approach can be defined.

## PREVALENCE

The prevalence of thyroid nodules depends on the modality used to examine the thyroid gland. In the general population, palpation detects nodules in 1 to 5% of individuals.[1,2] The prevalence of thyroid nodules in the Framingham study was 6.4% in females and 1.5% in males, aged 30 to 59.[3] Thyroid nodules are more common in women than in men.[1,4]

Ultrasonography discloses nodules in 20 to 40% of thyroid glands examined. Most of these nodules are small and not palpable but a few will be greater than 1 cm in diameter and escape palpation because of their deep and/or posterior location in the thyroid.[5-8] Routinely performed autopsies (in patients without known thyroid disease) can find thyroid nodules in as many as 50 to 60% of patients.[9] These statistics underlie the high prevalence of thyroid nodules and the disparity between palpation and the more sensitive methods used to examine the thyroid, such as ultrasonography. Given the fact that many patients have thyroid nodules that are of little clinical consequence, the critical issue is how best to approach patients with thyroid nodules to maximize the discovery of nodules that harbor thyroid cancer, while minimizing the use of expensive and time consuming procedures, including surgery. The prevalence of thyroid nodules in children is low: 0.05 to 1.8 %[10] and increases with age. Exposure to ionizing radiation increases the prevalence of thyroid nodules: 33% of Marshall Islanders who were exposed to nuclear fall-out were found to have nodules.[11,12] Another study found nodules in 43% of patients treated with cervical irradiation for malignancy when followed up for longer than 10 years.[13] Follow-up of subjects exposed to radiation at Chernobyl also has revealed a high incidence of thyroid nodules and cancer. Exposure to as little as 200 to 500 rads of ionizing radiation, particularly during infancy and childhood, causes nodules to develop at a rate of approximately 2% annually with a peak incidence in 15 to 25 years.[14]As many as 20 to 50% of patients found to have a solitary thyroid nodule on palpation harbor other nodules when examined by high-resolution ultrasonography.[5,15,16]

## DIFFERENTIAL DIAGNOSIS

The differential diagnosis of thyroid nodules includes a variety of benign and malignant conditions (Table 7–1). Some non-thyroid structures are also included in the differential given their proximate location to the thyroid gland. The majority of thyroid nodules are benign with only about 5 to 10% being malignant.[17,18]

*Benign colloid adenomas* are the most common type of thyroid nodules, accounting for 42 to 77%[1]; they are generally present in a multi-nodular gland. Most are hypo-functioning on thyroid scintigraphy. They may show high cellularity on fine-needle aspirate.[19]

*Follicular adenomas* represent 15 to 40% of thyroid nodules, the most common being macrofollicular adenoma. Follicular neoplasms, which are cellular adenomas, have about a 20% chance of malignancy. These nodules need to be excised and examined histologically in order to rule out malignancy.

*Autonomous thyroid nodules* are solitary nodules that secrete excessive thyroid hormones, typically suppressing serum TSH; they represent 5% of all nodules. They show normal or mild to moderate cellularity,[20,21] and they are almost always benign.[22]

*Thyroid cysts* represent 15 to 25% of nodules. We differentiate pure cysts from mixed solid-cystic lesions. A pure cyst contains no internal echoes on sonogram and has through transmission, which means that the sound wave accelerates through the cystic component and then intensifies in the tissue posterior to the cyst. Aspiration yields clear yellow fluid with few cells. Pure cysts are very rare. The majority of cystic nodules contain both cystic and solid components.[23] We believe that these lesions should be approached as solid thyroid nodules. When evaluating complex nodules with fine-needle aspiration, it is important to try and aspirate not only the cystic component, but also the solid portion of the cyst. The chance of malignancy in a purely cystic nodule is probably 2 to 4%,[24,25] whereas mixed lesions probably contain carcinoma about 14% of the time. The frequency with which thyroid carcinoma is found depends on various factors, including the thoroughness of the aspirate, the skill of the cytologist, and the success of efforts to assess both the solid and cystic components. The aspiration of bloody fluid could be seen in both benign and malignant cysts and, therefore, is not diagnostic.[24,25]

*Thyroglossal duct cysts* are generally diagnosed in infancy but may present in adults. They are usually midline and can occur anywhere along the primordial

**Table 7–1.** Causes of thyroid nodules

| Benign causes | Malignant causes |
|---|---|
| Colloid adenoma | Papillary cancer |
| Follicular adenoma | Follicular cancer |
| Hürthle cell adenoma | Medullary thyroid cancer |
| Cysts | Anaplastic cancer |
| Thyroiditis | Thyroid lymphoma |
| Infections | Metastatic cancer (renal, breast, melanoma, colon) |
| Infiltrative disease | |
| Thyroglossal duct cyst | |
| Teratoma | |

**Non-thyroid causes**
Parathyroid cyst or adenoma
Thymoma
Lipoma
Cystic hygroma
Brachial cyst

migration pathway of the thyroid gland. Classically, they tend to move in a cephadal direction when the patient sticks out his/her tongue. They rarely harbor thyroid cancer.[26]

*Parathyroid cysts* are rare. The aspiration of crystal clear fluid is highly suggestive but needs confirmation by cytologic assessment and by documenting an extremely high PTH level in this fluid.[27]

## HISTORY AND PHYSICAL EXAMINATION

Most patients with thyroid nodules are asymptomatic. However, several elements of the history and physical examination are associated with increased risk of malignancy and should be taken into account in the final therapeutic decision even when the cytological diagnosis is benign.

### History

*Age.* The risk of thyroid cancer increases with extremes of age; children with thyroid nodules have, in the absence of prior radiation exposure, a 10 to 15 % chance of malignancy.[28,29] Similarly, men over age 60, have a higher risk of cancer.[25]

*Gender.* Although thyroid nodules are more common in females, a nodule has a higher chance of malignancy in males. Of course, these are simply demographic features and the entire cytologic and clinical context must be considered.

*Exposure to ionizing radiation* during infancy and childhood increases the risk of both benign and malignant thyroid disease. In the past, radiation has been used to treat a variety of conditions, including cystic acne, tinea capitis, tonsils and adenoids and presently may still be used in the treatment of certain malignancies in the cervical area. To the extent possible, an effort should be made to determine the nature and the dose of radiation delivered. In general, the earlier the age at exposure the higher the likelihood of cancer. Cancer can occur as early as 3 years after exposure with a peak incidence between 15 and 30 years with up to 30–40% chance of malignancy.[30-33]

Exposure to radiation typically is associated with a lag time of several decades before nodules or cancer become manifest. In stark contrast, radiation exposure related to the Chernobyl accident is associated with tumor development much earlier, even within several years. Even without a history of radiation it has recently been reported that microscopic papillary thyroid cancers can occur in families, and, further, the likelihood of this type of tumor being more aggressive is increased in this circumstance. Rapid tumor growth in an elderly woman with a history of Hashimoto thyroiditis may indicate thyroid lymphoma.[34]

Controversy exists regarding the malignant risk of a thyroid nodule in a patient with Graves' disease; some authors suggest a higher risk in those nodules and recommend a surgical approach but this philosophy is not universal.[35-37]

Persistent hoarseness and dysphagia are infrequent and suggest an associated malignancy, although these findings may also be seen in benign thyroid disease.

The physician should also inquire about a family history of medullary or papillary thyroid cancer. Finally, the rare Gardner's syndrome (colonic polyps and other benign tumors) increases the likelihood that a thyroid nodule is malignant. Cowden's syndrome and Carney's syndrome also are associated with the development of thyroid nodules, and probably thyroid cancer.

### Physical Examination

Several findings on physical examination have been associated with increased risk of cancer; firm consistency, large size, fixation to adjacent structures, vocal cord paralysis and enlarged cervical lymph nodes. Although suggestive, they lack sensitivity and specificity when considered separately; for example, a calcified adenoma can be firm and some cystic papillary thyroid cancers are soft. Multi-nodular goiters have, it appears now incorrectly, been suggested to have less malignant risk than solitary nodules; based upon more recent analysis, the risk appears similar.[25,38] Attention should be given to those features suggestive of MEN-2, such as Marfanoid habitus, mucosal neuromas of the tongue.

## SERUM TESTING

Among the various available serum thyroid function tests, thyroid-stimulating hormone, TSH, is the most useful to assess gland dysfunction. Determination of the TSH with a sensitive assay and measurement of serum free $T_4$ and $T_3$, when appropriate, help determine the context in which thyroid nodules are diagnosed.[39] Most patients who present with thyroid nodules are euthyroid. We emphasize the difference between structural and functional abnormalities and that they may either occur concurrently or, more commonly, be dissociated. In the past, there have been numerous thyroid tests such as total $T_4$, resin $T_3$ uptake, and free $T_4$ Index. The total $T_4$ is a function test but is interfered with by any condition that alters thyroid binding proteins, such as estrogen or testosterone. Therefore, we only recommend the use of free $T_4$, which now can be measured in a cost effective, rapid manner and measures the clinically relevant unbound fraction of $T_4$. Indirect measures of binding protein such as the resin $T_3$ uptake should not be used any longer. They are obsolete because they can give confusing results, and improved techniques now exist to measure thyroid hormones in a more direct manner. Total $T_3$ can be measured easily but it too is affected by the concentration of binding proteins. Soon we will be able to measure free $T_3$ efficiently and rapidly and this will supplant the measurement of total $T_3$.

A low or suppressed TSH indicates overt or subclinical thyrotoxicosis; this could be the result of a solitary toxic adenoma (Plummer's syndrome ), Graves' disease or the early stage of thyroiditis (subacute, silent or postpartum). Exogenous thyroid hormone, HCG production, or multi-nodular goiter may also cause a suppressed TSH. Every patient with a suppressed TSH should also have serum free $T_4$ and $T_3$ measured to help assess the degree of biochemical disease. Of course, rarely, a suppressed TSH may be related to a pituitary tumor causing secondary hypothyroidism, and exogenous steroids and dopamine infusion may also decrease TSH.

An elevated TSH generally indicates hypothyroidism, usually resulting from chronic autoimmune thyroiditis. Measurement of TSH alone is reasonable for population screening studies, but the additional determination of free $T_4$ and $T_3$ is usually needed when patients are being assessed for the presence of thyroid disease.

Serum *thyroglobulin* is most useful in the follow-up of patients with thyroid cancer. In fact, the importance of routinely measuring serum thyroglobulin levels in patients with differentiated thyroid cancer cannot be over emphasized. Some authors have also recommended measuring thyroglobulin levels in patients with thyroid nodules and a history of head and neck irradiation, although we do not generally believe this is useful. Serum thyroglobulin levels have little sensitivity and specificity in the initial evaluation of thyroid nodules.[40] Serum thyroglobulin levels may be used, however, to help differentiate exogenous thyroid hormone administration from endogenous secretion, for example, in patients suspected of taking excessive L-thyroxine.

Neither the presence, nor the titer of *anti-thyroid peroxidase* and *anti-thyroglobulin* antibodies are helpful in distinguishing benign from malignant disease.

*Calcitonin* is secreted by the parafollicular or C cells of the thyroid and is a sensitive marker of medullary thyroid cancer (MTC). In patients with an intact thyroid gland, basal serum calcitonin determination, with or without provocative stimulation testing (eg, calcium/pentagastrin), has been advocated as part of the initial evaluation of patients with thyroid nodules in order to detect early stages of MTC that may be missed by fine-needle aspirate.[41-43] This approach should be balanced by the fact that MTC is rare, there are cases of false positive elevations of calcitonin not related to MTC, and the availability of pentagastrin is now limited.[44] In patients who have already had a thyroidectomy and have been diagnosed with medullary thyroid cancer, serum calcitonin levels are used as an important monitor to help assess the tissue burden. A patient considered to possibly have medullary thyroid cancer preoperatively should have the syndrome of MEN2 excluded (ie, pheochromocytoma, elevated calcium).

## THYROID SCINTIGRAPHY

Scintigraphy represents a mechanism to assess functional aspects of the thyroid gland. When evaluated by scintigraphy, thyroid nodules can be classified into hypo-functioning or photopenic ("cold"), or hyper-functioning ("warm" or "hot") based on their ability to concentrate the radioactive tracer.

The most commonly used radioisotopes are Technetium—Tc 99m Pertechnetate and radioactive iodine, either $I^{123}$ or $I^{131}$.[45] Technetium is less expensive and emits less radiation, however, there are a few nodules that appear "hot" on the technetium scan but are "cold" on the radioiodine scan: that is, they trap but do not organify iodine.[46] We prefer technetium or $I^{123}$ for scans and each institution should decide for itself what to use, based on cost, availability, and convenience.

Approximately 84% of nodules are "cold," 6% are "hot" and 10% are "warm."[39] Thyroid scintigraphy has historically been the initial test used to evaluate thyroid nodules until it was replaced by fine-needle aspiration. The principle underlying thyroid scintigraphy is that "hot" nodules are usually benign whereas "cold" nodules are more suspicious. In fact, only 5 to 15% of "cold" nodules are malignant, and nodules that trap isotope may harbor malignancy. As a result, scintigraphy is a poor predictor of malignancy and is not routinely used to evaluate thyroid nodules anymore.[47,48] Scintigraphy with assessment of the radioactive iodine uptake is most useful in patients with a low TSH with or without elevated $T_4$ and $T_3$; in this setting it can differentiate between a single toxic nodule, Graves' disease with a concomitant cold nodule and thyroiditis. It is important to differentiate thyroid scanning from uptake. When it is important to determine the capacity of the thyroid gland to trap radioactive iodine, (eg, hyperthyroidism), a radioactive iodine uptake test must be performed. Endogenous hyperthyroidism (eg, Graves' disease, multi-nodular goiter and toxic nodules) is associated with an elevated uptake, whereas destructive processes such as silent or subacute thyroiditis, as well as the administration of exogenous thyroid hormone, are associated with a very low uptake.

Other scintigraphic modalities have been evaluated in an attempt to improve the diagnostic accuracy of scanning. These tests include dynamic pertechnetate imaging,[49] Thallium 201,[50] or Technetium-labeled Sestamibi.[51] These different techniques do not offer a clear advantage over conventional thyroid scanning.

## THYROID ULTRASONOGRAPHY

High-resolution ultrasound is the method of choice to evaluate thyroid morphology and to determine the presence and volume of thyroid nodules.[52] The procedure is non-invasive and relatively inexpensive and can also be used to guide fine-needle aspiration when required. Thyroid nodules are classified by ultrasound into solid, cystic, and complex based on their structure and into hypo-echoic, iso-echoic and hyper-echoic based on their echogenicity relative to the surrounding thyroid tissue. Seventy percent of nodules are solid and pure cysts are very rare. Features that suggest benign nature of a nodule are: hyper-echogenicity; presence of a halo around the nodule; well defined margins; and "eggshell-like" calcifications. Features that suggest malignancy include: hypo-echogenicity; absence of a halo; poorly delineated nodule margins; and microcalcifications. There is, however, significant overlap between these features and overall, thyroid ultrasound certainly cannot accurately distinguish benign from malignant lesions.[52-55] In conjunction with isotope scans and serum thyroglobulin levels, thyroid ultrasound is a very useful tool in the monitoring for recurrence in patients who have had thyroidectomy for thyroid cancer, and who have evidence of recurrence.

Color Doppler ultrasonography evaluates the vascularity of a thyroid nodule but does not have an advantage over routine ultrasound in separating benign from malignant nodules.[56]

## FINE-NEEDLE ASPIRATION BIOPSY

Fine-needle aspiration biopsy, FNA, of the thyroid gland is the test of choice in evaluating thyroid nodules. It is a safe and accurate procedure and can be used in the office setting with minimum discomfort to the patient.[1,4,57,58] In order to maximize the advantages of FNA, it is important that the sample be interpreted by an experienced cytopathologist, that the aspiration be thorough, and that there be communication between the cytologist and the clinician to ensure that the meaning of the written report is mutually understood. The accuracy of thyroid FNA ranges from 70 to 97%. The false positive rate is 3 to 6% and false negative rate is 1 to 6% in experienced hands,[1,59] although the false negative rate critically depends on the features noted above as well as the size of the nodule. Despite the critical im-

portance of this procedure, it must be interpreted in the entire clinical context and worrisome clinical features may mandate that surgery be performed, regardless of a benign FNA interpretation.

Fine-needle aspiration, FNA, has also proved to be accurate in patients with irradiated nodules with a 95% positive predictive value for thyroid cancer.[60]

The use of FNA has resulted in about a 50% decrease in the number of patients requiring surgery and has led to doubling or tripling of malignancy yield at thyroidectomy.[1,61,62]

The results of fine-needle aspiration, FNA, can be subdivided into 4 categories:

1. Benign: includes colloid and macrofollicular adenomas.
2. Malignant: including papillary thyroid cancer, medullary thyroid cancer, anaplastic cancer, lymphoma and metastases (typically renal).
3. Suspicious: including follicular and Hürthle cell neoplasms and aspirates with features suggestive of papillary thyroid cancer.[39]
4. Insufficient cellularity.

A review of the results of large series of FNA showed the following distribution: 74% benign; 4% malignant; 11% suspicious; 11% insufficient.[14]

## Insufficient Aspirate

The adequacy of specimens collected by FNA depends on the operator's experience and the criteria used by the cytopathologist. Repeat aspiration can yield sufficient material in about 30 to 50% of cases.[4,17,63] Ultrasound-guided fine-needle aspirate can be helpful in this setting.[63,64] The malignancy yield in patients with insufficient FNAs, referred to surgery is 8 to 19%, underlying the importance of repeat efforts to obtain sufficient samples.[65-67] It is extremely important to try to obtain sufficient cellularity even by performing repeat aspirations or referral to others, who may be more experienced in this area. Further, the reading of cytology reports must be thorough. For example, a report that indicates that there are "no malignant cells seen" may be misleading if, in fact, there are no thyrocytes seen.

## Suspicious Results

Twenty percent ultimately turn out to be malignant.[54] Most of these are microfollicular neoplasms that cannot be distinguished cytologically from follicular cancers and require histologic examination of operative specimens in order to determine the presence or absence of malignancy. Follicular cancer cannot be diagnosed based on cytologic criteria alone.

## Ultrasound-Guided Fine-Needle Aspirate of the Thyroid

This is a valuable technique that can be used to evaluate non-palpable nodules, nodules that yield insufficient or suspicious results by palpation guided FNA, or to sample the solid component of a cystic lesion. The overall accuracy of US-FNA is 95% with a diagnostic rate of 68 to 98%.[64,68-70] Again, the experience of the person performing this aspiration is critical in determining the false negative and false positive rates.

## OTHER DIAGNOSTIC TESTS

The limitations of FNA, in particular the inability to distinguish between follicular cancer and follicular adenomas, has led to research for tumor markers, the presence of which in the aspirate may further improve the accuracy of FNA and the preoperative selection of patients. At present, none of these markers has shown sufficient reliability clinically. Among those markers, *Galectin-3*, is a beta-galactoside-binding protein expressed in malignancy. In two separate reports, immunohistochemical analysis of thyroid specimens and preoperative analysis of cytological samples obtained by FNA biopsy from non-selected patients with thyroid nodules showed that Galectin-3 was not expressed in benign lesions but was invariably detected in cancers of follicular origin.[71,72] The confirmation of those findings would represent another step forward in the management of thyroid nodules. Other potential useful markers that are under consideration include human telomerase reverse transcriptase, hTERT[73] and high mobility group I *HMGI(Y) protein.*[74]

## NATURAL HISTORY OF THYROID NODULES

Published data examining the natural history of benign thyroid nodules provide us with important information that is pertinent to the manner in which patients should be followed up clinically. In one study, patients with cytologically benign thyroid nodules were followed for 9 to 11 years: nodules disappeared or decreased in 43% of patients, were unchanged in 34% and increased in size in 14%. Papillary thyroid cancer was diagnosed in 0.7%.[75] Other studies found comparable results.[76,77] Therefore, most thyroid nodules that have an original benign aspirate remain benign. Further studies in this area are warranted; however, it is our practice at present to consider re-aspiration of all originally benign nodules, especially when larger than 3 cm. It is especially important to reassess patients who have worrisome signs or symptoms that have developed or whose nodules have grown. We believe that patients with an originally benign aspirate, and who do not have worrisome clinical features, should be monitored for changes in their clinical state and nodule size. In addition to periodic clinical examination and history, we think periodic thyroid sonograms are very useful.

The main exceptions to the comments noted above are autonomous thyroid nodules, which rarely harbor malignancy. We would emphasize that this category only applies, in our view, to patients who have an undetectable TSH with a nodule that solely traps iodine on scan. Autonomous thyroid nodules are usually caused by mutations of the TSH receptor or the G-protein.[78,79] Thyrotoxicosis develops in 20% and is more likely to occur in older patients with large nodule size.[80] Autonomous thyroid nodules are usually treated with 131-I or surgery.

## THERAPY

A detailed discussion of therapy of thyroid nodules is beyond the scope of this chapter but we would like to review several selected aspects.

The choice of therapy for a thyroid nodule depends on the cytological diagnosis, the presence of local compressive symptoms, cosmetic reasons and patient's preference. The physician's role is to integrate the information derived from the history and physical examination, the results of fine-needle aspiration and other tests and help make an appropriate decision. The decision to excise a nodule that appears benign on fine-needle aspirate may be justified if other risk factors are present, for example, a large nodule (5 cm) in an elderly man or a rapidly growing nodule with benign cytology. Obviously, all patients with a malignant cytology should have thyroid surgery. If the aspiration shows papillary thyroid cancer, we would prefer that the patient have a near total or total thyroidectomy. This procedure has the distinct advantages, over a lobectomy alone, that it not only allows appropriate isotope scanning and treatment with adequate doses of radioiodine, but it also allows appropriate monitoring with serum thyroglobulin levels and radiologic studies (eg, sonograms) in an attempt to detect cancer recurrence as early as possible. However, this issue is controversial and depends on the philosophy and experience of the surgeon and the desires of the patient. As mentioned above, the majority of nodules that have an originally benign aspirate, remain benign over time. Prolonged monitoring for worrisome clinical features and change in nodule size is important, and in addition to palpation, we prefer to utilize sonograms to assess for changes in morphology.

## Thyroxine Therapy

Suppressive therapy with thyroxine in the past had been widely used and remains an area of controversy mainly because of questionable efficacy and end points. Typical indications for suppressive therapy include distinguishing benign from malignant nodules, decreasing nodular size for cosmetic reasons, preventing benign nodular recurrence after partial thyroidectomy and preventing nodular growth in patients with history of head and neck irradiation who are at higher risk for malignancy.[81] However, recent studies, including double blind placebo controlled studies, have now indicated that the utility of administering L-thyroxine for suppressive purposes and to help distinguish benign from malignant nodules is low. A meta-analysis of randomized trials comparing suppressive therapy to placebo concluded that only a small percent of patients benefit from suppression with reduction in nodular size.[82] The highest shrinkage response rate appears to occur in areas of iodine deficiency,[83] and for nodules smaller than 2.5 cm. Colloid and degenerative nodules may respond reasonably well but hyperplastic or fibrotic nodules do not.[84,85] There is no consensus on the degree of TSH suppression that is desired, although most authors agree that TSH should not be suppressed to less than 0.1 mIU/L. The criteria used to define a positive response and the modalities used to verify those criteria vary in the different studies that have examined the effect of suppression.

Given the accuracy of FNA, the fact that benign nodules can spontaneously shrink, and the observation that up to 15% of thyroid cancers decrease in size with suppressive therapy,[39,86] we find it difficult to justify the indiscriminate use of suppression. For the noted reasons, the authors do not utilize L-thyroxine suppression for benign thyroid nodules. Basically, L-thyroxine suppression has not been proven to be useful to differentiate benign from malignant nodules, especially when one or more biopsies have been benign. The single exception is the subgroup of patients with irradiated nodules in whom the use of suppressive therapy after partial thyroidectomy for benign disease significantly reduced the development of new benign nodules but made no difference in the frequency of malignancy observed.[33]

## Autonomous Thyroid Nodules

Because of the potentially adverse effects of a suppressed TSH, including atrial fibrillation and enhanced bone loss, patients with autonomous nodules should typically be treated with radioactive iodine 131-I or lobectomy. Both surgery and 131-I therapy have excellent cure rates but do result in hypothyroidism in a few patients.[87,88] Accordingly, these patients should be followed for the development of hypothyroidism for life.

A less standard approach for the treatment of autonomous thyroid nodules is percutaneous ethanol injection. Alcohol injection is to be considered an experimental therapeutic modality that is presently used in several European centers to treat not only toxic nodules but also cysts and other cold benign nodules. It is performed under ultrasound guidance and is typically reserved for patients with contraindications to surgery or those who refuse 131-I. The major side effects related to the technique are local and generally self-limited but may occasionally be severe.[89,90] This technique has not been widely accepted yet in the United States, and, in our view, should not be used except in extremely rare circumstances and only by a group of physicians experienced in this technique.

## Indeterminate Lesions

Repeat aspiration, with or without ultrasound guidance, can yield sufficient sample in a significant percentage of cases. If the cytological findings remain indeterminate, particularly in the presence of features suggestive of malignancy in the history and/or physical exam, referral to surgery should be contemplated.[59,91]

## Patients with History of Head and Neck Irradiation

Given the increased frequency of benign and malignant thyroid disease in these patients, we believe these patients need routine sound ultrasonographic screening as well as routine careful palpation of the thyroid and the neck. FNA is reliable and relatively accurate in this subgroup. Our present approach is to try to aspirate all nodules greater than 1 cm in diameter. Assuming the aspiration is benign and there are no significant worrisome features, these patients can be monitored with clinical examination and history as well as with periodic sonograms. If worrisome clinical features develop or if the thyroid morphology changes, repeat aspiration and/or surgery can be considered. It should be remembered that thyroid malignancy in irradiated glands can occur outside the largest nodules and the disease is frequently mutifocal. Therefore, a near total or total thyroidectomy should be performed when surgery is contemplated.

## CONCLUSION

Thyroid nodules are common and can pose an interesting and difficult challenge to the physician. The majority of thyroid nodules are benign.

Fine-needle aspiration biopsy of the thyroid with or without ultrasound guidance is a proven technique with excellent diagnostic accuracy and few false negatives, and is the most useful initial diagnostic test. Scintigraphy and ultrasonography have limited indications. Molecular analysis of aspirate specimen are promising new tools and may decrease the false positive rate of FNA and further improve patient's selection for surgery. The physician's goal is to use the current data in a cost-effective and expeditious way that serves the best interest of the patient.

## References

1. Rojeski MT, Gharib H. Nodular thyroid disease: Evaluation and management. *N Engl J Med.* 1985; 313:428.

2. Tan GH, Gharib H. Thyroid incidentalomas: Management approaches to nonpalpable nodules discovered incidentally on thyroid imaging. *Ann Intern Med.* 1997; 126:226.

3. Vander JB, Gaston EA, Dawber TR. The significance of non-toxic thyroid nodules: Final report of 15-year study of the incidence of thyroid malignancy. *Ann Intern Med.* 1968; 69:537.

4. Gharib H. Changing concepts in the diagnosis and management of thyroid nodules. *Endocrinol Metab Clin North Am.* 1997; 26:777.

5. Brander A, Viikinkoski P, Tuuhea J, et al. Clinical versus ultrasound examination of the thyroid gland in common clinical practice. *J Clin Ultrasound.* 1992; 20:37.

6. Bruneton JN, Balu-Maestro C, Marcy PY, et al. Very high frequency ( 13 MHz ) ultrasonographic examination of normal neck: detection of normal lymph nodes and thyroid nodules. *J Ultrasound Med.* 1994; 13:87.

7. Ezzat S, Sarti DA, Cain DR, et al. Thyroid incidentalomas: prevalence by palpation and ultrasonography. *Arch Intern Med.* 1994; 154:1838.

8. Tomimori E, Pedrinola F, Cavaliere H, et al. Prevalence of incidental thyroid disease in a relatively low iodine intake area. *Thyroid.* 1995; 5:273.

9. Mortensen JD, Woolner LB, Bennet WA. Gross and microscopic findings in clinically normal thyroid glands. *J Clin Endocrinol Metab.* 1955; 15:1270.

10. Rallison ML, Dobyns BM, Keating FR, et al. Thyroid nodularity in children. *JAMA.* 1975; 233:1069.

11. Conrad RA, Dibyns BM, Sutow WW. Thyroid neoplasia as late effect of exposure to radioactive iodine fallout. *JAMA.* 1970; 214:316,

12. Hamilton TE, van Belle G, LoGerfo JP. Thyroid neoplasia in Marshall Islanders exposed to nuclear fallout. *JAMA.* 1987; 258:629.

13. Kaplan MM, Garnick MB, Gelber R, et al. Risk factors for thyroid abnormalities after neck irradiation for childhood cancer. *Am J Med.* 1983; 74:272.

14. Mazzaferri EL. Current concepts: management of a solitary thyroid nodule. *N Engl J Med.* 1993; 328:553.

15. Tan GH, Gharib H, Reading CC. Solitary thyroid nodule: comparison between palpation and ultrasonography. *Arch Intern Med.* 1995; 155:2418.

16. Walker J, Findlay D, Amar SS, et al. A prospective study of thyroid ultrasound scan in the clinically solitary thyroid nodule. *Br J Radiol.* 1985; 58:617.

17. Hall TL, Layfield LJ, Philippe A, et al. Sources of diagnostic error in fine needle aspiration of the thyroid. *Cancer.* 1989; 63:718.

18. Einhorn J, Franzen S. Thin-needle biopsy in the diagnosis of thyroid disease. *Acta Radiol (Stockh).* 1962; 58:321.

19. Murray D. The thyroid gland. In: Kovacs K, Asa SL, eds. *Functional Endocrine Pathology.* Cambridge, Mass: Blackwell Scientific 1991; 293.

20. Liel Y, Zirkin HJ, Sobel RJ. Fine-needle aspiration of the hot nodule. *Acta Cytol.* 1988; 32:866.

21. Jayaram G. Fine-needle aspiration cytologic study of the solitary thyroid nodule: profile of 308 cases with histologic correlation. *Acta Cytol.* 1985; 29:967.

22. Schlinkert RT, van Heerden JA, Goellner JR, et al. Factors that predict malignant thyroid lesions when fine-needle aspiration is "suspicious for follicular neoplasm." *Mayo Clin Proc.* 1997; 72:913.

23. Simeone JF, Daniels GH, Mueller PR, et al. High-resolution real-time sonography of the thyroid. *Radiology.* 1982; 145:431.

24. De Los Santos ET, Keyhani-Rofagha S, Cunningham JJ, et al. Cystic thyroid nodules: the dilemma of malignant lesions. *Arch Intern Med.* 1990; 150:1422.

25. Rosen IB, Provias JP, Walfish PG. Pathologic nature of cystic thyroid nodules selected for surgery by fine needle aspiration biopsy. *Surgery.* 1986; 100:606.

26. Ewing CA, Komblut A, Greeley C, et al. Presentation of thyroglossal duct cysts in adults. *Eur Arch Otorhinolaryngol.* 1999; 256:136.

27. Ginsberg J, Young JEM, Walfish PG. Parathyroid cysts—medical diagnosis and management. *JAMA.* 1978; 240:1506.

28. Belfiore A, Giuffrida D, LaRosa GL, et al. High frequency of cancer in cold thyroid nodules occurring at young age. *Acta Endocrinol (Copenh).* 1989; 121:197.

29. Hung W, August GP, Randolph JG, et al. Solitary thyroid nodules in children and adolescents. *J Pediatr Surg.* 1982; 17:225.

30. Favus MJ, Schneider AB, Stachura ME, et al. Thyroid cancer occurring as a late consequence of head-and-neck irradiation: Evaluation of 1056 patients. *N Eng J Med.* 1976; 294:1019.

31. Schneider AB. Thyroid nodules following childhood irradiation. A 1989 update. *Thyroid Today.* 1989; 12:1.

32. DeGeoot LJ, Reilly M, Pinnameneni K, et al. Retrospective and prospective study of radiation-induced thyroid disease. *Am J Med.* 1983; 74:852.

33. Fogelfeld L, Wiviot MBT, Shore-Freedman E, et al. Recurrence of thyroid nodules after surgical removal in patients irradiated in childhood for benign conditions. *N Engl J Med.* 1989; 320:835.

34. Compagno J, Oertel JE. Mailgnant lymphoma and other lymphoproliferative disorders of the thyroid gland. *Am J Clin Pathol.* 1980; 74:1.

35. Farbota LM, Calandra DB, Lawrence AM, et al. Thyroid carcinoma in Graves' disease. *Surgery.* 1985; 98:1148.

36. Hales IB, McElduff A, Crummer P, et al. Does Graves' disease or thyrotoxicosis affect the prognosis of thyroid cancer? *J Clin Endocrinol Metab.* 1992; 75:886.

37. Cantalamessa L, Baldini M, Orsatti A, et al. Thyroid nodules in Graves' disease and the risk of thyroid carcinoma. *Arch Intern Med.* 1999; 159:1705.

38. Mcall A, Jarosz H, Lawrence AM, et al. The incidence of thyroid carcinoma in solitary cold nodules and in multinodular goiters. *Surgery.* 1986; 100:1128.

39. Burch HB. Evaluation and management of the thyroid nodule: *Endocrinol Metab Clin North Am.* 1995; 24:663.

40. Christensen SB, Bondeson L, Ericsson UB, et al. Prediction of malignancy in the solitary thyroid nodule by physical examination, thyroid scan, fine-needle biopsy and serum thyroglobulin. *Acta Chir Scand.* 1984; 150:433.

41. Vierhapper H, Raber W, Bieglmayer C, et al. Routine measurement of plasma calcitonin in nodular thyroid diseases. *J Clin Endocrinol Metab.* 1997; 82:1589.

42. Niccoli P, Wion-Barbot N, Caron P, et al. Interest of routine measurement of serum calcitonin: study in a large series of thyroidectomized patients. The French Medullary Study Group. *J Clin Endocrinol Metab.* 1997; 82:338.

43. Rieu M, Lame MC, Richard A, et al. Prevalence of sporadic medullary thyroid carcinoma: the importance of routine measurement of serum calcitonin in the diagnostic evaluation of thyroid nodules. *Clin Endocrinol.* 1995; 42:453.

44. Lamb EJ, Heddle RM, Ellis A. Spuriously elevated plasma calcitonin in a patient with a thyroid nodule not associated with medullary thyroid carcinoma. *Postgrad Med.* 1999; 75:289.

45. Reading CC, Gorman CA. Thyroid imaging techniques. *Clin Lab Med.* 1993; 13:711.

46. Hays MT, Wesselossky B. Simultaneous measurement of thyroidal trapping(Tc99mO₄) and binding(I131): Clinical and experimental studies in man. *J Nucl Med.* 1973; 14:785.

47. Ashcraft MW, Van Herle AJ. Management of thyroid nodules. II. Scanning techniques, thyroid suppressive therapy, and fine needle aspiration. *Head Neck Surg.* 1981; 3:297.

48. Nelson RL, Wahner HW, Gorman CA. Rectilinear thyroid scanning as a predictor of malignancy. *Ann Intern Med.* 1978; 88:41.

49. Kleiger PS, Wilson GA, Greenspan BS. The usefulness of the dynamic phase in pertechnetate thyroid imaging for solitary hypofunctioning nodules. *Clin Nucl Med.* 1992; 17:617.

50. KoizumiM, Taguchi H, Goto M, et al. Thalium-201 scintigraphy in the evaluation of thyroid nodules: a retrospective study of 246 cases. *Ann Nucl Med.* 1993; 7:147.

51. Sundram FX, Mack PO. Investigation of thyroid nodules using technetium-99m sestamibi. *Ann Acad Med Singapore.* 1993; 22:560

52. Simeone JF. High-resolution real time sonography of the thyroid. *Radiology.* 1982; 145:43.

53. Thijs LG, Wiener JD. Ultrasonic examination of the thyroid gland: possibilities and limitations. *Am J Med.* 1976; 60:96.

54. Evans DM. Diagnostic discriminants of thyroid cancer. *Am J Surg.* 1987; 153:569.

55. Hayashi N, Tamaki N, Yamamoto K, et al. Real-time ultrasonography of thyroid nodules. *Acta Radiologica.* 1986; 27:403.

56. Shimamoto K, Endo T, Ishigaki T, et al. Thyroid nodules: evaluation with color Doppler ultrasonography. *J Ultrasound Med.* 1993; 12:673.

57. Gharib H, Goellner JR, Johnson DA. Fine-needle aspiration cytology of the thyroid: a 12-year experience with 11,000 biopsies. *Clin Lab Med.* 1993; 13:699.

58. Blum M. The diagnosis of the thyroid nodule using aspiration biopsy and cytology. *Arch Intern Med.* 1984; 144:1140.

59. Caruso D, Mazzaferri EL. Fine needle aspiration biopsy in the management of thyroid nodules. *Endocrinologist.* 1991; 1:194.

60. Ito M, Yamashita S, Ashizawa K, et al. Childhood thyroid diseases around Chernobyl evaluated by ultrasound examination and fine needle aspiration cytology. *Thyroid.* 1995; 5:365.

61. Mazzaferri EL, De Los Santos ET, Rofagha-Keyhari S. Solitary thyroid nodule: diagnosis and management. *Med Clin North Am.* 1988; 72:1177.

62. Hamburger B, Gharib H, Melton LJ III, et al. Fine needle aspiration of thyroid nodules: impact on thyroid practice and cost of care. *Am J Med.* 1982; 73:381.

63. Cochand-Priollet B, Guillausseau PJ, Chagnon S, et al. The diagnostic value of fine needle aspiration biopsy under ultrasonography in nonfunctional thyroid nodules: a prospective study comparing cytologic and histologic findings. *Am J Med.* 1994; 97:152.

64. Rosen IB, Azadian A, Walfish PG, et al. Ultrasound-guided fine-needle aspiration biopsy in the management of thyroid disease. *Am J Surg.* 1993; 166:346.

65. Caplan RH, Kisten WA, Strutt PJ, et al. Fine-needle aspiration biopsy of thyroid nodules: a cost-effective diagnostic plan. *Postgrad Med.* 1991; 90:183.

66. Gharib H. Diagnosis of thyroid nodules by fine-needle aspiration biopsy. *Current Opin Endocrinol.* 1996; 3:433.

67. Hamburger JI, Husain M, Nishiyama R, et al. Increasing the accuracy of fine-needle biopsy for thyroid nodules. *Arch Pathol Lab Med.* 1989; 113:1035.

68. Leenhardt L, Hejblum G, Franc B, et al. Indications and limits of ultrasound-guided cytology in the management of nonpalpable thyroid nodules. *J Clin Endocrinol Metab.* 1999; 84:24.

69. Yokozawa T, Miyauchi A, Kuma K, et al. Accurate and simple method of diagnosing thyroid nodules: the modified technique of ultrasound-guided fine needle aspiration biopsy. *Thyroid.* 1995; 5:41.

70. Sabel MS, Haque D, Velasco JM, et al. Use of ultrasound-guided fine needle aspiration biopsy in the management of thyroid disease. *Am J Surg.* 1998; 64:738.

71. Inohara H, Honjo Y, Yoshii T, et al. Expression of *galectin-3* in fine-needle aspirates as a diagnostic marker differentiating benign from malignant thyroid neoplasms. *Cancer.* 1999; 85:2475.

72. Gasbarri A, Martegani MP, Del Prete F, et al. Galectin-3 and CD44v6 isoforms in the preoperative evaluation of thyroid nodules. *J Clin Oncol.* 1999; 17:3494.

73. Saji M, Xydas S, Westra WH, et al. Human telomerase reverse transcriptase (hTERT) gene expression in thyroid neoplasms. *Clin Cancer Res.* 1999; 5:1483.

74. Kim SJ, Ryu JW, Choi DS. The expression of the high mobility group I(Y) mRNA in thyroid cancers: useful tool of differential diagnosis of thyroid nodules. *Korean J Intern Med.* 2000; 15:71.

75. Kuma K, Matsuzuka F, Yokozawa T, et al. Fate of untreated benign thyroid nodules: results of long-term follow-up. *World J Surg.* 1994; 18:495.

76. Erdogan MF, Kamel N, Aras D, et al. Value of re-aspiration in benign nodular thyroid disease. *Thyroid.* 1998; 8:1087.

77. Mittendorf EA, McHenry CR. Follow-up evaluation and clinical course of patients with benign nodular thyroid disease. *Am J Surg.* 1999; 65:653.

78. Lyons J, Landis CA, Harsh G, et al. Two G protein oncogenes in human endocrine tumors. *Science.* 1990; 249:655.

79. O'Sullivan C, Barton CM, Staddon SL, et al. Activating point mutations in human thyroid adenomas. *Mol Carcinog.* 1991; 4:345.

80. Hamburger JI. Evolution of toxicity in solitary nontoxic autonomously functioning thyroid nodules. *J Clin Endocrinol Metab.* 1980; 50:1089.

81. Gharib H, Mazzaferri EL. Thyroxine suppressive therapy in patients with nodular thyroid disease. *Ann Intern Med.* 1998; 128:386.

82. Zelmanovitz F, Genro S, Gross J. Suppressive therapy with levothyroxine for solitary thyroid nodules: a double-blind controlled clinical study and cumulative meta-analyses. *J Clin Endocrinol Metab.* 1998; 83:3881.

83. Celani MF, Mariani M, Mariani G. On the usefulness of levothyroxine suppressive therapy in the medical treatment of benign solitary, solid or predominantly solid, thyroid nodules. *Acta Endocrinol (Copenh).* 1990; 123:603.

84. La Rosa GL, Lupo L, Giuffrida D, et al. Levothyroxine and potassium iodide are both effective in treating benign solitary solid cold nodules of the thyroid. *Ann Intern Med.* 1995; 122:1.

85. La Rosa GL, Ippoliti AM, Lupo L, et al. Cold thyroid nodule reduction with L-thyroxine can be predicted by initial nodule volume and cytological characteristics. *J Clin Endocrinol Metab.* 1996; 81:4385.

86. Smith SA, Gharib G. Thyroid nodule suppression. *Ad Endocrinol Metab.* 1991; 2:107.

87. Messina G, Viceconti N, Trinti B. Diagnostic items and treatment of Plummer's disease: a study on 180 patients. *Clin Ter.* 1998; 149:191.

88. Burch HB, Shakir F, Fitzimmons TR, et al. Diagnosis and management of the autonomously functioning thyroid nodule: The Walter Reed Army Medical Center experience, 1976–1996. *Thyroid.* 1998; 8:871.

89. Monzani F, Caraccio N, Goletti O, et al. Treatment of hyperfunctioning thyroid nodules with percutaneous ethanol injection: eight years' experience. *Exp Clin Endocrinol Diabetes.* 1998; 4:S54.

90. Zingrillo M, Torlontano M, Chiarella R, et al. Percutaneous ethanol injection may be a definitive treatment for symptomatic thyroid cystic nodules not treatable by surgery: five year follow-up study. *Thyroid.* 1999; 9:763.

91. Gharib H, Goellner JR, Zinsmeister AR, et al. Fine-needle aspiration of the thyroid: the problem of suspicious cytologic findings. *Ann Intern Med.* 1984; 101:25.

# 8

# Fine Needle Aspiration Biopsy in Thyroid Disease

## Steven C. Meschter, M.D.

## PREVALENCE OF SOLITARY THYROID NODULES IN THE GENERAL POPULATION

Fine needle aspiration (FNA) biopsy is an important presurgical method for triaging solitary thyroid nodules. Palpable thyroid nodules are very prevalent in the North American population. The routine use of fine needle aspiration biopsy has resulted in a reduction of unnecessary thyroid surgeries, an increase in the surgical yield of thyroid malignancy and a reduction in the cost of managing these nodules.[1]

Palpable thyroid nodules (generally 1–1.5 cm or greater in diameter) occur in approximately 4.2% of the adult population in North America.[2-4] Nodules are more prevalent in adult females (6.4%) than adult males (1.5%).[2-4] Imaging techniques (sonography, CT scan, scintigraphy) detect nodules in 19–67% of examined thyroid glands.[5,6] These methods allow detection of nodules as small as 1–3 mm in diameter (those less than 1cm in diameter usually escape clinical detection through palpation).[5,7] Finally, autopsy studies showed 30–60% of examined glands contained nodules, many of which were an incidental finding.[5,7] Assuming the population of the United States is approximately 200,000,000 these figures translate into literally millions of thyroid nodules that potentially could require evaluation.

## INCIDENCE OF THYROID CANCER AND EXPECTED DEATHS FROM THYROID CANCER

Only 19,500 new thyroid cancer cases (1.5% of all new cancers) were expected in 2001[8] while 1,300 deaths from thyroid malignancy (0.2% of all cancer related deaths) were expected in 2001.[8] Only 6.6% of patients with thyroid cancer will die of their disease (1,300 deaths/ 19,500 new cases), making this a relatively indolent malignancy. Clearly a non-surgical means of detecting thyroid malignancy is indicated as the risk of surgical morbidity, while low, approximates the morbidity of the disease if left untreated.

## CLINICAL FACTORS INDICATING A MALIGNANT THYROID NODULE

Thyroid nodules are more common in females, are seen with increasing frequency with advancing age, increase in number in patients exposed to ionizing radiation, and are increased in frequency in patients with deficient dietary intake of iodine.[2,9-11] The risk of thyroid malignancy is associated with the formation of a nodule in the thyroid gland. Risk of malignancy is increased in patients less than 30 years of age, and greater than 60 years of age.[9-11] A family history of medullary carcinoma or a history of multiple endocrine neoplasia syndromes increases the risk of thyroid malignancy. Prior exposure to ionizing radiation increases the risk of thyroid malignancy. On physical exam a nodule greater than 4 cm in diameter, which is painless and rapidly enlarging, is cause for concern.[9-11] Findings of associated cervical adenopathy associated with a dominant thyroid mass, and or fixation of a firm, painless mass to skin or muscle increase the probability of thyroid malignancy. Hoarseness caused by unilateral vocal cord paralysis (suggesting involvement of the recurrent laryngeal nerve) is an ominous finding. A truly solitary thyroid nodule carries a higher risk of malignancy than one occurring in a multinodular gland.[11] These clinical findings are of low specificity for identifying thyroid malignancy, although they must be considered in the selection of patients for thyroid surgery.[9] In fact the majority of patients presenting with a thyroid nodule lack any of these clinical findings which increase their risk of malignancy.

## WHY USE FINE NEEDLE ASPIRATION?

### Purpose

The goal of sampling thyroid nodules with FNA is to identify malignant nodules and distinguish these from benign nodules that do not require surgery.[12,13]

### Safe, Accurate, Cost-Effective Procedure

FNA when used as the first test in the evaluation of thyroid nodules is the most accurate and cost-effective test available for identifying potential thyroid malignancy.[14,15]

Many studies have reviewed the use of fine-needle aspiration biopsy in evaluating thyroid nodules.[3,10,12,13,16-26] The conclusion is that FNA is accurate, sensitive, specific, safe and cost-effective. Modalities for evaluating the thyroid such as serum tests, sonography, and scintigraphy were employed in varying combinations prior to the use of FNA. They proved to be sensitive but lacked specificity.[14,16] These techniques led to high costs of thyroid nodule management as the majority of patients selected for surgery ultimately yielded benign thyroid disease. The goal of the ideal screening test is the safe, accurate, presurgical identification of thyroid malignancy, a relatively low incidence, indolent cancer occurring in a large population of thyroid nodules. FNA offers a sensitive means of accurately identifying these various cancers with essentially no significant morbidity.[27] The acceptable specificity of FNA allows selection of patients for thyroid surgery with an increased yield of thyroid malignancy.[12,14] The reduction in unnecessary surgery for benign nodules significantly reduces the cost of managing thyroid nodules.[14]

FNA is a safe, simple procedure that can be used in an outpatient setting to obtain diagnostic material from palpable and (using ultrasound guidance) non-palpable thyroid nodules. In institutions fortunate to have on-site cytopathology support, the results of the FNA can be available immediately. This provides a significant advantage for the surgeon as well as the patient. The satisfactory performance of the FNA with an accurate, immediate diagnosis is an impressive means of providing valuable patient service at remarkable savings of both medical resources and patient anxiety. The immediate availability of diagnostic information allows the surgeon the luxury of planning patient management potentially on the first visit, with direct patient involvement. Surgical therapies, additional consultations and appropriate imaging studies necessary for the prompt management of the patient can be initiated efficiently and quickly. The patient's perception of the surgeon's expertise in resolving the situation is markedly enhanced. The simplicity of the FNA makes it ideally suited to special circumstances. For example, patients presenting with rapidly enlarging thyroid nodules or neck masses with impending airway obstruction can be rapidly and safely triaged by FNA in an outpatient setting. The difference in management of a large cyst, anaplastic thyroid carcinoma and thyroid lymphoma is significant. Knowing at the outset of the patient's presentation, the correct diagnosis can save valuable time and expedite the patient's management. The savings in unnecessary procedures and tests can be significant.

## FNA Can Identify Malignancies Not Requiring Surgical Management

FNA cytomorphology is sufficiently specific that entities such as Hashimoto's thyroiditis and malignant lymphoma can be correctly diagnosed. These findings not only offer explanation for a thyroid enlargement or nodule, but would also suggest that surgery (thyroidectomy, partial or total) would not be indicated. Having a preliminary FNA result dramatically facilitates management of these patients. Cases of anaplastic carcinoma of the thyroid usually can be recognized on FNA[21,28,29] and depending on the extent of the process may not directly benefit from surgical therapy.

## FNA Results Can Reduce Patient Anxiety

Patients often present with heightened anxiety over the presence of any "lump." The immediate patient concern is cancer. Thyroid nodules are predominantly benign. Immediate information provided by an FNA can be extraordinarily helpful in calming those worries.[21] The patient's perception of service is markedly embellished.

## THE TECHNIQUE

## How Does the Procedure Work?

Despite the name of this procedure a fine needle aspiration is not an aspiration, it is a true tissue biopsy. The ultimate success of this procedure is critically dependent on the understanding of this concept. Cellular material is not "aspirated" from the target nodule. The movement of the needle cuts small cores of tissue. The application of negative pressure by the attached syringe is solely to maintain the cut tissue fragments within the needle barrel. Significant negative pressure with the syringe is not only unnecessary but also counterproductive as it frequently results in drawing of blood which dilutes the specimen. Using no negative pressure at all can sometimes enhance the cellular yield by reducing blood or fluid aspiration. The goal of the procedure is to cut fragments of tissue and transfer them to the surface of the slide for evaluation. Liquid materials such as blood or cyst contents simply serve to dilute these diagnostic fragments and tend to make the specimen unsatisfactory or non-diagnostic.

The fine needle aspiration is performed with a small bore, disposable needle, the 1.5 inch 25-gauge needle being the most commonly used.[18] Although it is difficult to imagine that such a small bore needle can obtain diagnostic material it is ideally suited for obtaining fragments of thyroid tissue. The size of the needle relative to the microscopic follicular structure of the thyroid is sufficient to obtain material that offers important architectural information to the interpreting cytopathologist. The small bore of the needle results in a minimum of induced hemorrhage in the target nodule.

The key to the procedure is the multiple rapid strokes of the needle through the target nodule. Each push of the needle through the nodule results in a coring of tissue into the barrel and hub of the needle. Multiple, short quick strokes into the nodule maximize the tissue yield. Redirection of the needle for each successive group of passes allows for thorough sampling of the target. This is a distinct advantage over large core biopsies (true cut needle) that are limited to a single core sample of the nodule. Sampling error is higher with the core biopsy, in spite of the larger volume of tissue obtained. Additionally, the core biopsy must be fixed and sectioned before the success of the sampling can be assessed. The FNA can be assessed real time, on site. This allows immediate recognition of sampling error when it can be most easily corrected by obtaining additional material.

The small-bore needles cause a minimum of trauma to the tissue being sampled. This keeps bleeding to a minimum. Blood serves only to dilute the diagnostic fragments of tissue and makes the specimen inadequate or non-diagnostic. The high vascularity of the thyroid makes tissue sampling more difficult because of frequent blood contamination of the specimen. This is one of the common causes of inadequate FNAs of the thyroid. The use of larger-bore needles (22-gauge and larger) simply exacerbates the problem and increases the frequency of inadequate FNAs because of blood contamination. This does not mean that these larger-bore needles are not indicated, however. Situations in which there is a high degree of fibrous tissue in the target nodule may make the use of the 22-gauge needle more efficacious in obtaining diagnostic tissue fragments. It is best, however, to start the procedure with a 25-gauge needle and then use a larger bore needle if necessary. Once bleeding within the target nodule is started subsequent passes yield less diagnostic material and are more likely to be contaminated with blood.

## Equipment

The supplies required for the performance of FNA, are simple, readily available, and inexpensive. 10 cc disposable plastic syringes and 25-gauge 1.5 in. disposable hypodermic needles are the minimum requirements. A syringe holder such as the 10 cc pistol grip made by Cameco (Precision Dynamics Corporation, 13880 Del Sur St., San Fernando, CA 91340-3490) is quite helpful, but not an absolute requirement. Alcohol preparation pads, 2 x 2 cm sterile gauze pads, and Band-Aids are usually readily available. Local anesthetic (1% lidocaine) and 1.0 cc TB syringes with 27-gauge needles for installation of the anesthetic are ideal but not absolutely necessary. Ninety-five percent ethanol spray fixative (the same as used for fixation of routine Pap smears) is required. Polished glass slides with a frosted end for slide labeling (Fisher Scientific) are necessary for smear preparation. 15 ml capped, sterile, plastic centrifuge tubes (Corning Incorporated, Corning, NY 14831) for 10% formalin, RPMI solution (Life Technologies Inc., Gibco BRLA, 3175 Staley Rd., Grand Island, NY 14072) or Hank's solution (Genetics and IVF Institute, 3025 Hamaker Court, Suite 201, Fairfax, VA 22031) are also necessary. Most of these supplies are available in a routinely stocked physician's office and usually do not require special ordering. Depending on the frequency of performance of the FNA procedure, it is advantageous to put all these supplies together in a kit or tray so they are always readily available during the procedure. The availability of each of these items should be checked before beginning the FNA as delay in processing because of the absence of one of the required items may result in loss or damage of the precious specimen.

## Examination and Positioning of the Patient

A thorough examination of the patient and the target area are critical to the success of the FNA. Identification of a palpable nodule within the thyroid will depend on the size of the nodule and the skill of the examiner. The FNA of palpable lesions is done totally by feel. Sampling errors are significantly reduced by an accurate delineation of the limits of the nodule both by physical examination and by the "feel" of the needle within the lesion. The advantage of the operator at the time of the FNA is confirmation that the nodule of interest was actually sampled. Knowing that the nodule is within the thyroid and not an adjacent structure is critical to the interpretation of the FNA. For example, an aspiration composed of a mixture of benign lymphocytes may indicate a Hashimoto's thyroiditis or represent an adjacent benign lymph node. The difference is obviously important and frequently can be determined by careful palpation. Multiple neck nodules in addition to nodules palpable within the thyroid gland may have clinical implications (metastatic disease, lymphoma) and may serve as more informative targets for aspiration than those identified in the thyroid itself. These determinations will depend on the combination of clinical information and results of the examination of the neck. Knowledge of location of the nodule relative to other vital structures within the neck will also be valuable in reducing sampling of adjacent structures and their attendant complications.

Positioning the patient with additional elevation of the shoulders and dropping the head back will bring the thyroid gland into a position of greater exposure and access (see Figure 8-1). This will enhance the examiner's ability to palpate even small thyroid nodules and will increase the success of FNA sampling. This patient position is usually well tolerated and offers particular advantages in patients with short or obese necks.

Assuring the patient and making him or her as comfortable as possible prior to performing the FNA is greatly helpful in the outcome as the patient will be able to cooperate and remain still and well-positioned for the duration of the procedure.

## Performing the Fine Needle Aspiration Biopsy

Once the patient is correctly positioned, and the nodule identified, the skin overlying the nodule is cleansed with circular motions using an alcohol preparation pad. The cleansing of the skin is similar to the technique for routine venipuncture. It is not necessary to develop a sterile, draped surgical field. The surgeon, as in routine venipuncture, should use appropriate barrier precau-

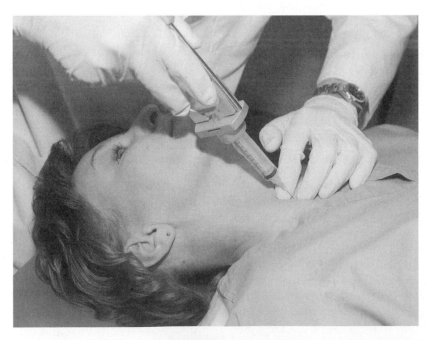

**Figure 8–1.** The patient is positioned with the shoulders elevated on a small pillow and the head dropped back, bringing the thyroid gland up into a more readily palpated position. The nodule is stabilized with firm pressure of the first and second fingers, stretching the skin overlying the nodule.

tions (gloves). 1 cc of 1% intradermal lidocaine may be administered in the skin overlying the nodule. This is optional and provides minimal anesthesia to the skin so the patient is spared the sensation of multiple needle sticks as most procedures will require 3–6 passes of the needle for adequate sampling.[18] After administering the anesthesia the biopsy needle (25-gauge 1.5 inch disposable hypodermic needle) is attached to the 10 cc disposable syringe and placed in the pistol grip. The nodule is stabilized between the first and second finger of the examining hand by stretching the overlying skin and applying pressure with the two fingers. The biopsy needle is then gently inserted into the target paying careful attention to any interfaces or changes in consistency that can be felt with the needle. Once the needle tip is in the target approximately 1cc of negative pressure is applied by gently retracting the syringe plunger. This is maintained throughout the FNA. The needle is then rapidly moved back and forth through the nodule with short quick strokes, redirecting the needle with each pass. It is important not to allow the needle tip to exit the skin in this process as air will be aspirated and the specimen lost in the syringe barrel. It is important to visually watch the needle hub. As soon as blood is detected in the transparent plastic hub of the needle, the aspiration should be stopped. The negative pressure is released before removing the needle from the target. The syringe plunger is allowed to passively move to its resting position. The needle is then removed from the target and pressure applied to the puncture site to prevent the formation of a hematoma.

Thorough sampling of the target is important to the accuracy of the aspiration as well as the adequacy. Sampling technique has been studied.[18,30] Specimen adequacy is maximized with multiple separate passes of the sampling needle. Three to six separate passes into the nodule are recommended,[18] particularly if the specimen is not being evaluated for adequacy on site. Nodules (1.0–4.0 cm) should be sampled in at least four regions, depending on the nodule size.[30] Sampling the middle region of a large nodule (4.0 cm or greater) may result in an increased inadequacy rate and increased false negative rate caused by degeneration or hemorrhage in the central region of the nodule. For larger nodules (4.0 cm or greater) sampling the edges of the nodule will improve the sensitivity and the specificity of the FNA procedure.

Finally, the quality of the needle action through the nodule will improve the results. Passing the tip of the needle from one margin of the nodule to the deep margin then withdrawing the needle tip to the proximal margin and redirecting through the nodule will improve the quality of fragments obtained.[18]

## Preparation of Slides

As soon as the specimen has been obtained, it must be quickly transferred to the slide, smeared, and then air-dried or alcohol-fixed. Each pass of the needle should result in two smears, one air-dried and one alcohol-fixed. The transfer is accomplished by detaching the needle, completely retracting the syringe plunger, reattaching the needle, firmly pressing the needle tip to the surface of the glass slide and forcefully pushing the air from the barrel through the needle to express the specimen fragments on the appropriately labeled (patient identification, target location, fixation) glass slide. The resulting drop of material is then smeared with a second glass slide. The first smear is allowed to air dry and the second is immediately alcohol-fixed. The needle and syringe are rinsed into the RPMI solution, and the needle disposed. This procedure is repeated for each pass into the nodule. It is critically important to stop the FNA when a drop of material is detected in the plastic needle hub. This will result in a single drop of cellular material for slide preparation. If excessive material or blood fills the needle hub and is present in the syringe barrel this should be transferred to the RPMI solution for cell block preparation. A single pass should not be smeared on multiple glass slides, as this frequently results in dilute, hypocellular specimens, which will be inadequate. If FNA of the nodule results in aspiration of cyst fluid, this fluid should be completely removed from the nodule and then placed directly in the RPMI solution. Any residual nodularity remaining after complete removal of the fluid should be sampled with subsequent passes.

After two or three passes, depending on the visual cellularity of the specimen, a final pass is expressed directly into RPMI solution for the production of a cell block. The rinsings of the needle subsequent to each smear preparation and the direct sampling placed in RPMI solution are important to the production of specimens for ancillary studies such as flow cytometry, immunocytochemistry, special stains, and molecular studies.

It is at this point that the materials obtained and smeared can be immediately evaluated. The Diff-Quick stain is ideally suited for this as it takes only one minute to perform. It is applied to the air-dried smear. An onsite interpretation based on a rapid Diff-Quick stain can determine the adequacy of the specimen. Any need for additional material for diagnosis or ancillary studies can be assessed at this time. This part of the process is dependent on the availability of dedicated cytopathologists or cytotechnologists to perform the interpretations. Their participation can significantly enhance the results of the procedure. Specimen adequacy is maximized and they can obtain ancillary materials for making the resulting diagnosis as specific as possible. In situations where such support is available the surgeon and the patient can be informed of the results of the fine needle aspiration. A management plan can be initiated immediately.

In situations where cytopathology support is not available on site, the slides and RPMI needle rinsings are submitted to the laboratory accompanied by the appropriate paperwork including complete history and clinical findings.

## Special Problems with FNA of the Thyroid

The thyroid gland is a very vascular structure. This complicates the performance of the FNA of the thyroid because blood dilutes the sample and is a frequent cause of inadequate aspiration specimens. As the FNA is truly a cutting biopsy it is important to keep blood contamination to a minimum. Several methods can be employed to accomplish this. First, excessive negative pressure in the syringe will serve only to draw blood as if in a venipuncture. Gentle (1 cc or less ) or even no negative pressure in the syringe barrel may improve results and decrease the amount of blood obtained. The smaller needle (25-gauge is recommended) causes less trauma to the tissue and improves the adequacy of the specimen. A larger needle (23–22 gauge) should be reserved for sclerotic targets such as fibrotic stages of chronic thyroiditis. Finally, some have advocated the use of a "aspirationless" biopsy using only the needle to pass through the target nodule. This technique while effective can be messy as there is no syringe attached to catch blood or cystic fluid. These fluids may leak onto the patient or gloves of the operator. An "aspirationless" technique can be utilized with the syringe attached but without any negative pressure applied. This is frequently helpful in improving the cellularity of the specimen.

Another problem frequently encountered in the thyroid are the presence of cysts filled with blood, colloid, debris or a combination of these. These are encountered in cystic nodular goiters, but may also be seen in neoplastic processes such as papillary carcinoma or even anaplastic carcinoma of the thyroid. The contents of the cyst are frequently not diagnostic and so may increase the proportion of inadequate specimens or contribute to falsely negative aspirations. It is important in these situations to attempt to sample the wall of the cyst. If the cyst is evacuated any solid palpable nodule that remains needs to be adequately sampled. Sonographic guidance of the needle may be necessary to adequately sample any intracystic masses. In some instances the concurrent use of a core needle biopsy

may provide supplemental material that can provide an adequately cellular sample reducing falsely negative diagnoses.

## Other Cervical Neck Nodules

A distinct advantage of the FNA is that it can be used to sample any palpable nodules whether they reside in the thyroid or adjacent to it. The procedure is sufficiently specific in that useful information as to the cause of the palpable nodule (enlarged lymph node, for example) or the presence of significant disease (metastatic papillary carcinoma, for example) can be obtained. These specimens are handled in a fashion identical to that described for aspirations of the thyroid nodule.

## Materials for Ancillary Studies

The use of FNA is rapidly becoming more specific as new ancillary studies are being developed. The use of materials submitted in the smears and in the RPMI solution has wide application including flow cytometry (lymphoma workup, ploidy analysis), immunocytochemical studies, and molecular studies. Cell block preparations can add valuable architectural information. All these studies if appropriately applied can contribute to the specificity of the final diagnosis.

## COMPLICATIONS

Complications of the FNA are minimal and usually equivalent to venipuncture. Local hematoma at the biopsy site is occasionally encountered. FNA is not a significant risk for implantation of tumor in the needle track.

## REPORTING THE RESULTS OF THE FNA PROCEDURE

### Diagnostic Categories for FNA of Thyroid Nodules

The interpretation of the FNA specimens can be assigned to the following categories.

### Satisfactory Cellularity for Interpretation
*Benign, non-neoplastic lesions*

Included in this group are entities such as thyroiditis, cystic goiter, nodular goiter, and colloid nodule. These entities will result in conservative therapy for the patient and exclude the need for surgery.

### Indeterminate lesions

**Cellular follicular lesions.** Included in this group are hyperplastic nodules, follicular adenoma, well-differentiated follicular carcinoma and some cases of follicular variant of papillary carcinoma.[12,28]

**Hürthle cell neoplasm.** This group includes Hürthle cell nodules in Hashimoto's thyroiditis, Hürthle cell adenoma and Hürthle cell carcinoma. Again, insufficient cytomorphologic criteria exist to separate benign from malignant lesions solely on the basis of an FNA.[12,28]

**Suspicious for malignancy.** FNA specimens that suggest malignancy, but lack criteria for unequivocally making the diagnosis are included in this group.[28]

### Malignant

This group includes all diagnoses of unequivocal malignancy. Entities such as papillary carcinoma, medullary carcinoma, anaplastic carcinoma, and lymphoma, are examples.[12,28]

## Unsatisfactory/non-diagnostic

### Non-diagnostic

FNA specimens with inadequate cellularity are regarded as non-diagnostic. This is not equivalent to the diagnosis of "negative for malignancy."

## Discussion

## Adequacy

The goal of the FNA procedure is to sample and obtain representative material from the target nodule in the thyroid gland. The predictive value of the test is critically dependent on obtaining an adequate sample.[11,16,18,31-33] Equally important is the discrimination by the cytopathologist of what constitutes an adequate specimen.[11,16,18] The dilemma is that malignancy can be diagnosed on very few cells. The exclusion of malignancy is more difficult and requires a larger number of cells.[11,16,18] An unsatisfactory or non-diagnostic specimen is not equivalent to a negative or benign FNA specimen. The number of cells required to deem the specimen adequate is debated but recommended cellularity is 6–10 clusters of follicular cells with 10–20 cells per cluster.[11,12,16,18,34] The stringency of the criteria will affect the false negative rate of the thyroid FNA.[32] The more stringent the criteria (greater amount of cellular material required to be satisfactory) the lower the false negative rate.[32] An additional criterion employed by some institutions is the identification of multiple clusters of follicular cells on at least two separate sampling passes of the needle.[18,32] The theory here is that similar material from multiple passes helps to assure that the needle was sampling the target nodule and not adjacent normal thyroid. The Papanicolaou Society of Cytopathology Task Force on Standards of Practice recommends[28] that several other judgments need to be included. First, if any malignant cells, regardless of the number, are identified, then the preparation is considered adequate. Secondly, aspirates yielding abundant colloid with few follicular cells should be interpreted as benign colloid nodule with the qualifier of low cellularity. Similarly, a cystic lesion that yields fluid with few follicular cells, numerous histiocytes and variable colloid may be interpreted as probable benign cystic goiter with limited cellularity. Large cysts (>4 cm) have a higher likelihood of malignancy and should be re-aspirated with recurrence. Any solid areas remaining after removal of cyst fluid should be sampled thoroughly.[28]

## Indeterminate Lesions

The indeterminate category represents one of the significant shortcomings of FNA of the thyroid.[13,24,34,35] There is significant overlap in the cytologic appearance of benign follicular lesions (adenomatous nodule, follicular adenoma, cellular nodular hyperplasia) and follicular carcinoma.[35] In fact, the diagnosis of follicular carcinoma requires the histologic identification of vascular or capsular invasion. This cannot be accomplished with the FNA. It is frequently difficult to achieve this diagnosis even on histologic sections. There is a significant degree of overlap between benign entities such as follicular adenoma and hyperplastic nodules in goiter.[35] Their discrimination would require the identification of a capsule. Again, this cannot be accomplished with an FNA. Hürthle cell neoplasms constitute another problematic area. Again, there is significant cytologic overlap between benign Hürthle cell metaplasia in nodular goiter, Hürthle cell changes seen in Hashimoto's thyroiditis, Hürthle cell adenomas and Hürthle cell carcinomas.[36] The result is that the findings of cellular follicular and Hürthle cell lesions by FNA lead to the recommendation of surgical management of the patient. If a method for making these discriminations could be identified the specificity and accuracy of the FNA could be significantly improved. Many have looked for markers that would assist in this discrimination. Attempts at using cell size measurements and nuclear ploidy studies have not been successfully applied. The search for molecular markers holds promise, however. In theory, a molecular marker specific to the follicular carcinoma might allow for accurate discrimination from benign proliferations. One such promising marker is galectin-3. Galectin-3 is a β-galactoside-binding protein with multiple physiologic and pathologic functions including cell growth, neoplastic transformation, and apoptosis.[37] It appears that malignant progression in the follicular cell may be associated with increased expression of galectin-3.[37] It has been shown that galectin-3 is overexpressed in thyroid malignancies. In particular, follicular carcinomas expressed galectin-3 in high level.[37,38] In contrast, benign thyroid adenomas, goiters, and normal thyroid follicular epithelium did not express high levels.[37] This measurement is ideally suited for application to FNA specimens, and immunocytochemical methods that can be applied to cellular FNA specimens have been developed. A second marker, CD44v6, a cell surface glycoprotein receptor for hyaluronic acid offers promise for separating benign from malignant follicular cells.[39,40] CD44v6 is expressed on proliferating thyroid follicular cells and up-regulated in follicular carcinomas.[39] This too has been developed as an immunocytochemical marker and appears well suited for application to FNA specimens. Using these markers holds promise for reliably separating benign follicular lesions from follicular carcinoma thus enhancing the presurgical evaluation of thyroid nodules.[40]

## FNA STATISTICS: THE BEST TEST TO ORDER FIRST

### Distribution of Cytologic Diagnoses

Several large series of thyroid nodule FNAs have been studied. The total of FNAs reviewed in these studies approximates 36,000 procedures.[12,16,34] These show a range of results for each of the diagnostic categories of the thyroid FNA. Seventy–80% of aspirates were diagnosed as satisfactory and benign.[12,16,34] Within this group the false negative rate ranged from 2.4–5.2%.[12,16,34] Aspirates diagnosed as malignant constituted 4% of the total with a false positive rate of 2.6–6%.[12,16,34] The category of indeterminate/suspicious was 11% of the total FNAs. The inadequate (non-diagnostic) FNAs ranged from 4.6–17%.[12,16,34]

### Sensitivity and Specificity

Sensitivity is a measure of the fraction of patients with a target disease who will have a positive FNA (total number of positive tests divided by the total number of positive tests plus the falsely negative tests). Specificity is the fraction of patients correctly identified by FNA who have no malignancy (total number of negative tests divided by the total number of negative tests plus the falsely positive tests). Large numbers of thyroid FNAs have been reviewed indicating a sensitivity range of 65–98% and a specificity range of 72–100%.[12,15,16,34,41] On average the sensitivity for FNA of thyroid nodules is 83% and specificity is 92%.[12,15,34] A major reason for the range of sensitivity and specificity is the method of incorporation of data from the suspicious or indeterminate category of the thyroid FNA.[12] If the suspicious FNA specimens are regarded as positive diagnoses then the sensitivity is increased but the specificity is decreased. Eliminating the suspicious diagnoses from the positive category decreases sensitivity and increases specificity. As the suspicious or indeterminate category is variable depending on the institution and the criterion utilized for placing cases in this diagnostic category, it can constitute from 5–23% (average of 10%) of cytologic diagnoses on thyroid FNAs.[12] Also significant as a reason for the range of sensitivity and specificity is the experience of the individual performing the FNA and the expertise of the cytopathologist interpreting the test.[3,31,32]

## False Negative Rate

The false negative rate is defined as the percentage of nodules diagnosed as benign by FNA which are found to contain malignancy at surgery. The aim of most screening or triaging methods is to minimize the false negative rate. The ideal test will accurately identify malignant nodules. At the same time a benign diagnosis should be equally as accurate to allow for confident exclusion of malignancy. In order to accurately calculate the false negative rate all thyroid nodules found to be benign with FNA would have to undergo surgery to confirm the absence of malignancy. This is impractical because of the large number of surgeries that would be required. Nodules, which are diagnosed as benign by FNA but sent to surgery, usually are selected for other reasons. These might include patient risk factors, rapid growth of the nodule, clinical signs of malignancy or patient anxiety. Those selected for surgery are typically not representatives of the entire group of nodules found to be benign by FNA. Thus it is difficult to know the true false negative rate of the thyroid FNA. In one reported series in which all benign nodules underwent excision the false negative rate was 2.6%.[16] Most believe that the false negative rate for the thyroid FNA is less than 5%.[12] In another large series[12] the false negative rate was 2.4%. However, only 26% of the thyroids felt to be benign by FNA were actually taken to surgery for histologic determination. Using the same data, if one were to assume that all those nodules that did not go to surgery were actually negative (no clinical or other signs of malignancy) then the recalculated false negative rate was 0.6%. Another method employed for determining the false negative rate is to follow patients with adequate FNA specimens diagnosed as benign over extended periods of time to see if they ever develop clinical or other evidence of malignancy. Using this approach benign cytologic diagnoses in a group of patients were followed for a period of 6.1 years and the false negative rate was determined to be 0.7%.[42] A second similar study found a 0.9% false negative rate with an average follow-up of 10 years.[43]

Given an adequately cellular FNA indicating a benign thyroid nodule, how should those patients be followed to assure that the nodule is truly benign? It has been suggested that repeat FNA has a role in the continued non-surgical management in these patients. However, studies that have evaluated this conclude that repeated FNA of the benign nodules continues to provide the same benign diagnosis in 93%–97% of these patients.[11,18,43-45] Most agree that repeat FNA appears necessary only if the nodule enlarges or other clinical features suggesting malignancy occur. Even in these instances the incidence of malignancy is extremely low and the causes of enlargement most frequently are hemorrhage, degeneration with hemorrhage, or unappreciated autonomous function in the nodule.[18] If on repeat FNA suspicious findings are identified the nodule should be treated surgically depending on the cytologic findings.

## Factors Contributing to the False Negative Rate

Multiple studies of the causes of the false negative rate have been performed. All agree that the two most important reasons for falsely negative FNA diagnoses of suspicious thyroid nodules are inadequate sampling and geographic misses of the target nodule.[30,31,32,46] In situations where a nodule is small or where the patient's anatomy makes palpation difficult, using ultrasound guidance of the biopsy needle can reduce geographic misses. Obtaining adequate material via FNA is operator dependent and shown to be significantly better with committed and experienced aspirators.[31,47] The best results are obtained when the cytopathologist performs the aspiration and can assess cellularity at the time of the procedure.[31] In institutions where this service is not available then the specimen is usually not immediately evaluated on site. In this situation the aspirator cannot be entirely certain of the success of each pass and the frequency of inadequate sampling becomes higher.[31] In this situation it has been demonstrated that multiple passes (4–6) improve cellularity.[18] One argument for using local anesthesia at the puncture site is to maintain the patient's cooperation with the multiple passes.[18] In addition the multiple passes should sample the nodule in different areas.[30] If the target is small (1-1.5 cm) then this is less readily accomplished. However, in nodules larger than 1.5 cm, sampling of four distinct regions provides improved cellularity and minimizes non-diagnostic results.[30] Very large targets (>4 cm)

cause yet another problem. These may undergo significant degenerative change in the central region of the nodule. Alternatively, they may contain hemorrhage or even macrophage-filled fluid. The aspiration of the center of these nodules yields the least information. Appropriately, cellular material is best obtained from the periphery of the nodule. Each separate pass should obtain only enough material to make one or two slides when smeared. Making multiple smears from a single pass is discouraged for the material is likely too diluted by blood, degenerated debris or fluid to be helpful. These specimens should not be discarded, but rinsed into RPMI for cell block preparation.[18]

The cytopathologist is very important in minimization of the false negative rate. This is accomplished by strict adherence to criteria for adequate cellularity before offering a benign diagnosis. Analysis of falsely negative FNA diagnoses of thyroid nodules showed that a significant proportion of these occurred when the diagnosis was made on an insufficiently cellular specimen.[32] For a benign diagnosis to be rendered at least 6 clusters of benign follicular cells should be identified on at least two slides prepared from separate passes of the needle.[32]

Finally, being constantly vigilant can reduce the false negative rate. A negative FNA in a patient with other significant risk factors for thyroid malignancy should prompt additional means of confirmation of the diagnosis. Repeat FNA, use of ultrasound guidance to assure the target was sampled, addition of a core needle biopsy or even referral for surgical management should all be considered in these situations.

## Unsatisfactory Specimens

The incidence of unsatisfactory specimens by FNA is minimized when an experienced aspirator performs the FNA and the specimen can be reviewed on-site. The on-site review allows the aspirator to continue sampling until adequate cellularity is obtained. Aspirates obtained in a situation where on-site review is not available may be deemed unsatisfactory because of insufficient cellularity. These FNAs should be repeated as the second procedure will obtain adequate cellularity in greater than 50% of the cases.[41,45,48] Other techniques for improving cellular adequacy should be attempted and include multiple passes to sample different areas of the nodule, sampling the periphery of the nodule, and the use of ultrasound to guide the sampling by the needle to solid areas. Nodules that continue to yield inadequate cellularity by FNA may be sampled with a large core biopsy.[46] The results of such a core biopsy may offer complementary diagnostic information that can impact on the decision for thyroid surgery. If all of these means to obtain adequate cellularity fail, the patient should be considered for thyroid surgery as the incidence of carcinoma occurring in this setting is 10–20%.[48]

## Cysts

Thyroid cysts constitute another technical problem in FNAs of thyroid nodules. When aspirating a cyst the character of the lesion will be evident to the aspirator, as fluid will be obtained. The fluid should be entirely removed and submitted for cytologic evaluation. In most instances the aspiration of cyst fluid results in the disappearance of the nodule. Any residual nodule remaining should be thoroughly sampled with additional needle passes. Evaluation of the cyst fluid usually reveals degenerative debris, blood and pigmented macrophages. These are technically unsatisfactory (non-diagnostic) specimens, as the required follicular cells to meet the criterion of adequacy are usually not obtained. If the cysts do not recur following aspiration the patient can be reassured. However, the presentation of thyroid malignancy can occur in the form of cystic or partially cystic nodules. These are technically challenging and contribute to the false negative rate unless sampled adequately. Criteria identified for selection of cysts for thyroid surgery include cysts yielding fluid-containing malignant cells, or suspicious cells (indeterminate), cysts which recur following at least two aspirations, cysts which do not completely decompress with aspiration and which yield unsatisfactory results with FNA of the residual mass.[49] Using these criteria for selection, up to 32% of these cystic nodules will reveal malignant lesions, 43% follicular adenomas, and 25% colloid nodules.[49] Of these criteria, the finding of malignant cells or suspicious cells in the aspirated fluid provides the most sensitive means of detecting malignancy.[50] The most frequently discovered malignancy in cystic nodules was papillary carcinoma,[50] although follicular carcinoma, medullary carcinoma and importantly anaplastic carcinoma all can present with a cystic component. Malignant lesions are identified at surgery in cystic nodules at a rate comparable to those discovered in solid lesions (14% vs. 23%).[50] However, cysts sent to surgery are selected from a much larger group of cysts that disappear with FNA or which yield diagnostic material confirming benign thyroid conditions. Using this rationale it appears that the incidence of carcinoma in all thyroid cysts is less than 9%.[16] The quality of the fluid aspirated (clear, bloody, thick, brown) bears no relationship to the presence of malignancy.[16,50] Sonography does not offer any specificity in identifying which lesions are malignant. The role of sonography is in guiding needle aspirations of residual nodules remaining after evacuation of cyst fluid. Sonography can assist in identifying mural nodules in the cyst wall, which serve as the target of aspiration.[50]

## False Positive Rate

False positive diagnoses in FNA of thyroid nodules range from 0–10% with most reporting the rate at 3%.[15,16,18,34] This statistic depends on the classification of suspicious/indeterminate FNAs as being equivalent to a malignant diagnosis. With this inclusion the false positive rate is larger, and without, it is reduced.

False positive diagnoses are caused by interpretive errors. Specimen adequacy usually is not a factor, as the specimens tend to be quite cellular. Differentiation of benign papillary fronds of nodular goiter from papillary carcinoma, differentiation of Hürthle cells from Hashimoto's thyroiditis and nodular goiter from Hürthle cell tumors, and the differentiation of benign follicular lesions from follicular carcinoma are all sources for this interpretive error.[18] Most accept the small false positive rate as the rate will be always greater than zero if the focus is on minimizing the false negative rate. The false positive rate, of course, contributes to the total cost of management as these few patients receive surgery for benign lesions. The diagnostic overlap between benign adenomas (follicular and Hürthle cell) and follicular carcinomas and Hürthle cell carcinomas remains as a limitation to FNA diagnosis in the thyroid. Until this discrimination can be refined the false positive rate will remain finite.

## Accuracy

Overall the accuracy of the FNA is quite high (95–97%).[15] When looking at malignant diagnoses the accuracy of the FNA is equivalent to core biopsy and frozen section.[16,51,52]

## How Does the FNA Compare to a Core Biopsy?

Comparison of accuracy rates, false negative rates, false positive rates and yield of insufficient material show that FNA is very comparable to a variety of core biopsy techniques.[16] The major difference between these techniques is the complication rate of the FNA is significantly lower than the core biopsy. It is also cheaper to perform than the core biopsy, and allows for immediate results. However, there are instances where these modalities can be used in conjunction to complement the information provided. On occasion a core biopsy may provide a diagnostic specimen where the FNA result was inadequate. Another valuable combination is in situations where the additional tissue may be used for ancillary studies such as immunocytochemical studies to add specificity to FNA diagnosis.

## How Does the FNA Compare to a Frozen Section?

FNA compares favorably with frozen section diagnosis. Diagnostic accuracy of FNA in benign lesions is 98% while intraoperative frozen section is 97%; for suspicious FNAs the accuracy is 12% while frozen section is 96% and for malignant nodules FNA is close to 98% while intraoperative frozen section is 76%.[51] These results suggest that frozen section may not add any useful information when the FNA diagnosis is benign or malignant. Frozen section is complementary in situations of indeterminate (suspicious) or unsatisfactory FNA results. The use of FNA can generate cost savings by reducing some of the frozen sections performed.

## COST-EFFECTIVENESS

Of the modalities currently available FNA is the most sensitive, accurate and cost-effective method of screening thyroid nodules.[1,11,14-16,18,24,34] Studies have compared management algorithms prior to the advent of routine FNA to those utilizing FNA as the first test for evaluating thyroid nodules. All have demonstrated that the use of FNA has resulted in a 45% decrease in the number of thyroid nodules being referred for surgery and a doubling of the yield of thyroid malignancy in those with thyroidectomies.[1,11,14,15] This was calculated to be equivalent to a 25% reduction in the cost of managing a thyroid nodule. In centers using on-site evaluation of thyroid FNAs, preliminary diagnoses can be used to schedule management and eliminate unnecessary tests. A reduction in the total number of actual patient visits can also be achieved. The impact on the patient's perception of the service provided is significant. Patients can be informed of results immediately and involved in the decisions necessary for subsequent management. Finally, FNA can significantly reduce the need for intraoperative frozen sections, again contributing to its cost-effectiveness.[11,15,52]

## PALPABLE NODULES VERSUS NON-PALPABLE NODULES

Ultrasonography is a sensitive method for detecting thyroid nodules and is superior to palpation.[53] Palpation is most reliable when the nodule is 1.0 cm in diameter or greater and located in a region readily accessible to palpation. Ultrasound can resolve non-palpable nodules as small as 1–3 mm in diameter.[5,53] However because of the high prevalence of benign, asymptomatic thyroid nodules in the general population (up to 67% of patients prospectively studied with ultrasound[5]) general screening with ultrasound is not recommended. On occasion, ultrasound or CT scan studies of the neck (performed for reasons other than evaluation of the thyroid) may demonstrate a thyroid nodule.[5,6] These asymptomatic "incidentalomas" are usually less than 1.0–1.5 cm in dimension. The prevalence of occult malignancy in these non-palpable nodules is low (3.9%).[5] Most of the occult thyroid malignancy that does occur is papillary carcinoma, a very indolent cancer.[5,11] If on retrospective clinical exam the incidentaloma is palpable, then routine FNA of the nodule is recommended. If the nodule is nonpalpable and the patient has a history of multiple endocrine neoplasia or has had prior radiation of the neck, then the FNA under ultrasound guidance is recommended as the first means of analysis.[5] Otherwise the incidentaloma can be followed conservatively and sampled if it becomes palpable or if there are other clinical or ultrasonic evidence of potential malignancy.

## THE ROLE OF THE CYTOPATHOLOGIST

The successful screening of thyroid nodules for infrequent malignancies is clearly a team effort. It is predicated upon accurate clinical evaluation, skillful FNA of the nodule and accurate interpretation of the cytologic specimen. The sensitivity and specificity, the accuracy and the false negative rates are all critically dependent on the expertise of this team. Communication between all members of the team is important to interpretation of the results of the FNA and their application to the accurate and successful management of the patient. The cytopathologist who is trained in the performance and interpretation of the thyroid FNA offers one of the best methods for maximizing the success and application of this technique.

## References

1. Hamberger B, Gharib H, Melton LJ et al. Fine-needle aspiration biopsy of thyroid nodules: impact on thyroid practice and cost of care. *Am J Med.* 1982;73:381–384.
2. Vander JB, Gatson EA, Dawber TR. The significance of nontoxic thyroid nodules. Final report of a 15 year study of the incidence of thyroid malignancy. *Ann Intern Med.* 1968;69:537.
3. Rojeski MT, Gharib H. Nodular thyroid disease evaluation and management. *N Engl J Med.* 1985;313(7):428.
4. Gharib H, Goellner JR. Evaluation of nodular thyroid disease. *Endocrinol Metab Clin North Am.* 1988;17:511–527.
5. Tan GH, Gharib H. Thyroid incidentalomas: management approaches to nonpalpable nodules discovered incidentally on thyroid imaging. *Ann Intern Med.* 1997;126:226–231.
6. Yousem DM, Huang T, Loevner LA, et al. Clinical and economic impact of incidental thyroid lesions found with CT and MR. *Am J Neuroradiol.* 1997;18:1423–1428.
7. Ezzat S, Sarti DA, Cain DR, et al. Thyroid incidentalomas prevalence by palpation and ultrasonography. *Arch Intern Med.* 1994; 154:1838–1840.

8. Greenlee RT, Hill-Harmon MB, Murray T et al. Cancer statistics, 2001. *CA Cancer J Clin.* 2001;51:15–36.

9. Caplan RH, Kisken WA, Strutt PJ, et al. Fine-needle aspiration biopsy of thyroid nodules: a cost-effective diagnostic approach. *Postgrad Med.* 1991;90:183–190.

10. Wool MS. Thyroid nodules: the place of fine-needle aspiration biopsy in management. *Postgrad Med.* 1993;94:111–122.

11. Mazzaferri EL, Santos ET, Rofagha-Keyhani S. Solitary thyroid nodule: diagnosis and management. *Med Clin North Am.* 1988;72(5):1177–1210.

12. Gharib H, Goellner JR. Fine-needle aspiration biopsy of the thyroid: an appraisal. *Ann Intern Med.* 1993;118:282–289.

13. Gharib H. Fine-needle aspiration biopsy of thyroid nodules: advantages, limitations, and effect. *Mayo Clin Proc.* 1994;69:44–49.

14. Van Herle AJ, Rich P, Ljung BE, et al. The thyroid nodule. *Ann Intern Med.* 1982;96:221–232.

15. Gharib H. Changing Concepts in the diagnosis and management of thyroid nodules. *Endocrin Metabol Clin N Am.* 1997;26(4):777–800.

16. Ashcraft MW, Van Herle AJ. Management of thyroid nodules. II: scanning techniques, thyroid suppressive therapy, and fine needle aspiration. *Head Neck Surg.* 1981;3:297–322.

17. Akerman M, Tennval J, Biorklund A, et al. Sensitivity and specificity of fine needle aspiration cytology in the diagnosis of tumors of thyroid gland. *Acta Cytol.* 1985;29(5):850–854.

18. Hamburger JI, Hamberger SW. Fine needle biopsy of thyroid nodules: avoiding the pitfalls. *NY State J Med.* 1986;86:241–249.

19. Hawkins F, Bellido D, Bernal C, et al. Fine needle aspiration biopsy in the diagnosis of thyroid cancer and thyroid disease. *Cancer.* 1987;59(6):1206–1209.

20. Gagneten CB, Roccatagliata G, Lowenstein A, et al. The role of fine needle aspiration biopsy cytology in the evaluation of the clinically solitary thyroid nodule. *Acta Cytol.* 1987;31(5):595–598.

21. Anderson JB, Webb AJ. Fine-needle aspiration biopsy and the diagnosis of thyroid cancer. *Br J Surg.* 1987;74:292–296.

22. Wetzig NR, Giddings AE. Solitary thyroid nodule: audit shows improved care requires cytological diagnosis. *Ann R Coll Surg Engl.* 1989;71:316–319.

23. Mazzaferri E. Management of a solitary thyroid nodule. *N Engl J Med.* 1993;328(8):553–559.

24. Gharib H, Goellner JR, Johnson DA, et al. Fine-needle aspiration cytology of the thyroid: a 12-year experience with 11,000 biopsies. *Clin Lab Med.* 1993;13(3):699–709.

25. Woeber K. Cost-effective evaluation of the patient with a thyroid nodule. *Surg Clin N Amer.* 1995;75(3):357–363.

26. Lioe TF, Elliott H, Allen DC, et al. A 3-year audit of thyroid fine needle aspirates. *Cytopath* 1998;9:188–192.

27. Nguyen G, Ginsberg J, Crockford PM, et al. Fine-needle aspiration biopsy cytology of the thyroid its value and limitations in the diagnosis and management of solitary thyroid nodules. *Pathol Ann.* 1991;26(1):63–91.

28. Suen K, Abdul-Karim FW, Kaminsky DB, et al. FNA of the thyroid: Guidelines of the Papanicolaou Society of Cytopathology for the examination of fine-needle aspiration specimens from thyroid nodules. *Modern Path.* 1996;9(6):710–715.

29. Ramacciotti CE, Pretorius HT, Chu EW, et al. Diagnostic accuracy and use of aspiration biopsy in the management of thyroid nodules. *Arch Intern Med.* 1984;144:1169–1173.

30. Musgrave YM, Davey DD, Weeks JA, et al. Assessment of fine-needle aspiration sampling technique in thyroid nodules. *Diag Cytopath.* 1998;18(1):76–80.

31. Hall, TL, Layfield LJ, Philippe A, et al. Sources of diagnostic error in fine needle aspiration of the thyroid. *Cancer.* 1989;63:718–725.

32. Hamburger JI, Husain M, Nishiyama R, et al. Increasing the accuracy of fine-needle biopsy for thyroid nodules. *Arch Pathol Lab Med.* 1989;113:1035–1041.

33. Burch HB, Burman KD, Reed HL, et al. Fine needle aspiration of thyroid nodules. Determinants of insufficiency rate and malignancy yield at thyroidectomy. *Acta Cytol.* 1996;40(6):1176–1183.

34. Caruso D, Mazzaferri EL. Fine needle aspiration biopsy in the management of thyroid nodules. *Endocrinologist.* 1991;1(3):194–202.

35. Ravinsky E, Safneck JR. Fine needle aspirates of folliclar lesions of the thyroid gland the intermediate-type smear. *Acta Cytol.* 1990;34(6):813–820.

36. Caraway NP, Sneige N, Samaan NA. Diagnositc pitfalls in thyroid fine-needle aspiration: a review of 394 cases. *Diag Cytopath.* 1993;9(3):345–350.

37. Inohara H, Honjo Y, Yoshii T, et al. Expression of galectin-3 in fine-needle aspirates as a diagnostic marker differentiating benign from malignant thyroid neoplasms. *Cancer.* 85(11) 2000;2475–2484.

38. Orlandi F, Saggiorato E, Pivano G, et al. Galectin-3 is a presurgical marker of human thyroid carcinoma *Cancer Res.* 1998;58:3015–3020.

39. Bartolaszzi A. Improving accuracy of cytology for nodular thyroid lesions. *Lancet.* 2000;355:1661–1662.

40. Gasbarri A, Martegani MP, Prete FD et al. Galectin-3 and CD44v6 isoforms in the preoperative evaluation of thyroid nodules. *J Clin Oncol.* 1999;17(11):3494–3502.

41. Goellner JR, Gharib H, Grant CS, et al. Fine needle aspiration cytology of the thyroid, 1980 to 1986. *Acta Cytol.* 1987;31(5):587–590.

42. Grant CS, Hay ID, Gouch IR, et al. Long-term follow-up of patients with benign thyroid fine-needle aspiration cytologic diagnoses. *Surgery.* 1989;106(6):980–986.

43. Kuma K, Matsuzuka F, Yokozawa T, et al. Fate of untreated benign thyroid nodules: results of long-term follow-up. *World J Surg.* 1994;18, 495–499.

44. Dwarakanthan AA, Staren ED, D'Amore MJ, et al. Importance of repeat fine-needle biopsy in the management of thyroid nodules. *Am J Surg.* 1993;166:350–352.

45. Van Hoeven KH, Gupta PK, LiVolsi VA. Value of repeat fine needle aspiration (FNA) of the thyroid. *Mod Path.* 1994;7:43A.

46. Boey J, Hsu C, Collins RJ, et al. False-negative errors in fine-needle aspiration biopsy of dominant thyroid nodules: a prospective follow-up study. *World J Surg.* 1986;10:623-630.

47. Dwarakanthan AA, Ryan WG, Staren ED, et al. Fine-needle aspiration biopsy of the thyroid: diagnostic accuracy when performing a moderate number of such procedures. *Arch Intern Med.* 1989;149;2007–2009.

48. McHenry CR, Walfish PG, Rosen IB, et al. Non-diagnostic fine needle aspiration biopsy: a dilemma in management of nodular thyroid disease. *Am Surg.* 1993;59:415–419.

49. Rosen IB, Provias JP, Walfish PG, et al. Pathologic nature of cystic thyroid nodules selected for surgery by needle aspiration biopsy. *Surgery.* 1986;100(4):606–613.

50. De los Santos ET, Keyhani-Rofagha S, Cunningham JJ, et al. Cystic thyroid nodules: the dilemma of malignant lesions. *Arch Intern Med.* 1990;150:1422–1427.

51. Rodriguez JM, Parrilla P, Sola J, et al. Comparison between preoperative cytology and intraoperative frozen-section biopsy in the diagnosis of thyroid nodules. *Br J Surg.* 1994;81:1151–1154.

52. Bugis SP, Young JE, Archibald SD, et al. Diagnostic accuracy of fine-needle aspiration biopsy versus frozen section in solitary thyroid nodules. *Am J Surg.* 1986;152:411–416.

53. Tan GH, Gharib H, Reading CC, et al. Solitary thyroid nodule comparison between palpation and ultrasonography. *Arch Intern Med.* 1995;155:2418–2423.

# 9

# Thyroidectomy

John I. Song, M.D.
Eugene N. Myers, M.D., F.A.C.S.

## HISTORICAL BACKGROUND

The thyroid gland derives its name from the Greek *thyreos* or shield because of its shape. By the mid-1800s, physicians including Graves, von Basedow, and Curling began describing the classic symptoms of hyper- and hypothyroidism and began associating them with abnormalities of the thyroid gland. The importance of this gland in the disease process was subsequently proven by the work of surgeons who produced experimental myxedema in dogs by thyroidectomy and treated this condition successfully with thyroid extracts[1].

It was not until the 19th century that thyroidectomy became safe to perform as a result of the development of reliable general anesthesia. Billroth and his associates began performing thyroidectomy in the 1860s, but it is Theodor Kocher, who did not operate on the thyroid gland until years after Billroth, who is regarded as the founder of modern thyroid surgery. He performed several thousand thyroidectomies in the late 1800s with an astonishingly low mortality rate of less than 5%. In 1909, Kocher received the Nobel Prize for his pioneering work in this challenging field. In fact, the demands of this operation were such that surgical giants such as Crile, Lahey, and the Mayo brothers made their respective reputations based, in large part, on their ability to perform thyroidectomy safely.

Despite tremendous advances in surgical technique in the last century, the technical challenges of this operation continue to demand that the surgeon be familiar with the anatomy of the gland and its associated neurovascular structures, in order to manage the surgical problems of the thyroid gland successfully. In this chapter we will review the pertinent surgical anatomy of the gland and its surrounding structures, describe the surgical techniques for several commonly performed thyroid procedures, and discuss some of the pitfalls of operating in this area.

## SURGICAL ANATOMY

A complete review of the embryology and anatomy of the thyroid gland can be found elsewhere in this text. Anatomic highlights pertinent to the successful performance of a thyroidectomy will be discussed:

1. The average gland weighs 15–20 grams and is covered by a thick fibrous capsule (true capsule) that sends septae into the substance of the gland to form pseudo-lobulations. A thinner fascia (false capsule) derived from the pretracheal layer of deep cervical fascia can also be found covering the gland.

2. The sternohyoid and sternothyroid muscles overlie the thyroid gland in the midline. These muscles are fused to the medial border of the sternocleido mastoid muscle (SCM) by the superficial layer of deep cervical fascia. Exposure of the thyroid gland requires dividing the midline fascia between the strap muscles. Additional exposure may be required in some cases and is obtained by dividing the attach-

ment between the strap muscles and SCM, or by dividing the strap muscles. If division of the strap muscles is required, this should be done superiorly so as to preserve the motor supply (ansa hypoglossus) that enters the muscles inferiorly.

3. The fascial covering of the thyroid gland is thickened posteriorly to form a posterior suspensory ligament [(PSL) or Berry's ligament]. The PSL extends from an area between the cricoid cartilage and the first two tracheal rings to the posteromedial aspect of each lobe and forms an attachment of the thyroid gland to the larynx and trachea. The PSL has several important relationships with the neurovascular bundle with which the surgeon must be familiar in order to avoid injuring these structures. The recurrent laryngeal nerve (RLN) will often pass deep to the PSL, but may sometimes pass between the main ligament and its lateral leaf. Any traction on the PSL may therefore cause inadvertent injury to the nerve.

4. The anterior jugular veins overlie the sternohyoid muscles and may send communicating branches to either side and to the external jugular veins laterally. The anterior jugular veins may be quite engorged in some patients and great care should be taken when dividing the midline fascia between the strap muscles in order to maintain optimal hemostasis.

5. The deep veins of the thyroid gland have an inconsistent relationship to the arterial system. Numerous deep veins anastomose within the substance of the thyroid gland and form a large plexus on the capsule. The inferior thyroid vein often has several branches that form a plexus near the posterior suspensory ligament and recurrent laryngeal nerve. The wall of these veins can be extremely thin, especially in older patients, and can bleed easily risking injury to the recurrent nerve while attempting to obtain hemostasis. Once clamped and transected, these fragile veins may be avulsed if the hemostat is pulled too hard. This may lead to bleeding in the postoperative period.

6. The inferior thyroid artery (ITA) has an intimate but variable relationship to the recurrent laryngeal nerve. The ITA will often branch before entering the gland and one or both branches may pass deep to the PSL or just inferior to it. Injury to the RLN can occur while attempting to achieve hemostasis. The PSL may itself contain thyroid tissue or a posteromedial portion of the gland may be located deep to the ligament. Attempting to remove this thyroid tissue can also result in injury to the nerve.

7. The superior thyroid artery (STA) will descend over the inferior constrictor muscle to enter the superior pole of the thyroid at its anteromedial surface. The superior laryngeal nerve (SLN) will divide into an internal sensory branch and an external motor branch at the level of the cornu of the hyoid. The SLN will have a variable relationship with the STA but tends to run medially and superiorly to the artery or may be intertwined with it. Approximately 1 cm cephalad to the entry of the STA into the thyroid, the SLN will enter the larynx to innervate the cricothyroid muscle. Attempts to ligate the STA above its site of entry into the superior pole may result in injury to the SLN.

8. The thyroid ima artery occurs in 10% of patients and arises either from the aorta or the innominate artery to provide the blood supply to the inferior portion of the thyroid gland. The thyroid ima artery can cause significant and troublesome hemorrhage if encountered inferiorly in the sternal notch.

9. The RLN passes posterior to the carotid sheath after arising from the vagus nerve bilaterally. At the level of the ITA, the RLN can pass into the tracheoesophageal (TE) groove or lie 1–2 cm lateral to the trachea. In one study, the right RLN was found in the TE groove in 64% of the patients, while the left RLN was in the TE groove in 77%.[1] The RLN was lateral to the trachea in 33% of patients on the right side while only 22% of patients on the left.[1]

10. The RLN will pass posterior to the ITA but can be anterior to the artery in a third of the patients. The RLN enters the larynx between the cricoid cartilage and the inferior cornu of the thyroid cartilage. In most cases, the RLN does not divide below the level of the ITA. In rare instances where the RLN is not recurrent because of an abnormal retroesophageal subclavian artery, the laryngeal nerve will emerge from the vagus in close proximity to the superior thyroid artery.[2]

## SURGICAL TECHNIQUE

The successful thyroid surgeon should have in his/her armamentarium at least four techniques for addressing thyroid disease. These techniques include:

1. Thyroid lobectomy
2. Subtotal thyroidectomy
3. Total thyroidectomy
4. Substernal thyroidectomy

In addition, the neck must be addressed when there is evidence of cervical metastasis or if the primary thyroid tumor is a high grade malignancy.

### Airway Management

We perform these operations under general anesthesia after appropriate preoperative evaluation and consultation by the anesthesia and medical teams. In the case of a very large goiter or a substantial thyroid gland, the airway may be partially narrowed by compression or the trachea may be displaced because of mass effect[3]. Despite these concerns, endotracheal intubation can be safely and effectively carried out in the vast majority of cases, and we discourage the routine use of more complex anesthetic techniques as unnecessarily time-consuming and increasing the risk to the patient.

One exception to our airway philosophy involves a new technique currently being used at the Department of Otolaryngology, University of Pittsburgh School of Medicine, for selected cases. This technique utilizes laryngeal mask anesthesia (LMA) and a fiberoptic endoscope[4]. The endoscope is placed through the slot in the laryngeal mask just superior to the level of the glottis. The true vocal cords are visualized on a monitor placed opposite the surgeon. During the procedure, structures that may represent recurrent laryngeal nerves can be stimulated while the glottis is visualized. Identification and preservation of the recurrent laryngeal nerve is enhanced with this approach because, unlike other systems that rely upon completing electric contacts on the surface of a modified endotracheal tube, the LMA technique allows direct visualization of the true vocal cords while the recurrent laryngeal nerve is being stimulated.

## Operative Preparation

After endotracheal intubation, the patient is placed in a supine position. The planning of the incision takes into account the size and position of the thyroid mass and the length and width of the patient's neck. Incision planning should be done prior to placing the patient into extension in order to have the scar in the neck rather than being placed on top of the clavicle or on the chest. We prefer an incision approximately one finger-breath above the clavicle so that the scar does not come to rest below the clavicle where it can cause a stretched or prominent scar that will not be successfully camouflaged (Figure 9–1). In a patient with a longer, slender neck, the incision will have to be placed more superiorly to gain access to the gland. In these cases, it is even more important that a suitable natural skin crease be used in order to maximize cosmesis. The incision is designed to extend approximately 1–2 cm lateral to the medial border of the sternocleidomastoid muscle.

Placing a rolled sheet under the shoulder blades places the patient's neck into moderate extension thereby bringing the thyroid gland into a more accessible position in the neck. The head is placed into a soft donut holder to ensure stability of the head during surgery. The surgical area is then prepped with povidone-iodine solution and sterile drapes are stapled to the surgical field.

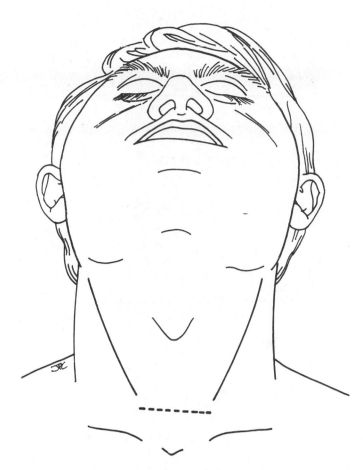

**Figure 9–1.** The incision is placed approximately one finger-breath above the clavicle. (Reprinted with permission—Myers EN [ed]: *Operative Otolaryngology Head and Neck Surgery.* 1997; Philadelphia: WB Saunders, p. 542.)

## Elevation of Flaps

The incision is carried through the platysma muscle and the flaps are elevated superiorly and inferiorly between the platysma and strap muscles. The anterior jugular veins and their midline anastomosing plexus are encountered in this plane. Great care should be taken to avoid injuring these structures in order to maintain optimal hemostasis. Small vessels can be electrocoagulated and larger vessels should be clamped, transected and ligated with 2-0 silk sutures. The strap muscles are separated in the midline and undermined to give adequate exposure laterally (Figures 9–2 and 9–3). A thyroid or Mayhorner retractor together with Wheatlander retractors is used to retract the flaps (Figure 9–2) and Green retractors are used to retract the strap muscles laterally.

This approach provides excellent exposure to the thyroid gland and surrounding structures. The strap muscles can be divided to provide additional expo-

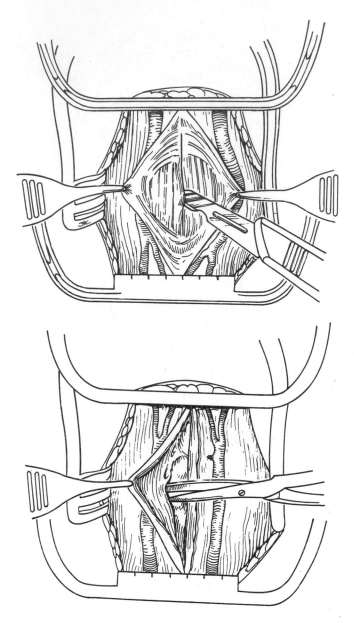

**Figures 9–2 and 9–3.** The strap muscles are divided in the midline and undermined bilaterally. (Reprinted with permission—Myers EN [ed]: *Operative Otolaryngology Head and Neck Surgery.* 1997; Philadelphia: WB Saunders, p. 543.)

sure, although in our experience this is rarely required. When it is necessary, the strap muscles are divided in their superior aspect to avoid injuring the ansa hypoglossus nerve that enters the muscle inferiorly. This maneuver preserves the innervation of the strap muscles. Additional exposure can be gained by dividing the superficial layer of deep cervical fascia between the strap muscles and medial border of the SCM allowing further lateral retraction of the SCM.

## Thyroid Lobectomy

After the flaps are elevated, the thyroid gland is carefully palpated to determine if any other additional masses are present in both the ipsilateral and contralateral lobes. The trachea is identified and the area of the cricothyroid membrane is bluntly dissected to reveal the superior extent of the thyroid isthmus (Figure 9–4). We divide the isthmus at this point to provide increased mobility of the gland; however, the isthmus can also be divided after the lobectomy has been completed. The isthmus is cross-clamped, divided, and the edges over sewn with 2-0 silk sutures. In cases where the nodule is arising from the isthmus, only the isthmus is removed if frozen sections indicate a benign process. Otherwise, the isthmus should be ligated toward the contralateral lobe. The thyroid lobe is dissected free from the surrounding strap muscles and pretracheal fascia bluntly using a Kittner sponge. The lobe is carefully mobilized into the surgical field (Figure 9–5). Continued blunt dissection along the lateral and posterior surface of the lobe is used to identify the parathyroid glands.

The parathyroid glands can be differentiated from the surrounding areolar fat and thyroid tissue by its brownish, caramel, or tan appearance (quail's egg) and its oblong and flattened shape. When placed in saline the denser parathyroid glands will sink while adipose tissue will float. This is a helpful differential point in identification of the parathyroid glands. Both the superior and inferior parathyroid glands receive their blood supply from branches of the inferior thyroid artery, although the superior glands may receive an additional supply from the superior thyroid artery.[5] The terminal branches of the inferior thyroid artery must be preserved to the level of the thyroid capsule in order to avoid devascularizing the parathyroid glands. A devascularized gland will become very dark in appearance. If this occurs, the parathyroid gland should be confirmed by frozen section before being reimplanted to avoid inadvertently seeding thyroid tumor. Once the parathyroid glands have been identified they are gently separated from the thyroid gland and preserved. This is facilitated by dissecting soft tissues away from the capsule of the thyroid gland. Once the lobe is delivered into the field, the carotid artery is identified by blunt dissection.

The safest approach at this point is to identify the RLN inferiorly in the triangle created by the trachea, carotid artery and inferior pole of the thyroid lobe just superior to the thoracic inlet (Figure 9–6).[5] The RLN can be reliably found in this area. We are staunch advocates of the routine identification of the RLN. Studies have shown that injury to the RLN is higher

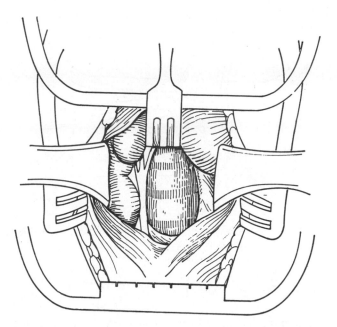

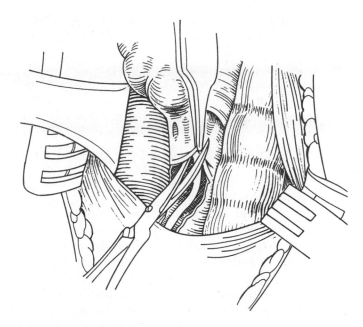

**Figure 9–4.** The trachea is identified and the area of the cricothyroid membrane is bluntly dissected to reveal the superior extent of the thyroid isthmus. The isthmus is divided to increase the mobility of the thyroid lobe. (Reprinted with permission—Myers EN [ed]: *Operative Otolaryngology Head and Neck Surgery.* 1997; Philadelphia: WB Saunders, p. 544.)

**Figure 9–6.** The recurrent laryngeal nerve is most reliably found in the area bordered by the trachea, carotid artery, and the inferior thyroid lobe. Dissection is continued superiorly to the level of the cricothyroid muscle. (Reprinted with permission—Myers EN [ed]: *Operative Otolaryngology Head and Neck Surgery.* 1997; Philadelphia: WB Saunders, p. 546.)

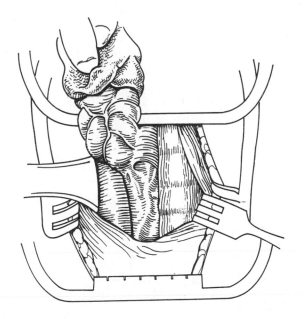

**Figure 9–5.** The thyroid lobe is mobilized into the surgical field. Great care is taken not to place excessive tension on the posterior suspensory ligament as injury to the recurrent laryngeal nerve can occur with this maneuver. (Reprinted with permission—Myers EN [ed]: *Operative Otolaryngology Head and Neck Surgery.* 1997; Philadelphia: WB Saunders, p. 545.)

when routine identification of the nerve is not performed.[6–9] There are many advantages of identifying the nerve inferiorly. As it is traced superiorly, the relationship of the RLN to the inferior thyroid artery and Berry's ligament can be appreciated. The recurrent laryngeal nerve will run from the carotid artery toward the tracheoesophageal sulcus within this triangle.[5] The inferior thyroid artery, on the other hand, tends to have an inconsistent and variable relationship to the nerve and is not a reliable surgical landmark.

Another advantage of identifying the nerve inferiorly is that a non-recurrent laryngeal nerve can be anticipated if the nerve is not found inferiorly. A non-recurrent nerve occurs rarely (less than 1% of patients).[2] The nerve will arise directly from the vagus nerve and may pass anterior to Berry's ligament. On the right, it is associated with an absent innominate artery and a right subclavian artery that arises from the aortic arch and follows a retroesophageal course. A left-sided non-recurrent nerve is associated with Kartagener's syndrome.[10] Some of these patients can be identified preoperatively by barium swallow if a history of dysphagia is elicited, or on the CT scan, which may be performed to visualize the mass in the thyroid gland.

The RLN is dissected free using the closed tip of a dissecting scissors. Overlying small branches of the inferior thyroid vein, as well as branches of the inferior thyroid artery, should be clamped, divided and suture ligated to prevent subsequent hemorrhage that can result in inadvertent injury to the RLN in the process of obtaining hemostasis. Some authors advocate the use of a bipolar electrocautery to divide the small venous branches near the nerve.[11] We feel that this technique unnecessarily introduces the risk of thermal or electrical injury to the nerve even at low power. Careful dissection and ligation of the appropriate vessels provides the safest method of achieving hemostasis around the nerve.

The recurrent laryngeal nerve is dissected in a superior direction by dividing the overlying tissue over closed scissors until the nerve can be seen entering the larynx at the level of the cricoid cartilage and the inferior cornu of the thyroid cartilage. The lobe is gently retracted medially to provide traction on the posterior suspensory ligament (Berry's ligament). This maneuver can be done safely only after the RLN is completely identified, otherwise the traction placed on Berry's ligament can injure the nerve. When dissecting around the posterior suspensory ligament, one should keep in mind the relationship of the RLN and inferior thyroid vessels to the ligament. The RLN usually passes posterior (deep) to Berry's ligament, but this relationship is variable and the nerve can pass anterior to, inferior to, or even through the ligament. The ligament is transected close to the posterior thyroid capsule, freeing the gland from the trachea. This will greatly increase the mobility of the lobe.

Dissection along the true capsule of the thyroid is now continued superiorly until the lobe is pedicled on the superior thyroid vessels (Figure 9–7). The artery and vein are bluntly dissected from the surrounding tissues close to the true capsule of the thyroid. The superior laryngeal nerve usually enters the larynx 1 cm cephalad to the entrance of the artery, and keeping the dissection close to the thyroid capsule will ensure that the nerve is not injured. Indiscriminate clamping of the superior vessels will result in injury to the superior laryngeal nerve. The superior thyroid vessels are individually dissected and identified near the thyroid capsule before they are clamped with a right-angle clamp, divided, and doubly-ligated with 2-0 silk sutures. Injury to the superior laryngeal nerve is minimized with this technique by ligating the vessels at the level of the thyroid capsule and leaving the dissection of the superior vessels as the last step prior to delivering the thyroid lobe.

The pathologist is invited into the operating room and the lobe is delivered for frozen section analysis. Closure of the wound should begin at this point if there is a strong suspicion of a benign nodule based upon intraoperative evaluation. By the time the wound is

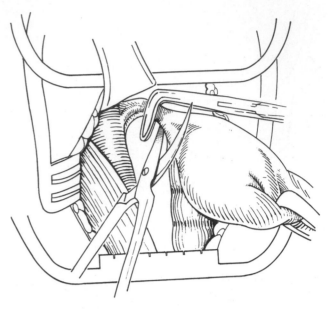

**Figure 9–7.** The thyroid lobe is pedicled to the superior thyroid vessels. Ligation of the superior vessels is done close to the thyroid capsule to avoid injuring the superior laryngeal nerve. (Reprinted with permission—Myers EN [ed]: *Operative Otolaryngology Head and Neck Surgery.* 1997; Philadelphia: WB Saunders, p. 547.)

closed, the results of the frozen section diagnosis should be available. If the diagnosis is benign the operation is complete. If the diagnosis is malignant the wound can be reopened in seconds, and the total thyroidectomy completed. This is much more "time efficient" than waiting for the diagnosis before closing.

Hemostasis is achieved and the surgical field is copiously irrigated with saline solution. Maintenance of meticulous hemostasis during thyroidectomy cannot be overemphasized. It is our policy to carefully clamp and tie all bleeding vessels prior to proceeding with the next step. The use of electrocautery, even bipolar electrocautery, should be avoided near the RLN. Small amounts of oozing near the recurrent laryngeal nerve is best managed conservatively at this point to prevent injury. Rather than attempting to use a bipolar electrocautery or clamping near the exposed nerve, gelfoam, surgi-cel or Avitene can be used over the area. Most oozing from small veins will stop spontaneously, and we strongly discourage steps that put the nerve at risk.

We routinely drain all wounds with Hemovac drains, although some authors have not reported any differences in postoperative complications in groups without drains.[12] A small Hemovac drain is placed through a separate stab incision 1 cm lateral to the surgical incision and brought into the thyroid compartment. The overlying strap muscles are reapproximated at the midline with chromic suture. This will prevent adhesions from forming between the flap and the larynx that will cause an unsightly tethering of the skin which will move with deglutition. The incision is closed with chromic suture subcutaneously and a continuous 6-0 mild chromic suture. Mastisol adhesive is applied and the incision is covered with Steri-Strip surgical tapes. A compressive dressing may be applied if the thyroid compartment (dead space) is significant or if the patient has a large neck. Otherwise, a small, light dressing is sufficient. The patient is recovered from general anesthesia with a minimum of bucking, extubated, and taken to the recovery room.

## Subtotal Thyroidectomy

The indications for a total vs. subtotal thyroidectomy are somewhat controversial. Most surgeons agree that a total thyroidectomy should be performed when there is obvious bilateral involvement, extrathyroidal or metastatic disease, or a significant history of head and neck irradiation.[11,13–14] But the extent of surgery for a well-differentiated tumor that is limited to the unilateral thyroid lobe is the subject of much debate. A subtotal or near-total thyroidectomy can at least theoretically decrease the risk of injury to the recurrent laryngeal nerve and parathyroid glands by minimizing the dissection in the contralateral tracheoesophageal groove.[15] The goal of this procedure is to remove all but a few grams of thyroid tissue along the posterior aspect of the contralateral lobe and to protect the integrity of the nerve.

Advocates of subtotal thyroidectomy argue that overall survival and recurrence rates for well-differentiated thyroid carcinomas are not different for total vs. subtotal procedures. They also argue that contralateral small (< 1.5 cm) occult foci of papillary carcinoma do not have clinical significance and are not likely to be the focus of recurrent disease.[16–18] While these are interesting points, we feel the advantages of a total thyroidectomy outweigh the potential risks of this procedure.

By removing the gland en bloc, total thyroidectomy will reduce the chance of recurrent disease. Although the recurrence rates may arguably be small in the majority of well-differentiated thyroid carcinomas, complication rates for re-exploration and reoperation remain significant. Also, removal of all residual thyroid tissue facilitates the detection and treatment of metastatic disease with radioiodine and allows the use of thyroglobulin as a marker in follow-up.[19] Finally, in experienced hands, complication rates for a total thyroidectomy are no different than for subtotal procedures. We have not used the technique of subtotal thyroidectomy in our department.

## Total Thyroidectomy

Frozen section diagnosis of a well-differentiated thyroid carcinoma necessitates that a total thyroidectomy is carried out. The technique is identical to the unilateral lobectomy, but special attention must be placed in identifying and preserving the parathyroid glands. The inferior thyroid artery and recurrent laryngeal nerve can serve as useful landmarks in identifying the inferior parathyroid glands. The inferior thyroid artery can also be used to identify the superior parathyroid glands, although it can also get arterial supply from the superior thyroid artery.

In cases of FNA-proven thyroid carcinoma or total thyroidectomy for hyperthyroidism, the technique for a total thyroidectomy is modified to include the entire gland as an en bloc resection. The isthmus is not divided (as described for a lobectomy) and the recurrent laryngeal nerve is identified as previously described. The inferior thyroid artery is ligated and the lobe is mobilized by identifying and ligating the posterior suspensory ligament. The superior thyroid artery is then ligated. The entire procedure is repeated on the contralateral side. The dissection is carried medially over the trachea to connect to the opposite side and the entire gland is removed en bloc.

A central compartment (zone VI) node dissection is performed routinely in cases of differentiated thyroid carcinoma. If there is no palpable nodal disease beyond zone VI, no further neck dissection is needed in the treatment of well-differentiated carcinomas. Any palpable or radiographically suspicious cervical nodes should be addressed by a modified neck dissection sparing all normal structures.

The goal of a total thyroidectomy for thyroid carcinoma is to remove as thoroughly as possible any vestiges of thyroid tissue that may harbor residual thyroid cancer or act as an "iodine sink" which makes postoperative $^{121}$I or $^{131}$I scanning and treatment more complex.[20–22] Studies have shown that as little as 5 mg of thyroid tissue can effectively sequester standard doses of radioiodine scanning.[20,21] Aggressive management of medullary carcinoma including total laryngectomy, sacrifice of involved recurrent laryngeal nerves and sternotomy to resect mediastinal disease is more likely to result in a cure.[23,24] Similarly, the rare circumstance of undifferentiated carcinomas less than 2 cm without extracapsular spread can be effectively treated with aggressive surgical management.[25]

The management of well-differentiated thyroid carcinoma with local invasion into the trachea, larynx, esophagus or recurrent laryngeal nerve remains controversial. In patients with limited involvement of the tracheal cartilage, there is no consensus as to how much of the involved trachea should be resected.

Some authors have advocated a cartilage-shaving technique.[25,26] In one study of 124 patients with laryngotracheal invasion by well-differentiated thyroid carcinoma, the survival rates of patients who underwent shave excision were not different from those who had radical resection if gross tumor did not remain.[27] The authors advocated a shaving technique if there was minimal tumor invasion, but recommended complete resection if gross intraluminal involvement was seen.[27] Others have advocated a more aggressive resection of the trachea arguing that locally invasive thyroid carcinoma probably has a more aggressive biological nature and will have a greater tendency to recur. In cases of invasion of the larynx, we feel a partial laryngeal resection should be employed whenever possible, but the surgeon should have the patient's permission to remove the entire larynx in advanced cases. Management of recurrent disease with postoperative radioiodine therapy, external beam radiation, and salvage surgery has had disappointing results so we recommend an initial aggressive surgical approach whenever feasible.

Managing the recurrent laryngeal nerve that is infiltrated or surrounded by tumor should take into consideration the age of the patient, the function of both recurrent nerves, and tumor type. For medullary carcinoma, any nerves involved with tumor should be sacrificed in order to obtain complete excision.[24] With well-differentiated tumors in children, an attempt should be made to preserve a functioning recurrent nerve.[11] Any residual tumor in these cases can be treated with postoperative radioiodine therapy. In adults, a recurrent nerve that is encased by tumor should be sacrificed after the function of the opposite nerve has been verified. We advocate thyroplasty at the time of resection in order to preserve the voice and swallowing. If both nerves are involved with tumor, an effort should be made to preserve one functioning nerve with the goal of treating any residual tumor with radioiodine therapy. With anaplastic cancer heroic measures including the sacrifice of normal structures should be discouraged, since more aggressive surgery which may result in loss of function cannot be justified by an improvement in overall survival rates.

## Substernal Thyroidectomy

Most substernal thyroid glands can be removed from a cervical approach. Preoperative imaging and FNA tissue diagnosis should be used to anticipate a thyroid carcinoma that may be adherent to surrounding vital structures. In these cases, median sternotomy should be used to gain access and control of major vascular structures.

Whenever possible, the patient with a substernal goiter should be placed into extreme extension in order to facilitate mobilizing the gland superiorly out of the mediastinum. The gland is mobilized and the recurrent laryngeal nerves are identified bilaterally. Both superior and inferior thyroid arteries are ligated. Before attempting to mobilize the substernal goiter, the entire gland must be freed from the underlying larynx and trachea by ligating the posterior suspensory ligament bilaterally. In some instances, dividing the isthmus in the midline can also facilitate mobilizing the cervical thyroid.

The surgeon then places his/her finger or a Kittner sponge into the superior mediastinum with the mobilized gland being used to place superior traction on the substernal goiter. Careful dissection around the capsule of the thyroid will free the inferior extent of the gland and allow it to be retracted out of the mediastinum. Additional retraction with ring forceps can facilitate dissection of the inferior-most aspect of the thyroid gland. In some large goiters, the inferior pole of the thyroid may need to be freed from the substernal component and the mediastinal mass removed as a separate specimen.

## SUMMARY

In many ways, the challenges of thyroid surgery remain the same since the time that surgeons first successfully removed the gland in the early 19th century. Key points in preventing complications in thyroid surgery include: thorough preoperative evaluation and radiographic assessment; a thorough understanding of the anatomy of the thyroid gland, including the relationships of the thyroid vessels, recurrent laryngeal nerve, and posterior suspensory ligament; routine identification of the recurrent laryngeal nerve inferiorly within the supra-sternal triangle; maintaining the surgical plane close to the thyroid capsule; identification and preservation of parathyroid glands; and achieving meticulous hemostasis.

When these details are followed, the complication rates will be quite low and risks for a total thyroidectomy will not differ significantly from a less than total procedure. We feel that the oncologic advantages of an en bloc resection warrants the complete removal of all thyroid tissue whenever possible. Having said this, there is no substitute for experience and each surgeon operating on the thyroid gland must make his/her own clinical assessment of the risks involved. The risks of a total thyroidectomy are very real in inexperienced hands. If there is any possibility that the laryngeal nerves or parathyroid glands would be at increased risk if a total thyroidectomy were per formed, a less than total procedure would be the better part of valor. Unfortunately, this kind of surgical decision-making cannot be taught and can only come from years of carefully treading where surgical giants like Kocher have already walked.

## References

1. Schwartz SI. The thyroid gland. In: *Principles of Surgery*, ed. 7. 1999; New York: McGraw-Hill.
2. Wijetilaka SE. Non-recurrent laryngeal nerve. *Br J Surg.* 1978;65(3):179–81.
3. Hinnie J, Lafferty M, Vasey P, Milroy R. A case of acute respiratory failure due to tracheal compression by a thyroid cyst. *Scot Med J.* 1993;38(2):49–50.
4. Carrau RL, Herlich A, Rosen CA. Visualization of the glottis through a laryngeal mask during medialization laryngoplasty. *Laryngoscope.* 1998;108(5):769–71.
5. Lore JM. The thyroid gland. In: *An Atlas of Head and Neck Surgery*, ed. 3. 1988; Philadelphia: WB Saunders.
6. Shaha A, Jaffe BM. Complications of thyroid surgery performed by residents. *Surgery.* 1988;104(6):1109-14.
7. Reeve TS, Curtin A, Fingleton L et al. Can total thyroidectomy be performed as safely by general surgeons in provincial centers as by surgeons in specialized endocrine surgical units? Making the case for surgical training. *Arch Surg.* 1994;129(8):834–6.
8. Ready AR, Barnes AD. Complications of thyroidectomy. *Br J Surg.* 1994;81(11):1555-6.
9. Shindo ML, Sinha UK, Rice DH. Safety of thyroidectomy in residency: a review of 186 consecutive cases. *Laryngoscope.* 1995;105(11):1173–5.
10. Miller RD, Divertie MB. Kartagener's syndrome. *Chest.* 1972;62(2):130–5.
11. Friedman M, Pacella BL Jr. Total versus subtotal thyroidectomy. Arguments, approaches, and recommendations. *Otolaryngo Clin North Am.* 1990;23(3):413–27.
12. Schoretsanitis G, Melissas J, Sanidas E, Christodoulakis M, Vlachonikolis JG, Tsiftsis DD. Does draining the neck affect morbidity following thyroid surgery? *Am Surgeon.* 1998;64(8): 778–80,
13. Pappalardo G, Guadalaxara A, Frattaroli FM, Illomei G, Falaschi P. Total compared with subtotal thyroidectomy in benign nodular disease: personal series and review of published reports. *Eur J Surg.* 1998;164(7):501–6.
14. Hoffman E. Carcinoma of the thyroid: review of 304 cases. *So Med J.* 1987;80(6):741–52.
15. Schroeder DM, Bors A, France CJ. Operative strategy for thyroid cancer: is total thyroidectomy worth the price? *Cancer.* 1986;58:2320–2328.
16. Yamamoto Y, Maeda T, Izumi K, Otsuka H. Occult papillary carcinoma of the thyroid. A study of 408 autopsy cases. *Cancer.* 1990;65(5):1173–9.
17. Harach HR, Franssila KO, Wasenius VM. Occult papillary carcinoma of the thyroid. A "normal" finding in Finland. A systematic autopsy study. *Cancer.* 1985;56(3):531–8.
18. Schroder S, Pfannschmidt N, Bocker W, Muller HW, de Heer K. Histopathologic types and clinical behaviour of occult papillary carcinoma of the thyroid. *Path Res Pract.* 1984;179(1):81–7.
19. Attie JN, Bock G, Moskowitz GW. Postoperative radioactive iodine evaluation of total thyroidectomy for thyroid carcinoma: reappraisal and therapeutic interventions. *Head Neck.* 1992;14: 297–302.
20. Clark OH, Hoelting T. Management of patients with differentiated thyroid cancer who have positive serum thyroglobulin levels and negative radioiodine scans. *Thyroid.* 1994;4(4):501–5.
21. Dralle H, Schwarzrock R, Lang W et al. Comparison of histology and immunohistochemistry with thyroglobulin serum levels and radioiodine uptake in recurrences and metastases of differentiated thyroid carcinomas. *Acta Endocrinol.* 1985;108(4): 504–10.
22. Ericsson UB, Tegler L, Lennquist S, Christensen SB, Stahl E, Thorell JI. Serum thyroglobulin in differentiated thyroid carcinoma. *Acta Chir Scand.* 1984;150(5):367–75.
23. Pender S, Little DM, Burke P, Broe P. Treatment of medullary carcinoma of the thyroid by laryngo-pharyngo-esophagectomy—a case report. *Irish J Med Sci.* 1992;161(7):450–1.
24. Block MA. Surgical treatment of medullary carcinoma of the thyroid. *Otolaryngol Clin North Am.* 1990;23(3):453–73.
25. Rossotto P, Durante E, Cavallini G, Pampolini M. Anaplastic adenocarcinoma of the thyroid gland: a study of ten cases. *Ital J Surg Sci.* 1986;16(3):205–7.
26. Park CS, Suh KW, Min JS. Cartilage-shaving procedure for the control of tracheal cartilage invasion by thyroid carcinoma. *Head Neck.* 1993;15:289-291.
27. Czaja JM, McCaffrey TV. The surgical management of laryngo-tracheal invasion by well-differentiated papillary thyroid carcinoma. *Arch Otolaryngol-Head Neck Surg.* 1997;123(5):484-90.

# 10

# Mechanisms of Thyroid Oncogenesis

## Michael T. McDermott, M.D.

## INTRODUCTION

Carcinomas of the thyroid gland are generally classified into four major categories: papillary, follicular, anaplastic and medullary. Papillary, follicular and anaplastic carcinomas arise from thyroid follicular cells that normally synthesize and secrete thyroid hormones. Papillary and follicular cancers are referred to as differentiated thyroid carcinomas because they retain some morphological and functional features of normal follicular cells and tend to follow a relatively benign course with low potential for local invasion and distant metastases. Anaplastic carcinomas, in contrast, are highly malignant tumors that exhibit aggressive local invasiveness and metastatic spread to distant sites. Tumors are referred to as being poorly differentiated or undifferentiated when their histologic appearance and biological behavior lie somewhere between that of differentiated and anaplastic carcinomas. Medullary carcinomas arise from the calcitonin-producing parafollicular C cells; their biological behavior is more aggressive than papillary and follicular cancers but less so than anaplastic carcinomas.

Malignant tumors of the thyroid gland develop as a result of one or more mutations in genes known as oncogenes and tumor suppressor genes. Study of these genetic aberrations in thyroid tumor cells has given us exciting new insights into the pathobiology of thyroid tumor development. While we are far from understanding the complete set of molecular events that transform benign thyroid cells into malignant ones, the information gleaned so far has already proven to be of significant diagnostic and prognostic value and will hopefully lead to therapeutic advances in the near future.

The intent of this chapter is to propose a general model of thyroid cell growth, to describe the basic mechanisms by which various well-characterized cancer causing genes promote tumor growth, to highlight some of the most promising areas of ongoing research and to discuss the current and potential clinical applications of this prolific field of study.

## ONCOGENES AND TUMOR SUPPRESSOR GENES—GENERAL PRINCIPLES

The human organism begins as a single cell. This cell is ultimately transformed into a mature human being composed of approximately 100 trillion cells, all having an identical genotype but exhibiting a highly diverse array of morphological and functional phenotypes. For this metamorphosis to occur, multiple simultaneous and sequential events must transpire. Cells must proliferate by repetitive cell division. Cells must differentiate to acquire the size, shape and internal components necessary to carry out the specific functions of their ultimate phenotype. And finally, they must eventually undergo age-appropriate programmed cell death or apoptosis. This enormously complex series of events is orchestrated by a diverse set of proteins that serve as signals, receptors, messengers and effectors. The spatial and temporal expression of these proteins is precisely regulated by the genes that encode them.

The human genome consists of approximately 100,000 genes and contains about 3 billion nucleotide base pairs. The inherent nucleotide sequences must be duplicated faithfully with each cell division. It is estimated that nearly 6,000 nucleotide mutations occur in each cell every time it replicates. Environmental mutagens, such as viruses, radiation and chemicals may cause additional mutations to occur. More than 99% of such mutations are detected and repaired by a complex set of DNA repair proteins but some mutations persist and may result in disease.

Certain genes, known as proto-oncogenes, encode the proteins that promote normal cell division. An oncogene is a proto-oncogene that has developed an activating (gain of function) mutation, causing it to produce proteins that are quantitatively increased or qualitatively overactive and that consequently stimulate the excessive cellular proliferation characteristic of neoplastic tissue.[1-7] Gain of function mutations tend to be dominantly expressed and thus produce biological effects even when only one allele is affected (heterozygous state). Tumor suppressor genes are genes that encode proteins that normally restrain cell division, enhance cell differentiation or promote apoptosis.[7-11] Inactivating (loss of function) mutations of tumor suppressor genes can also lead to neoplasia; these mutations tend to produce disease only when both alleles are affected (homozygous state). Cells that are undergoing unregulated cell division as a result of an activated oncogene or an inactivated tumor suppressor gene are said to be transformed. Transformed cells have survival advantages conferred by the mutation that allow them to expand monoclonally and thereby to develop into a tumor.

Gene mutations may be either somatic or germline. Somatic mutations are those that develop any time after fertilization. They are usually limited to only one tissue or to one cell and generally predispose to sporadic solitary tumors. Germline mutations, in contrast, are passed from parent to offspring through a germ cell and are thus present in all cells of the recipient. Affected offspring may thus be susceptible to the development of multiple tumors in a given organ or to tumors in multiple sites throughout the body. Inherited cancer syndromes most commonly result from germline inactivating mutations of tumor suppressor genes. Affected individuals are heterozygous for the mutations and thus initially have a normal gene at the homologous locus that makes some of the normal tumor suppressor protein. If a somatic mutation later inactivates this normal locus, however, the individual develops a complete deficiency of the suppressor protein and becomes highly susceptible to tumor development.

Although a single genetic mutation may transform a cell, one mutation alone probably cannot produce the highly malignant behavior characteristic of most cancers. Rather, the unregulated replication of transformed cells predisposes them to develop additional mutations, which, in turn, lead to ever-accelerating cell proliferation, tissue invasion and distant metastases.

Indeed, highly malignant and metastatic tumors have been demonstrated to harbor multiple oncogenes and inactivated tumor suppressor genes.[12,13]

The precise mechanisms whereby cells are directed to divide, differentiate or die vary considerably among the different tissues throughout the body. Nonetheless, a general model of signal transduction is useful for understanding the basic mechanisms by which gene mutations lead to the development of cancer (Figure 10–1). The initial signal for normal cellular change is often an extracellular protein generated from a nearby or distant site. This signal protein binds to a membrane-bound receptor on the target cell, leading to the generation of cytoplasmic messengers, which then activate appropriate transcription factors within the nucleus. These nuclear proteins bind to the promoter regions of target genes where they govern the production of cell cycle regulatory proteins that are the effectors of cell division, differentiation or apoptosis. Activated oncogenes and inactivated tumor suppressor genes that cause or permit abnormal regulation of these pathways can generally be classified according to their site of function as being abnormal signals, receptors, messengers, transcription factors or cell cycle regulatory proteins. Multiple examples of each class have been reported to be involved in the development of thyroid neoplasms.[14-22]

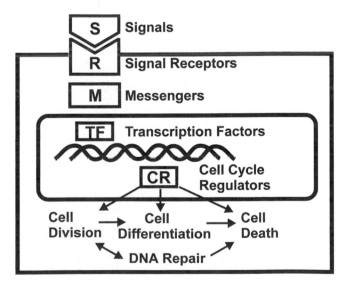

**Figure 10–1.** A model of signal transduction for cellular growth. An extracellular signal molecule binds to a specific membrane receptor, generating intracellular messengers that relay the signal to the nucleus by activating transcription factors. These nuclear proteins then bind to target genes where they alter the production of cell cycle regulatory proteins that are the effectors of cell proliferation, differentiation or apoptosis (cell death).

## THYROID RELATED ONCOGENES AND TUMOR SUPPRESSOR GENES

### Extracellular Signal Proteins

The major known extracellular signal for thyroid cells is thyrotropin (TSH). This hormone is a glycoprotein that consists of a specific beta subunit (TSHβ) and a common alpha subunit that is also present in luteinizing hormone (LH), follicle stimulating hormone (FSH) and human chorionic gonadotropin (HCG). TSH is secreted into the circulation by the pituitary gland and subsequently binds to TSH receptors (TSH-R) present on thyroid follicular cell membranes, where it activates a signaling pathway that promotes thyroid function and, to a lesser extent, thyroid growth.[23] Other systemic and local growth factors activate additional signaling pathways that promote growth but not function; these include insulin-like growth factor-1 (IGF-1), epidermal growth factor (EGF), fibroblast growth factors (FGF), platelet-derived growth factor (PDGF), interleukin-1 (IL-1), transforming growth factor-α (TGF-α), TGF-β, and likely others that have not yet been identified.[24–27]

There is strong evidence that growth factors play a significant role in the pathogenesis of thyroid tumors. TSH, for example, promotes both the growth and invasiveness of thyroid cancer cells *in vitro*.[28] Furthermore, the incidence of follicular thyroid carcinoma is increased in geographic areas of endemic iodine deficiency, which is associated with chronic TSH hypersecretion.[29] Although serum TSH levels are normal in the majority of patients with thyroid cancer in the United States, it is believed that even physiological serum TSH levels may promote the growth of existing thyroid cancers. This principle is the basis for the administration of TSH suppressive doses of levothyroxine in patients with differentiated thyroid carcinoma.[30,31]

The thyroid stimulating immunoglobulins (TSI) produced aberrantly by B lymphocytes in patients with Graves' disease also appear to have mitogenic effects. This notion is suggested by *in vitro* studies demonstrating that Graves' autoantibodies stimulate thyroid cell growth and activate the c-*fos* proto-oncogene.[32] Further support comes from clinical reports that Graves' disease is associated with an increased risk of developing thyroid cancer[33–36] and that thyroid cancer may be more aggressive in patients with underlying Graves' disease.[36–39]

The most impressive body of evidence, however, concerns the effects of the other extracellular thyroid growth factors on the development and propagation of thyroid cancer cells. Overexpression of various growth factors including IGF-1, EGF, FGF, PDGF, IL-1, TGF-α and TGF-β as well as receptors for IGF-1, EGF, FGF,

PDGF and estrogen has been reported in multiple thyroid tumor types.[24–27,40–75] The mechanisms responsible for this enhanced expression have not been fully elucidated. Nonetheless, it is becoming increasingly apparent that one or more growth factors may act either as primary mitogenic stimuli or serve significant supportive roles in the development, maintenance and progression of thyroid tumor growth.[24–27]

### TSH Receptor-Gs Alpha Signal Pathways

The TSH receptor (TSH-R) is a protein that consists of a large extracellular domain for TSH binding, a membrane associated region with seven transmembrane spanning segments and a short domain that extends into the cytoplasm (Figure 10–2). The latter is coupled to a guanine nucleotide binding stimulatory protein (Gs) that is composed of three subunits—alpha, beta and gamma—and an alpha bound guanosine diphosphate (GDP) molecule. The Gs alpha subunit has several distinctive characteristics: it is inactive when bound to

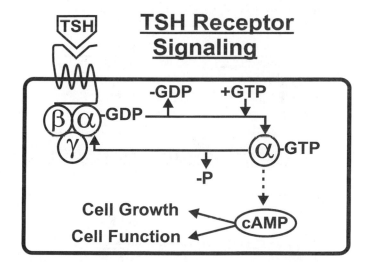

**Figure 10–2.** TSH signal transduction in thyroid cells. The TSH receptor (TSH-R) is a 7 transmembrane receptor protein present only on thyroid follicular cells. TSH binding to the large extracellular domain of the TSH-R causes dissociation of an intracellular guanine nucleotide binding stimulatory protein (Gs) into alpha, beta and gamma subunits; simultaneously, the alpha subunit releases a bound guanosine diphosphate (GDP) molecule. Free alpha then binds to a guanosine triphosphate (GTP) molecule, forming an active dimer that enhances cyclic adenosine monophosphate (cAMP) production. The alpha subunit then deactivates itself by using intrinsic GTPase activity to convert its bound GTP back to GDP. TSH activation of this pathway promotes normal cellular proliferation and thyroid hormone production.

GDP; it is activated by binding to guanosine triphosphate (GTP); and it possesses intrinsic GTPase activity that converts GTP to GDP. When TSH binds to the TSH-R extracellular domain, Gs dissociates into its individual subunits and the alpha subunit releases its bound GDP. The free alpha subunit then attaches to GTP, forming an active alpha-GTP dimer that stimulates adenylate cyclase to generate cyclic adenosine monophosphate (cAMP). The cAMP burst activates protein kinase A to further propagate this messenger cascade that ultimately promotes thyroid cell proliferation and function.[23] The intrinsic GTPase activity of the alpha subunit subsequently deactivates the alpha-GTP dimer by converting its bound GTP back to GDP, thus terminating the signal pulse.

Autonomously functioning follicular adenomas are benign thyroid neoplasms that synthesize and secrete thyroid hormone independent of TSH stimulation. Activating point mutations in the TSH-R gene, that produce TSH-independent constitutively active TSH-R (Figure 10–3), have been reported to underlie the majority of these hormone secreting neoplasms in most[76–81] but not all[82–84] studies from various locations around the world. Activating mutations of the Gs alpha subunit gene have also been detected in up to 25% of autonomously functioning follicular adenomas.[83–86] These mutations encode alpha subunits that lack intrinsic GTPase activity, rendering them unable to convert GTP back to GDP to terminate signal pulses (Figure 10–4). As a result, the active alpha-GTP dimers persist, causing continuous and excessive generation

of cAMP. Since the TSH-R and the Gs alpha subunit are components of a signaling pathway that normally stimulates both thyroid cell growth and function, it follows that gene mutations resulting in constitutively active TSH-R or Gs alpha subunits produce neoplasms that exhibit both autonomous growth and hormone secretion (functioning adenomas).[87] Neither type of mutation, however, appears to play a significant role in the development of malignant thyroid neoplasms.[83,84,87,88]

## *Ras* Signal Pathways

Growth factors other than TSH also bind to their specific receptors on thyroid cells to initiate various growth signaling pathways. *Ras* proteins are important components of many such pathways (Figure 10–5). *Ras* proteins are functionally similar to Gs alpha subunits: they are inactive when bound to GDP, they are active when associated with GTP, and they possess intrinsic GTPase activity. Basally, *ras* is bound to GDP in an inactive *ras*-GDP dimer that is attached to the inner aspect of the cell membrane. Extracellular growth factor binding activates membrane receptors, causing them to combine with adjacent receptors (dimerization) and to acquire phosphate groups on tyrosine residues on the receptor's intracellular domain (tyrosine phosphorylation).

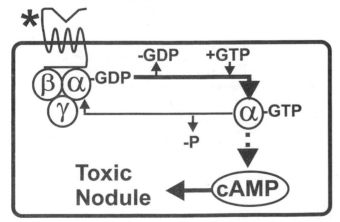

**Figure 10–3.** Activating TSH receptor (TSH-R) mutations. Mutations of the TSH-R gene may produce a TSH-R that is constitutively active, independent of TSH binding. Gain of function TSH-R mutations promote excessive cell growth and function, leading to the development of autonomously functioning follicular adenomas (functioning nodules).

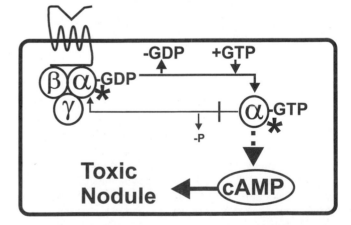

**Figure 10–4.** Activating Gs alpha subunit mutations. Mutations of the Gs alpha subunit gene produce an alpha protein that can become normally activated by binding to GTP but that cannot subsequently deactivate itself because it lacks intrinsic GTPase activity to convert GTP back to GDP. This persistently active alpha-GTP dimer generates a continuous signal that promotes excessive thyroid cell proliferation and function, leading to the development of autonomously functioning follicular adenomas (functioning nodules).

The activated receptor then recruits additional proteins, such as grb-2 and sos, which cooperate to dissociate *ras* from GDP. Liberated *ras* proteins immediately bind to GTP, forming active *ras*-GTP dimers that initiate a multi-step protein phosphorylation cascade that promotes thyroid cell proliferation but has little or no effect on hormone secretory function. The intrinsic GTPase activity of *ras* subsequently converts its bound GTP back to GDP, deactivating the *ras* protein and terminating the signal pulse.

Gene mutations producing constitutively active *ras* proteins have been detected in 20–80% of non-functioning follicular adenomas and differentiated thyroid carcinomas.[89–100] The mechanism for this constitutive *ras* overactivity is similar to that described above for Gs alpha subunit mutations. Mutated *ras* proteins can be normally activated by forming *ras*-GTP dimers but lack the intrinsic GTPase activity necessary to deactivate themselves by converting GTP back to GDP (Figure 10–6). In contrast to Gs alpha mutations, however, *ras* mutations participate only in growth stimulating pathways and therefore promote the development of non-functioning thyroid tumors.

## Ret Signal Pathways

The Ret protein is a receptor that is normally expressed in the calcitonin producing parafollicular C cells but not in the thyroid hormone producing follicular thyroid cells. Ret consists of an extracellular ligand binding domain, a single transmembrane segment and an intracellular domain that possesses intrinsic tyrosine kinase activity. Glial derived neurotropic factor (GDNF), a growth factor for cells of neural crest origin, is the normal cognate ligand for the Ret receptor.[101–104] GDNF binding to the Ret receptor causes receptor dimerization and significant augmentation of its tyrosine kinase activity. This activates a *ras* signaling pathway of downstream messengers that promote parafollicular C cell proliferation (Figure 10–7).

Medullary carcinoma of the thyroid (MCT), a malignancy of the parafollicular C cells, may be familial (~ 10%) or sporadic (~ 90%). Familial MCT is transmitted as an autosomal dominant disorder that may be present as part of the MEN II A syndrome (MCT, pheochromocytoma, hyperparathyroidism), the MEN II B syndrome (MCT, pheochromocytoma, multiple mucosal neuromas) or as familial isolated MCT. Activating single base mutations in the Ret gene (Ret/MCT), affecting discrete segments of the transmembrane and intracellular domains of the Ret receptor, have been reported to be present in over 90% of patients with these familial forms of MCT.[105–116] The resultant Ret receptors exhibit

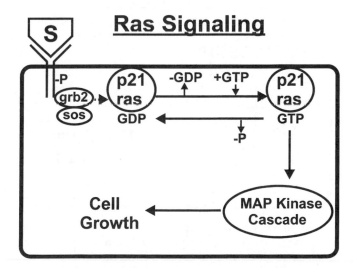

**Figure 10–5.** The *ras* signaling proteins. *Ras* proteins are located on the inner aspect of the cell membrane, where they are bound in an inactive state to GDP molecules. Growth signals that utilize *ras* bind to specific membrane receptors, resulting in receptor dimerization and phosphorylation; proteins such as grb-2 and sos then complex with the receptor and promote dissociation of GDP from *ras*. *Ras* then binds to GTP, forming an active *ras*-GTP dimer that initiates a multistep downstream protein phosphorylation cascade that promotes primarily cell proliferation. The intrinsic GTPase activity of *ras* then deactivates the *ras*-GTP dimer by converting GTP back to GDP.

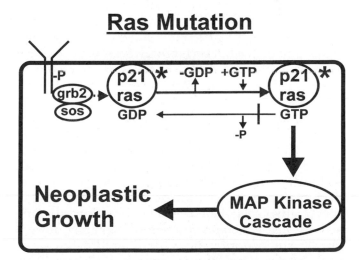

**Figure 10–6.** Activating *ras* mutations. Mutations of *ras* genes may produce *ras* proteins that can be normally activated by GTP binding but that cannot deactivate themselves because they lack intrinsic GTPase activity. These persistently active *ras*-GTP dimers continuously stimulate the downstream growth signaling cascade, resulting in excessive cell proliferation. This predisposes to the development of non-functioning follicular neoplasms (cold nodules).

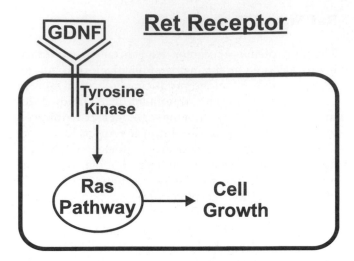

**Figure 10–7.** The Ret receptor. The Ret receptor is a single transmembrane protein that is normally present in thyroid parafollicular C cells but not in follicular cells. Glial derived neurotropic factor (GDNF) binds to the receptor's extracellular domain, resulting in receptor dimerization and augmentation of the intrinsic tyrosine kinase activity of the intracellular domain. This activates a *ras* mediated downstream signaling cascade that promotes normal C cell proliferation.

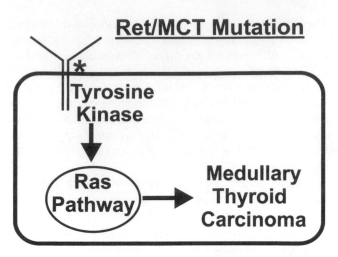

**Figure 10–8.** Activating Ret mutations (Ret/MCT) in medullary carcinoma of the thyroid. Germline point mutations in the Ret gene may produce Ret receptors with enhanced basal tyrosine kinase activity. This results in continuous activation of a growth stimulating pathway that eventually leads to the development of C cell hyperplasia and multifocal medullary carcinoma. This same mutation underlies the development of familial pheochromocytomas.

high level GDNF-independent tyrosine kinase activity, which incessantly drives the downstream *ras* signaling cascade, eventually leading to C cell hyperplasia and multifocal MCT (Figure 10–8). The Ret/MCT oncogene is also present in some sporadic MCTs,[105,108–111] suggesting that these tumors, which tend to be unifocal, may arise from a somatic Ret mutation in a single cell; in contrast, familial MCT results from a germline Ret mutation affecting all cells. Both familial[105,106,110,112] and some sporadic[117,118] pheochromocytomas have also been found to harbor the Ret/MCT oncogene. Interestingly, mutations in this gene have also been detected in patients with Hirschsprung's disease.[106,115]

Ret mutations of a different type, expressed aberrantly in thyroid follicular cells, have been discovered in papillary thyroid carcinomas. These mutations produce a deletion of the receptor's extracellular domain and interposition of an activating segment proximal to the intracellular tyrosine kinase domain. This results in constitutive GDNF-independent tyrosine kinase hyperactivity that generates continuous signaling down a growth stimulatory pathway leading to the development of papillary thyroid carcinoma (Figure 10–9). Approximately 20–50% of papillary carcinomas harbor these Ret/PTC mutations.[119–125] The two most common forms are Ret/PTC-1 and Ret/PTC-3. Ret/PTC-1, which is the predominant type found in sporadic papillary carcinomas in adults, appears to have a long latency period between mutation and neoplasm development. Ret/PTC-3, in contrast, has a shorter latency

## Ret/PTC Mutation

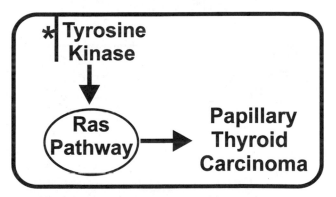

**Figure 10–9.** Activating Ret mutations (Ret/PTC) in papillary thyroid carcinoma. Acquired deletion/rearrangement mutations of the Ret gene produce a truncated receptor that has enhanced basal tyrosine kinase activity and that is aberrantly expressed in thyroid follicular cells. This promotes excessive follicular cell proliferation and leads to the development of papillary thyroid carcinoma.

period and has been found more often in children with papillary carcinoma and in thyroid cancer following radiation exposure, such as occurred following the Chernobyl nuclear accident.[125]

NTRK1 is another receptor that exhibits ligand-dependent intracellular tyrosine kinase activity. Like Ret,

NTRK1 is normally expressed in tissues of neural crest origin. Sequence variations in NTRK1 have recently been discovered in sporadic MCT.[126] Furthermore, NTRK1 rearrangements similar to those seen in the Ret/PTC oncogene have been described in sporadic papillary carcinoma[123,127,128] and in children exposed to radiation at Chernobyl.[129]

Met is a high affinity receptor for hepatocyte growth factor (HGF), which is a widely distributed cytokine that stimulates epithelial cell proliferation, motility and invasion. Although the mechanism is not yet clear, overexpression of Met has been reported in a high percentage of papillary thyroid carcinomas[130–137] and has been associated with increased invasiveness, lymph node metastases and advanced pathological stage.[131,137,138] Constitutive activation of Met has also been reported in anaplastic thyroid carcinoma cell lines.[139]

## Transcription Factors

Transcription factors are nuclear proteins that bind to the regulatory regions of genes to enhance or inhibit their transcription of messenger RNA (mRNA). Two important transcription factors, *myc* and *fos*, regulate the production of cell cycle regulatory proteins that are distal components of the growth and differentiation signaling pathways described above.[140] Although the causes have not been clearly determined, overexpression of *myc* and *fos* has been reported frequently, though not invariably, in thyroid tumors and has tended to be associated with more aggressive tumor behavior.[141–153]

The p53 protein is a unique transcription factor that has important anti-proliferative effects on cells; the p53 gene is therefore a tumor suppressor gene.[154,155] Normal p53 protein enters the nucleus and binds to specific DNA sequences in the promoter regions of p53-regulated genes, where it augments the production of cell cycle regulatory proteins that inhibit cell division or that promote DNA repair and/or age-appropriate apoptosis (Figure 10–10).[156–160] Inactivating mutations of the p53 gene produce p53 proteins that are unable to enter the nucleus and bind normally to DNA and which thereby predispose cells to undergo progressive malignant growth by failure to perform these normal functions (Figure 10–11). Because the mutant proteins tend to accumulate in the cell, p53 gene mutations are often detected by finding increased tissue levels of p53 protein. p53 gene mutations have been found in 20–100% of anaplastic and poorly differentiated thyroid cancers and in nearly 20% of radiation-induced thyroid tumors, but they are rare in sporadic papillary and follicular carcinomas.[161–169] Interestingly, p53 mutations have been detected in up to 50% of all human malignancies,[156–160] making them among the most common of all cancer causing gene mutations.

# p53 Function

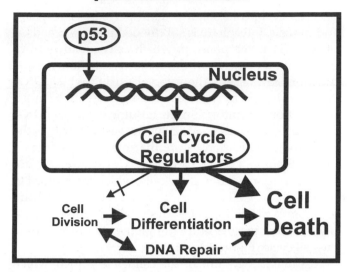

**Figure 10–10.** The p53 protein. The normal p53 protein enters the nucleus and binds to target genes where it governs the production of cell cycle regulatory proteins that inhibit cell proliferation and promote cell differentiation, DNA repair and age-appropriate apoptosis. The p53 gene is thus a tumor suppressor gene.

# p53 Mutation

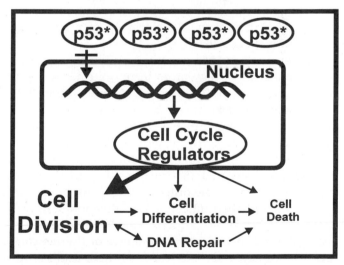

**Figure 10–11.** Inactivating p53 mutations. Mutations of the p53 gene in thyroid cells generally occur only after the cells have been transformed by a primary oncogene mutation. Inactivating p53 mutations produce p53 proteins that do not enter the nucleus or bind to DNA; this results in unrestrained cellular proliferation without cell differentiation, DNA repair or apoptosis. The appearance of p53 mutations heralds transformation of thyroid tumors to the more aggressive undifferentiated and anaplastic types.

## Cell Cycle Regulatory Proteins

The cell cycle consists of 2 main periods—interphase and mitosis. Interphase is subdivided into G1, S and G2 phases. G1 is the phase in which cells spend most of their time and perform the majority of their normal functions. S phase is the interval during which DNA synthesis occurs as chromosomes replicate in the initial preparation for mitosis. In the ensuing G2 phase, DNA repair proteins detect and repair the vast majority of the nucleotide replication errors that may have occurred during S phase. The cell then proceeds to undergo mitosis, dividing into 2 daughter cells, which then return to the G1 phase. Cell cycle regulatory proteins, which are effectors of the various growth signaling pathways, regulate cellular progression through the various phases of the cell cycle (Figure 10–12).[11,170]

A major regulator of the cell cycle is pRB, which acts as a master brake, preventing cells from progressing past G1. pRB itself is subject to multiple regulatory influences. The cyclins, for example, bind to cyclin dependent kinases (CDKs), forming complexes that inactivate pRB, thereby promoting passage of the cell into S phase.[11,170–172] Other proteins, such as p15, p16, p21 and p27, counteract the cyclins by inactivating CDK to prevent its inhibition of pRB. Accordingly, pRB, p15, p16, p21 and p27 have anti-proliferative activity, while cyclins and CDKs are pro-proliferative. Mutations affecting genes encoding proteins that regulate critical checkpoints in the cell cycle have been shown to be important events in the development of various human malignancies.[11,159,173–175]

Extensive research investigating the roles played by these cell cycle regulators in thyroid neoplasia is currently underway. Reduced pRB expression in thyroid cancers has been observed in some studies[176] but not in others[177]; loss of pRB, however, has been shown to be associated with a worsened prognosis.[178] Overexpression of cyclins in thyroid cancer has also been variably reported[179–183] and has similarly been related to a less favorable outcome.[183] Finally, abnormal expression and aberrant cellular localization of p15,[184] p16,[184,188] p21[169,186,187] and p27[181,182,188,189] have also been detected in variable percentages of thyroid cancers. The causes and significance of these findings remain to be determined.

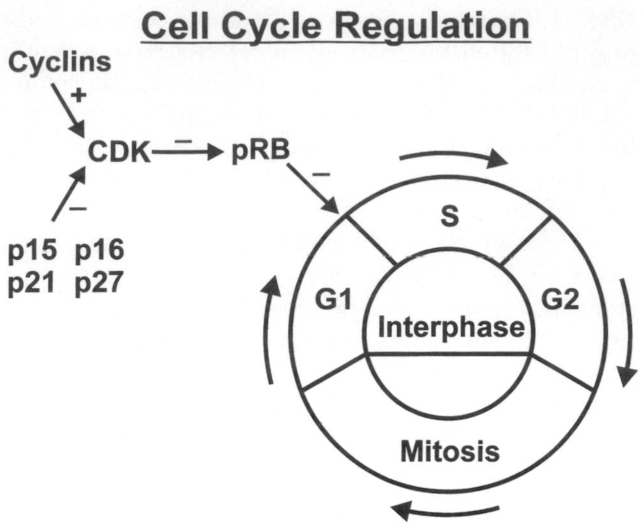

## Apoptosis

A critical aspect of the cell cycle is apoptosis, or programmed cell death. Apoptosis maintains tissue health by ridding organisms of senescent cells; it also serves as a means of self-destruction of emerging neoplastic cells.

## Cell Cycle Regulation

**Figure 10–12.** The cell cycle. The cell cycle consists of two major stages: interphase and mitosis. Interphase is subdivided into G1, S and G2 phases. The G1 phase is the time during which most normal cellular functions occur. S phase is the brief interval during which DNA replication results in doubling of the number of chromosomes in the cell as it moves toward mitosis. During the G2 phase, DNA replication errors are repaired. The cell then enters into mitosis, or cell division, when the cell splits to form two daughter cells, each having the normal number of chromosomes. Certain proteins have critical roles in the regulation of the cell cycle. pRB is a master cycle regulator that inhibits cellular proliferation by halting the cell cycle in the G1 phase. pRB, in turn, is regulated by both stimulatory and inhibitory pathways. Cyclins drive the cell cycle forward by forming active complexes with cyclin dependent kinases (CDKs) that inactivate pRB. Other proteins, such as p15, p16, p21 and p27, inhibit the cycle by inactivating CDKs, thereby restoring the restraining influence of pRB on the cell cycle.

Malignant growth in thyroid tumors is characterized by an imbalance between cellular proliferation and apoptosis.[190] The importance of apoptosis in oncogenesis has been amply demonstrated by the high prevalence of mutations of p53, a pro-apoptotic transcription factor, in a wide variety of human malignancies and by the increased aggressiveness of tumors bearing this mutation.[154–169] Several of the aforementioned signaling pathways activate proteins that are directly involved in apoptosis. Abnormal expression of these effectors may lead to failure of apoptosis, resulting in immortalization of clones of malignant cells.

A model of a general signaling pathway for apoptosis is shown in Figure 10–13. The signal for cell death may originate from sources external to the cell or from within the cell itself. External signals include proteins such as the *fas* ligand (*fas*-L), tumor necrosis factor alpha (TNF-α) and tumor necrosis factor-related apoptosis inducing ligand (TRAIL). Binding of one or more of

## Apoptosis Signaling

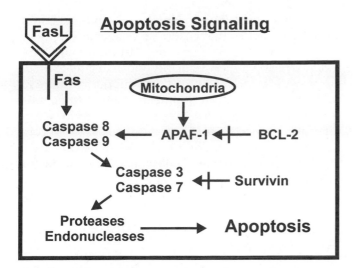

**Figure 10–13.** Apoptosis signaling pathways. Apoptosis, or programmed cell death, may be initiated by extracellular or intracellular signals. There are numerous extracellular apoptosis signals including the *fas* ligand (*fas* L), tumor necrosis factor alpha (TNFα and tumor necrosis factor related apoptosis inducing ligand (TRAIL). When these signals bind to their specific membrane receptors, they activate an intracellular signal cascade that sequentially utilizes caspases 8, 9, 3 and 7 to activate proteases and endonucleases that induce cell death by digesting cellular proteins and nucleic acids (DNA and RNA). Apoptosis can also be initiated internally by intracellular signals that stimulate apoptotic protease activating factor-1 (APAF-1), which activates the same caspase cascade. Apoptosis can be inhibited by factors such as BCL-2, which inactivates APAF-1, and survivin, which interrupts the signal cascade further downstream.

these signals to their membrane receptors results in initiation of an intracellular signaling cascade that involves sequential participation of caspases 8, 9, 7 and 3, with eventual activation of proteases and endonucleases that destroy the cell through enzymatic breakdown of proteins and nucleic acids (DNA and RNA), respectively. This same pathway can also be provoked intrinsically through an intracellular signal that stimulates apoptotic protease activating factor-1 (APAF-1) to initiate the same caspase cascade. BCL-2 is an anti-apoptotic factor[191,192] that inhibits the intracellular apoptosis signal by selectively inactivating APAF-1. Altered expression of BCL-2 has been observed in some, but not all, thyroid carcinomas;[191–201] it is not clear, however, if these changes are primary or whether they may arise secondarily in response to other events that alter apoptotic activity. Other proteins, such as survivin, interrupt both the intracellular and extracellular apoptosis signals by interacting with and disabling caspases 3 and/or 7. Survivin has recently been reported to be expressed at high concentrations in thyroid carcinomas compared to benign nodules and normal thyroid tissue;

furthermore, its level of expression was shown to correlate with tumor aggressiveness.[202]

Telomerase is an anti-apoptotic protein that functions to preserve the integrity of telomeres, the chromosomal caps that prevent chromosomes from sticking together or forming otherwise unstable configurations.[203,204] Every time a cell divides, some of its terminal telomeric sequences are lost. Shortening of telomeres to a critical length triggers the cell to undergo apoptosis. Germ cells avoid this fate by producing telomerase, an enzyme that rebuilds telomeres after each cycle; normal somatic cells, in contrast, do not express telomerase and eventually undergo age-appropriate apoptosis. Malignant tissues commonly reacquire the ability to express telomerase activity, an event that is believed to play an important role in the immortalization of cancer cells by preventing tumor cell apoptosis (Figure 10–14A and B). Accordingly, telomerase activity has now been demonstrated in 20–100% of all thyroid carcinomas[205–215] and has been shown to be associated with increased tumor invasiveness.[205,208,213]

## Maintenance Proteins

Growing tissue must also produce ancillary proteins to maintain the integrity of existing tissue and to support further tissue growth. A multitude of proteins are involved in this maintenance and support role. For this discussion however, we will highlight only two specific groups: the cell adhesion molecules and the angiogenesis factors.[216–219]

Cell adhesion molecules serve primarily to attach cells to one another (cell-cell adhesion molecules) and to the intercellular matrix (cell-matrix adhesion molecules) in order to maintain normal tissue architecture. Cadherins are an important class of cell-cell adhesion molecules; these membrane spanning proteins form critical complexes with intracellular proteins called catenins that are necessary for normal cadherin function. Integrins are cell-matrix adhesion molecules that bind to extracellular basement membrane components known as laminins. Loss of normal adhesion molecule function in cancer cells can lead to the disorganized tissue architecture characteristic of tumors and enable malignant cells to migrate from their site of origin to invade adjacent tissues or metastasize to distant sites.[220,221] Consistent with this concept, E-cadherin expression is reportedly reduced in the majority of differentiated thyroid carcinomas, while complete loss of E-cadherin is associated with tumor de-differentiation, local invasiveness and metastatic spread.[222–232] Down-regulation of cadherin expression does not appear to result from alterations of cadherin genes[228] but instead may be caused by deactivation of cadherin molecules

## Somatic Cell

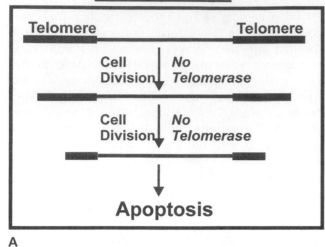

**A**

## Cancer Cell

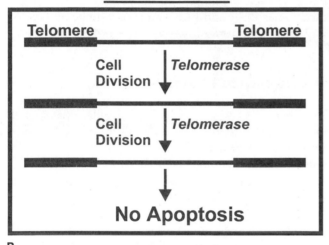

**B**

**Figure 10–14.** Telomerase. Telomeres are the protective caps on the ends of chromosomes. As somatic cells undergo repetitive cycles of cell division, telomeres progressively shorten; when telomeres reach a critical length, a signal is generated instructing the cell to undergo apoptosis (A). Telomerase is an enzyme that rebuilds telomeric ends after each cell division, preventing their progressive shortening and thus forestalling apoptosis; normal somatic cells do not express telomerase although germ cells do. Malignant thyroid cells also frequently express telomerase. This anti-apoptotic enzyme contributes to the immortalization of telomerase expressing neoplastic cells (B).

by the addition of multiple methyl groups (methylation).[229] Abnormal integrin expression is also associated with thyroid tumor development and progression.[225,232] Other adhesion molecules that may play a role in the malignant behavior of thyroid neoplasms include catenins,[27,230,231] laminins,[225,233] Muc1,[234] oncofetal fibronectin,[235] metalloproteinase-1 and tissue metalloproteinase inhibitor-1.[236]

Angiogenesis factors stimulate the production of vascular networks that ensure an adequate supply of nutrients and oxygen to growing tissues. Tumors commonly develop hypervascularity, indicating that vascular growth factors likely play key supportive roles at some point in the development of most tumors.[219] Angiogenesis factors that have been reported to be significantly overexpressed in and that are likely to contribute to the growth of thyroid cancers include basic FGF[57–60] and vascular endothelial growth factor (VEGF).[237–243]

## Multiple Mutations Contribute to Thyroid Cancer

I have thus far described numerous individual oncogene and tumor suppressor gene mutations that have been reported to be involved in various types of thyroid neoplasia. Some mutations (TSH-R and Gs alpha) have been found predominantly in benign functioning follicular adenomas while others (*ras*) have been found in both benign and malignant non-functioning tumors. Certain mutations have been observed primarily or exclusively in specific tumor types (Ret/PTC and Met in papillary carcinomas; Ret/MTC in medullary carcinomas; p53 in undifferentiated and anaplastic carcinomas) while others occur more generally. As with other malignancies, thyroid cancer probably does not result from a single mutation. Rather, it is becoming increasingly apparent that malignant thyroid neoplasms result from multiple sequential gene mutations that result in progressive degrees of abnormal tumor behavior.[12,13,16,17] A proposed scheme for molecular events underlying the development of thyroid tumors is illustrated in Figure 10–15.

## CLINICAL APPLICATIONS

While the study of oncogenes has afforded us tremendous insights into the pathobiology of cancer development, oncogene measurement techniques are already proving to be useful clinically as well. The most important diagnostic application in the thyroid field so far has been preclinical testing for familial MCT by screening for the Ret/MCT mutation. Familial MCT is an autosomal dominant disorder that will, on average, develop in 50% of an affected individual's siblings and offspring. Preclinical screening of family members is therefore recommended in order to detect disease before it is clinically apparent. Traditional screening has involved measurement of plasma calcitonin levels before and after stimulation with pentagastrin, calcium or both. These tests, however, only become positive when C cell

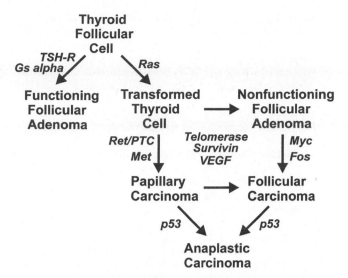

**Figure 10–15.** Multiple genetic mutations in thyroid neoplasia. Gene mutations producing constitutively active TSH-R and Gs alpha proteins promote both thyroid cell proliferation and function, leading to the development of functioning follicular adenomas with a low potential for malignant degeneration. Activating *ras* mutations stimulate growth but not function and thereby lead to the formation of non-functioning follicular tumors that are prone to incur further genetic alterations. Acquired mutations of the Ret receptor (Ret/PTC) or the hepatocyte growth factor receptor (Met) may then lead to the development of papillary carcinomas while those causing overexpression of *myc* and/or *fos* may transform follicular adenomas into follicular carcinomas. Malignant growth may be further enhanced by mutations that increase expression of anti-apoptosis factors, like survivin and telomerase, or that increase angiogenesis factors, such as vascular endothelial growth factor (VEGF). Inactivating p53 mutations may eventually promote transformation to more aggressive undifferentiated and anaplastic carcinomas.

hyperplasia or frank MCT has already developed. Furthermore, they must be performed annually until the age of 35 years, after which the likelihood of appearance of this condition diminishes. Testing for the Ret/MCT mutation, in contrast, can be performed on a single blood sample, needs to be done only once, and has a sensitivity of over 99% even before the disease has had time to develop.[107,115]

When cancers arise from somatic mutations, tissue samples of the tumor itself must be used for oncogene screening. This technology is still in the investigational stages and not yet available clinically. Nonetheless, the prospect of using oncogene panels to screen fine needle aspiration (FNA) samples and surgical specimens holds great promise for more accurate preoperative and postoperative diagnostic testing in the future. Similarly, oncogene screening of the primary tumor or of recurrent lesions may permit more accurate estimations of prognosis based on the types of genetic mutations detected. This information could help identify those patients whose tumors are more likely to follow an aggressive course, and thereby serve as a guide to providers when making decisions regarding the desired extent of surgery, the use and dose of radioactive iodine, and the optimal degree of levothyroxine suppression.

Finally, oncogene studies may lead to the development and use of treatments directed at the specific molecular aberrations found in individual cancers. Chemotherapy, immune modulation and even gene therapy could be tailored specifically to retard thyroid cell proliferation, to promote cell differentiation, to restore normal apoptosis, to maintain normal cell adhesiveness or to impair tumor angiogenesis.[218,219,243–245] Such advances may soon usher in a new era of more specific and more effective management of patients with thyroid cancer.

## References

1. Weinberg RA. How cancer arises. *Scientific American.* 1996; 275:62–70.
2. Cline MJ, Slamom DJ, Lipsick JS. Oncogenes: Implications for the diagnosis and treatment of cancer. *Ann Intern Med.* 1984; 101:223–233.
3. Gordon H. Oncogenes. *Mayo Clin Proc.* 1985; 60:697–713.
4. Druker BJ, Mamon HJ, Roberts TM. Oncogenes, growth factors, and signal transduction. *N Engl J Med.* 1989; 321:1383–1391.
5. Krontiris TG. Molecular medicine: oncogenes. *N Engl J Med.* 1995; 333:303–306.
6. Latchman DS. Transcription factor mutations and disease. *N Engl J Med.* 1995; 334:28–33.
7. Friend SH, Dryja TP, Weinberg RA. Oncogenes and tumor suppressing genes. *N Engl J Med.* 1988; 318:618–622.
8. Weinberg RA. Tumor suppressor genes. *Science.* 1991;254: 1138–1145.
9. Marshall CF. Tumor suppressor genes. *Cell.* 1991; 64:313–326.
10. Knudson AG. Antioncogenes and human cancer. *Proc Natl Acad Sci.* 1993; 90:10914–10921.
11. Hartwell LH, Kastan MB. Cell cycle control and cancer. *Science.* 1994; 266:1821–1828.
12. Vogelstein B, Kinzler KW. The multistep nature of cancer. *Trends in Genetics.* 1993; 9:138–141.
13. Bishop JM. Cancer: The rise of the genetic paradigm. *Genes and Development.* 1995; 9:1309–1315.
14. Melmed S. Oncogenes and the thyroid. *Thyroid Today.* 1988;11: 1–7.
15. Frauman AG, Moses AC. Oncogenes and growth factors in thyroid carcinogenesis. *Endocrinol Metab Clin NA.* 1990; 19:479–492.
16. Fagin JA. Genetic basis of endocrine disease 3: Molecular defects in thyroid gland neoplasia. *J Clin Endocrinol Metab.* 1992;5: 1398–1400.
17. Fagin JA. Molecular pathogenesis of human thyroid neoplasms. *Thyroid Today.* 1994; 17:1–6.
18. Farid NR, Shi Y, Zou M. Molecular basis of thyroid cancer. *Endocrine Rev.* 1994; 15:202–232.
19. Farid NR, Zou M, Shi Y. Genetics of follicular thyroid cancer. *Endocrinol Metab Clin NA.* 1995; 24:865–883.
20. Williams ED. Mechanisms and pathogenesis of thyroid cancer in animals and man. *Mutat Res.* 1995; 333:123–129.

21. Robinson BG. Molecular genetics of thyroid and parathyroid neoplasia. *Aust N Z J Surg.* 1995; 65:77–79.

22. Gagel RF. An overview of molecular abnormalities leading to thyroid carcinogenesis: a 1993 perspective. *Stem Cells.* 1997; 15:7–13.

23. Vassart G, Dumont JE. The thyrotropin receptor and the regulation of thyrocyte function and growth. *Endocrine Rev.* 1992; 13:596–611.

24. Lewinski A, Pawlikowski M, Cardinali DP. Thyroid growth-stimulating and growth-inhibiting factors. *Biol Signals.* 1993;2:313–351.

25. Eggo MC, Pratt MAC, Becks G, Burrow GN. Regulation of growth and of differentiation in thyroid follicular cells. *Adv Exp Med Biol.* 1990; 261:327–340.

26. Dumont JE, Maenhaut C, Pirson I, Baptist M, Roger PP. Growth factors controlling the thyroid gland. *Balliere Clin Endocrinol Metab.* 1991; 5:727–754.

27. Goretzki PE, Frilling A, Simon D, Roeher HD. Growth regulation of normal thyroids and thyroid tumors in man. *Recent Results Cancer Res.* 1990; 118:48–54.

28. Hoelting T, Tezelman S, Siperstein AE, Duh QY, Clark OH. Biphasic effects of thyrotropin on invasion and growth of papillary and follicular thyroid cancer in vitro. *Thyroid.* 1995; 5:35–40.

29. Cuello C, Correa P, Eisenberg H. Geographic pathology of thyroid carcinoma. *Cancer.* 1969; 23:230–238.

30. Burmeister LA, Goumaz MO, Mariash CN, Oppenheimer JH. Levothyroxine dose requirements for thyrotropin suppression in the treatment of differentiated thyroid cancer. *J Clin Endocrinol Metab.* 1992; 75:344–350.

31. Pujol P, Daures J-P, Nsakala N, Baldet L, Bringer J, Jaffiol C. Degree of thyrotropin suppression as a prognostic determinant in differentiated thyroid cancer. *J Clin Endocrinol Metab.* 1999; 81:4318–4323.

32. Huber GK, Safirstein R, Neufeld D, Davies TF. Thyrotropin receptor autoantibodies induce human thyroid cell growth and c-fos activation. *J Clin Endocrinol Metab.* 1991; 72:1142–1147.

33. Pemberton JD, Black BM. The association of carcinoma of the thyroid gland and exophthalmic goiter. *Surg Clin NA.* 1948;28:935–952.

34. Farbota LM, Calandra DB, Lawrence AM, Paloyan E. Thyroid carcinoma in Graves' disease. *Surgery.* 1985; 98:1148–1152.

35. Filetti S, Belfiori A, Amir SM et al. The role of thyroid-stimulating antibodies of Graves' disease in differentiated thyroid cancer. *N Engl J Med.* 1988; 318:753–759.

36. Pacini F, Elisei R, DiCoscio GC. Thyroid carcinoma in thyrotoxic patients treated by surgery. *J Endocrinol Invest.* 1988; 11:107–112.

37. Ozaki O, Ito K, Kobayashi K. Thyroid carcinoma in Graves' disease. *World J Surg.* 1990; 14:437–441.

38. Belfiori A, Garofalo MR, Giuffrida D, Runello F. Increased aggressiveness of thyroid cancer in patients with Graves' disease. *J Clin Endocrinol Metab.* 1990; 70:830–835.

39. Hales IB, McElduff A, Crummer P, Clifton-Bligh P, Delbridge L. Does Graves' disease or thyrotoxicosis affect the prognosis of thyroid cancer? *J Clin Endocrinol Metab.* 1992; 75:886–889.

40. van Der Laan BFAM, Freeman JL, Asa SL. Expression of growth factors and growth factor receptors in normal and tumorous thyroid tissue. *Thyroid.* 1995; 5:67–73.

41. Eggo MC, Bachrach LK, Burrow GN. Interaction of TSH, insulin and insulin-like growth factors in regulating thyroid growth and function. *Growth Factors.* 1990; 2:99–109.

42. Tramontano D, Cushing GW, Moses AC, Ingbar SH. Insulin-like growth factor-1 stimulates the growth of rat thyroid cells in culture and synergizes the stimulation of DNA synthesis induced by TSH and Graves'-IgG. *Endocrinology.* 1986; 119:940–945.

43. Bachrach LK, Eggo MC, Hintz RL. Insulin-like growth factors in sheep thyroid cells: action, receptors and production. *Biochem Biophys Res Comm.* 1988; 154:861–867.

44. Minuto F, Barreca A, Del Monte P, Cariola G, Torre GC, Giordano G. Immunoreactive insulin-like growth factor 1 (IGF-1) and IFG-1 binding protein content in human thyroid tissue. *J Clin Endocrinol Metab.* 1989; 68:621–626.

45. Williams DW, Williams ED, Wynford-Thomas D. Evidence for autocrine production of IGF-1 in human thyroid adenomas. *Mol Cell Endocrinol.* 1989; 61:139–143.

46. Vannelli GB, Barni T, Modigliani U. Insulin-like growth factor-1 receptors in nonfunctioning thyroid nodules. *J Clin Endocrinol Metab.* 1990; 71:1175–1182.

47. Maciel RMB, Moses AC, Villone G, Tramontano D, Ingbar SH. Demonstration of the production and physiological role of insulin-like growth factor 2 in rat thyroid follicular cells in culture. *J Clin Invest.* 1988; 82:1546–1553.

48. Westermark K, Karlsson FA, Westermark B. Epidermal growth factor modulates thyroid growth and function in culture. *Endocrinology.* 1983; 112:1680–1686.

49. Waters MJ, Tweedale RC, Whip TA. Dedifferentiation of cultured thyroid cells by epidermal growth factor: Some insights into the mechanism. *Mol Cell Endocrinol.* 1987; 49:109–117.

50. Duh QY, Siperstein AE, Miller AE, Sancho JJ, Demeure MJ, Clark OH. Epidermal growth factor receptors in normal and neoplastic thyroid tissue. *Surgery.* 1985; 98:1000–1007.

51. Kanamori A, Abe Y, Yajima Y, Manabe Y, Ito K. Epidermal growth factor receptors in plasma membranes of normal and diseased human thyroid glands. *J Clin Endocrinol Metab.* 1989; 68:899–903.

52. Myamoto M, Sugawa H, Mori T. Epidermal growth factor receptors in cultured neoplastic human thyroid cells and effects of epidermal growth factor and thyroid stimulating hormone on their growth. *Cancer Res.* 1988; 48:3652–3656.

53. Masuda H, Sugenoya A, Kobayashi S, Kasuge Y, Iida F. Epidermal growth factor receptor on human thyroid neoplasms. *World J Surg.* 1988; 12:616–622.

54. Hoelting T, Siperstein AE, Clark OH, Duh QY. Epidermal growth factor enhances proliferation, migration and invasion of follicular and papillary thyroid cancer in vitro and in vivo. *J Clin Endocrinol Metab.* 1994; 79:401–408.

55. Emoto M, Isozaki O, Arai M. Identification and characterization of basic fibroblast growth factor in porcine thyroids. *Endocrinology.* 1991; 128:58–64.

56. Logan A, Black EG, Gonzalez A-M, Buscaglia M, Sheppard MC. Basic fibroblast growth factor: an autocrine mitogen of rat thyroid follicular cells. *Endocrinology.* 1992; 130:2363–2372.

57. Daa T, Kodama M, Kashima K, Yokoyama S, Nakayama I, Noguchi S. Identification of basic fibroblast growth factor in papillary carcinoma of the thyroid. *Acta Pathol Jpn.* 1993; 43:582–589.

58. Kodama M, Daa T, Kashima K, Yokoyama S, Nakayama I, Noguchi S. Immunohistochemical localization of acidic and basic fibroblast growth factors in human benign and malignant thyroid lesions. *Jpn J Clin Oncol.* 1994; 24:66–73.

59. Shingu K, Sugenoya A, Itoh N, Kato R. Expression of basic fibroblast growth factor in thyroid disorders. *World J Surg.* 1994; 18:500–505.

60. Eggo MC, Hopkins JM, Franklyn JA, Johnson GD, Sanders SA, Sheppard MC. Expression of fibroblast growth factors in thyroid cancer. *J Clin Endocrinol Metab.* 1995; 80:1006–1011.

61. Shingu K, Fujimori M, Ito K et al. Expression of fibroblast growth factor-2 and fibroblast growth factor receptor-1 in thyroid diseases: difference between neoplasms and hyperplastic lesions. *Endocr J.* 1998; 45:35–43.

62. Emoto N, Onose H, Sugihara H, Minami S, Shimizu K, Wakabayashi I. Fibroblast growth factor-2 free from extracellular matrix is increased in papillary thyroid carcinomas and Graves' thyroids. *Thyroid.* 1998; 8:491–497.

63. Onose H, Emoto N, Sugihara H, Shimizu K, Wakabayashi I. Overexpression of fibroblast growth factor receptor 3 in a human thyroid carcinoma cell line results in overgrowth of the confluent cultures. *Eur J Endocrinol.* 1999; 140:169–173.

64. Taylor AH, Millatt LJ, Whitley GStJ, Johnstone AP, Nussey SS. The effect of basic fibroblast growth factor on the growth and function of human thyrocytes. *J Endocrinol.* 1999; 136:339–344.

65. Heldin N-E, Gustavsson G, Claesson-Welsh L. Aberrant expression of receptors for platelet-derived growth factor in an anaplastic thyroid carcinoma cell line. *Proc Natl Acad Sci.* 1988;85: 9302–9306.

66. Matsuo K, Tang S, Sharifi B, Rubin SA, Schreck R, Fagin JA. Growth factor production by human thyroid carcinoma cells: Abundant expression of a platelet-derived growth factor-β-like protein by a human papillary carcinoma cell line. *J Clin Endocrinol Metab.* 1993; 77:996–1004.

67. Tsushima T, Arai M, Saji M. Effects of transforming growth factor-beta on deoxyribonucleic acid synthesis and iodine metabolism in porcine thyroid cells in culture. *Endocrinology.* 1988; 123:1187–1194.

68. Coletta G, Cirafici AM, DiCarlo A. Dual effects of transforming growth factor beta on rat thyroid cells: inhibition of thyrotropin-induced proliferation and reduction of thyroid-specific differentiation markers. *Cancer Res.* 1989; 49:3457–3462.

69. Grubeck-Loebenstein B, Buchan G, Sadeghi R. Transforming growth factor beta regulated thyroid growth: role in the pathogenesis of nontoxic goiter. *J Clin Invest.* 1989; 83:764–770.

70. Hoelting T, Zielke A, Siperstein AE, Clark OH, Duh QY. Transforming growth factor beta 1 is a negative regulator for differentiated thyroid cancer: studies of growth, migration, invasion and adhesion of cultured follicular and papillary thyroid cancer cell lines. *J Clin Endocrinol Metab.* 1994; 79:806–813.

71. Mine M, Tramontano D, Chin WW. Interleukin-1 stimulates thyroid cell growth and increases the concentration of the c-myc proto-oncogene mRNA in thyroid follicular cells in culture. *Endocrinology.* 1987; 120:1212–1214.

72. Zakarija M, McKenzie JM. Influence of cytokines on growth and differentiated function of FRTL5 cells. *Endocrinology.* 1989;125: 1260–1265.

73. Kawabe Y, Eguchi K, Shimomura C. Immunohistochemical study of estrogen receptors and the responsiveness to estrogen in papillary thyroid carcinoma. *J Clin Endocrinol Metab.* 1989;68:1174–1183.

74. Inoue H, Oshimo K, Miki H. Immunohistochemical study of estrogen receptors and the responsiveness to estrogen in papillary thyroid carcinoma. *Cancer.* 1993; 72:1364–1368.

75. Hoelting T, Siperstein AE, Duh QY. Tamoxifen inhibits growth, migration and invasion of human follicular and papillary thyroid cancer cells in vitro and in vivo. *J Clin Endocrinol Metab.* 1995; 80:308–313.

76. Paschke R, Tonacchera M, Van Sande J, Parma J, Vassart G. Identification and functional characterization of two new somatic mutations causing constitutive activation of the thyrotropin receptor in hyperfunctioning autonomous adenomas of the thyroid. *J Clin Endocrinol Metab.* 1994; 79:1785–1789.

77. Porcellini A, Ciullo I, Laviola L, Amabile G, Fenzi G, Avvedimento VE. Novel mutations of thyrotropin receptor gene in thyroid hyperfunctioning adenomas. Rapid identification by fine needle aspiration biopsy. *J Clin Endocrinol Metab.* 1994; 79:657–661.

78. Russo D, Arturi F, Wicker R, Chazenbalk GD. Genetic alterations in thyroid hyperfunctioning adenomas. *J Clin Endocrinol Metab.* 1995; 80:1347–1351.

79. Ohno M, Endo T, Ohta K, Gunji K, Onaya T. Point mutations in the thyrotropin receptor in human thyroid tumors. *Thyroid.* 1995; 5:97–100.

80. Parma J, Duprez L, Van Sande J, Paschke R. Constitutively active receptors as a disease-causing mechanism. *Mol Cell Endocrinol.* 1994; 100:159–162.

81. Van Sande J, Parma J, Tonacchera M, Swillens S, Dumont J, Vassart G. Somatic and germline mutations of the TSH receptor gene in thyroid diseases. *J Clin Endocrinol Metab.* 1995;80: 2607–2611.

82. Takeshita A, Nagayama Y, Yokoyama N, Ishikawa N. Rarity of oncogenic mutations in the thyrotropin receptor of autonomously functioning thyroid nodules in Japan. *J Clin Endocrinol Metab.* 1995; 80:2607–2611.

83. Matsuo K, Friedan E, Gejman PV, Fagin JA. The thyrotropin receptor (TSH-R) is not an oncogene for thyroid tumors: Structural studies of the TSH-R and the alpha subunit of Gs in human thyroid neoplasms. *J Clin Endocrinol Metab.* 1993; 76:1446–1451.

84. Esapa C, Foster S, Johnson S. G protein and thyrotropin receptor mutations in thyroid neoplasia. *J Clin Endocrinol Metab.* 1997; 82:493–496.

85. Lyons J, Landis CA, Harsh G, Vallar L, Grunewald K. Two G protein oncogenes in human endocrine tumors. *Science.* 1990; 249:655–658.

86. Dumont JE. Thyroid adenoma, Gsa expression and the cyclic adenosine monophosphate mitogenic cascade: a complex relationship (Editorial). *J Clin Endocrinol Metab.* 1995; 80:1518–1520.

87. Tonacchera M, Vitti P, Agretti P et al. Functioning and nonfunctioning thyroid adenomas involve different molecular pathogenetic mechanisms. *J Clin Endocrinol Metab.* 1999; 84:4155–4158.

88. Spalmberg D, Sharifi N, Elisei R. Structural studies of the thyrotropin receptor and Gsa in human thyroid cancers: Low prevalence of mutations predicts infrequent involvement in malignant transformation. *J Clin Endocrinol Metab.* 1996; 81:3898–3901.

89. Suarez HG, Du Villard JA, Calliou B. Detection of activated ras oncogenes in human thyroid carcinomas. *Oncogene.* 1988;2: 403–406.

90. Lemoine NR, Mayall ES, Wyllie FS. Activated ras oncogenes in human thyroid cancers. *Cancer Res.* 1988; 48:4459–4463.

91. Hashimoto T, Matsubara F, Mizukami Y, Miyazaki I, Michigishi T, Yanaihara N. Tumor markers and oncogene expression in thyroid cancer using biochemical and immunohistochemical studies. *Endocrinol Jpn.* 1990; 37:247–254.

92. Namba H, Gutman RA, Matsuo K, Alvarez A, Fagin JA. H-Ras proto-oncogene mutations in human thyroid neoplasms. *J Clin Endocrinol Metab.* 1990; 71:223–229.

93. Namba H, Rubin SA, Fagin JA. Point mutations of ras oncogenes are an early event in thyroid tumorigenesis. *Mol Endocrinol.* 1990; 4:1474–1479.

94. Schark C, Fulton N, Jacoby RF, Westbrook CA, Straus FH, Kaplan EL. N-ras 61 oncogene mutations in benign and malignant thyroid neoplasms. *Surgery.* 1990; 108:994–1000.

95. Karga H, Lee J-K, Vickery AL, Thor A, Gaz RD, Jameson JL. Ras oncogene mutations in benign and malignant thyroid neoplasms. *J Clin Endocrinol Metab.* 1991; 73:832–836.

96. Schark C, Fulton N, Tashiro T, Stanislav G, Jacoby RF. The value of measurement of RAS oncogenes and nuclear DNA analysis in the diagnosis of Hurthle cell tumors of the thyroid. *World J Surg.* 1992; 16:745–752.

97. Goretzki PE, Lyons J, Stac-Phipps S, Rosenau W. Mutational activation of RAS and GSP oncogenes in differentiated thyroid cancer and their biological implications. *World J Surg.* 1992;16: 576–582.

98. Masood S, Auguste LJ, Westerband A, Belluco C, Valderama E, Attie J. Differential oncogenic expression in thyroid follicular and Hurthle cell carcinomas. *Am J Surg.* 1993; 166:366–388.

99. Basolo F, Pinchera A, Fugazzola L et al. Expression of p21 ras protein as a prognostic factor in papillary thyroid cancer. *Eur J Cancer.* 1994; 30A:171–174.

100. Ezzat S, Zheng L, Kolenda J. Prevalence of activating ras mutations in morphologically characterized thyroid nodules. *Thyroid.* 1996; 5:409–416.
101. Trupp M, Arenas E, Fainzilber M. Functional receptor for GDNF encoded by the c-ret proto-oncogene. *Nature.* 1996; 381:785–789.
102. Durbec P, Marcos-Gutierrez CV, Kilkenney C. GDNF signalling through the ret receptor tyrosine kinase. *Nature.* 1996; 381: 789–793.
103. Jing S, Wen D, Yu Y. GDNF-induced activation of the ret protein tyrosine kinase is mediated by GDNF-a, a novel receptor for GDNF. *Cell.* 1996; 85:1113–1124.
104. Treanor JJS, Goodman L, de Sauvage F. Characterization of a multicomponent receptor for GDNF. *Nature.* 1996; 382:80–83.
105. Hofstra RMW, Landspater RM, Checherini I, Stulp RP, Stelwagen TE. A mutation in the RET proto-oncogene associated with multiple endocrine neoplasia type 2B and sporadic medullary thyroid carcinoma. *Nature.* 1994; 367:375–376.
106. Smith DP, Eng C, Ponder BAJ. Mutations of the RET proto-oncogene in the multiple endocrine neoplasia type 2 syndromes and Hirschsprung disease. *J Cell Science.* 1994; 18 (suppl):43–49.
107. Lips CJM, Landsvater RM, Hoppener JWM, Geerdink RA, Blijham G. Clinical screening as compared with DNA analysis in families with multiple endocrine neoplasia type 2A. *N Engl J Med.* 1994; 31:828–835.
108. Zedenius J, Larsson C, Bergholm U et al. Mutations of codon 918 in the RET proto-oncogene correlate to poor prognosis in sporadic medullary thyroid carcinomas. *J Clin Endocrinol Metab.* 1995; 80:3088–3090.
109. Romei C, Elisei R, Pinchera A et al. Somatic mutations of the ret proto-oncogene in sporadic medullary thyroid carcinoma are not restricted to exon 16 and are associated with tumor recurrence. *J Clin Endocrinol Metab.* 1996; 81:1619–1622.
110. Jhiang SM, Fithian L, Weghorst CM et al. RET mutation screening in MEN2 patients and discovery of a novel mutation in a sporadic medullary thyroid carcinoma. *Thyroid.* 1996; 6:115–121.
111. Wohllk N, Cote G, Bugalho MMJ. Relevance of ret proto-oncogene mutations in sporadic medullary thyroid carcinoma. *J Clin Endocrinol Metab.* 1996; 81:3740–3745.
112. Frank-Raue K, Hoppner W, Frilling A et al. Mutations of the ret proto-oncogene in German multiple endocrine neoplasia families: relation between genotype and phenotype. *J Clin Endocrinol Metab.* 1996; 81:1780–1783.
113. Quadro L, Panariello L, Salvatore D, Carlomagno F. Frequent RET proto-oncogene mutations in multiple endocrine neoplasia type 2A. *J Clin Endocrinol Metab.* 1994; 79:590–594.
114. Mulligan LM, Ponder BAJ. Genetic basis of endocrine disease: Multiple endocrine neoplasia type 2. *J Clin Endocrinol Metab.* 1995; 80:1989–1995.
115. Eng C. The ret proto-oncogene in multiple endocrine neoplasia type 2 and Hirschsprung's disease. *N Engl J Med.* 1996; 335: 943–951.
116. Russo D, Arturi F, Chiefari E et al. A case of metastatic medullary thyroid carcinoma: early identification before surgery of an Ret proto-oncogene somatic mutation in fine-needle aspirate specimens. *J Clin Endocrinol Metab.* 1997; 82:3378–3382.
117. Lindor NM, Honchel R, Khosla S, Thibodeau SN. Mutations in the RET proto-oncogene in sporadic pheochromocytomas. *J Clin Endocrinol Metab.* 1995; 80:627–629.
118. Beldjord C, Desclaux-Arramond F, Raffin-Sanson M et al. The RET proto-oncogene in sporadic pheochromocytomas: frequent MEN 2-like mutations and new molecular defects. *J Clin Endocrinol Metab.* 1995; 80:2063–2068.
119. Grieco M, Santoro M, Berlingieri MT et al. PTC is a novel rearranged form of the ret proto-oncogene and is frequently detected in vivo in human thyroid papillary carcinomas. *Cell.* 1990; 60:557–563.
120. Santoro M, Carlomagno F, Hay ID, Herrmann MA, Grieco M. Ret oncogene activation in human thyroid neoplasms is restricted to the papillary cancer subtype. *J Clin Invest.* 1992; 89: 1517–1522.
121. Jhiang SM, Mazzaferri EL. The ret/PTC oncogene in papillary thyroid carcinoma. *J Lab Clin Med.* 1994; 123:331–337.
122. Sugg S, Zheng L, Rosen IB. Ret/PTC-1, -2, and -3 oncogene rearrangements in human thyroid carcinomas: implications for metastatic potential? *J Clin Endocrinol Metab.* 1996; 81:3360–3365.
123. Bongarzone I, Fugazzola L, Vigneri P et al. Age-related activation of the tyrosine kinase receptor proto-oncogenes ret and ntrk1 in papillary thyroid carcinoma. *J Clin Endocrinol Metab.* 1996; 81:2006–2009.
124. Lee C-H, Hsu L-S, Chi C-W, Chen G-D, Yang A-H, Chen J-Y. High frequency of rearrangement of the RET proto-oncogene (RET/PTC) in Chinese papillary thyroid carcinomas. *J Clin Endocrinol Metab.* 1998; 83:1629–1632.
125. Thomas GA, Bunnell H, Cook HA et al. High prevalence of RET/PTC rearrangements in Ukrainian and Belarussian post-Chernobyl thyroid papillary carcinomas: a strong correlation between RET/PTC3 and the solid-follicular variant. *J Clin Endocrinol Metab.* 1999; 84:4232–4238.
126. Gimm O, Greco A, Hoang-Vu C, Dralle H, Pierotti MA, Eng C. Mutation analysis reveals novel sequence variants in NTRK1 in sporadic human medullary thyroid carcinoma. *J Clin Endocrinol Metab.* 1999; 84:2784–2787.
127. Bongarzone I, Vigneri P, Mariani L, Collini P, Pilotti S, Pierotti MA. RET/NTRK1 rearrangements in thyroid gland tumors of the papillary carcinoma family: correlation with clinicopathological features. *Clin Cancer Res.* 1998; 4:223–228.
128. Pierotti MA, Vigneri P, Bongarzone I. Rearrangements of RET and NTRK1 tyrosine kinase receptors in papillary thyroid carcinomas. *Recent Results Cancer Res.* 1998; 154:237–247.
129. Beimfohr C, Klugbauer S, Demidchik EP, Lengfelder E, Rabes HM. NTRK1 re-arrangement in papillary thyroid carcinomas of children after the Chernobyl reactor accident. *Int J Cancer.* 1999; 80:842–847.
130. Di Renzo MF, Olivero M, Ferro S. Overexpression of the c-MET/HGF receptor gene in human thyroid carcinomas. *Oncogene.* 1992; 7:2549–2553.
131. Belfiori A, Gamgemi P, Santomocito MG. Prognostic value of c-MET expression in papillary thyroid carcinoma. *Thyroid.* 1995; 5(1):5–13.
132. Ruco LP, Ranalli T, Marzullo A et al. Expression of Met protein in thyroid tumours. *J Pathol.* 1996; 180:266–270.
133. Belfiori A, Gangemi P, Costantino A et al. Negative/low expression of the Met/hepatocyte growth factor receptor identifies papillary thyroid carcinomas with high risk of distant metastases. *J Clin Endocrinol Metab.* 1997; 82:2322–2328.
134. Trovato M, Villari D, Bartolone L et al. Expression of the hepatocyte growth factor and c-met in normal thyroid, non-neoplastic, and neoplastic nodules. *Thyroid.* 1998; 8:125–131.
135. Oyama T, Ichimura E, Sano T, Kashiwabara K, Fukuda T, Nakajima T. c-Met expression of thyroid tissue with special reference to papillary carcinoma. *Pathol Int.* 1998; 48:763–768.
136. Zanetti A, Stoppacciaro A, Marzullo A et al. Expression of Met protein and urokinase-type plasminogen activator receptor (uPA-R) in papillary carcinoma of the thyroid. *J Pathol.* 1998; 186:287–291.
137. Chen BK, Ohtsuki Y, Furihata M et al. Overexpression of c-Met protein in human thyroid tumors correlated with lymph node metastasis and clinicopathologic stage. *Pathol Res Pract.* 1999; 195:427–433.
138. de Luca A, Arena N, Sena LM, Medico E. Met overexpression confers HGF-dependent invasive phenotype to human thyroid carcinoma cells in vitro. *J Cell Physiol.* 1999; 180:365–371.

139. Bergstrom JD, Hermansson A, Diaz de Stahl T, Heldin NE. Non-autocrine, constitutive activation of Met in human anaplastic thyroid carcinoma cells in culture. *Br J Cancer.* 1999; 80:650–656.

140. Kelly K, Siebenlist U. The role of c-myc in the proliferation of normal and neoplastic cells. *J Clin Immunol.* 1985; 5:65–77.

141. Del Senno L, Gambari L, Degli UE et al. C-myc oncogene alterations in human thyroid carcinomas. *Cancer Detection and Prevention.* 1987; 10:159–166.

142. Terrier P, Sheng Z-M, Schlumberger M et.al. Structure and expression of c-myc and c-fos proto-oncogenes in human thyroid carcinomas. *Br J Cancer.* 1988; 57:43–47.

143. Boultwood J, Wyllie FS, Williams ED et.al. N-myc expression in neoplasia of human thyroid C-cells. *Cancer Res.* 1988; 48:4073–4077.

144. Vierbuchen M, Schroder S, Uhlenbruck G, Ortmann M, Fischer R. CA50 and CA19-9 antigen expression in normal, hyperplastic, and neoplastic thyroid tissue. *Lab Invest.* 1989; 60:726–731.

145. Yamasaki Y, Mori K, Naito M, Akagi M, Takahashi K. Histochemical determination of iodide peroxidase activity in various thyroid tissues. *Am J Surg.* 1990; 160:271–276.

146. de Micco C, Ruf J, Chrestian MA, Gros N, Henry JF, Carayon P. Immunohistochemical study of thyroid peroxidase in normal, hyperplastic and neoplastic human thyroid tissues. *Cancer.* 1991; 67:3036–3041.

147. Brabant G, Maenhaut C, Kohrle J et al. Human thyrotropin receptor gene: expression in thyroid tumors and correlation to markers of thyroid differentiation and dedifferentiation. *Mol Cell Endocrinol.* 1991; 82(1):R7–R12

148. Mizukami Y, Nonomura A, Hashimoto T et al. Immunohistochemical demonstration of epidermal growth factor and c-myc oncogene product in normal, benign and malignant thyroid tissues. *Histopathology.* 1991; 18:11–18.

149. Hoang-Vu C, Dralle H, Scheumann G et al. Gene expression of differentiation and dedifferentiation markers in normal and malignant human thyroid tissues. *Exp Clin Endocrinol.* 1992; 100(1–2):51–56.

150. Auguste LJ, Masood S, Westerband A, Belluco C, Valderama E, Attie J. Oncogene expression in follicular neoplasms of the thyroid. *Am J Surg.* 1992; 164:592–593.

151. Wallin G, Bronnegard M, Grimelius L, McGuire J, Torring O. Expression of the thyroid hormone receptor, the oncogenes c-myc and H-ras, and the 90 kD heat shock protein in normal, hyperplastic and neoplastic human thyroid tissue. *Thyroid.* 1992, 2(4):307–313.

152. Shi Y, Zou M, Farid NR. Expression of thyrotrophin receptor gene in thyroid carcinoma is associated with a good prognosis. *Clin Endocrinol Oxf.* 1993; 39:269–274.

153. Romano MI, Grattone M, Karner MP et al. Relationship between the level of c-myc mRNA and histologic aggressiveness in thyroid tumors. *Horm Res.* 1993; 39:161–165.

154. Lane DP. p53, guardian of the genome. *Nature.* 1992; 358:15–16.

155. Marx J. How p53 suppresses cell growth. *Science.* 1993; 262:1644–1645.

156. Frebourg T. Cancer risks from germline p53 mutations. *J Clin Invest.* 1992; 90:1637–1641.

157. Harris CC. Medical progress: clinical implications of the p53 tumor suppressor gene. *N Engl J Med.* 1993; 329:1318–1327.

158. Greenblat MS, Bennet WP, Hollstein M et.al. Mutations in the p53 tumor suppressor gene: clues to cancer aetiology and molecular pathogenesis. *Cancer Res.* 1994; 54:4855–4878.

159. Hooper ML. The role of the p53 and Rb-1 genes in cancer, development and apoptosis. *J Cell Science.* 1994; 18:13–17.

160. Cho Y, Gorina S, Jeffrey PD, Pavletich NP. Crystal structure of a p53 tumor suppressor-DNA complex: understanding tumorigenic mutations. *Science.* 1994; 265:346–355.

161. Nakamura T, Yana I, Kobayashi T et al. p53 gene mutations associated with anaplastic transformation of human thyroid carcinomas. *Jpn J Cancer Res.* 1992; 83(12):1293–1298.

162. Ito T, Seyma T, Mizuno T et.al. Unique association of p53 mutations with undifferentiated but not with differentiated carcinoma of the thyroid. *Cancer Res.* 1992; 52:1369–1371.

163. Fagin JA, Matsuo K, Karmakar A, Chen DL, Tang S-H, Koeffler HP. High prevalence of mutations of the p53 gene in poorly differentiated human thyroid carcinomas. *J Clin Invest.* 1993; 91:179–184.

164. Donghi R, Longoni A, Pilotti S, Michieli P, Porta GD, Pierotti MA. Gene p53 mutations are restricted to poorly differentiated and undifferentiated carcinomas of the thyroid gland. *J Clin Invest.* 1993; 91:1753–1760.

165. Dobashi Y, Sakamoto A, Sugimura H et al. Overexpression of p53 as a possible prognostic factor in human thyroid carcinoma. *Am J Surg Pathol.* 1993; 17:375–381.

166. Zou M, Shi Y, Farid NR. p53 mutations in all stages of thyroid carcinomas. *J Clin Endocrinol Metab.* 1993; 77:1054–1058.

167. Dobashi Y, Sugimura H, Sakamoto A et al. Stepwise participation of p53 gene mutation during dedifferentiation of human thyroid carcinomas. *Diagn Mol Pathol.* 1994; 3:9–14.

168. Fogelfeld L, Bauer TK, Schneider AB, Swartz JE, Zitman R. p53 gene ribonucleic acid in normal, hyperplastic, and neoplastic human thyroid tissue. *J Clin Endocrinol Metab.* 1994; 79:384–389.

169. Zedenius J, Larsson C, Wallin G et al. Alterations of p53 and expression of WAF1/p21 in human thyroid tumors. *Thyroid.* 1996; 6:1–9.

170. Pestell RG, Albanese C, Reutens AT, Segall JE, Lee RJ, Arnold A. The cyclins and cyclin-dependent kinase inhibitors in hormonal regulation of proliferation and differentiation. *Endocrine Rev.* 1999; 20:501–534.

171. Doree M, Galas S. The cyclin-dependent protein kinases and the control of cell division. *FASEB J.* 1994; 8:1114–1121.

172. Morgan DO. Principles of CDK regulation. *Nature.* 1995;374: 131–134.

173. Hartwell LH. Defects in the cell cycle checkpoint may be responsible for genomic instability of cancer cells. *Cell.* 1992;71: 543–546.

174. Kamb A, Gravis S, Weaver-Feldheus J et.al. A cell cycle regulator potentially involved in genesis of many tumor types. *Science.* 1994; 264:436–440.

175. Cyrus VL, Thor A, Xu H-J et.al. Loss of the retinoblastoma tumor-suppressor gene in parathyroid carcinoma. *N Engl J Med.* 1994; 330:757–761.

176. Figge J, Bakst G, Weisheit D, Solis O, Ross JS. Image analysis quantitation of immunoreactive retinoblastoma protein in human thyroid neoplasms with a streptavidin-biotin-peroxidase staining technique. *Am J Pathol.* 1991; 139:1213–1219.

177. Holm R, Nesland JM. Retinoblastoma and p53 tumour suppressor gene protein expression in carcinomas of the thyroid gland. *J Pathol.* 1994; 172:267–272.

178. Omura K, Nagasato A, Kanehira E et al. Retinoblastoma protein and proliferating-cell nuclear antigen expression as predictors of recurrence in well-differentiated papillary thyroid carcinoma. *J Clin Oncol.* 1997; 15:3458–3463.

179. Zou M, Shi Y, Farid NR, al-Sedairy ST. Inverse association between cyclin D1 overexpression and retinoblastoma gene mutation in thyroid carcinomas. *Endocrine.* 1998; 8:61–64.

180. Lazzereschi D, Sambuco L, Carnovale Scalzo C et al. Cyclin D1 and Cyclin E expression in malignant thyroid cells and in human thyroid carcinomas. *Int J Cancer.* 1998; 76:806–811.

181. Baldassarre G, Belletti G, Bruni P et al. Overexpressed cyclin D3 contributes to retaining the growth inhibitor p27 in the cytoplasm of thyroid tumor cells. *J Clin Invest.* 1999; 104:865–874.

182. Wang S, Wuu J, Savas L, Patwardhan N, Khan A. The role of cell regulatory proteins, cyclin D1, cyclin E, and p27 in thyroid carcinogenesis. *Hum Pathol.* 1998; 29:1304–1309.

183. Muro-Cacho CA, Holt T, Klotch D, Mora L, Livingston S, Futran N. Cyclin D1 expression as a prognostic parameter in papillary carcinoma of the thyroid. *Otolaryngol Head Neck Surg.* 1999; 120:200–207.

184. Elisei R, Shiohara M, Koeffler HP, Fagin JA. Genetic and epigenetic alterations of the cyclin-dependent kinase inhibitors p15INK4b and p16INK4a in human thyroid carcinoma cell lines and primary thyroid carcinomas. *Cancer.* 1998; 83:2185–2193.

185. Jones CJ, Shaw JJ, Wyllie FS, Gaillard N, Schlumberger M, Wynford-Thomas D. High frequency deletion of the tumour suppressor gene P16INK4a (MTS1) in human thyroid cancer cell lines. *Mol Cell Endocrinol.* 1996; 116:115–119.

186. Ito Y, Kobayashi T, Takeda T et al. Expression of p21 (WAF1/CIP1) protein in clinical thyroid tissues. *Br J Cancer.* 1996; 74:1269–1274.

187. Shi Y, Zou M, Farid NR, al-Sedairy ST. Evidence of gene deletion of p21 (WAF1/CIP1), a cyclin-dependent protein kinase inhibitor, in thyroid carcinomas. *Br J Cancer.* 1996; 74:1336–1341.

188. Erickson LA, Jin L, Wollan PC, Thompson GB, van Heerden J, Lloyd RV. Expression of p27kip1 and Ki-67 in benign and malignant thyroid tumors. *Mod Pathol.* 1998; 11:169–174.

189. Resnick MB, Schacter P, Finkelstein Y, Kellner Y, Cohen O. Immunohistochemical analysis of p27/kip1 expression in thyroid carcinoma. *Mod Pathol.* 1998; 11:735–739.

190. Yoshida A, Nakamura Y, Imada T, Asaga T, Shimizu A, Harada M. Apoptosis and proliferative activity in thyroid tumors. *Surg Today.* 1999; 29(3):204–208.

191. Reed JC. Bcl-2 and the regulation of programmed cell death. *J Cell Biol.* 1994; 124:1–6.

192. Hockenbery DM. bcl-2 in cancer, development and apoptosis. *J Cell Science.* 1994; 18:51–55.

193. Pilotti S, Collini P, Rilke F, Cattoretti G, Del Bo R, Pierotti MA. Bcl-2 protein expression in carcinomas originating from the follicular epithelium of the thyroid gland. *J Pathol.* 1994;172:337–342.

194. Brocker M, de Buhr I, Papageorgiou G, Schatz H, Derwahl M. Expression of apoptosis-related proteins in thyroid tumors and thyroid carcinoma cell lines. *Exp Clin Endocrinol Diab.* 1996; 104:20–23.

195. Basolo F, Pollina L, Fontanini G, Fiori L, Pacini F, Baldanzi A. Apoptosis and proliferation in thyroid carcinoma: correlation with bcl-2 and p53 protein expression. *Br J Cancer.* 1997; 75:537–541.

196. Manetto V, Lorenzini R, Cordon-Cardo C et al. Bcl-2 and Bax expression in thyroid tumours. an immunohistochemical and western blot analysis. *Virchows Arch.* 1997; 430:125–130.

197. Moore D, Ohene-Fianko D, Garcia B, Chakrabarti S. Apoptosis in thyroid neoplasms: relationship with p53 and bcl-2 expression. *Histopathology.* 1998; 32:35–42.

198. Wang DG, Liu WH, Johnston CF, Sloan JM, Buchanan KD. Bcl-2 and c-Myc, but not bax and p53, are expressed during human medullary thyroid tumorigenesis. *Am J Pathol.* 1998; 152:1407–1413.

199. Pollina L, Pacini F, Fontanini G, Vignati S, Bevilacqua G, Basolo F. bcl-2, p53 and proliferating cell nuclear antigen expression is related to the degree of differentiation in thyroid carcinomas. *Br J Cancer.* 1996; 73:139–143.

200. Lombardi L, Frigerio S, Collini P, Pilotti S. Immunocytochemical and immunoelectron microscopical analysis of BCL2 expression in thyroid oxyphilic tumors. *Ultrastruct Pathol.* 1997; 21:33–39.

201. Muller-Hocker J. Immunoreactivity of p53, Ki-67, and Bcl-2 in oncocytic adenomas and carcinomas of the thyroid gland. *Hum Pathol.* 1999; 30:926–933.

202. Haugen BR, Smart A, Shroyer KR, Pugazhenthi U. Survivin, an inhibitor of apoptosis, is overexpressed in thyroid carcinoma. *72nd Annual Meeting of the American Thyroid Association 1999*; Abstract #7.

203. Haber DA. Telomeres, cancer and immortality. *N Engl J Med.* 1995; 332:955–956.

204. Greider CW, Blackburn EH. Telomeres, telomerase and cancer. *Scientific American.* 1996; 274(2):92–97.

205. Haugen BR, Nawaz S, Markham N et al. Telomerase activity in benign and malignant thyroid tumors. *Thyroid.* 1997; 7(3):337–342.

206. Umbricht CB, Saji M, Westra WH, Udelsman R, Zeiger MA, Sukumar S. Telomerase activity: a marker to distinguish follicular thyroid adenoma from carcinoma. *Cancer Res.* 2000; 57: 2144–2147.

207. Brousset P, Chaouche N, Leprat F et al. Telomerase activity in human thyroid carcinomas originating from the follicular cells. *J Clin Endocrinol Metab.* 1997; 82:4214–4216.

208. Okayasu I, Osakabe T, Fujiwara M, Fukuda H, Kato M, Oshimura M. Significant correlation of telomerase activity in thyroid papillary carcinomas with cell differentiation, proliferation and extrathyroidal extension. *Jpn J Cancer Res.* 1997; 88: 965–970.

209. Saji M, Westra WH, Chen H et al. Telomerase activity in the differential diagnosis of papillary carcinoma of the thyroid. *Surgery.* 1997; 122:1137–1140.

210. Yashima K, Vuitch F, Gazdar AF, Fahey TJ. Telomerase activity in benign and malignant thyroid diseases. *Surgery.* 1997; 122: 1141–1145.

211. Cheng AJ, Lin JD, Chang T, Wang TC. Telomerase activity in benign and malignant human thyroid tissues. *Br J Cancer.* 1998; 77:2177–2180.

212. Aogi K, Kitahara K, Buley I et al. Telomerase activity in lesions of the thyroid: Application to diagnosis of clinical samples including fine-needle aspirates. *Clin Cancer Res.* 1998; 4:1965–1970.

213. Onoda N, Ishikawa T, Yoshikawa K et al. Telomerase activity in thyroid tumors. *Oncol Rep.* 1998; 5:1447–1450.

214. Saji M, Xydas S, Westra WH et al. Human telomerase reverse transcriptase (hTERT) gene expression in thyroid neoplasms. *Clin Cancer Res.* 1999; 5:1483–1489.

215. Aogi K, Kitahara K, Urquidi V, Tarin D, Goodison S. Comparison of telomerase and CD44 expression as diagnostic tumor markers in lesions of the thyroid. *Clin Cancer Res.* 1999; 5:2790–2797.

216. Bernstein LR, Liotta LA. Molecular mediators of interactions with extracellular matrix components in metastasis and angiogenesis. *Curr Opin Oncol.* 1994; 6:106–113.

217. Ruoslahti E, Reed JC. Anchorage dependence, integrins and apoptosis. *Cell.* 1994; 77:477–478.

218. Oliff A, Gibbs JB, McCormick F. New molecular targets for cancer therapy. *Scientific American.* 1996; 275:144–149.

219. Folkman K. Fighting cancer by attacking its blood supply. *Scientific American.* 1996; 275:150–154.

220. Ruoslahti E. How cancer spreads. *Scientific American.* 1996; 275:72–77.

221. Akiyama SK, Olden K, Yamada KM. Fibronectin and integrins in invasion and metastasis. *Cancer and Metastasis Reviews.* 1996; 14:173–189.

222. Scheumann GFW, Hoang-Vu C, Cetin Y et al. Clinical significance of E-cadherin as a prognostic marker in thyroid carcinomas. *J Clin Endocrinol Metab.* 1995; 80:2168–2172.

223. Brabant G, Hoang-Vu C, Cetin Y et al. E-cadherin: A differentiation marker in thyroid malignancies. *Cancer Res.* 1993; 53: 4987–4993.

224. Scheumann GF, Hoang-Vu C, Cetin Y et al. Clinical significance of E-cadherin as a prognostic marker in thyroid carcinomas. *J Clin Endocrinol Metab.* 1995; 80:2168–2172.

225. Serini G, Trusolino L, Saggiorato E et al. Changes in integrin and E-cadherin expression in neoplastic versus normal thyroid tissue. *J Natl Cancer Inst.* 1996; 88:442–449.

226. von Wasielewski R, Rhein A, Werner M et al. Immunohistochemical detection of E-cadherin in differentiated thyroid carcinomas correlates with clinical outcome. *Cancer Res.* 1997;57: 2501–2507.

227. Cerrato A, Fulciniti F, Avallone A, Benincasa G, Palombini L, Grieco M. Beta- and gamma-catenin expression in thyroid carcinomas. *J Pathol.* 1998; 185:267–272.

228. Soares P, Berx G, van Roy F, Sobrinho-Simoes M. E-cadherin gene alterations are rare events in thyroid tumors. *Int J Cancer.* 1997; 70:32–38.

229. Graff JR, Greenberg VE, Herman JG et al. Distinct patterns of E-cadherin CpG island methylation in papillary, follicular, Hurthle's cell, and poorly differentiated human thyroid carcinoma. *Cancer Res.* 1998; 58:2063–2066.

230. Huang SH, Wu JC, Chang KJ, Liaw KY, Wang SM. Distribution of the cadherin-catenin complex in normal human thyroid epithelium and a thyroid carcinoma cell line. *J Cell Biochem.* 1998; 70:330–337.

231. Husmark J, Hedlin NE, Nilsson M. N-cadherin-mediated adhesion and aberrant catenin expression in anaplastic thyroid-carcinoma cell lines. *Int J Cancer.* 1999; 83:692–699.

232. Dahlman T, Grimelius L, Wallin G, Rubin K, Westermark K. Integrins in thyroid tissue: upregulation of alpha2beta1 in anaplastic thyroid carcinoma. *Eur J Endocrinol.* 1998; 138:104–112.

233. Montuori N, Müller F, De Riu S, Fenzi G, Sobel ME, Rossi G, et al. Laminin receptors in differentiated thyroid tumors: restricted expression of the 67-kilodalton laminin receptor in follicular carcinoma cells. *J Clin Endocrinol Metab.* 1999; 84:2086–2092.

234. Bièche I, Ruffet E, Zweibaum A, Vildé F, Lidereau R, Franc B. MUC1 mucin gene, transcripts, and protein in adenomas and papillary carcinomas of the thyroid. *Thyroid.* 1997; 7:725–731.

235. Higashiyama T, Takano T, Matsuzuka F et al. Measurement of the expression of oncofetal fibronectin mRNA in thyroid carcinomas by competitive reverse transcription-polymerase chain reaction. *Thyroid.* 1999; 9:235–240.

236. Aust G, Hofmann A, Laue S, Rost A, Köhler T, Scherbaum WA. Human thyroid carcinoma cell lines and normal thyrocytes: expression and regulation of matrix metalloproteinase-1 and tissue matrix metalloproteinase inhibitor-1 messenger-RNA and protein. *Thyroid.* 1997; 7:713–724.

237. Viglietto G, Maglione D, Rambaldi M et al. Upregulation of vascular endothelial growth factor (VEGF) and downregulation of placenta growth factor (PlGF) associated with malignancy in human thyroid tumors and cell lines. *Oncogene.* 1995; 11:1569–1579.

238. Soh EY, Sobhi SA, Wong MG et al. Thyroid-stimulating hormone promotes the secretion of vascular endothelial growth factor in thyroid cancer cell lines. *Surgery.* 1996; 120:944–947.

239. Soh EY, Duh QY, Sobhi SA et al. Vascular endothelial growth factor expression is higher in differentiated thyroid cancer than in normal or benign thyroid. *J Clin Endocrinol Metab.* 1997; 82:3741–3747.

240. Klein M, Picard E, Vignaud JM et al. Vascular endothelial growth factor gene and protein: Strong expression in thyroiditis and thyroid carcinoma. *J Endocrinol.* 1999; 161:41–49.

241. Katoh R, Miyagi E, Kawaoi A et al. Expression of vascular endothelial growth factor (VEGF) in human thyroid neoplasms. *Hum Pathol.* 1999; 30:891–897.

242. Belletti B, Ferraro P, Arra C et al. Modulation of in vivo growth of thyroid tumor-derived cell lines by sense and antisense vascular endothelial growth factor gene. *Oncogene.* 1999; 18: 4860–4869.

243. Kebebew E, Wong MG, Siperstein AE, Duh Q-Y, Clark OH. Phenylacetate inhibits growth and vascular endothelial growth factor secretion in human thyroid carcinoma cells and modulates their differentiated function. *J Clin Endocrinol Metab.* 1999; 84:2840–2847.

244. Bassi V, Vitale M, Feliciello A, De Riu S, Rossi G, Fenzi G. Retinoic acid induces intercellular adhesion molecule-1 hyperexpression in human thyroid carcinoma cell lines. *J Clin Endocrinol Metab.* 1995; 80:1129–1135.

245. Old LJ. Immunotherapy for cancer. *Scientific American.* 1996; 275:136–143.

# 11

# Risk and Prognostic Factors in Thyroid Cancer

## Ashok R. Shaha, M.D., F.A.C.S.

Although there are several controversies in the management of thyroid cancer, prognostic factors and risk groups are extremely important in the understanding of its biology. Most controversies in the management of thyroid cancer related to the extent of thyroidectomy could be easily resolved by prognostic factors and risk group analysis. Thyroid cancer can be divided into good (low) and poor (high) risk groups. Survival in the good-risk group is excellent, while the thyroid cancer is quite aggressive in poor-risk groups. The decisions regarding extent of thyroidectomy and adjuvant therapy related to radioactive iodine and external radiation therapy should be based on prognostic factors and risk groups. The outcome in good-risk thyroid cancer is excellent and there is no specific role for adjuvant therapy. Conservative surgical resection will render the same long-term results as total thyroidectomy with reduced risk of overall complications. However, in the high-risk group, one needs to be surgically aggressive along with postoperative radioactive iodine and external radiation therapy in selected cases.

## INTRODUCTION

Although thyroid disease and thyroid nodules are extremely common in the United States, the incidence of thyroid cancer in relation to overall thyroid pathology is not very high. Approximately 10% to 15% of patients with solitary thyroid nodules are likely to have thyroid cancer. Thyroid cancer can be divided into two distinct groups pathologically—well-differentiated thyroid cancer (including papillary, follicular, mixed and Hürthle cell) and the other group, which consists of medullary and anaplastic thyroid cancers. The rare forms of thyroid cancer are also included in this latter group such as lymphoma, sarcoma, and metastatic tumors to the thyroid. The overall prognosis and outcome depend on the histologic variety and the extent of the disease at initial presentation. The tumors most commonly metastatic to thyroid primarily originate in lung, breast, kidney, and melanoma.

The discussion on thyroid cancer generates considerable controversy and more than 2,000 peer-reviewed papers are published every year on the subject of thyroid disease, of which approximately 500 are related to thyroid cancer. The major controversies revolve around the diagnostic workup and the extent of surgery. There appear to be two strong groups, one firmly believing in routine total thyroidectomy, and the other group believing that the extent of thyroidectomy should be based on prognostic factors, risk groups, and extent of disease.

Thyroid cancer is a unique neoplasm that encompasses a wide spectrum of diseases. At one end of the spectrum there is well-differentiated thyroid cancer—which has an excellent outcome, while at the other end of the spectrum there is anaplastic thyroid cancer—which has the worst outcome and the average survival is counted in months. It is quite interesting that the clinical and histologic presentations of the disease in the same organ are so variable.

The American Cancer Society estimates approximately 20,000 new patients with thyroid cancer in the year 2002.[1] There appears to be a steady increase in the incidence of thyroid cancer in the United States, with approximately 8,000 cases seen in 1974 to the current number of 20,000 in the year 2002. There also appears to be a steady increase in the incidence of thyroid cancer in women. However, it is interesting to note that the overall mortality from thyroid cancer has essentially remained unchanged, with approximately 1,300 individuals dying of thyroid cancer every year in the United States. Of this mortality, approximately 500 patients die of anaplastic thyroid cancer, while 200 to 300 die of medullary thyroid cancer. Interestingly, death from well-differentiated thyroid cancer is quite rare, as a majority of patients with well-differentiated thyroid cancer do extremely well. However, there is a certain group of well-differentiated thyroid cancers where the incidence of mortality is quite high. It is very important to define this group and to treat them more aggressively along with adjuvant therapies.

Samuel Gross, back in 1866, considered thyroid surgery to be "butchery" and went on to write, "no honest and sensible surgeon would ever engage in thyroid surgery."[2] Toward the turn of the last century, there was considerable progress in thyroid surgery. Theodore Kocher from Vienna was at the forefront in thyroid surgery by perfecting the technique of the surgery and describing the physiology of thyroid diseases. He was the first surgeon to win the Nobel Prize in Medicine for his contributions in thyroidology. Of course, our understanding of thyroid cancer has improved considerably in the last two decades with the definition of major prognostic factors and risk groups. The clinical parameters are now supplemented with histologic parameters and molecular markers, while the role of the pathologist is paramount in describing the well-differentiated, poorly differentiated, and undifferentiated thyroid cancers. Our understanding of molecular markers in thyroid cancer also appears to be still in its infancy, although P-53 mutation appears to be an important factor. Other molecular markers are being studied in a very small number of cases, but it is difficult to make any meaningful determinations from these studies. The comparative genomic hybridization and DNA arrays will definitely add to our understanding of the molecular biology of thyroid cancer in the next few years. Hundahl et al reported a large series of patients with thyroid cancer from the National Cancer Data Base, which collected a series of 53,856 patients with thyroid cancer from 1985 to 1995.[3,4] The histologic distribution of various types of thyroid cancers included papillary (79%), follicular (14.2%), medullary (3.7%), Hürthle cell (2.7%) and undifferentiated or anaplastic thyroid cancers (1.6%). The ten-year overall relative survival rates for patients with papillary, follicular, Hürthle cell, medullary, and undifferentiated anaplastic carcinoma were 99%, 85%, 76%, 75%, and 14%, respectively.

Thyroid cancer has many unique features, which makes it very different from other human cancers. Age continues to be the most important prognostic indicator. Young patients with thyroid cancer do extremely well in comparison to older people. The mortality in young patients with thyroid cancer is extremely low. In younger individuals (generally below the age of 20), thyroid cancer clinically may appear more aggressive, even with distant metastasis, but the prognosis in this group of patients is very good. It is interesting to note that this is the only human cancer where the AJCC-UICC Staging System has included age as an important parameter[5] (Table 11–1). There is no Stage III or IV cancer below the age of 45. Another unique feature of this tumor is that nodal metastasis has minimal prognostic bearing. No other human cancer parallels this particular feature. Even in patients with nodal metastasis, there is no survival difference. Clearly, this relates mainly to the biology of thyroid cancer, and it is important for treating physicians to understand this biology rather than to make uniform treatment decisions for all patients with thyroid cancer. In patients over the age of 45, there may be some deleterious effect of nodal metastasis, mainly in relation to multiple neck recurrences.[6] A third unique feature of this tumor is recognition of poorly differentiated varieties such as tall cell and insular pathology.[7,8] The histopathologic understanding of this entity is extremely important in distinguishing between well-differentiated and poorly differentiated thyroid cancer. The relationship of previous external radiation therapy to the neck and development of thyroid cancer is also a unique feature. Patients who were radiated during childhood for acne, enlarged tonsil, enlarged thymus, or skin lesions, have a very high incidence of subsequent development of thyroid cancer—most of which are papillary thyroid cancers. A similar effect was noted with the nuclear accident in Chernobyl where there is an almost 12- to 34-fold rise in the development of thyroid cancer in surrounding regions such as Belarus, Ukraine, and Russia. Most of these are in the pediatric age group and include a high incidence of poorly differentiated thyroid cancers.

Completeness of resection of the tumor is extremely important for better local control.[9–11] The presence of extra-thyroidal extension is deleterious and there is a high incidence of local recurrence in patients with extra-thyroidal extension.[12] The mortality in patients who have recurred locally in the thyroid bed is quite high; therefore, every effort should be made to remove all gross tumor at the time of surgery. The role of external radiation therapy is quite limited in thyroid cancer, particularly in the United States where thyroid cancer used to be considered resistant to external radiation therapy. However, reports from other parts of the world have concluded that external radiation therapy does reduce

**Table 11–1.** Cancer staging for papillary, follicular and medullary thyroid carcinoma

---

**Definition of TNM**

| | | |
|---|---|---|
| Primary Tumor (T) | T0 | = No evidence of primary tumor |
| | T1 | = Tumor 1.0 cm or less in greatest dimension limited to the thyroid. |
| | T2 | = Tumor more than 1.0 cm but not more than 4.0 cm in greatest dimension limited to the thyroid. |
| | T3 | = Tumor more than 4.0 cm in greatest dimension limited to the thyroid. |
| | T4 | = Tumor of any size extending beyond the thyroid capsule. |
| Regional Lymph Nodes (N) | N0 | = No regional lymph node metastasis |
| | N1 | = Regional lymph node metastasis |
| | N1a | = Metastasis in ipsilateral cervical lymph node(s) |
| | N1b | = Metastasis in bilateral, midline or contralateral cervical or mediastinal lymph node(s). |
| Distant Metastasis (M) | M0 | = No distant metastasis |
| | M1 | = Distant metastasis |

**Papillary or Follicular**

| | *Age < 45 Years* | *Age 45 or Older* |
|---|---|---|
| Stage I | Any T, any N, M0 | Any T1, N0, M0 |
| Stage II | Any T, any N, M1 | T2 or 3, N0, M0 |
| Stage III | — | T4, N0, M0 or any T, N1, M0 |
| Stage IV | — | Any T, any N, M1 |

**Medullary**

| | |
|---|---|
| Stage I | T1, N0, M0 |
| Stage II | T2–4, N0, M0 |
| Stage III | Any T, N1, M0 |
| Stage IV | Any T, any N, M1 |

**Undifferentiated**

| | |
|---|---|
| Stage IV (all cases) | Any T, any N, any M |

---

Based on data from American Joint Committee on Cancer Staging.

the incidence of local recurrence and may control the tumor for a considerable duration of time in an inoperable situation.[13] Radioactive iodine is considered to be one of the mainstays in the adjuvant treatment of thyroid cancer after surgical resection.[14,15] The thyroid gland and its metastases have a high affinity for radioactive iodine that can be utilized both for diagnostic purposes after surgical intervention and for therapeutic purposes.

Although Hürthle cell tumors of the thyroid are considered to be a variation of follicular thyroid cancer, these tumors behave in an unique fashion. Histologically they are distinct oncocytic tumors with a high incidence of distant metastasis. It is interesting to note that Hürthle cell tumors generally do not pick up radioactive iodine. The recent interest in PET scan has defined a group of patients who are nonradio-avid, but recurrent or metastatic disease will be easily seen on PET scan and are generally poorly differentiated tumors. From a histopathologic standpoint, it is important to remember that the distinction between a benign follicular adenoma

and follicular carcinoma is made by reviewing the entire capsule of the thyroid tumor.[16,17] If there is capsular or vascular invasion, the diagnosis of follicular adenoma is changed to follicular carcinoma. As a result, it is important for the pathologist to review multiple sections of the thyroid mass to evaluate the status of the capsule. If the tumor is larger than 3 cm, there is an almost 30% chance that the diagnosis of follicular adenoma may be changed into follicular carcinoma by review of the entire capsule for capsular or vascular invasion.

## PROGNOSTIC FACTORS IN THYROID CANCER

A variety of patient-related and tumor-related prognostic factors have been studied in different institutions in a retrospective fashion.[18-33] Unfortunately, there are no prospective randomized trials in thyroid cancer in relation to treatment approaches, as a trial would require a large number of patients to be followed for a substantial period of time. In spite of this, there is minimal survival difference to make any definite or statistical conclusions regarding overall outcome. The treatment of thyroid cancer also depends on the institutional policy and the philosophy of the treating physician, because there clearly are differences between the philosophies of surgeons, nuclear physicians, and endocrinologists. The American College of Surgeons Oncology Group (ACOSOG) is currently reviewing certain proposed randomized prospective trials in thyroid cancer, mainly related to postoperative radiation therapy.

The following prognostic factors are studied in detail in various retrospective studies:

## Age

Age continues to be the most important prognostic factor in thyroid cancer.[5] Patients below the age of 45 (as divided by AJCC Staging System) continue to show excellent prognosis. The mortality in patients below the age of 45 is 1–2% while the mortality in individuals above the age of 60 is quite high. The Mayo Clinic series of papillary carcinoma of more than 1,500 patients revealed mortality rates less than 1% in patients below the age of 50, 7% for those between the ages of 50 and 59, 20% for those between the ages of 60 and 69, and 46% for patients above the age of 70. The SEER (Surveillance Epidemiology and End Results) reporting of the National Cancer Institute reported a significantly high mortality in the 7th decade of life. Most of the patients dying of thyroid cancer generally are in the 6th and 7th decades of life.[4] The mortality in the younger age group is quite rare, and most of the patients who die at a young age have either poor histologic parameters or very advanced distant metastatic disease.

## Size

Tumors less than 1 cm are considered to be micro-carcinomas, and the mortality in this group is less than 1% in the long-term follow-up.[34] A specific condition of occult primary carcinoma with regional or distant metastasis is well known. However, this is a rare condition and mostly occurs with metastatic neck nodes. The experience from Memorial Sloan-Kettering Cancer Center showed that there was no survival difference in tumors less than 3 cm.[2,25,31] However, the follicular cancers greater than 4 cm had higher incidence of long-term mortality and in papillary carcinoma, the tumors greater than 3 cm had a higher incidence of nodal metastasis, even though there was no survival difference up to 4 cm. The AJCC UICC Staging system has

used T1–T2 as tumors less than 2 cm and 2–4 cm, respectively, as the staging classification.

## Extra-Thyroidal Invasion

Probably the most important prognostic factor for local recurrence is extra-thyroidal tumor extension.[2,12] Various retrospective studies have reviewed this prognostic factor critically with extension of the disease into surrounding structures such as strap muscles, recurrent laryngeal nerve, trachea or esophagus. There is considerable debate regarding the resection of the upper aerodigestive tract versus shaving-off procedures. It is extremely important for treating physicians to document the extent of the disease. One may require additional imaging studies such as ultrasound, CT scan or MRI. Direct laryngoscopy, bronchoscopy and tracheoscopy may be helpful to rule out any intraluminal disease. If the tumor extends through to the lumen, appropriate resection and anastomosis of the trachea is necessary. If the tumor invades the cartilaginous structures of the larynx, partial laryngectomy or resection of the cartilage may be performed. If the tumor invades the esophagus, generally the esophageal musculature can be resected. It is quite rare that the tumor will invade the esophageal mucosa. Primary laryngectomy, even in advanced local disease, is rarely indicated and every attempt is made to preserve the laryngeal function. If the tumor invades the tracheal lumen, the procedure of choice is resection of the segment of the trachea with end-to-end anastomosis. The mucosal involvement of the tumor can lead to intraluminal bleeding and occasionally respiratory distress. The surgical procedure in patients with extra-thyroidal invasion should be quite aggressive to remove all gross tumor. The surgical technique can make a difference in the local control by removing all macroscopic disease. Again, in patients below the age of 45 with extra-thyroidal extension, if all gross tumor is removed, then there is no survival difference. This indicates that the resection of all gross tumor is extremely important in patients with extra-thyroidal invasion.[35–37] If the recurrent laryngeal nerve is functioning preoperatively and the tumor encircles the recurrent laryngeal nerve, every attempt should be made to preserve the nerve. However, it is important not to leave any gross tumor behind. If one nerve is involved, it may be sacrificed with preservation of satisfactory laryngeal function. If both nerves seem to be involved by the tumor, every attempt should be made to preserve at least one functioning nerve to avoid tracheotomy. Again, the principle of thyroid surgery is to make every effort to preserve the functioning laryngeal nerve. In view of this, it is vitally important to evaluate the vocal cord function preoperatively in every patient undergoing thyroidectomy and also during the postoperative follow-up. Preoperative imaging studies such as CT scan will better define the extent of the disease.

## Distant Metastasis

Most of the patients with distant metastasis are generally diagnosed with tumor in the lung followed by bone and other structures such as brain, liver, and so forth. Young patients with pulmonary metastasis do remarkably well with appropriate adjuvant treatment such as radioactive iodine. Most of the patients with papillary and follicular carcinoma have radio-avid metastatic disease. One of the major advances in the management of these patients is early detection of pulmonary metastasis, which is generally considered in intermediate or high-risk patients postoperatively after appropriate total thyroidectomy and paratracheal clearance. Radioactive iodine dosimetry should be performed. Most of the time this is done in the hypothyroid state. One of the major recent advances is the use of recombinant TSH or thyrogen. With two injections of thyrogen, the TSH can be raised without making patients hypothyroid and subsequent radioactive iodine dosimetry and ablation can be performed. The procedure may be repeated in 6–12 months depending upon the initial findings of radioactive iodine ablation. In the low-risk patient, 29 mCi of radioactive iodine may be used to ablate the residual thyroid tissue. However, in high-risk patients, a large dose of radioactive iodine (ranging between 100 to 200 mCi or more) may be required to ablate any gross residual disease or distant metastasis. The pulmonary metastases that are not seen on chest X-ray, but which are detected by radioactive iodine, are much easier to control with appropriate dosage of radioactive iodine. A second dose may be required after a few months. Patients with metastatic disease to the bones have much poorer long-term survival with mortality of almost 80% in 10 years. Patients with metastatic disease to lung and bone generally have a poor outcome. However, the worst prognosis is associated with brain metastasis—with a median survival of only one year.

## Lymph Node Metastasis

The incidence of metastatic cervical nodal disease in papillary thyroid cancer is approximately 50%. However, it has very little prognostic implication. In young patients with nodal metastasis, there is no survival difference. However, in older patients, there may be some impact of metastatic neck nodes, especially in relation to the multiple cervical recurrences.[38] The radical neck

dissection is rarely undertaken, even with bulky nodal disease. However, the old surgical procedure of "berry picking" is rarely used today as there is a high incidence of local recurrence in the neck after "berry picking" procedures. The classical modified neck dissection preserving the sternomastoid muscle, internal jugular vein, and accessory nerve is routinely performed with removal of all the lymph nodes in the neck except Level I. The incidence of metastatic disease to Level I is quite rare in thyroid cancer, and the submandibular salivary gland is rarely removed in the management of metastatic neck disease. The critical area for nodal clearance is the central compartment in the region of the paratracheal area and superior mediastinum. Every attempt should be made to remove all gross tumor in the central compartment and to achieve adequate and appropriate central compartment clearance from removal of the lymph nodes including the superior mediastinum. However, one has to keep in mind that that there is a high incidence of temporary and permanent hypoparathyroidism in this surgical procedure. Every attempt should be made to identify the parathyroid glands and preserve them with their own blood supply. If a parathyroid gland or its blood supply is compromised it is important to autotransplant the parathyroid, preferably in the strap muscles of the neck or the sternomastoid muscle.

## Multifocality of the Tumor

Papillary carcinoma of the thyroid is well-known to have multifocal extension, although whether this is a truly multifocal disease or microscopic lymphatic spread of the tumor is difficult to confirm. The presence of microscopic multifocal disease, classically called "laboratory cancer," has no prognostic bearing. Approximately 50% of these individuals have microscopic thyroid cancer, but as long as it is not clinically significant, it has little prognostic significance. The decision regarding the extent of thyroidectomy should be based on many other prognostic factors rather than the consideration of microscopic multifocal thyroid cancer. In the series published from Memorial Sloan-Kettering Cancer Center, the multifocality had no prognostic bearing.[31] The incidence of local recurrence in the contralateral lobe after unilateral thyroid lobectomy in patients presenting with solitary thyroid nodule is between 5 and 10%.

## Gender

Thyroid disease is more common in women; however, thyroid cancer is more common in men. In elderly males, thyroid cancer is more aggressive than in the female population, even though in many series there was no major statistical difference in the outcome with respect to gender. Clearly thyroid disease is considered to be much more aggressive in the elderly male population. The incidence of thyroid cancer is slightly higher in male patients presenting with thyroid masses compared to women.

## OTHER PROGNOSTIC FACTORS

The delay between the initial presentation and clinical manifestation of the disease is also considered to be an important prognostic factor. The completeness of resection as popularized by the Mayo Clinic is another important prognostic factor for local recurrence and long-term control. Associated conditions such as Graves' disease, coexisting thyroiditis or Hashimoto's disease do not seem to have major impact on the long-term outcome.

### Molecular Markers

The immunohistochemical studies, although not studied in detail, seem to have an effect in the local control and long-term survival. The increased tumor vascularity, expression of epidermal growth factor receptors, RET, PTC, P-53, and ploidy seem to have definite impact in the overall outcome.[2,14] The aneuploid tumors do much worse compared to diploid tumors. The postoperative thyroglobulin levels may be used as a marker of tumor activity, especially with a rising thyroglobulin level after total thyroidectomy heralding the possibility of recurrent tumor. The role of radioactive iodine ablation in persistently elevated thyroglobulin still remains to be defined.

### Clinical Staging and Risk Group Analysis

Based on these prognostic factors, various risk groups have been characterized. The Mayo Clinic and Lahey Clinic divided their patients into low- and high-risk groups. The mortality in their low-risk group was less than 2% while the mortality in the high-risk group was approximately 46%. The studies from Memorial Sloan-Kettering Cancer Center with 1,038 patients followed for a long period of time revealed important and significant prognostic factors.[2] These prognostic factors include grade of the tumor, age, presence or absence of distant metastasis, extra-thyroidal extension and size of the tumor (GAMES).[31] The prognostic factors were divided into patient-related factors such as age and gender and the tumor-related factors such as histology, size of the tumor, extra-thyroidal extension, grade of the tumor and presence of distant metastasis. The data from Memorial Sloan-Kettering Cancer Center was reanalyzed and the risk groups were stratified, dividing the patients into low-, intermediate-, and high-risk groups. Patients in the low-risk groups included low-risk patients generally below the age of 45 with low-risk tumors, while the high-risk group included high-risk patients above the age of 45 with high-risk tumors. The intermediate-risk group included young patients with more aggressive tumors or elderly patients with less aggressive tumors. The survival in this latter group generally depends on the aggressiveness of the thyroid tumor. Even though the overall survival in differentiated thyroid carcinoma is excellent, the mortality in the high-risk group is very high with long-term survival of only 57% in the Memorial Sloan-Kettering series.

## AGES (Mayo Clinic)

The Mayo Clinic identified important prognostic factors as age, grade of the tumor, extra-thyroidal extent of the disease, and size of the tumor.[9] The Mayo Clinic developed a prognostic score for individual factors (Table 11–2). Based on their AGES prognostic scoring system, patients below the score of 3.99 had a 20-year survival of 99%, while the survival decreased to 80% for patients with a score of 4 to 4.99. The survival was 67% for patients with a score of 5 to 5.99 and only 13% for patients with score above 6. Even though the Mayo Clinic popularized grade as the important prognostic factor, it is not universally applicable, as many pathologists do not agree with the exact grade of the tumor and on many occasions grade is not routinely described in the histologic report.

**Table 11–2.** AGES

Prognostic score = 0.05 × age (if age ≥ 40)
    +1 (if grade 2)
    +3 (if grade 3 or 4)
    +1 (if extra-thyroid)
    +3 (if distant spread)
    +0.2 × tumor size (cm maximum diameter)

Survival by AGES score (20 years)
    < 3.99 = 99%
    4–4.99 = 80%
    5–5.99 = 67%
    > 6.00 = 13%

Based on data from the Mayo Clinic.

## MACIS (Mayo Clinic)

The Mayo Clinic re-reviewed their data base and developed a prognostic system of MACIS.[10] The most important distinction in this group compared to AGES was completeness of resection (Table 11–3). Again, based on their prognostic scoring system, patients were divided into four categories with scores less than 6 (99% survival), scores between 6 to 6.99 (89% survival), 7 to 7.99 (56% survival), and patients with a MACIS score of more than 8 (24% survival) for a period of 20 years. From a surgical standpoint, completeness of resection of the tumor is probably the most important prognostic factor, both for local recurrence, nodal disease and eventually, in the long-term, distant metastasis.

## AMES

Cady et al from the Lahey Clinic divided their patients into low-risk and high-risk groups.[18,20,22] They separated men at the age of 40 and women at the age of 50

**Table 11–3.** MACIS

---

SCORE = 3.1 (if age < 40 years) or 0.08 x age (if age ≥ 40 years)

      + 0.3 x tumor size (cm maximum diameter)

      + 1 (if incompletely resected)

      + 1 (if locally invasive)

      + 3 (if distant spread)

Survival by MACIS score (20 years)

        < 6 = 99%

      6–6.99 = 89%

      7–7.99 = 56%

        ≥ 8 = 24%

---

Based on data from the Mayo Clinic.

(Table 11–4). They also divided their patients by tumor size into less than or greater than 5 cm groups. Again, in their series of a large number of patients followed for an average 20-year period, 89% were classified as low-risk and 11% as high-risk. The mortality in the low-risk group was 1.8% compared to 46% for patients in the high-risk group. The data from the M.D. Anderson Cancer Center and University of Chicago were analyzed based on the AMES classification and similar outcomes were reported.

## EORTC

Probably one of the earliest scoring systems and prognostic factors was developed by EORTC.[19] A very complex coding system was described; however, it again confirmed that patients with a low score did extremely well in comparison to those in the high score group. The European Organization for Research and Treatment of Cancer (EORTC) Thyroid Cancer Cooperative Group studied prognostic factors in approximately 507 patients in 1979. They developed a prognostic index based on multivariate analysis. The concept of prognostic factors was initially described by Sloan and McDermott in 1954. However, the EORTC study also included patients with medullary and anaplastic thyroid cancer. These two more aggressive forms of thyroid cancer should not be included in any risk group analysis of well-differentiated thyroid cancer, particularly because their behavior is strikingly different compared to well-differentiated thyroid cancer.

## TNM Classification

The AJCC-UICC developed a TNM classification based on tumor size, presence or absence of nodal metastasis, and distant metastasis.[5] They included age as an important prognostic factor with absence of Stage III and IV

**Table 11–4.** AMES

---

Low risk:  Younger patients (men ≤ 40, women ≤ 50) with no metastases)
          Older patients (intrathyroid papillary, minor capsular invasion for follicular lesions)
          Primary cancers < 5.0 cm
          No distant metastases

High risk:  All patients with distant metastases
           Extra-thyroid papillary, major capsular invasion follicular
           Primary cancers ≥ 5.0 cm in older patients (men > 40, women > 50)

Survival by AMES risk groups (20 years):
     Low risk = 99%
     High risk = 61%

---

Based on data from the Lahey Clinic.

cancers in patients below the age of 45 indicating that young patients do remarkably well. The nodal status was divided into presence or absence of neck nodes and the N1 disease was divided into N1a indicating ipsilateral cervical nodes and N1b defining bilateral, contralateral or mediastinal nodes (see Table 11–1).

## IMPLICATIONS OF PROGNOSTIC FACTORS IN THE MANAGEMENT OF WELL-DIFFERENTIATED THYROID CANCER

It is extremely important to understand the biology of thyroid cancer, the prognostic factors and risk group analysis. Based on an understanding of these elements, appropriate management of patients with thyroid cancer may be administered with great potential for cure and miminal treatment-related morbidity. A limited surgical procedure may be performed in low-risk patients where the overall mortality is less than 2%, while a more aggressive surgical approach (including adjuvant therapy) is necessary in high-risk patients where the potential for disease-related mortality exceeds 45%. The risk groups are based on important prognostic factors—including age of the patient, grade of the tumor, size of the tumor, extra-thyroidal extension and presence or absence of distant metastasis. The reports from Memorial

Sloan-Kettering Cancer Center divide their patients based on the prognostic factors into patient-related and tumor-related factors (Table 11–5). The patients were divided into low-, intermediate-, and high-risk groups. The unique intermediate-risk group consisted of two categories: low-risk patients under the age of 45 with high-risk tumors and high-risk patients above the age of 45 with low-risk tumors. Based on these three risk group categories, the long-term survival was 99% in the low-risk group, 87% in the intermediate-risk group and 57% in the high-risk group (Table 11–6). Decisions regarding extent of thyroidectomy in the intermediate-risk group should be based mainly on the tumor-related factors (Table 11–7, Table 11–8). Rosai et al[7] reviewed differentiated thyroid cancers more critically, reviewing a large number of patients for histologic grade; a separate entity of poorly differentiated carcinoma was identified. Poorly differentiated tumors, which are more aggressive and have a higher likelihood of extra-thyroidal spread and distant metastasis, are more commonly seen in elderly patients. The histologic variants include tall cell, insular, trabecular, solid pattern, scirrhous, and undifferentiated areas. Elderly patients with poorly differentiated thyroid cancer show much less radioactive iodine avidity. Even though radioactive iodine is commonly used in this group of patients, its role remains undefined at this stage. In addition, the role of external radiation therapy in the management of thyroid cancer remains unclear at this time.

**Table 11–5.** Risk groups in thyroid cancer

| | |
|---|---|
| Low Risk | Low-risk patient/Low-risk tumor |
| Intermediate Risk | Low-risk patient/High-risk tumor |
| | High-risk patient/Low-risk tumor |
| High Risk | High-risk patient/High-risk tumor |
| Patient Factors | Age, Gender |
| Tumor Factors | Grade, Size, Extra-thyroidal extension, Distant metastasis |

**Table 11–6.** Risk-group definitions in differentiated carcinoma of the thyroid

| | *Low Risk* | *Intermediate Risk* | *Intermediate Risk* | *High Risk* |
|---|---|---|---|---|
| Age (Years) | < 45 | < 45 | > 45 | > 45 |
| Distant Metastasis | M0 | M+ | M0 | M+ |
| Tumor Size | T1, T2 (< 4 cm) | T3, T4 (> 4 cm) | T1, T2 (< 4 cm) | T3, T4 (> 4 cm) |
| Histology and Grade | Papillary | Follicular and/or high-grade | Papillary | Follicular and/or high-grade |
| 5-Year Survival | 100% | 96% | 96% | 72% |
| 20-Year Survival | 99% | 85% | 85% | 57% |

**Table 11–7.** Differentiated carcinoma of the thyroid: Impact of risk groups on survival

|  | *Number* | *Percent* | *Death Rate* |
|---|---|---|---|
| Memorial |  |  |  |
| Low Risk | 364 | 40% | 1% |
| Intermediate Risk | 357 | 38% | 15% |
| High Risk | 210 | 22% | 54% |
| Mayo |  |  |  |
| Low Risk | 737 | 86% | 2% |
| High Risk | 121 | 14% | 46% |
| Lahey |  |  |  |
| Low Risk | 277 | 89% | 1.8% |
| High risk | 33 | 11% | 46% |

**Table 11–8.** Well-differentiated thyroid cancer: Prognostic factors referenced by system

| System | Institution | | | | |
|---|---|---|---|---|---|
| **AGES** (1987) | Mayo Clinic | **A**ge | **G**rade | **E**xtra capsular tumor | **S**ize |
| **AMES** (1990) | Lahey Clinical Group I–III | **A**ge | **M**etastasis regional and distant | **E**xtra capsular tumor | **S**ize |
| **DAMES** (1993) | Swedish Akslen Group | **D**NA Ploidy | **A**ge | **M**etastasis | **E**xtent of primary **S**ize |
| **GAMES** (1992) | MSKCC | **G**rade | **A**ge | **M**etastasis | **E**xtra capsular tumor **S**ize |
| **MACIS** (1993) | Mayo Clinic | **M**etastasis | **A**ge | **C**ompleteness | **I**nvasion **S**ize |
| **EORTC** (1979) |  | Age | Histology | Invasion | Metastasis |

The interest in external radiation therapy in the United States is limited at this time. However, radiation therapy is an appropriate choice in patients with poorly differentiated thyroid cancer or locally aggressive thyroid cancer where gross or microscopic tumor might have been left in the central compartment.

In understanding the overall considerations in the management of thyroid cancer, it is important to note that 80% of patients do well with lobectomy alone, 15% will require a total thyroidectomy (based on the extent of the disease and the need for radioactive iodine or external radiation therapy), and 5% of the patients will die regardless of the extent of thyroidectomy or adjuvant treatment. This last group mainly includes elderly patients with locally aggressive thyroid cancer and poorly differentiated histologies. There clearly are specific indications for total thyroidectomy such as high-risk patients with high-risk tumors, young individuals with bulky nodal metastasis where there is a high incidence of microscopic metastatic disease to the lungs, patients with gross disease in both lobes of the thyroid, gross extra-thyroidal extension requiring radioactive iodine ablation, or patients with a preoperative diagnosis of poorly differentiated tumors.

Although these prognostic factors and risk groups are very important in the management of thyroid cancer, attention should be focused on identifying molecular tumor markers preoperatively (via FNA), which may guide both the extensiveness of surgery and postoperative adjuvant therapy. Until such indicators are identified and their detection refined so as to be clinically applicable, the identification of risk stratification for patients with thyroid cancer will be extremely important in guiding appropriate surgical and adjuvant management.

## References

1. Jemal A, Thomas A, Murray T, Thurg M. *Cancer statistics*, 1999. *CA.* 2002;52(1):23–47.
2. Shaha AR. Controversies in the management of thyroid nodule. *Laryngoscope.* 2000;110(2 part 1):183–193.

3. Hundahl SA, Fleming ID, Fremgen AM, et al. A National Cancer Data Base report on 53,856 cases of thyroid carcinoma treated in the US, 1985–1995. *Cancer.* 1998;83:2638–2648.

4. Gilliland FD, Hunt WC, Morris DM, et al. Prognostic factors for thyroid carcinoma: a population-based study of 15,698 cases from the Surveillance, Epidemiology and End Results (SEER) program, 1973–1991. *Cancer.* 1997;79:564–573.

5. Fleming ID, Cooper JS, Henson DE, et al, eds. *AJCC Cancer Staging Manual.* 5th ed. American Joint Committee on Cancer. Philadelphia, PA: Lippencott-Raven; 1997.

6. Hughes CJ, Shaha AR, Shah JP, Loree TR. Impact of lymph node metastasis in differentiated carcinoma of the thyroid—a matched pair analysis. *Head & Neck.* 1996;18:127–132.

7. Rosai J, Carcangiu ML, DeLellis RA. *Tumors of the Thyroid Gland. Atlas of Tumor Pathology,* Third Series, Vol 5, Fascicle 5. Washington, DC: Armed Forces Institute of Pathology; 1992.

8. Carcangiu ML, Zampi G, Pupi A, et al. Papillary carcinoma of the thyroid: a clinicopathologic study of 241 cases treated at the University of Florence, Italy. *Cancer.* 1985;55(4):805–828.

9. Hay ID, Grant CS, Taylor WF, et al. Ipsilateral lobectomy versus bilateral lobar resection in papillary thyroid carcinoma: a retrospective analysis of surgical outcome using a novel prognostic scoring system. *Surgery.* 1987;102:1088–1095.

10. Hay ID, Bergstralh EJ, Goellner JR, et al. Predicting outcome in papillary thyroid carcinoma: development of a reliable prognostic scoring system in a cohort of 1779 patients surgically treated at one institution during 1940 through 1989. *Surgery.* 1993;104:947–953.

11. Hay ID, Grant CS, Bergstralh EJ, et al. Unilateral total lobectomy: is it sufficient surgical treatment for patients with AMES low-risk papillary thyroid carcinoma? *Surgery.* 1998;124:958-966.

12. Andersen PE, Kinsella J, Loree TR, et al. Differentiated carcinoma of the thyroid with extrathyroidal extension. *Am J Surg.* 1995; 170(5):467-470.

13. Brierley JD, Panzarella T, Tsang RW, et al. Review. A comparison of different staging systems predictability of patient outcome: thyroid carcinoma as an example. *Cancer.* 1997;79:2414–2423.

14. Sherman SI, Brierley JD, Sperling M, et al. Prospective multicenter study of thyroid carcinoma treatment: initial analysis of staging and outcome. National Thyroid Cancer Treatment Cooperative Study Registry Group. *Cancer.* 1998;83:1012–1021, .

15. Clark OH. Total thyroidectomy: the treatment of choice for patients with differentiated thyroid cancer. *Ann Surg.* 1982;196: 361–370.

16. van Heerden JA, Hay ID, Goellner JR, et al. Follicular thyroid carcinoma with capsular invasion alone: a non-threatening malignancy. *Surgery.* 1992;112:1130–1136.

17. Shaha AR, Loree TR, Shah JP. Prognostic factors and risk group analysis in follicular carcinoma of the thyroid. *Surgery.* 1995;118: 1131–1138.

18. Cady B. Staging in thyroid carcinoma. *Cancer.* 1998;83:844–847.

19. Byar DP, Green SB, Dor P, et al. A prognostic index for thyroid carcinoma: a study of the EORTC Thyroid Cancer Cooperative Group. *Eur J Cancer.* 1979;15:1033–1041.

20. Cady B. Hayes Martin Lecture. Our AMES is true: how an old concept still hits the mark, or risk group assignment points the arrow to rational therapy selection in differentiated thyroid cancer. *Am J Surg.* 1997;174:462–468.

21. Mazzaferri EL, Jhiang SM. Long-term impact of initial surgical and medical therapy on papillary and follicular thyroid cancer. *Am J Med.* 1994;97:418–428.

22. Cady B, Rossi R. An expanded view of risk-group definition in differentiated thyroid carcinoma. *Surgery.* 1988;104:947–953.

23. Cohn KH, Backdahl M, Forsslund G, et al. Biologic considerations and operative strategy in papillary thyroid carcinoma: arguments against the routine performance of total thyroidectomy. *Surgery.* 1984;96:957–991.

24. Pasieka JL, Zedenius J, Auer G, et al. Addition of nuclear DNA content to the AMES risk-group classification for papillary thyroid cancer. *Surgery.* 1992;112:1154–1160.

25. Shaha AR, Shah JP, Loree TR. Low-risk differentiated thyroid cancer: the need for selective treatment. *Ann Surg Oncol.* 1997;4:328–333.

26. Mazzaferri EL. Review. Papillary thyroid carcinoma: factors influencing prognosis and current therapy. *Semin Oncol.* 1987;14:315–332.

27. Akslen LA, Myking AO, Salvesen H, Varhaug JE. Prognostic importance of various clinicopathological features in papillary thyroid carcinoma. *Eur J Cancer.* 1993;29A:44–51.

28. Cunningham MP, Duda RB, Recant W, et al. Survival discriminants for differentiated thyroid cancer. *Am J Surg.* 1990;160(4): 344–347.

29. Noguchi M, Mizokami Y, Michigishi T, et al. Multivariate study of prognostic factors of differentiated thyroid carcinoma: the significance of histologic subtype. *Int Surg.* 1993;78:10–15.

30. Schindler AM, van Melle G, Evequoz B, Scazziga B, et al. Prognostic factors in papillary carcinoma of the thyroid. *Cancer.* 1990; 68(2):324–330.

31. Shah JP,Loree TR, Dharker D, et al. Prognostic factors in differentiated carcinoma of the thyroid gland. *Am J Surg.* 1992;164(6): 658–661.

32. Simpson WJ, McKinney SE, Carruthers JS, et al. Papillary and follicular thyroid cancer: prognostic factors in 1578 patients. *Am J Med.* 1987;83(3):479–488.

33. Tubiana M, Schlumberger M, Rougier P, et al. Long-term results and prognostic factors in patients with differentiated thyroid carcinoma. *Cancer.* 1985;55(4):794–804.

34. Hay ID, Grant CS, van Heerden JA, et al. Papillary thyroid microcarcinoma: a study of 535 cases observed in a 50-year period. *Surgery.* 1992;112(6):1139–1147.

35. Czaja JM, McCaffrey TV. The surgical management of laryngotracheal invasion by well-differentiated papillary thyroid carcinoma. *Arch Otolaryngol Head Neck Surg.* 1997;123:484–490.

36. Grillo HC, Zannini P. Resectional management of airway invasion by thyroid carcinoma. *Ann Thorac Surg.* 1986;42:287–298.

37. McCaffrey TV, Bergstralh EJ, Hay ID. Locally invasive papillary thyroid carcinoma: 1940-1990. *Head Neck.* 1994;16:165–172.

38. Coburn MC, Wanebo HJ. Prognostic factors and management considerations in patients with cervical metastases of thyroid cancer. *Am J Surg.* 1992;164:671–676.

# 12

# Papillary Carcinoma of the Thyroid

## Thomas V. McCaffrey, M.D.

## INTRODUCTION

The estimated incidence of clinical thyroid carcinoma in the United States for the year 2000 was 18,400 cases.[1] This represents approximately 1.5% of all cancers excluding skin cancers. The majority of thyroid cancers are papillary carcinoma, which represent approximately 80% of all thyroid neoplasms (see Table 12–1).

The true incidence of papillary thyroid carcinoma is not reflected in the clinical incidence. A study published in 1954 by Mortensen et al demonstrated thyroid carcinoma in 2.8% of 1,000 consecutive postmortem examinations of thyroid glands performed at the Mayo Clinic.[2] The majority of these tumors were found in otherwise clinically normal thyroid glands. The term "occult" carcinoma was used to refer to this type of cancer. Currently the term microcarcinoma is used to refer to these clinically unapparent tumors. International studies have consistently demonstrated an occult tumor in-

cidence of 2 to 10%. Almost all these occult carcinomas are papillary carcinomas smaller than 1 cm in diameter. The relationship of occult cancers to clinically significant disease is unclear. The incidence of occult tumors is not increased where high rates of clinical disease are seen, and the marked female predominance for clinical disease is not reflected in the sex ratio of occult tumor, which is nearly equal.

## HISTOPATHOLOGY

The typical histopathologic appearance of papillary carcinoma is an invasive neoplasm with ill-defined margins, and a granular appearing cut surface, occasionally with calcifications. The World Health Organization (WHO) defines papillary carcinoma as a malignant epithelial tumor showing evidence of follicular cell differentiation, typically with papillary and follicular structures as well as characteristic nuclear changes.[3] Most papillary carcinomas contain complex branching papillae that are fibrovascular and have a fibrovascular core covered by a single layer of tumor cells. The distinctive nuclear features have taken on more importance in the diagnosis of papillary carcinoma with the increased use of fine needle aspiration (FNA). Distinctive nuclear features include large, pale staining nuclei, termed "Orphan Annie-eyed" nuclei. Another nuclear characteristic is the presence of a deep nuclear groove seen in at least 88% of papillary carcinomas.[4] Because of the frequent use of fine needle aspiration biopsy for the diagnosis of thyroid carcinoma, nuclear features are of particular importance. These characteris-

**Table 12–1.** Relative incidence of malignant thyroid tumors

| Cell Type | Relative Incidence (%) |
|-----------|------------------------|
| Papillary | 80 |
| Follicular | 10 |
| Hürthle Cell | 3 |
| Medullary | 5 |
| Anaplastic | 1 |
| Others | 1 |

**141**

tic features permit the accurate diagnosis of these lesions based on cytologic specimens. In the older literature, mixed papillary follicular carcinomas have been described and occasionally confused with follicular carcinomas. Currently, it is known that tumors that have both papillary and follicular features exhibit biologic behavior typical of papillary carcinoma and should be classified as such. The typical papillary carcinomas comprise 70 to 75% of all papillary carcinomas. The remaining tumors are subtypes or variant forms. Several subtypes of papillary carcinoma with distinct biologic behaviors have been described.[4]

## VARIANTS OF PAPILLARY CARCINOMA

### Papillary Microcarcinoma

This tumor usually measures 1 cm or less in diameter and is found incidentally in up to 10% of population based autopsy studies and 6% of surgical specimens. Hay reported a series of 535 patients with papillary microcarcinoma followed for a mean of 17.5 years. There were no deaths in patients without metastases and only a 1% local or regional recurrence rate.[5]

### Follicular Variant

As mentioned previously, the follicular variant of papillary thyroid carcinoma may appear identical to a follicular adenoma, except for the presence of the characteristic nuclear features of papillary carcinoma. This variant was described in 1977 by Chen and Rosai.[6] This tumor is usually non-encapsulated and grows in a microfollicular pattern. The follicular variant constitutes approximately 8–13% of papillary thyroid carcinomas. The characteristic nuclear features, however, are diagnostic and these tumors should be considered papillary carcinomas with a prognosis identical to the usual papillary carcinoma.

### Tall Cell Variant

Hawk and Hazzard first characterized the tall cell variant of papillary carcinoma in 1976.[7] They defined these tumors as having features of tall columnar cells with a height at least twice the width. The tall cell variant represents approximately 10% of all papillary carcinomas. These tumors have been shown to have a higher incidence of extra-thyroidal invasion, distant metastasis, and higher mortality rates than age and sex matched patients with typical papillary thyroid carcinoma. A characteristic clinical feature of these tumors is

that nearly all the primary tumors are large and have extra-thyroidal invasion at presentation. One-third of patients present with pulmonary metastasis and loss of iodine uptake, and locally persistent or recurrent disease occurs in half of these patients. This extremely aggressive behavior conveys a much poorer prognosis than the usual papillary carcinoma.

## PROGNOSTIC SCORING SYSTEMS

In order to predict risk of mortality in patients with well-differentiated thyroid carcinoma and as a guide to the aggressiveness of the treatment, several prognostic scoring systems have been devised. The most widely used scoring system is the TNM Classification. Among the other systems that have shown utility in assessing prognosis are the AMES, AGES, and MACIS classification systems.

### TNM System

The TNM classification is widely used to stage cancer.[8] Microcarcinomas are classified as T1, T2 tumors are >1cm and ≤4cm, T3 tumors are >4cm, and T4 tumors invade beyond the thyroid capsule. Nodes are classified as N0 if not present and N1 if present. Distant metastases are M0 if not present and M1 if present. Table 12–2 demonstrates that the stage category depends on a patient's age, greater or less than 45 years of age, and reflects the influence of age on prognosis for this tumor. The limitations of the TNM system for establishing prognosis for thyroid tumors has led to other systems which may be more predictive of disease free survival.

### AMES System

The AMES prognostic system proposed by Cady and Rosai is based on age, distant metastasis, extent of primary tumor, and size of primary tumor.[9] In this system, mortality in the lowest risk group was 1.8% and the system was predictive of mortality.

### AGES and MACIS Systems

The AGES system as proposed by Hay et al is based on a multiple regression analysis of a large cohort of Mayo Clinic patients with papillary carcinoma.[10] It predicts risk based on age, tumor grade, tumor extent and primary tumor size. Risk group is based on a weighted scoring system of these clinical features and correlates with disease specific mortality.

Hay et al later improved on the AGES system by developing the MACIS scoring system following a re-analysis of the prognostic variables of the AGES system.[11] The new system was based on metastasis, age, completeness of the surgery, invasion of extra-thyroidal tissues, and size of primary tumor. This system was no longer dependent upon histologic grading and did not require DNA ploidy analysis. Recently Brierley et al evaluated 382 patients with differentiated thyroid cancer and found no significant differences among AGES, TMN, AMES, and MACIS systems in predicting the prognosis of patients with papillary thyroid cancer.[12] A thorough discussion of risk scoring systems as well as other prognostic factors characteristic of thyroid carcinoma may be found in Chapter 11 of this text.

## MANAGEMENT

### Surgery

The diagnosis of papillary thyroid carcinoma is usually known prior to surgery as a result of fine needle aspiration biopsy cytology, the results of which are usually diagnostic.[13] The clinical assessment often provides information regarding the likelihood of local invasion as well as regional nodal metastasis. If cervical lymphadenopathy is noted, some form of neck dissection is indicated in addition to thyroidectomy. Extra-thyroidal extension of the tumor with invasion of strap muscles or adjacent aero-digestive viscera is suggested by fixation or dense adherence to underlying structures or vocal cord paralysis. Intraluminal invasion of the larynx or trachea is uncommon in papillary thyroid carcinoma and is suggested by airway obstruction dysphagia or hemoptysis. CT scanning is helpful in assessing the extent of extra-thyroidal extension by demonstrating soft tissue invasion, intraluminal invasion of the trachea, or destruction of laryngeal cartilages.

Invasion of laryngotracheal structures as the presenting finding of thyroid carcinoma is uncommon. Therefore, the most likely surgical consideration is thyroidectomy with or without node dissection. When considering thyroidectomy, the primary decision is to determine the extent of resection, ie subtotal vs. total thyroidectomy.

### Extent of Thyroidectomy

Determining the extent of thyroidectomy in the management of differentiated thyroid carcinoma, particularly papillary carcinoma, is a matter of controversy.[14] Since most patients with papillary thyroid carcinoma present in a low-risk category, it can be predicted that survival will be excellent. Therefore, it may be difficult to determine the influence of the extent of surgery on the eventual outcome for these patients. In addition, it is known that the greater the extent of surgery from lobectomy proceeding to total thyroidectomy, the more likely the potential for significant complications of surgery to be incurred, the most important of which are permanent hypoparathyroidism and injury to recurrent laryngeal nerves. Both of these complications produce significant morbidity. Therefore when considering the extent of surgery, both the likelihood of improved survival and the probability of complications must be weighed.

Some guidance helpful in determining the extent of thyroidectomy may be obtained from the various risk assessment scores that have been recorded in the literature. These include the TNM, AMES, AGES, and MACIS systems.[9,11,15] Each of these prognostic scoring systems has been shown to have predictive value in assessing the outcome of treatment.[16] Low risk patients may be suitably treated with less than total thyroidectomy and still have an excellent outcome with a lower possibility of morbidity, while high risk patients with poor prognostic characteristics would most likely benefit most from more extensive surgery.

Proponents for routine total thyroidectomy cite several factors to support their preference for this procedure: 1) high incidence of microscopic disease in the opposite thyroid lobe; 2) improved potential for the use of radioiodine ablation postoperatively; 3) better monitoring of recurrence with radioiodine scan and serum thyroid binding globulin levels; 4) decreased risk of development of undifferentiated thyroid cancer in the thyroid remnant; and, 5) increased sensitivity of early detection of pulmonary metastasis.[17] These factors are logical reasons to perform total thyroidectomy if the likelihood of benefit is reasonably high. In the case of high risk patients, this is no doubt the case. However, in low risk patients, which comprise the majority of thyroid cancer patients, prolonged survival is in excess of 99%, making the use of total thyroidectomy controversial and subjective.[18] With regard to low risk patients, a significant survival benefit has not been demonstrated for patients undergoing total thyroidectomy over those receiving less extensive resection. Survival results for lobectomy with isthmusectomy have been shown to be comparable to total resection in low risk patients. A principal factor arguing for total thyroidectomy is the possible presence of microscopic disease in the opposite lobe. Although this has been shown to occur in between 40–70% of cases, the presence of microscopic disease may not by itself convey increased risk for recurrence. Clinically evident disease recurring in the opposite lobe of patients undergoing initial lobectomy and isthmusectomy is noted to occur in less than 5% of these patients. Therefore, the incidence of multifocal microscopic disease may represent the same clinically insignificant disease as is noted for occult microcarcinoma identified incidentally in otherwise normal thyroid glands. Based on these considerations, the author's indications for total thyroidectomy in patients with papillary cancer include: 1) high risk patients with high risk tumor, 2) young patients with bulky nodal disease requiring postoperative radioiodine ablation, 3) patients with gross disease in both lobes of the thyroid gland, 4) gross extra-thyroidal tumor requiring radioiodine ablation, 5) poorly differentiated tumors, 6) cytologic evidence of tall cell variant of papillary carcinoma, 7) carcinoma arising with a history of radiation, and 8) patients with known distant metastasis requiring radioiodine ablation.

Although it is no doubt true that highly skilled surgeons with a practice focused on thyroid carcinoma can perform total thyroidectomy on a routine basis safely, the use of total thyroidectomy in all situations is an individual surgical decision and at the present time cannot be supported by strong clinical evidence.

## Nodal Metastases

Microscopic cervical nodal disease can occur in 30–50% of papillary thyroid cancers. In low risk patients, microscopic nodal disease does not appear to influence survival. In general, elective neck dissection is not recommended in patients with papillary thyroid carcinoma in the absence of detectable lymphadenopathy. Cervical node metastases have a minimal effect on local recurrence rate in the neck in low risk patients and only a modest effect in high risk patients above the age of 45. However, if nodal disease is identified in the lateral neck, selective node dissection is indicated. In addition, the surgeon should visualize the tracheoesophageal grove and upper and superior mediastinum to assess for nodes in these regions and any obviously large nodes should be removed. Level 1 and submandibular lymph nodes are rarely involved in patients with thyroid cancer, and submandibular gland excision and level 1 node dissection is not indicated in these patients. A thorough discussion on the risk of neck dissection in managing thyroid carcinoma may be found elsewhere in this text.

## Radioiodine Therapy

Post surgery therapy with $I^{131}$ has continued to arouse controversy among clinicians. Recently a growing number of studies have demonstrated decreased recurrence of papillary thyroid carcinoma and reduced disease specific mortality when radioiodine therapy is used to ablate any remnant of thyroid tissue postoperatively. The use of postoperative radioiodine therapy requires surgical removal of the majority of the thyroid gland and therefore total thyroidectomy. The use of radioiodine ablation, in the author's opinion, is therefore confined to patients with a high risk of recurrence as determined by the operative staging.

## Ablation of the Thyroid Remnant

Radioiodine therapy is recommended for most patients with high-risk, differentiated thyroid carcinoma, including papillary cancer. Following thyroidectomy, the patient is given Cytomel®, 25 µg 2 or 3 times daily for four weeks then discontinued for two weeks. Alternatively, complete removal from thyroid hormone or, more recently, the use of thyrogen may be chosen to prepare the patient for radioiodine treatment. Serum TSH and thyroglobulin are measured prior to ablation. A whole body scan is performed with a tracer dose of 15 millicuries of $I^{131}$ to determine extent of disease. If there is minimum residual thyroid present on scan, an ablation dose of 100 millicuries of radioiodine is given as the ablating dose. More extensive uptake may require a dose of 150 millicuries. If distant pulmonary metastases are noted on scanning, the appropriate $I^{131}$ dose is calculated based on dosimetry studies.

Following ablation, the patient is placed on thyroid hormone (Thyroxine) at a dose adjusted to achieve a TSH level suppression of less than 0.1 mU/L. Approximately twelve months after the initial ablation, the patient is once again withdrawn from thyroid hormone, the thyroglobulin is measured and a diagnostic scan is performed with 5 millicuries of radioiodine. If there is a negative scan outside the thyroid and thyroglobulin is less than 2 nanograms per milliliter, the patient is resumed on thyroid hormone and followed on a yearly basis. If the scan is positive outside the thyroid gland or thyroglobulin is greater than 5–10 nanograms per milliliter, another ablative dose of $I^{131}$ is administered and patient follow-up is resumed.

## Recurrence and Progression of Disease

Progression of disease is noted by either palpable recurrence within the thyroid bed, increasing thyroglobulin levels, or detectable iodine uptake outside the thyroid bed. With any of these scenarios, treatment is based on the site and extent of disease. Local gross recurrence requires surgical resection, whereas pulmonary metastatic disease is best treated with radioiodine ablation.

In some cases, the tumor fails to concentrate iodine. These tumors are not detectable by radioiodine scanning. PET scanning is useful for detecting tumors that do not concentrate radioiodine.[19] Localized tumor that does not concentrate iodine may respond to surgical resection or external beam radiotherapy.[20]

## Invasive Disease

Invasion of local aero-digestive tract structures by papillary thyroid carcinoma can offer a therapeutic dilemma.[21] As with other aspects of the management of thyroid cancer, the treatment of locally invasive papillary thyroid cancer is controversial. Treatment options include radical resection, including resection of the trachea and larynx, if necessary, to achieve complete tumor removal.[22] These procedures, in most cases, produce significant morbidity. For this reason, alternative treatment plans including shave excision and ablation with radioiodine or external beam radiotherapy have been advocated.[20] This procedure can benefit some cases; however, the treatment of locally invasive disease must be individualized to a particular patient's situation with consideration of risk factors, overall medical condition and patient choice representing issues important in decision-making. The management of locally invasive thyroid carcinoma is comprehensively addressed in a later chapter.

## References

1. Greenlee RT, Murry T, Bolder S, Wingo PA. Cancer Statistics, 2000. *CA Cancer J Clin.* 2000;50:7–33.
2. Mortensen JD, Bennett WA, Woolner LB. Incidence of carcinoma in thyroid glands removed in 1000 consecutive routine necropsies. *Surg Forum.* 1954;5:659.
3. Hedinger CE, Williams ED, Sobin LH. *Histological Typing of Thyroid Tumors.* Berlin: Springer-Verlag; 1988.
4. Muro-Cacho CA, Ku NNK. Tumors of the thyroid gland: Histologic and cytologic features—Part 1. *Cancer Control.* 2000;7:276–287.
5. Hay ID, Grant CS, van Heerden JA, Goellner JR, Ebersold JR, Bergstralh EJ. Papillary thyroid microcarcinoma: a study of 535 cases observed in a 50-year period. *Surgery.* 1992;112:1139–46; discussion 1146–7.
6. Chen KTK, Rosai J. Follicular variant of thyroid papillary carcinoma: a clinicopathological study of six cases. *Am J Surg Pathol.* 1977;1:123.
7. Hawk WA, Hazard JB. The many appearances of papillary carcinoma of the thyroid. *Clev Clin Q.* 1976;43:207.
8. Fleming ID, Cooper JS, Hensen DE, et al. *AJCC Cancer Staging Manual.* Philadelphia: Lippincott-Raven; 1997.
9. Cady B, Rosai R. An expanded view of risk-group definition in differentiated thyroid carcinoma. *Surgery.* 1988;104:947–953.
10. Hay ID, Grant CS, Taylor WF, McConahey WM. Ipsilateral lobectomy versus bilateral lobar resection in papillary thyroid carcinoma: a retrospective analysis of surgical outcome using a novel prognostic scoring system. *Surgery.* 1987;102:1088–95.
11. Hay ID, Bergstralh EJ, Goellner JR, Ebersold JR, Grant CS. Predicting outcome in papillary thyroid carcinoma: development of a reliable prognostic scoring system in a cohort of 1779 patients surgically treated at one institution during 1940 through 1989. *Surgery.* 1993;114:1050-7; discussion 1057–8.
12. Brierley JD, Panzarella T, Tsang RW, et al. A comparison of different staging systems' predictability of patient outcome: thyroid carcinoma as an example. *Cancer.* 1997;79:2414–2423.
13. Gharib H. Fine-needle aspiration biopsy of thyroid nodules: advantages, limitations, and effect. *Mayo Clin Proc.* 1994;69:44.
14. Shaha AR. Thyroid cancer: extent of thyroidectomy. *Cancer. Control.* 2000;7:240–245.
15. Hay ID. Papillary thyroid carcinoma. *Endocrinol Metab Clin North Am.* 1990;19:545–76.
16. Dean DS, Hay ID. Prognostic indicators in differentiated thyroid carcinoma. *Cancer Control.* 2000;7:229–239.
17. Clark OH. Total thyroidectomy: the treatment of choice for patients with differentiated thyroid cancer. *Ann Surg.* 1982;196:361–370.
18. Shaha RR, Shah JP, Loree TR. Low risk differentiated thyroid cancer: the need for selective treatment. *Ann Surg Oncol.* 1997;4:328–333.
19. Alnafisi NS, Driedger AA, Coates G, Moote DJ, Raphael SJ. FDG PET of recurrent or metastatic 131I-negative papillary thyroid carcinoma. *J Nucl Med.* 2000;41:1010–5.
20. Farahati J, Reiners C, Stuschke M, et al. Differentiated thyroid cancer. Impact of adjuvant external radiotherapy in patients with perithyroidal tumor infiltration (stage pT4). *Cancer.* 1996;77:172–80.
21. Czaja JM, McCaffrey TV. The surgical management of laryngotracheal invasion by well-differentiated papillary thyroid carcinoma. *Arch Otolaryngol Head Neck Surg.* 1997;123:484–90.
22. McCaffrey TV, Bergstralh EJ, Hay ID. Locally invasive papillary thyroid carcinoma: 1940-1990 [see comments]. *Head Neck.* 1994;16:165–72.

# 13

# Thyroid Follicular Neoplasms

## Roger J. Levin, M.D., F.A.C.S.

The contents of this chapter provide a concise and current review of follicular neoplasms of the thyroid gland. Attention is focused on the clinical characteristics of these tumors, including a discussion of some of the controversies surrounding the role of frozen section analysis to determine extent of surgery and the post-surgical management of low-grade, completely resected disease. The philosophy of the author's institution will be presented during the discussion of these controversies. In order to be thorough, there will be some overlap with topics covered in other chapters. A detailed evaluation of current studies into the molecular oncogenesis of follicular adenomas and carcinomas is provided. The chapter is divided into several segments: 1) An overview of the histology and general clinical features of follicular neoplasms; 2) risk factors for the development of these tumors; 3) molecular biology; 4) diagnosis and treatment; and 5) prognosis and follow-up. A comprehensive bibliography is provided for further study.

## FOLLICULAR NEOPLASMS OF THE THYROID GLAND—HISTOPATHOLOGIC DEFINITION

The majority of thyroid neoplasms are derived from the follicular epithelium of the thyroid gland. The term *follicular neoplasm*, however, is primarily used to describe follicular adenomas and follicular carcinomas of the thyroid gland. This term, therefore, should not be used synonymously with other follicular-derived neoplasms, which include malignancies, such as papillary and Hürthle cell carcinomas, and benign disorders, such as hyperplastic nodules and goiter. Furthermore, mixed follicular/papillary carcinoma or follicular-variant of papillary thyroid carcinoma should not be included under true follicular neoplasms.

The distinction between follicular adenoma and follicular carcinoma is possible only through recognition of the presence of histologic capsular and/or vascular invasion or metastasis.[1-3] Follicular adenomas are non-invasive neoplasms, whereas invasion is a *sine qua non* for the diagnosis of follicular carcinomas. On gross exam, adenomas are solitary, encapsulated, and have a homogeneous cut surface.[3] Histologically, follicular adenomas have a complete fibrous capsule containing vessels (Figure 13–1). Follicular adenomas may have a trabecular/solid, microfollicular, macrofollicular, or mixed architectural pattern.[2,3] While these have no clinical importance, more cellular tumors should be diligently searched for evidence of capsular/vascular invasion to absolutely exclude malignancy (Figure 13–2). Degenerative changes, such as hemorrhage, cystic change, fibrosis, calcification and metaplastic ossification may occur in adenomas. Mitoses are usually absent. The adjacent thyroid is normal or compressed in larger tumors.

Two types of follicular carcinomas are recognized grossly, the minimally invasive (encapsulated) type and the widely invasive type.[3] Since the minimally invasive follicular carcinomas are well defined and encapsulated, they resemble follicular adenomas on gross examination. Some authors have emphasized a thicker capsule in minimally invasive carcinomas when compared to adenomas.[9] Histologically, the cytoarchitectural features of follicular carcinoma resemble those of adeno-

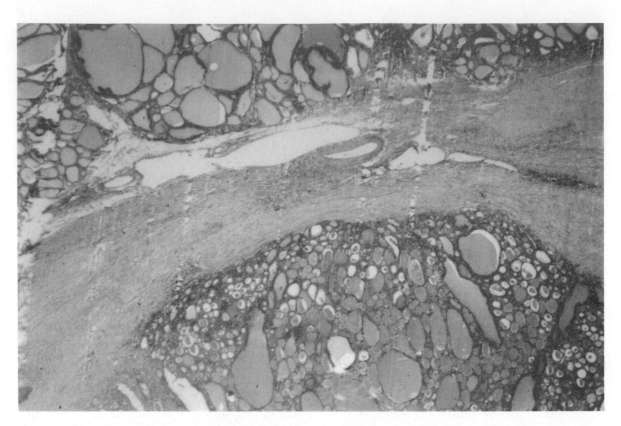

**Figure 13–1.** Photomicrograph (150×) of a well-encapsulated follicular adenoma of the thyroid gland, with the adenoma adjacent to normal thyroid parenchyma (hematoxylin and eosin). (Courtesy of Silloo Kapadia, MD.)

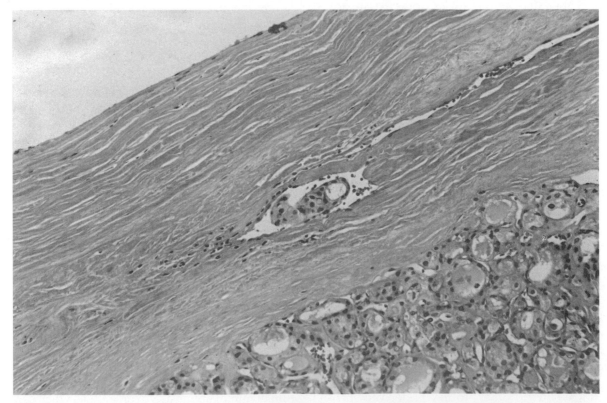

**Figure 13–2.** Photomicrograph (150×) of follicular thyroid epithelium within the capsule of a neoplasm. This case was ultimately determined to be a minimally-invasive follicular thyroid carcinoma, though it would be difficult to call on this one section only (hematoxylin and eosin). (Courtesy of Silloo Kapadia, MD.)

mas.[3] Minimally invasive follicular carcinomas tend to be hypercellular with a solid, trabecular, microfollicular or atypical pattern of growth and demonstrate focal capsular and/or vascular invasion. The capsular invasion should be not only into but through the capsule outside the bulk of the lesion (Figure 13–3). The vascular invasion should show tumor plugs in the lumen of veins within or beyond the capsule and attach at some point to the vessel wall.[2-9] Vascular invasion appears to be of greater importance diagnostically than capsular invasion, since the latter is more difficult to define. Tumor nests seen only within the capsule, as demonstrated in Figure 13–2, may conceivably represent trapping or distortion by fibrosis.[10] Widely invasive follicular carcinomas are rare and show extensive invasion on gross and microscopic exam. Microscopically, some have features similar to minimally invasive tumors. Most show cytoarchitectural features of malignancy, high mitotic activity and necrosis in addition to extensive invasion.[2,3]

Extreme caution should be exercised in attempting to evaluate a follicular lesion in a patient who has had a prior fine-needle aspiration biopsy (FNAB). Histologic alterations following FNAB may include hemorrhage, granulation tissue, hemosiderin-laden macrophages, reactive atypia of follicular epithelium, capsular distortion, pseudocapsular or pseudovascular invasion, and focal necrosis or infarction of the entire nodule.[3]

## FOLLICULAR NEOPLASMS OF THE THYROID—GENERAL CLINICAL FEATURES

The "classic" presentation of a *follicular adenoma* is a painless thyroid mass in a middle-aged woman.[3] Most patients are euthyroid when evaluated serologically. Pressure related symptoms, such as tracheal compression or dysphagia, occur with larger tumors. Intratumoral hemorrhage may cause sudden enlargement and pain. On radionuclide thyroid scanning, adenomas are usually "cold" (hypofunctional) or "warm" (functional), but rarely "hot" (hyperfunctional).[3]

*Follicular carcinomas* typically occur more frequently in women with an average age one decade older than in those patients developing an adenoma or a papillary thyroid carcinoma. These tumors present as solitary thyroid nodules unaccompanied by cervical adenopathy.[2,3] Patients with the minimally invasive type of follicular carcinoma can usually be cured surgically without concern for recurrence or regional lymph node metastases. Patients with widely invasive carcino-

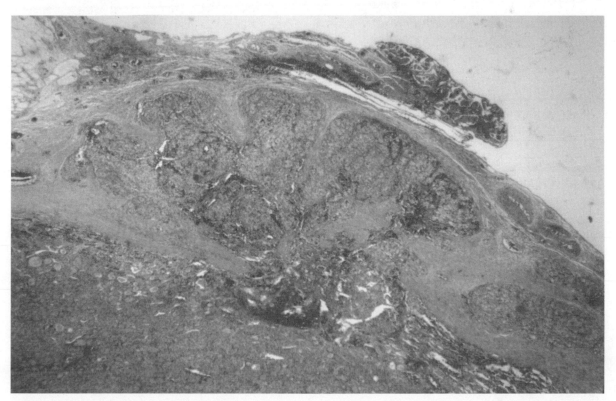

**Figure 13–3.** Photomicrograph (40×) of obvious capsular invasion in a follicular thyroid carcinoma (hematoxylin and eosin). (Courtesy of Silloo Kapadia, MD.)

mas have a less favorable prognosis, with death from cancer occurring in 20–50% of patients and 80% developing metastases, mainly to lung and bone.[2,3] Other sites include brain, liver, and skin.[4-7] In both the minimally invasive and the widely invasive type of follicular thyroid carcinomas (FTC), lymph node involvement at presentation or later is uncommon, usually less than 10%.[8]

The relationship of follicular neoplasms and *Hürthle cell neoplasms* must be mentioned briefly, though a more detailed discussion of Hürthle cell tumors can be found in Chapter 14. Hürthle (oxyphilic) cells are nothing more than follicular cells with eosinophilic, granular cytoplasm in the majority of their cells. For this reason, Hürthle cell neoplasms will often be classified under the broader rubric of follicular neoplasms. Hürthle cells have this eosinophilic appearance because of an abundance of mitochondria in the cytoplasm.[11] Hürthle cell neoplasms of the thyroid have been found to be more aggressive in behavior by several groups of authors,[12-18] though others have disputed this.[11,19-22] A recent review addressing the question of whether Hürthle cell neoplasms are simply a histologic variant of follicular neoplasms concluded that these tumors were not more virulent in behavior. Furthermore, among patients with encapsulated Hürthle cell neo-

plasms, there were no distant metastases and no deaths, in contradistinction to patients with encapsulated follicular carcinomas (minimally invasive), who had an appreciable distant metastasis rate.[11] A final study examined the risk factors suggestive of malignancy in Hürthle cell neoplasms. As with follicular neoplasms, size greater than 4 cm strongly predicted malignancy; hence, these authors felt that all patients with large Hürthle cell tumors should undergo total thyroidectomy, although smaller nodules required only a hemithyroidectomy.[23]

A second histologic subtype of follicular neoplasm that warrants review is *insular cell carcinoma*. These tumors consist of well-defined rounded nests of small, poorly-differentiated cells, with only occasional microfollicle formation (Figure 13–4).[3] Abundant mitotic figures and extensive vascular invasion are nearly always present, and, hence, there is some overlap with the "widely invasive" growth pattern of "ordinary" follicular carcinoma. These tumors are at the most de-differentiated end of the spectrum of follicular carcinoma; they may well represent transitional forms towards anaplastic cancers. Immunohistochemical analysis may be required for accurate classification (Figure 13–5). Insular carcinomas, not surprisingly, are associated with a worse prognosis than typical follicular carcinomas.[24,25]

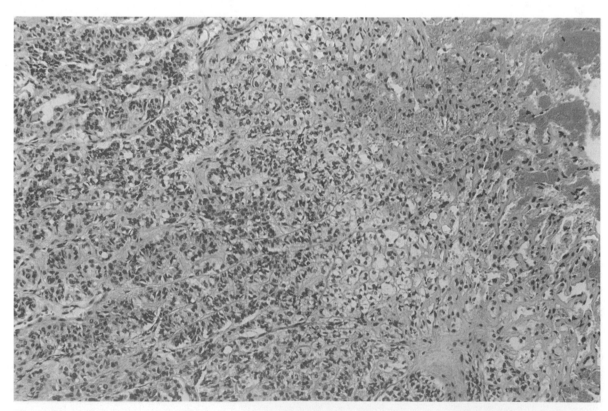

**Figure 13–4.** Photomicrograph (150×) of an insular thyroid carcinoma with necrotic focus and solid nests (insulae) mixed with small follicles. Nuclei are small and uniform (hematoxylin and eosin). (Courtesy of Silloo Kapadia, MD.)

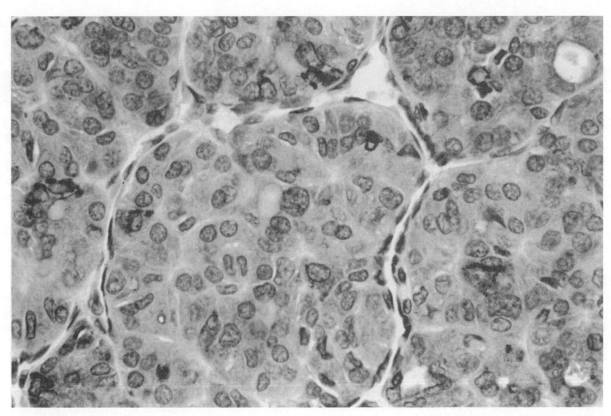

**Figure 13–5.** Photomicrograph (400×) of insular thyroid carcinoma demonstrating solid nests of small uniform cells separated by clefts. Immunohistochemical stain for thyroglobulin is positive (shown) though a stain for calcitonin was negative (not shown). (Courtesy of Silloo Kapadia, MD.)

## RISK FACTORS FOR THE DEVELOPMENT OF FOLLICULAR NEOPLASMS

As mentioned above, follicular neoplasms are most commonly identified in middle aged to elderly female patients, with carcinomas seen more frequently in the advanced age group. Follicular thyroid carcinomas (FTC) also tend to be found in endemic goiter areas. Starting in the late 1970s, several case-control studies strongly suggested that dietary iodine content was the main variable causing this relative shift in frequencies of histologic types.[26,27] Not surprisingly, dietary iodine supplementation has since been shown to decrease the relative frequency of follicular carcinoma.[28,29] In fact, there is a reciprocal relationship between the ratio of follicular/papillary thyroid carcinoma (PTC) and dietary iodide intake.[29] One possible explanation is that a state of chronic low-grade hypothyroidism, ie, a continuously elevated thyrotropin (TSH) level, is partly responsible for this development of follicular thyroid cancer. The fact that thyroid cancer, in general, is no more common in hypothyroid subjects versus euthyroid subjects (and the proportion of FTC to PTC is unchanged in these two groupings) suggests that iodine deficiency,

per se, is the major factor determining the ratio of FTC to PTC. Another factor contributing to the decrease of FTC in general has been the narrower definition of FTC recently. Previously, follicular variants of papillary carcinoma, as well as some benign lesions, such as partially encapsulated hyperplastic nodules and adenomas showing pseudoinvasion following needle aspiration biopy, were included as follicular carcinomas.[30]

A second well-known factor responsible for the development of follicular thyroid neoplasms, both benign and malignant, is childhood radiation exposure. While papillary carcinoma is the most frequent histology associated with ionizing radiation, several studies suggest that the follicular type may also be affected.[31-36]

The female preponderance of patients with FTC has led to speculation about the role of estrogens as a risk factor. Interestingly, it has been observed that breast cancer and thyroid cancer occur more frequently in the same individual than expected by chance.[37,38] Experimental evidence has demonstrated that follicular cells of the thyroid express estrogen receptors; furthermore, estrogen stimulates the growth of thyrocytes, and the partial estrogen antagonist, tamoxifen, inhibits follicular-derived cancer cells both *in vitro* and *in vivo*.[39,40] The effect of tamoxifen on these cells, however, is not reversed by estrogen, suggesting an estrogen-independent mechanism. Clinically, the role of sex hormones as a risk factor for the development of follicular-derived thyroid cancer must still be considered unresolved. For example, epidemiologic data on common risk factors for breast cancer and thyroid cancer have shown that those risk factors for breast cancer which lead to increased estrogen exposure (such as low parity and absence of breast feeding), with the exception of increased body weight, are not associated with an increased risk for thyroid cancer.[20,37] Case-control studies, on the other hand, have suggested a correlation between pregnancy, an extremely high estrogen state, and the onset of thyroid cancer.[41] Since increased parity seems to increase thyroid cancer risk, it may be that the pregnant state itself, rather than its accompanying elevated estrogen levels, is associated with increased thyroid cancer risk. Finally, given that FTC tends to occur in an elderly population, it seems unlikely that there is a major contribution from sex steroids (even with the long latency period for tumorigenic estrogen effects).[42]

Lastly, genetic factors may have some role in predisposing to FTC. For example, aggregation of FTC cases in families with dyshormonogenesis has been described.[43] As well, certain HLA types may also predispose to FTC. Studies have suggested an association between follicular carcinoma and DR1, Drw6, and DR7. Ethnic background and environmental iodine content may determine which HLA association is relevant in a given population. The study implicating DR1 was conducted in eastern Hungary (an endemic goiter area), the study suggesting an association with Drw6 is from a moderate iodine intake area in Germany, and the study finding DR7 to be a risk factor for FTC was conducted in iodine-rich Chicago.[44-46] Overall, however, the role of HLA type in predisposing to FTC remains disputed.

## MOLECULAR BIOLOGY OF FOLLICULAR NEOPLASMS

In recent years, evidence has mounted to suggest an adenoma-to-carcinoma multi-step pathogenesis similar to that in colon cancer and other adenocarcinomas.[47-51] Although this model for tumor progression has its limitations and detractors, it can serve as a useful working hypothesis. It has been asserted that tumors of the thyroid follicular cell are proving to be one of the most informative models for "dissecting" the molecular genetics of multi-stage human tumorigenesis.[49]

Adult thyroid follicular cells are classified from a cell kinetic standpoint as a "stable" or "conditional renewal" cell population. This implies a normal basal state characterized by a very low rate of both cell proliferation and cell death, but in which a significant (if transient) proliferative response can occur given the appropriate stimulus (eg, elevation of the extracellular concentration of TSH).[49,52,53] Therefore, unlike many other highly specialized cells, follicular cells are not irreversibly terminally differentiated. When they proliferate in response to certain growth signals, they temporarily lose the ability to concentrate iodide and to synthesize thyroglobulin.[47] Not surprisingly, TSH stimulation of the adenyl cyclase/protein kinase A pathway has been suggested as an early event in thyroid follicular neoplasia.[48] *In vitro* evidence exists that TSH does stimulate adenyl cylcase activity in thyroid follicular cell derived neoplasms, and that this activity can be inhibited by somatostatin.[50] Nonetheless, tissue growth factors other than TSH must also be involved in the development and growth of thyroid follicular neoplasms or there would be uniform growth of the thyroid gland. Furthermore, it is now known that the majority of thyroid follicular neoplasms, benign and malignant, are of monoclonal origin.[54]

Numerous studies have documented that the H-, K-, and N-*ras* proteins are present in thyroid neoplasms.[55-57] *Ras* proteins are small GTP-binding proteins involved in signaling from the cell membrane to the nucleus. Mutations of codon 12, 13, and 61 are activating mutations that increase the duration of GTP binding, thus keeping adenylate cyclase activated. *Ras* mutations are thought to be early mutations because they are found in both benign and malignant follicular neoplasms. Lemoine et al and Wright et al documented *ras* mutations in approximately 20% of follicular adenomas and 60% of follicular carcinomas.[55,56] Namba et al, however, identified *ras* mutations in only 25% of all benign and malignant follicular neoplasms.[57] At the molecular level, introduction of mutant *ras* into normal follicular cells in monolayer culture results in a dramatic stimulation of proliferation and can even give rise in an artificial tissue culture matrix to three-dimensional clones containing structures highly reminiscent of some types of human follicular adenoma.[58]

Cytogenetic abnormalities and evidence of genetic losses are far more frequent in FTC than in PTC, and are also observed with modest frequency in follicular adenomas.[59-66] These findings suggest that cell cycle control, mitotic spindle formation, DNA repair, or several of these mechanisms may be impaired in these neoplasms, possibly even at a relatively early stage. Follicular adenomas display abnormal karyotypes in about 30% of cases, with a wide range of chromosomes being involved.[67-75] Interestingly, translocations involving chromosome band 19q13 have been observed repeatedly.[70,74,75] The fact that these translocations involving chromosome 19q13 seem identical to those occurring in some benign hyperplastic nodules suggests that the events associated with this translocation could be among the earliest steps in follicular tumorigenesis.[76]

It appears likely that an oncogene, or less likely, a tumor suppressor gene of pathogenetic importance is located between chromosome bands 19q13.3 and 19q13.4. Among known genes in this region, potential candidate genes, which may act as oncogenes if mutated or constitutively activated, include two genes encoding zinc finger proteins (ZNF83 and ZNF160), as well as the gene coding for the gamma subunit of protein kinase C.[77]

In FTC, losses have been particularly associated with chromosomes 3, 10, and 11.[61,63,65] Deletions, partial deletions and deletion/rearrangements involving the p arm of chromosome 3 have been the most commonly observed changes in FTC.[65,78] Loss of heterozygosity (LOH) studies have corroborated the cytogenetic studies, with frequently observed LOH on 3p loci.[60] Because LOH at 3p has also been found in both a primary tumor and its metastasis, it appears that loss of genetic material on the p arm of chromosome 3 is a non-random, inheritable property of certain follicular thyroid cancers and, hence, of possible etiological and prognostic significance.[65] One possible gene, located on 3p, which has been examined for activity in follicular carcinomas, is the gene for von Hippel-Lindau (VHL) syndrome. This gene is responsible for tumorigenesis in VHL and clear cell carcinoma of the kidney. However, in several follicular thyroid cancers exhibiting LOH on chromosome 3p, no mutations in the VHL gene were found, suggesting that this particular gene is not involved in follicular thyroid carcinogenesis.[79]

Interestingly, LOH on chromosome 3p seems to be limited to follicular thyroid carcinomas. Matsuo et al were unable to detect LOH using probes from a relatively small region between 3p21.2 and 3p21.3 in 27 follicular adenomas.[63] Mapping a larger region of chromosome 3p, Hermann et al found no evidence of LOH among six papillary carcinomas and three follicular adenomas, but did identify it in all six follicular carcinomas.[60] These studies suggest that loss of a tumor suppressor on 3p could be specific for follicular thyroid carcinomas and might be viewed as a key event in the adenoma to carcinoma progression. For FTC tumorigenesis, it therefore appears that a tentative sequence of events, starting with TSH stimulation and/or 19q13 rearrangement in hyperplastic nodules, followed by *ras* activation in some adenomas, and finally tumor suppressor loss on 3p, culminating in established FTC, can be proposed.[77]

## DIAGNOSIS OF FOLLICULAR NEOPLASMS

The presentation of most follicular neoplasms of the thyroid will be an asymptomatic thyroid mass. When promptly referred to a head and neck surgeon, further evaluation simply consists of a fine needle aspiration biopsy (FNAB). Oftentimes, however, the patient will already have had several other studies done prior to referral to the surgeon, including thyroid ultrasound and/or nuclear scan. These studies are rarely helpful in deciding whether surgery is warranted. High-resolution ultrasonography will detect nodular thyroid disease in approximately 35% of normal volunteers.[80] Furthermore, the criteria used to rule out malignancy on ultrasound, such as echofree (cystic) and homogeneously hyperechoic lesions, are not very accurate in their predictive power.[81] Isotopic scanning of the gland with $Tc^{99}m$, $I^{131}$, or $I^{123}$ is somewhat more reliable in that almost all malignancies will be "cold" on scintiscanning. As is well known, however, this is neither a highly specific nor a totally sensitive test for malignancy. Only between 15% and 30% of cold nodules will actually prove malignant at the time of surgery.[82-84]

As alluded to above, FNAB is an extremely valuable tool in diagnosing thyroid nodular disease, and often will dictate whether surgery is indicated. The majority of benign hyperplastic nodules, degenerative cysts, and papillary neoplasms can accurately be diagnosed this way.[20] Unfortunately, on cytologic examination, malignant follicular thyroid neoplasms are frequently indistinguishable from benign adenomas.[3] Several studies have examined morphometric parameters in order to improve the predictive value in FNAB of follicular neoplasms. Nuclear size and shape, patterns of cellular aggregation, and the presence of marginal vacuoles have been identified as helpful to the cytopathologist in interpreting these specimens.[85-87] Another study used reverse transcription polymerase chain reaction to identify high mobility group 1 (HMG1-Y) protein in thyroid cancer aspirates. This protein is rarely identified in benign adenomas.[88] Despite these encouraging studies, no absolute way yet exists to distinguish a benign from malignant follicular neoplasm on FNAB.

## TREATMENT OF FOLLICULAR NEOPLASMS

The treatment of follicular neoplasms of the thyroid engenders some controversy. The ostensible reason for removing a discrete thyroid mass, aside from cosmetic or mass effect reasons, is to treat malignancy. Surgical excision is generally recommended for any thyroid nodule that has been diagnosed as a follicular neoplasm on FNAB. As detailed above, the reason for this is that it is currently impossible to differentiate benign adenoma from a carcinoma on needle biopsy. For a benign adenoma, a thyroid lobectomy with isthmusectomy is the recommended procedure. Unfortunately, it is difficult to be absolutely sure that a lesion is benign until permanent microscopic analysis is performed. Frozen section analysis can be beneficial, although its usefulness has been disputed. In experienced hands, frozen section analysis has a high degree of accuracy. For example, in a series from the University of Innsbruck, Austria, between 1976 and 1985, only 4.5% of frozen section analyses (48/1079) had to be revised after examination of paraffin-embedded tissue.[89] Others have not found frozen section analysis to be helpful in the diagnosis of follicular neoplasm when used alone.[90] Whether this reflects differences in patient population or in histopathologic expertise remains uncertain. At our institution, frozen section analysis of follicular neoplasms is almost always deferred, unless there are obvious findings of follicular-variant of papillary carcinoma (eg, intranuclear grooving) or widespread vascular and capsular invasion.

The extent of surgical resection for follicular carcinomas also elicits vigorous discussion. It seems apparent that removal of all cancerous tissue is the minimum that should be undertaken. All studies in which data on FTC have been analyzed with respect to the completeness of surgery have found substantially better survival of patients rendered tumor-free by the procedure.[20,91-95] At follow-up (between 2 and 30 years), mortality was between 10% and 50% lower for patients without residual disease. However, none of the studies presented a multivariate analysis on this aspect of the data. Lesser mortality in completely operated tumors may therefore reflect the fact that patients with smaller and less invasive tumors are more likely to have neoplasms that can be completely removed. Consequently, final confirmation of the importance of complete tumor removal must await the results of multivariate studies on relatively large numbers of patients with FTC.[20]

Frequently, follicular carcinomas are limited to one lobe of the thyroid gland. Unlike papillary carcinoma, the incidence of multifocality and intrathyroid metastasis in FTC is quite low. For this reason, several authors have suggested that lobectomy and isthmusectomy is an adequate resection in the majority of follicular carcinomas.[96-98] Further evidence for this approach derives from a review of 250 patients with FTC treated at the Mayo Clinic. The authors failed to find a significant relationship between the extent of primary surgery and cause-specific survival or recurrence.[20] Other authors, however, persuasively argue for total thyroidectomy in most cases.[99-102] Mazzaferri and Jhiang performed a multivariate analysis on the treatment of a group of well-differentiated thyroid cancers (278 were FTC). They found that patients who underwent at least a near-total thyroidectomy (defined as removal of all tissue except a small rim attached to the posterior capsule) had a

significantly lower mortality than patients undergoing a lesser procedure.[103] Another study focusing exclusively on follicular thyroid carcinoma found a trend toward better survival in 101 patients who were treated more aggressively (more than a lobectomy) as compared to 68 patients treated with lobectomy or a lesser procedure.[104]

It is the author's preference to perform total thyroidectomy in all cases of follicular thyroid carcinoma. This aggressive approach facilitates the effectiveness of adjuvant radioiodine therapy and allows for long-term follow-up with serial thyroglobulin levels. When a follicular carcinoma is finally identified on permanent analysis after a hemithyroidectomy, it is the author's preference to perform a completion thyroidectomy. This approach will occasionally result in a second surgical procedure, often with a normal lobe being removed. Again, the reason for this is to improve the efficacy of adjuvant therapy with radioiodine and tumor marker surveillance. Radioablation of the entire remaining thyroid lobe can be considered, but it requires a substantial radiation dosage and may not be as effective oncologically as a straightforward surgical procedure. The benefit of a second surgery, or more comprehensive initial surgery, in the author's opinion, outweighs the risk of recurrent laryngeal nerve paralysis and permanent hypocalcemia/hypoparathyroidism (which occurs in less than 1% of cases).

For patients with tumors that cannot be resected completely, surgery should still be undertaken. A substantial number of these patients will succumb to local vascular and airway complications, which can be ameliorated by surgical debulking. This can result in a 60% 2-year survival in this patient group.[105] The role of neck dissection in addition to thyroidectomy for well-differentiated thyroid cancer will be addressed in Chapter 18. Because of the low rate of cervical metastases in follicular thyroid cancer, however, neck dissection is rarely indicated with this pathology.

All patients treated for FTC at the author's institution will be treated with post-operative radioiodine (RAI) and serial thyroglobulin measurements. Several studies have shown improved outcome when postoperative RAI is used.[93-95] In one study, the benefit was primarily limited to those patients who had also undergone a total thyroidectomy, although there was a tendency toward improved outcomes for patients who had lesser procedures performed.[93] Two other studies demonstrated improved outcomes even for patients who had undergone incomplete or limited surgery.[94,95] Contradictory studies have also been published, however, failing to show any benefit from postoperative RAI—one of these actually showed a slight detrimental effect.[106,107]

After radioablation, patients at our institution will also be maintained on suppressive doses of thyroxine, aimed at keeping the TSH in the range of 0.1 to 0.3 mIU/L. The rationale for this approach is also not entirely clear-cut. Two studies have found a significant reduction in recurrence rate and mortality, respectively, for patients treated with thyroxine.[104,108] Other studies have not corroborated these findings.[93,95] Nonetheless, thyroxine treatment aimed at modestly suppressing TSH (range of 0.1 to 0.3 mIU/L) is most likely beneficial. Furthermore, it is unlikely to be any more "toxic" (particularly with regard to bone physiology) than simple replacement doses.

## PROGNOSIS FOR PATIENTS WITH FOLLICULAR CARCINOMA

A large number of retrospective studies have focused on prognostic factors in differentiated thyroid cancer. The majority of these studies combine papillary and follicular carcinoma, although some focus exclusively on FTC.[12,14,21,104,108-113] In the majority of studies examining both papillary and follicular cancer in the same population, FTC has been associated with a greater overall and cause-specific mortality than papillary cancer.[93,96,106,114-123] One study examined 49 patients for an average of 10.7 years, and showed that the cause-specific deaths from follicular carcinoma were twice that of papillary carcinoma.[124] Other studies have shown increased mortality only in certain subgroups of patients with follicular carcinoma, namely, for patients with widely invasive cancers, poorly differentiated histology,[125,126] and/or widespread metastatic disease at presentation.[103,127] Furthermore, five of the studies demonstrating a detrimental prognostic effect of follicular histology (as compared to papillary) showed that this effect was very slight when other factors such as age, sex, and stage were adjusted for in multivariate models.[106,114,116,121,122]

Overall, therefore, it appears that the differences in outcome between PTC and FTC are slight, perhaps to the point of being nonexistent. It seems reasonable, then, to apply the prognostic criteria to follicular carcinoma that have been helpful in papillary thyroid carcinoma. Recently, therefore, several prognostic scoring systems have been applied to FTC.[128] These include EORTC (European Organization for Research and Treatment of Cancer), AGES (age, grade, extent, size) and AMES (age, metastasis, extent, size). The authors of this review concluded that the AGES and EORTC scoring systems best defined low- and high-risk groups of patients with pure follicular carcinoma, although the separation between groups was low.[128] Another study divided follicular thyroid cancer patients into three groups, high-, intermediate-, and low-risk, and reviewed their 10- and 20-year survival.[16] In this study, 228 patients were studied; however, 59 of the patients

had Hürthle cell histology. The authors identified several well-known risk factors including age >45 years, extrathyroidal extension, tumor size greater than 4 cm, and the presence of distant metastases. Hürthle cell histology was a separate risk factor. Low-risk factors included age <45, early T-stage, low-grade pathology, and no distant metastases. The intermediate group had a mixture of these parameters, eg, age <45 years or small T-stage, but distant metastases. The 10-year survival for the low-, intermediate-, and high-risk groups was 98%, 88%, and 56%, respectively, while the 20-year survival was 97%, 87%, and 49%. Importantly, gender, focality, and presence of lymph node metastases had no significant bearing on the outcome.[16] A similar study out of the Mayo Clinic found that distant metastasis at presentation, patient age greater than 50 years, tumor size of 4 cm or more, marked vascular invasion, and higher-grade histology predicted a poor outcome. If two or more of these factors were present, the 5-year survival rate was only 47%, and the 10-year survival rate was 8%.[12]

Applying the same prognostic criteria to FTC as for PTC does seem useful. The specific risk factors can therefore be stratified in the following descending order of importance: distant metastases at initial presentation, increasing patient age, larger tumor size, and the presence of local (extrathyroidal) invasion. To a lesser degree, male sex is associated with increased mortality, as is higher-grade (less well-differentiated) primary tumors. In addition, vascular invasiveness or insular histology can be identified as further potential prognostic variables unique to follicular cancer.[20] Lymphatic involvement at presentation and DNA aneuploidy may also have some prognostic significance.

The prognostic impact of vascular invasion in FTC has been studied extensively. Seven studies have found marked vascular invasiveness to be of prognostic relevance,[21,108-113] and only one found it to be irrelevant on multivariate analysis.[91] Furthermore, all but one of the studies questioning the impact of the degree of vascular invasiveness in both papillary and follicular cancer found this to be a predictor of poor outcome in FTC.[20,103,115,122,123,129] The importance of the degree of vascular invasiveness is underscored further by a Mayo Clinic study that showed that a small cohort of patients with FTC with minimal capsular invasion and no evidence of vascular invasion had a cause-specific mortality of 0% at 5- and 10-year follow-up.[130]

The role of lymphatic involvement and DNA aneuploidy as prognostic factors in follicular carcinoma of the thyroid is unclear. Unlike papillary carcinoma, where the presence of lymph node metastases does not impact the long-term survival of the patient, the presence of regional node metastases may have minor significance in FTC in terms of a worse outcome.[8] DNA status appears to have a major prognostic role in Hürthle cell carcinoma, where nearly all patients who die of the disease are aneuploid.[59] Its role in pure follicular carcinoma remains debatable.[59,61,62]

## FOLLOW-UP OF PATIENTS WITH FOLLICULAR CARCINOMA

It is widely assumed that life-long follow-up is required in thyroid cancer given the propensity for differentiated thyroid cancer to recur decades after its initial treatment. On detailed analysis of longitudinal studies of differentiated thyroid cancer, however, it appears that the majority of recurrences and deaths occur within the first five years of treatment.[20,21,106,109,110,114-117,131,132] Several studies have demonstrated that between 50% and 80% of all events occur within the first 1 to 2 years.[20,21,106,114,115,131,132] Given the marked differences in the risk of death or progressive disease between low-risk and high-risk patients, as defined above, the frequency and intensity of follow-up can be tailored to the individual patient's risk.[20] Some low-risk patients could therefore have relatively minimal post-surgical follow-up, while a thyroid cancer specialist should manage high-risk patients at least every 6 months for the first several years. After five years of diligent follow-up, it might be reasonable for the specialist to see the patients yearly. The intermediate-risk group should also be followed relatively closely (every 6 months to a year), though it may be reasonable to consider returning their long-term surveillance to the primary care physician.

Given the low rate of cervical node metastases for patients with FTC, little attention needs to be focused on this anatomic region. Chest X-rays may be useful on a yearly basis, since the lungs are at risk for distant metastasis. Diagnostic radioiodine scanning will often detect systemic spread before clinical exam or less sensitive and specific screening tests such as chest radiograph. Different scanning conditions can result in widely variable detection rates of metastasis, and tumor foci which do not concentrate iodine will be missed.[133] Furthermore, patients with significant residual thyroid tissue in the neck will probably not show uptake in metastases. MRI imaging may overcome some of these problems with regard to loco-regional recurrence, although it obviously will be less useful for monitoring systemic spread.[134,135]

Judicious use of serum thyroglobulin measurements is warranted in any patient with high- or intermediate-risk follicular thyroid carcinoma. At the author's primary institution, it is also used in low-risk patients, the majority of whom will have had a total thyroidectomy. Traditionally, measurements of serum thyroglobulin have been performed after the patient

has discontinued thyroxine replacement for four to six weeks. It has been well documented, however, that serum thyroglobulin levels obtained while the patient is taking thyroxine will probably only miss the occasional metastasis.[136] Undetectable serum thyroglobulin levels during treatment are very useful, because they are virtually never associated with recurrent or metastatic tumors.[137,138] Even detectable levels less than 5 ng/ml are extremely rare in disseminated or recurrent differentiated tumors.[138] Finally, there is evidence that FTC only rarely, and much less commonly than PTC, leads to false negative serum thyroglobulin measurements while the patient is taking thyroxine.[139] The presence of anti-thyroglobulin antibodies, which can occur in as many as 25% of patients, may render serum thyroglobulin measurements less reliable.[140-142] Obviously, when evidence of metastasis or recurrence is found, either on radioiodine scanning or by thyroglobulin measurement, further disease-specific treatment is warranted. Once detected, management will of course depend on size, location, and whether it is solitary or multicentric. Whether the few patients with potential occult metastatic disease, as suggested by elevated serum thyroglobulin levels accompanied by negative diagnostic scans, should receive empiric radioiodine therapy remains uncertain.[137,143]

## SUMMARY

While the majority of thyroid neoplasms are derived from follicular epithelium, the term *follicular neoplasm* usually refers to follicular adenomas and carcinomas. Sometimes Hürthle cell and insular cell tumors will be included under the heading of follicular neoplasms, although more often they are considered unique histologic subtypes with different clinical behavior. The incidence of follicular thyroid carcinoma, as compared to papillary thyroid carcinoma, has decreased in recent years because of dietary iodine supplementation. Further contributing to the declining incidence, the histologic subtype follicular-variant of papillary carcinoma is now accurately characterized under the heading of papillary cancer. Recently, a model of thyroid carcinogenesis has been proposed in which normal thyroid follicular epithelium can progress to adenomatous epithelium and then, ultimately, to follicular carcinoma. Mutations of the genes encoding for the *ras* proteins occur in both follicular adenomas and carcinomas, and, therefore, may be an early molecular event. Cytogenetic evaluation has revealed translocations involving chromosome band 19q13, which may be another early event. Loss of heterozygosity on chromosome 3p may be a late event, given the frequency at which it is seen in follicular carcinoma. The diagnosis and treatment of follicular neoplasms, in general, is similar to the management of other thyroid tumors. The role of molecular technology to ferret out which FNABs are follicular carcinomas is promising, although still experimental. Careful frozen section analysis of lobectomy specimens may accurately diagnose minimally invasive follicular carcinoma, allowing for more comprehensive surgery at the initial setting. A trend toward improved loco-regional control and long-term survival is seen when more thorough surgery is performed and followed-up with radioiodine ablation. Prognosis for follicular neoplasms can reliably be determined using criteria proposed for papillary thyroid carcinoma—patients can be stratified into low-, intermediate-, and high-risk groups, based on the age of the patient, size of the primary tumor, extrathyroid spread, and distant metastases. Monitoring thyroglobulin levels is useful for long-term surveillance in those patients with follicular thyroid carcinoma who have undergone total thyroidectomy and postoperative radioablation.

# References

1. Hedinger C, Williams ED, Sobin LH. *Histologic Typing of Thyroid Tumors.* Second ed. Berlin: Springer-Verlag; 1988. (International histologic classification of tumors, World Health Organization).
2. LiVolsi V. *Surgical Pathology of the Thyroid. Major Problems in Pathology.* Philadelphia: W.B. Saunders; 1990: 367–384.
3. Rosai J, Carcangiu ML, DeLellis RA. *Atlas of Tumor Pathology, 3rd Series, Fascicle 5. Tumors of the Thyroid Gland. Thyroid Tumors-General Considerations.* Washington, DC: Armed Forces Institute of Pathology; 1992: 327–338.
4. Casara D, Rubello D, Saladini G et al. Distant metastases in differentiated thyroid cancer. long-term results of radioiodine treatment and statistical analysis of prognostic factors in 214 patients. *Tumori.* 1991; 77:432.
5. Mizukami Y, Michigisi T, Nonomura A et al. Distant metastases in differentiated thyroid carcinomas. a clinical and pathologic study. *Hum Pathol.* 1990; 21:283.
6. Ruegemer JJ, Hay ID, Bergstrahl EJ et al. Distant metastases in differentiated thyroid carcinoma. A multivariate analysis of prognostic variables. *J Clin Endocrinol Metab.* 1988; 67:501.
7. Schlumberger M, Tubiana M, De Vathaire F et al. Long-term results of treatment of 283 patients with lung and bone metastases from differentiated thyroid carcinoma. *J Clin Endocrinol Metab.* 1986; 63:960.
8. Grebe SKG, Hay ID. Thyroid cancer nodal metastases. Biological significance and therapeutic considerations. *Surg Oncol Clin North Am.* 1996; 5:43–63.
9. Yamashina M. Follicular neoplasms of the thyroid. total circumferential evaluation of the fibrous capsule. *Am J Surg Pathol.* 1992; 16:392–400.
10. Lang W, Georgii G, Stauch G, et al. The differentiation of atypical adenomas and encapsulated follicular carcinomas in the thyroid gland. *Virch Arch Pathol Anat.* 1980; 385:125–141.
11. Evans HL, Vassiloopoulou-Sellin R. Follicular and Hurthle cell carcinomas of the thyroid. a comparative study. *Am J Surg Pathol.* 1998; 22(12):1512–1520.
12. Brennan MD, Bergstralh EJ, van Heerden JA, McConahey WM. Follicular thyroid cancer treated at the Mayo Clinic, 1946 through 1970. *Mayo Clin Proc.* 1991; 66:11–22.
13. Carcangiu ML, Bianchi S, Savino D et al. Follicular Hurthle cell tumors of the thyroid gland. *Cancer.* 1991; 68:1944–53.
14. Crile G, Pontius KI, Hawk WA. Factors influencing the survival of patients with follicular carcinoma of the thyroid gland. *Surg Gynecol Obstet.* 1985; 160:409–13.
15. McDonald MP, Sanders LE, Silverman ML et al. Hurthle cell carcinoma of the thyroid gland. *Surgery.* 1996; 120:1000–5.
16. Shaha AR, Loree TR, Shah JP. Prognostic factors and risk group analysis in follicular carcinoma of the thyroid gland. *Surgery.* 1995; 118:1131–8.
17. Shaha AR, Shah JP, Loree TR. Patterns of nodal and distant metastasis based on histologic varieties in differentiated carcinoma of the thyroid. *Am J Surg.* 1996; (Volume #) 692–4.
18. Watson RG, Brennan MD, Goellner JR et al. Invasive Hurthle cell carcinoma of the thyroid. *Mayo Clin Proc.* 1984; 59:851–5.
19. Grant CS. Operative and post-operative management of the patient with follicular and Hurthle cell carcinoma. Do they differ? *Surg Clin North Am.* 1995; 71:395–403.
20. Grebe SKG, Hay ID. Follicular thyroid cancer. *Endocrinol Metab Clin North Am.* 1995; 24:761–801.
21. Lang W, Choritz H, Hundeshagen H. Risk factors in follicular thyroid carcinomas. *Am J Surg Pathol.* 1986; 10:246–55.
22. Reiners C, Herrmann H, Schaffer R, Borner W. Incidence and prognosis of thyroid cancer with special regard to oncocytic carcinoma of the thyroid. *Acta Endocrinol.* 1983; (suppl 252):18.
23. Chen H, Nicol TL, Zeiger MA et al. Hurthle cell neoplasms of the thyroid: are there factors predictive of malignancy? *Ann Surg.* 1998; 227:542–6.
24. Carcangiu ML, Zampi G, Rosai J. Poorly differentiated ('insular') thyroid carcinoma. A reinterpretation of langerhans' 'Wuchernde Struma'. *Am J Surg Pathol.* 1984; 8:655–668.
25. Flynn SD, Forman BH, Stewart AF, Kinder BK. Poorly differentiated ('insular') carcinoma of the thyroid gland: an aggressive subset of differentiated thyroid neoplasms. *Surgery.* 1988; 104: 963–970.
26. Williams ED, Doniach I, Bjarnason O et al. Thyroid cancer in an iodide rich area: histopathological study. *Cancer.* 1977; 39:215.
27. Franceschi S, Levi F, Negri E et al. Diet in thyroid cancer: a pooled analysis of four European case-control studies. *Int J Cancer.* 1991; 48:395.
28. Harach HR, Escalante DA, Onativia A et al. Thyroid carcinoma and thyroiditis in an endemic goitre region before and after iodine prophylaxis. *Acta Endocrinol.* 1985; 108:55.
29. Harach HR, Williams ED. Thyroid cancer and thyroiditis in the goitrous region of Salta, Argentina, before and after iodine prophylaxis. *Clin Endocrinol.* 1995; 43:701–706.
30. LiVolsi VA, Asa SL. The demise of follicular carcinoma of the thyroid gland. *Thyroid.* 1994; 4:233–6.
31. Auguste LJ, Sako K. Radiation and thyroid carcinoma: Radiotherapy, head and neck regions, thyroid carcinoma. *Head Neck Surg.* 1985; 7:217.
32. McTiernan A, Weiss NS, Daling JR. Incidence of thyroid cancer in women in relation to previous exposure to radiation therapy and history of thyroid disease. *J Natl Cancer Inst.* 1984; 73:575.
33. Mehta MP, Goetowski PG, Kinsella TJ. Radiation induced thyroid neoplasms 1920 to 1987: a vanishing problem? *Int J Radiat Oncol Biol Phys.* 1989; 16: 1471.
34. Paloyan E, Lawrence AM. Thyroid neoplasms after radiation therapy for adolescent acne vulgaris. *Arch Dermatol.* 1978; 114:53.
35. Samaan NA, Schultz PN, Ordonez NG et al. A comparison of thyroid carcinoma in those who have and have not had head and neck irradiation in childhood. *J Clin Endocrinol Metab.* 1987; 64:219.
36. Schneider AB, Recant W, Pinsky SM et al. Radiation-induced thyroid carcinoma: clinical course and results of therapy in 296 patients. *Ann Intern Med.* 1986; 105:405.

37. McTiernan A, Weiss NS, Daling JR. Incidence of thyroid cancer in women in relation to known or suspected risk factors for breast cancer. *Cancer Res.* 1987; 47:292.

38. Ron E, Curtis R, Hoffman DA et al. Multiple primary breast and thyroid cancer. *Br J Cancer.* 1984; 49:87.

39. Hoelting T, Siperstein AE, Duh, QY et al. Tamoxifen inhibits growth, migration, and invasion of human follicular and papillary thyroid cancer cells in vitro and in vivo. *J Clin Endocinol Metab.* 1995; 80:308.

40. Van Hoeven KH, Menendez-Botet CJ, Strong EW et al. Estrogen and progesterone receptor content in human thyroid disease. *Am J Clin Pathol.* 1993; 99:175.

41. Ron E, Kleinerman RA, Boice JD Jr et al. A population-based case control study of thyroid cancer. *J Natl Cancer Inst.* 1987; 79:1.

42. Kravdal O, Glattre E, Haldorsen T. Positive correlation between parity and incidence of thyroid cancer. new evidence based on complete Norwegian birth cohorts. *Int J Cancer.* 1991; 49:831.

43. Cooper DS, Axelrod L, DeGroot LJ et al. Congenital goiter and the development of metastatic follicular carcinoma with evidence for a leak of non-hormonal iodine. clinical, pathological, kinetic, and biochemical studies and a review of the literature. *J Clin Endocrinol Metab.* 1994; 52:294.

44. Juhasz F, Boros P, Szegedi G et al. Immunogenetic and immunological studies of differentiated thyroid cancer. *Cancer.* 1989; 63: 1318.

45. Dralle H, Robin-Winn M, Reilman L et al. HLA and Schilddrusencarcinom. *K Wochenschr.* 1986; 64:522.

46. Sridima V, Hara Y, Fauchet R et al. Association of differentiated thyroid carcinoma with HLA-DR7. *Cancer.* 1985; 56:1086.

47. Farid NR, Shi Y, Zou M. Molecular basis of thyroid cancer. *Endocrin Rev.* 1994; 15:202–232.

48. Farid NR, Zou M, Shi Y. Genetics of follicular thyroid cancer. *Endocrinol Metab Clin North Am.* 1995; 24:865–881.

49. Wynford-Thomas D. Origin and progression of thyroid epithelial tumors. cellular and molecular mechanims. *Hormon Res.* 1997; 47:145–157.

50. Clark OH. Thyroid cancer: predisposing conditions, growth factors, signal transduction and oncogenes. *Aust N Z J Surg.* 1998; 68:469–477.

51. Fagin JA, Matsuo K, Karmakar A et al. High prevalence of mutations of the p53 gene in poorly differentiated human thyroid carcinomas. *J Clin Invest.* 1993; 91:179–84.

52. Smith P, Wynford-Thomas D. Control of thyroid follicular cell proliferation: cellular aspects. In Wynford-Thomas D, Williams ED, eds. *Thyroid Tumors: Molecular Basis of Pathogenesis.* Edinburgh: Churchill Livingston, 1989; 66–90.

53. Coclet J, Foureau F, Ketelbant P et al. Cell population kinetics in dog and human adult thyroid. *Clin Endocrinol.* 1989; 31:655–665.

54. Hicks DG, LiVolsi VA, Neidich JA et al. Clonal analysis of solitary follicular nodules in the thyroid. *Am J Pathol.* 1990; 137:553–561.

55. Lemoine NR, Mayall ES, Wyllie FS et al. Activated *ras* oncogenes in human thyroid cancers. *Cancer Res.* 1988; 48:4459–4463.

56. Wright PA, Williams ED, Lemoine NR, Wynford-Thomas D. Radiation-associated and "spontaneous" human thyroid carcinomas show a different pattern of *ras* oncogene mutation. *Oncogene.* 1991; 6:471–3.

57. Namba H, Gutman RA, Matsuo K et al. H-*ras* protooncogene mutations in human thyroid neoplasms. *J Endocrinol Metab.* 1990; 71:223–9.

58. Bond JA, Wyllie FS, Rowson J et al. In vitro reconstruction of tumor initiation in a human epithelium. *Oncogene.* 1994;9:281–290.

59. Hay ID. Cytometric DNA ploidy analysis in thyroid cancer. *Diagn Oncol.* 1991; 1:181.

60. Hermann MA, Hay ID, Bartlet DH et al. Cytogenetic and molecular genetic studies of follicular and papillary thyroid cancers. *J Clin Invest.* 1991; 88:1596–1604.

61. Jonasson JG, Hrafnkelsson J. Nuclear DNA analysis and prognosis in carcinoma of the thyroid gland: a nationwide study in Iceland on carcinomas diagnosed 1955-1990. *Virchows Arch [A].* 1994; 425:349.

62. Lukacs GL, Balazs G, Zs-Nagy I et al. Clinical meaning of DNA content in long-term behavior of follicular thyroid tumors: a 12–year follow-up. *Eur J Surg.* 1994; 160:417.

63. Matsuo K, Tang SH, Fagin JA. Allelotype of human thyroid tumors: loss of chromosome 11q13 sequences in follicular neoplasms. *Mol Endocrinol.* 1991; 5:1873.

64. Oyama T, Vickery AL Jr, Preffer RI et al. A comparative study of flow cytometry and histopathologic findings in thyroid follicular carcinomas and adenomas. *Hum Pathol.* 1994; 25:271.

65. Roque L, Castedo S, Clode A et al. Deletion of 3p25 pter in a primary follicular thyroid carcinoma and its metastasis. *Genes Chromosom Cancer.* 1993; 8:199.

66. Zedenius J, Auer G, Backdahl M et al. Follicular tumors of the thyroid gland: diagnosis, clinical aspects and nuclear DNA analysis. *World J Surg.* 1992; 16:589.

67. Bondeson L, Bengtsson A, Bondeson AG et al. Chromosome studies in thyroid neoplasia. *Cancer.* 1989; 64:680–685.

68. Taruscio D, Carcangiu ML, Ried T, Ward DC. Numerical chromosomal aberrations in thyroid tumors detected by double fluorescence in situ hybridization. *Genes Chromosom Cancer.* 1994; 9:180–185.

69. Teyssier JR, Liautaud-Roger F, Ferre D, et al. Chromosomal changes in thyroid tumors. relation with DNA content, karyotypic features, and clinical data. *Cancer Genet Cytogenet.* 1990; 50:249–263.

70. Barnitzke S, Herrmann ME, Lobeck H et al. Cytogenetic findings on eight follicular thyroid adenomas including one with a t(10:19). *Cancer Genet Cytogenet.* 1989; 39:65–68.

71. Roque L, Castedo S, Gomes P et al. Cytogenetic findings in 18 follicular thyroid adenomas. *Cancer Genet Cytogenet.* 1993; 67:1–6.

72. Sozzi G, Miozzo M, Cariani TC et al. A t(2:3)(q12–13:p24–25) in follicular thyroid adenomas. *Cancer Genet Cytogenet.* 1992; 64:38–41.

73. Herrmann MA, Hay ID, Bartelt DH Jr et al. Cytogenetics of six follicular thyroid adenomas including a case report of an oxyphil variant with t(8:14)(q13;q24.1). *Cancer Genet Cytogenet.* 1991; 56:231–235.

74. Roque L, Castedo S, Clode A, Soares J. Translocation t(5:19): A recurrent change in follicular thyroid adenoma. *Genes Chromosom Cancer.* 1992; 4:346–347.

75. Dal Cin P, Sneyers W, Aly MS et al. Involvement of 19q13 in follicular thyroid adenoma. *Cancer Genet Cytogenet.* (year?); 60:99–101.

76. Belge G, Thode B, Bullerdiek J, Barnitzke S. Aberrations of chromosome 19. Do they characterize a subtype of benign thyroid adenomas? *Cancer Genet Cytogenet.* 1992; 60:23–26.

77. Grebe SKG, Hay ID. Follicular cell-derived thyroid carcinomas. In: Arnold A, ed. *Endocrine Neoplasms.* Kluwer Academic Publications; 1997; 91–140.

78. Jenkins RB, Hay ID, Herath JF et al. Frequent occurrence of cytogenetic abnormalities in non-medullary thyroid carcinoma. *Cancer.* 1990; 66:1213–1220.

79. Linehan WM, Lerman MI, Zbar B. Identification of the von Hippel-Lindau (VHL) gene. its role in renal cancer. *JAMA.* 1995; 273:564–570.

80. Bruneton JN, Balu-Maestro C, Marcy PY et al. Very high-frequency (13Mhz) ultrasonographic examination of the normal neck: detection of normal lymph nodes and thyroid nodules. *J Ultrasound Med.* 1994; 13:87.

81. Seya A, Oeda T, Terano T et al. Comparative studies on fine-needle aspiration cytology with ultrasound scanning in the assessment of thyroid nodules. *Jpn J Med.* 1990; 29:478.

82. Christensen SB, Ljungberg O, Tibblin S. Prediction of malignancy in the solitary nodule by physical examination, thyroid scan, fine-needle biopsy, and serum thyroglobulin: a prospective study of 100 surgically treated patients. *Acta Chir Scand.* 1984; 150:433.

83. Cutfield RG, Croxson MS. A clinico-pathological study of 100 patients with solitary 'cold' thyroid nodules. *NZ Med J.* 1981; 93:331.

84. Oommen R, Walter NM, Tulasi NR. Scintigraphic diagnosis of thyroid cancer: correlation of thyroid scintigraphy and histopathology. *Acta Radiol.* 1994; 35:222.

85. Nagashima T, Suzuki M, Oshida M et al. Morphometry in the cytologic evaluation of thyroid follicular lesions. *Cancer Cytopathol.* 1998; 84:115–8.

86. Deshpande V, Kapila K, Sai KS, Verma K. Follicular neoplasms of the thyroid: decision tree approach using morphologic and morphometric parameters. *Acta Cytol.* 1997; 41:369–176.

87. Das DK, Jain S, Tripathi RP et al. Marginal vacuoles in thyroid aspirates. *Acta Cytol.* 1998; 42:1121–1128.

88. Chiapetta G, Tallini G, De Biasio MC et al. Detection of high mobility group 1 HMG1(Y) protein in the diagnosis of thyroid tumors: HMG1(Y) expression represents a potential diagnostic indicator of carcinoma. *Cancer Res.* 1998; 58:4193–4198.

89. Schmid KW, Ladurner D, Zechman W et al. Clinicopathologic management of tumors of the thyroid gland in an endemic goiter area: combined use of preoperative fine needle aspiration biopsy and intraoperative frozen section. *Acta Cytol.* 1989; 33:27.

90. Emerick GT, Duh QY, Siperstein AE et al. Diagnosis, treatment, and outcome in follicular thyroid carcinoma. *Cancer.* 1993; 72:3287.

91. Ladurner D, Seeber G. Das follikulare schilddrusenkarzinom: eine multivariate analyse. *Schweiz Med Wochenschr.* 1984; 114:1087.

92. Ladurner D, Seeber G, Hofstadter F et al. Das differenziete schilddrusenkarzinom in endemiegebiet. *Dtsch Med Wochenschr.* 1985; 110:333.

93. Rosler H, Birrer A, Luscher D et al. Langzeitverlaufe beim differenzierten schilddrusenkarzinom. *Schweiz Med Wochenschr.* 1992; 122:1843.

94. Shaw JH, Dodds P. Carcinoma of the thyroid gland in Auckland, New Zealand. *Surg Gynecol Obstet.* 1990; 171:27.

95. Simpson WJ, Panzarella T, Carruthers JS et al. Papillary and follicular thyroid cancer: impact of treatment in 1578 patients. *Int J Radiat Oncol Biol Phys.* 1988; 14:1063.

96. Cady B, Rossi R. An expanded view of risk-group definition in differentiated thyroid carcinoma. *Surgery.* 1988; 104:947.

97. Christensen SB, Ljungberg O, Tibblin S. Surgical treatment of thyroid carcinoma in a defined population, 1960-1977. evaluation of the results after a conservative surgical approach. *Am J Surg.* 1983; 146:349.

98. Crile G Jr, Pontius KI, Hawk WA. Factors influencing the survival of patients with follicular carcinoma of the thyroid gland. *Surg Gynecol Obstet.* 1985; 160:409.

99. Clark OH, Levin K, Zeng QH et al. Thyroid cancer. the case for total thyroidectomy. *Eur J Cancer Clin Oncol.* 1988; 24:305.

100. Hamming JF, van de Velde CJH, Goslings BM et al. Prognosis and morbidity after total thyroidectomy for papillary, follicular, and medullary thyroid cancer. *Eur J Clin Oncol.* 1989; 25:1317.

101. Ley PB, Roberts JW, Symmonds RE Jr et al. Safety and efficacy of total thyroidectomy for differentiated thyroid carcinoma. a 20-year review. *Am Surg.* 1993; 59:110.

102. Marchegiani C Lucci S, De Antoni E et al. Thyroid cancer. surgical experience with 322 cases. *Int Surg.* 1985; 70:121.

103. Mazzaferri EL, Jhiang SM. Long-term impact of initial surgical and medical therapy on papillary and follicular thyroid cancer. *Am J Med.* 1994; 97:418.

104. Szanto J, Ringwald G, Karika Z et al. Follicular cancer of the thyroid gland. *Oncology.* 1991; 48:483.

105. Rossi RL, Cady B, Silverman ML et al. Surgically incurable well-differentiated thyroid carcinoma. *Arch Surg.* 1988; 123:569.

106. Jensen MH, Davis RK, Derrick L. Thyroid cancer: a computer-assisted review of 5287 cases. *Otolaryngol Head Neck Surg.* 1990; 102:51.

107. Schumichen CE, Schmitt E, Scheufele C et al. Einflu des Therapiekonzepts auf die prognose des schilddrusenkarzinoms. *Nucl Med.* 1983; 22:97.

108. Young RI, Mazzaferri EL, Rahe et al. Pure follicular carcinoma: impact of therapy in 214 patients. *J Nucl Med.* 1980; 21:733.

109. Bottger T, Klupp J, Sorger K et al. Prognostisch relevante Faktoren beim follikularen Schilddrusenkarzinom. *Langenbecks Arch Chir.* 1990; 375:266.

110. Jorda M, Gonzalez-Campora R, Mora J et al. Prognostic factors in follicular carcinoma of the thyroid. *Arch Pathol Lab Med.* 1993; 117:631.

111. Mueller-Gartner HW, Brzac HT, Rehpenning W. Prognostic indices for tumor relapse and tumor mortality in follicular thyroid carcinoma. *Cancer.* 1991; 67:1903.

112. Schroder S, Baisch H Rehpenning W et al. Morphologie und prognose des follikularen Schilddrusenkarzinom—Eine klinisch-pathologische und DNS-cytometrische Unterschung an 95 tumoren. *Langenbecks Arch Chir.* 1987; 370:3.

113. Segal K, Arad A, Lubin E et al. Follicular carcinoma of the thyroid gland. *Head Neck.* 1994; 16:533.

114. Akslen LA, Haldorsen T, Thoresen S et al. Survival and causes of death in thyroid cancer: a population based study of 2479 cases from Norway. *Cancer Res.* 1991; 51:1234.

115. Franssila KO. Prognosis in thyroid carcinoma. *Cancer.* 1975; 36:1138.

116. Joensuu H, Klemi PJ, Paul R et al. Survival and prognostic factors in thyroid carcinoma. *Acta Radiol Oncol.* 1986; 25:243.

117. Kerr DJ, Burt AD, Boyle P et al. Prognostic factors in thyroid tumors. *Br J Cancer.* 1986; 54:475.

118. Russell MA, Gilbert EF, Jaeschke WF. Prognostic features of thyroid cancer. *Cancer.* 1975; 36:553.

119. Schelfhout LJDN, Creutzberg CL, Hamming JF et al. Multivariate analysis of survival in differentiated thyroid cancer. the prognostic significance of the age factor. *Eur J Cancer Clin Oncol.* 1988; 24:331.

120. Selzer G, Kahn LB, Albertyn L. Primary malignant tumors of the thyroid gland: a clinicopathological study of 254 cases. *Cancer.* 1977; 40:1501.

121. Shah JP, Dharker D, Strong EW et al. Prognostic factors in differentiated carcinoma of the thyroid gland. *Am J Surg.* 1992; 164:658.

122. Simpson WJ, McKinney SE, Carruthers JS et al. Papillary and follicular thyroid cancer: prognostic factors in 1578 patients. *Am J Med.* 1987; 83:479.

123. Tenvall J, Biorklund A, Moller T et al. Prognostic factors of papillary, follicular and medullary carcinomas of the thyroid gland. *Acta Radiol Oncol.* 1985; 24:17.

124. DeGroot LJ, Kaplan EL, Shukla MS et al. Morbidity and mortality in follicular thyroid cancer. *J Clin Endo Metab.* 1995; 80:2946–2953.

125. Tesarek T, Kissova D. Clinical analysis of 43 surgically treated patients with thyroid carcinoma. *Neoplasma.* 1975; 22:329.

126. Tubiana M, Schlumberger M, Rougier P et al. Long-term results and prognostic factors in patients with differentiated thyroid carcinoma. *Cancer.* 1985; 56:2298.

127. Glanzmann C, Horst W. Behandlung und prognose des follicularen und papillaren schilddreusenkarzinomas. *Strahlentherpie.* 1979; 155:515.

128. Davis NL, Bugis SP, McGregor GI, Germann E. An evaluation of prognostic scoring systems in patients with follicular thyroid cancer. *Am J Surg.* 1995; 170:476–480.

129. Torres J, Volpato RD, Power EG et al. Thyroid cancer: survival in 148 cases followed for 10 years or more. *Cancer.* 1985; 56:2298.

130. Van Heerden JA, Hay ID, Goellner JR et al. Follicular thyroid carcinoma with capsular invasion alone: a non-threatening malignancy. *Surgery.* 1992; 112:1130.

131. Cunningham MP, Duda RB, Recant W et al. Survival discriminants for differentiated thyroid cancer. *Am J Surg.* 1990; 160: 344.

132. Ruiz de Almodovar JM, Ruiz-Garcia J, Olea N et al. Analysis of risk of death from differentiated thyroid cancer. *Radiother Oncol.* 1994; 31:199.

133. Maxon HR III, Smith HS. Radioiodine-131 in the diagnosis and treatment of metastatic well-differentiated thyroid cancer. *Endocrinol Metab Clin North Am.* 1990; 19:685.

134. Chaudhuri R, Bingham JB, Clarke SE et al. MRI evaluation of thyroid malignancies. comparison with scintigraphy. *Nucl Med Commun.* 1991; 12:284.

135. Mallin WH, Elgazzar AH, Maxon HR. Imaging modalities in the follow-up of non-iodine avid thyroid carcinoma. *Am J Otolaryngol.* 1994; 15:417.

136. Ericsson UB, Tegler L, Lennquist S et al. Serum thyroglobulin in differentiated thyroid carcinoma. *Acta Chir Scand.* 1984; 150:367.

137. Clark OH, Hoelting T. Management of patients with differentiated thyroid cancer who have positive serum thyroglobulin levels and negative radioiodine scans. *Thyroid.* 1994; 4:501.

138. Ozata M, Suzuki S, Miyamoto T et al. Serum thyroglobulin in the follow-up of patients with differentiated thyroid cancer. *J Clin Endocrinol Metab.* 1994; 19:98.

139. Szanto J, Vincze B, Sinkovics I et al. Postoperative thyroglobulin level determination to follow-up patients with highly differentiated thyroid cancer. *Oncology.* 1989; 46:99.

140. Kumar A, Shah DH, Shrihari U et al. Significance of antithyroglobulin autoantibodies in differentiated thyroid carcinoma. *Thyroid.* 1994; 4:199.

141. Pacini F, Mariotti S, Formica N et al. Thyroid autoantibodies in thyroid cancer: incidence and relationship with tumor outcome. *Acta Endocrinol.* 1988; 119:373.

142. Rubello D, Casara D, Girelli ME, et al. Clinical meaning of circulating antithyroglobulin antibodies in differentiated thyroid cancer: a prospective study. *J Nucl Med.* 1992; 33:1478.

143. Mazzaferri EL. Treating high thyroglobulin with radioiodine—a magic bullet or a shot in the dark. *J Clin Endocrinol Metab.* 1995; 80:1485.

# 14

# Hürthle Cell Neoplasms of the Thyroid

## William B. Farrar, M.D.

The spectrum of thyroid cancer ranges from very favorable well-differentiated papillary cancer to poorly differentiated anaplastic cancer. There continues to be considerable controversy over many aspects of thyroid cancer management, especially in terms of diagnosis and treatment. One of the most controversial types is the Hürthle cell neoplasm.

Hürthle cell tumors account for 4–10% of thyroid neoplasms, although only 1% of thyroid cancers.[1] Historically, there has been considerable controversy regarding the ability to differentiate benign from malignant Hürthle cell tumors. Some authors have advocated that all Hürthle cell tumors be considered malignant and, therefore, should be aggressively treated with total thyroidectomy. Others believe that these tumors are truly variants of follicular tumors and should be managed as you would any other follicular tumor. This chapter will update the present information available concerning many of these issues.

## HISTORICAL

The term Hürthle Cell Tumor is actually a misnomer. Hürthle, in 1894, initially described an interfollicular cell in the canine thyroid which was actually a parafollicular C cell and not the cells which today bear his name.[2] The Hürthle cell was first described by Askanazy in 1898 in a patient with thyrotoxicosis.[3] The first Hürthle cell tumor was described by Langhans in 1907.[4] Ewing, in 1919, described a true Hürthle cell tumor and gave it the name of Hürthle, although Askanazy and Langhans made the original descrip-

tion.[5] Even today, these tumors maybe referred to as Askanazy or Langhans tumors.

## PATHOLOGY

There is strong evidence that Hürthle cell neoplasms actually arise from the follicular cells of the thyroid.[6] Hürthle cells are characterized by large polygonal cells with hyperchromatic, often bizarre, nuclei and eosinophilial cytoplasm, containing a large number of mitochondria. The individual Hürthle cells are 10–15 microns in diameter and can vary in shape and size from small dumbbells to bizarre giant cells.[7] These cells can be found in a variety of thyroid conditions including Hashimoto's thyroiditis, Graves' disease, nodular goiters, and thyroid neoplasm[1] (see Figure 14–1).

## CLINICAL PRESENTATION

The presentation of the Hürthle cell tumor is not different from any other thyroid tumor. There are no specific factors in the history or physical exam that would lead one to suspect a Hürthle cell tumor.[7] The initial evaluation of the thyroid nodule is well-discussed in other chapters of this book. FNA is the initial test and can lead to the diagnosis of Hürthle cell neoplasm. One controversy is what is actually called a Hürthle cell neoplasm. If one includes in the diagnosis of Hürthle cell neoplasms all nodules with any Hürthle cells present, then most Hürthle cell neoplasms would be benign, up to 80%.[8] If one is careful to not include the Hürthle cells

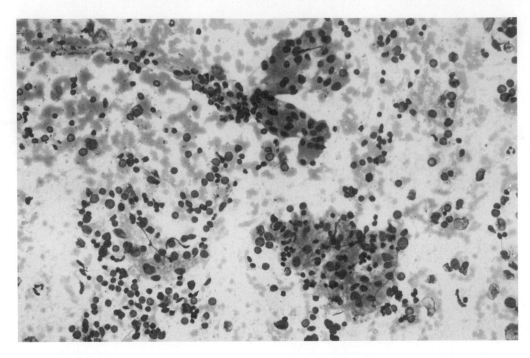

**Figure 14–1.** Aspiration cytology of a thyroid nodule showing Hürthle cells with thyroiditis.

that are found in the background of other thyroid diseases, then the incidence of benign neoplasms becomes much lower. Some pathologists feel strongly that you can differentiate between Hürthle cells associated with other thyroid disorders and true Hürthle cell neoplasms. Hürthle cell neoplasms have a much higher percentage of Hürthle cells, cellular dyshesion, large nucleoli, nuclear pleomorphism, and the absence of macrophages, plasma cells, and lymphocytes.[9,10] Hürthle cells can be associated with thyroiditis, hyperthyroidism, and other benign thyroid conditions.[11,12]

Hürthle cell neoplasms should be managed the same way that you would manage follicular neoplasms, although most clinicians would be more aggressive toward surgical resection of Hürthle cell neoplasms. Some advocate that all Hürthle cell neoplasms should be surgically resected while others would obtain a thyroid scan and only operate if the nodule is "cold." Fine needle aspiration biopsy cannot distinguish between benign adenomas and malignant. As in follicular neoplasms, to make the diagnosis of benign versus malignant, one needs to demonstrate capsular and/or vascular invasion that can only be seen on multiple tissue sections. This can be very difficult in some cases. The debate about Hürthle cell neoplasms being benign or malignant has been going on for a long time. In 1974, Thompson et al[12] reported on 26 patients with a histologic diagnosis of benign Hürthle cell adenoma in which 3 patients died of thyroid cancer. They concluded that these neoplasms should always be considered malignant irrespective of size. Grant et al[13] reported in

1988 a review of 272 patients with a diagnosis of benign Hürthle cell adenoma. Evidence of malignancy, ie, local recurrence, only occurred in one patient and no one died of thyroid cancer. They also looked at 20 other published reports of 642 patients with benign Hürthle cell adenomas. Only 6 (0.9%) were diagnosed incorrectly.[13] By careful pathologic review, Hürthle cell neoplasms should be correctly diagnosed. Considerations concerning treatment options should be made on an accurate diagnosis.

Most pathologists now agree that these tumors should be classified as a subclassification of follicular tumors. The criteria to make the diagnosis of benign or malignant should be the same for Hürthle cell neoplasms as follicular neoplasms. That criterion is based on the demonstration of capsular and/or vascular invasion. To document capsular invasion one needs to see tumor penetration of the capsule of the neoplasm (see Figures 14–2 and 14–3). Vascular invasion requires the demonstration of tumor cells penetrating blood vessels within or outside the capsule of the neoplasm. The need for this criterion to be seen makes the diagnosis of malignancy on FNA or frozen section at the time of surgery very unlikely. This has led many clinicians to not recommend frozen section analyses at the time of surgical resection and remains a controversial point. There are surgeons who do not do frozen sections because of the inability of the pathologists to distinguish between benign versus malignant. On the other hand, other surgeons send their thyroids for frozen sections to identify the small number of patients who may have

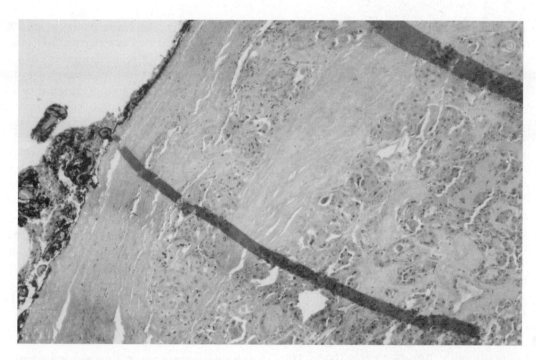

**Figure 14–2.** Clinical presentation. Thyroid nodule showing a Hürthle cell neoplasm with invasion into the capsule. No other invasions were noted. Final pathology: Minimal invasive Hürthle cell carcinoma.

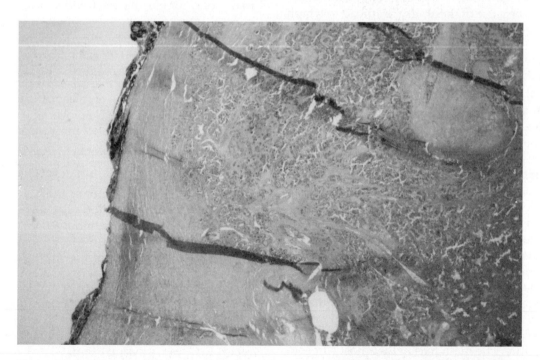

**Figure 14–3.** Clinical presentation. Thyroid nodule showing a Hürthle cell neoplasm with extension of Hürthle cell through the capsule. Final pathology: Invasive Hürthle cell carcinoma.

a papillary cancer that is easy to diagnose at frozen section. In that small number of patients, having to do a completion thyroidectomy at a later time is often avoided.

## SURGICAL MANAGEMENT

The decision to perform a thyroidectomy by most surgeons is similar to the decision process in deciding about follicular neoplasms. The pathologic criteria for malignancy are seen much more frequently in Hürthle cell neoplasms than in non-Hürthle cell neoplasms. Only 2–3% of solitary follicular neoplasms are malignant while 30% of Hürthle cell neoplasms are malignant.[8] Most surgeons would discuss with the patient that the initial procedure would be a total lobectomy and removal of the isthmus. There is never an indication to perform anything less than a total lobectomy. Intraoperative decision between total lobectomy versus total thyroidectomy includes a number of clinical findings: 1) extent of any extrathyroidal tumor spread; 2) any nodules or abnormalities of the contralateral lobe; 3) central compartment or cervical lymph nodes that are positive; 4) history of head and neck radiation treatment in the past. Any of the above would indicate the need for a total thyroidectomy. Most surgeons would also advocate total thyroidectomy for tumors over 2–3 cm in size. There are not enough available data to answer the specific question about size in Hürthle cell neoplasm. McLeod and Thompson did recommend a total thyroidectomy in patients with tumors greater than 5 cm and patients with tumors between 3–5 cm with aneuploid DNA.[1]

Hürthle cell carcinomas are different from follicular carcinomas because of the ability to spread to lymph nodes. Rarely do follicular cancers spread to lymph nodes while Hürthle cell carcinomas spread as often as 30%.[3,14,15] A central neck dissection should be performed at the initial surgery if the diagnosis of carcinoma is established. The lateral neck should also be palpated to be sure that there is no involvement and any suspicious nodes should be sampled. One should be prepared to perform a modified neck dissection if positive nodes are found.

If the diagnosis of carcinoma is made on the final pathology report, a completion thyroidectomy should be performed. This continues to be a very controversial subject, which is well-outlined in the chapters on papillary and follicular cancer. I will not discuss it in this chapter because there are not enough data to make any firm conclusions and there are no prospective randomized data to help in the decision process. The decision should include the characteristics of the tumor, the age of the patient, the risk factors for recurrence and mortality, and the experience of the surgeon who is performing the procedure. The main reason that most surgeons would advocate total thyroidectomy is recognized multifocal and bilateral disease as well as regional lymph node involvement. As most of these tumors are also reported to be more aggressive than the other well-differentiated tumors, aggressive surgical management provides better local control. At the definitive surgery, a central neck dissection should be performed.

Dr. Hundahl et al recently published data from the National Cancer Data Base evaluating 53,856 patients with thyroid cancer between the years 1985 and 1995. These retrospective data permit analysis of care patterns and survival for large numbers of contemporaneous U.S. patients with relatively rare neoplasms. In looking specifically at the Hürthle cell carcinomas, there were 1,310 patients. Approximately 60% had near-total or some other combination of total thyroidectomy and neck dissection. There were 25% who had only a lobectomy and 15% who had a procedure that could not be clearly identified. These data suggest that most surgeons perform more aggressive surgery for this pathologic diagnosis. What they found in regard to survival was that at 5-years overall stage-stratified relative survival for patients with Hürthle cell carcinoma closely matched patients with follicular carcinoma; however, the overall survival at 10 years was 9% lower suggesting a marginally worse prognosis.[16] Figure 14–4 summarizes the treatment of the thyroid nodule as it pertains to Hürthle cell tumors.

## POSTOPERATIVE MANAGEMENT

Postoperative management of patients following thyroidectomy for Hürthle cell tumors includes the options of RAI, thyroid suppressive therapy, and the use of serum thyroglobulin as a tumor marker. Historically, Hürthle cell cancers do not take up RAI. There are a lot of data to evaluate this. Reports show that only about 10% of patients with Hürthle cell carcinoma take up RAI while approximately 75% of follicular carcinoma do.[15,17] However, as this tumor has an overall worse prognosis than other thyroid cancers,[15,17] most clinicians would try RAI as a means of initial post-operative treatment.

The use of TSH-suppressive doses of thyroid hormone has been shown to reduce recurrence rates in patients with follicular carcinoma and may also improve survival.[18,19] Hürthle cell carcinoma has also been shown to have TSH receptor-adenylate cyclase system and should respond the same as follicular carcinoma.[6] The goal of hormone therapy is to keep the TSH level just below the lower limits of normal. Serum thyroglobulin is an excellent tumor marker and can be helpful in detecting recurrent disease.[20] When the serum thyroglobulin remains elevated after complete thyroidectomy or becomes elevated after therapy, workup with repeat RAI scan, physical exam, CT scans, and possible PET scans may be helpful to identify metastatic or recurrent local disease. If the disease is amenable to surgical resection, this should be accomplished prior to any further RAI therapy. The goal of treatment with patients is to reduce their tumor burden as much possible and then treat with any additional therapy such as RAI or possibly external radiation therapy.

Hürthle cell carcinoma tends to be more aggressive than the other types of differentiated thyroid can-

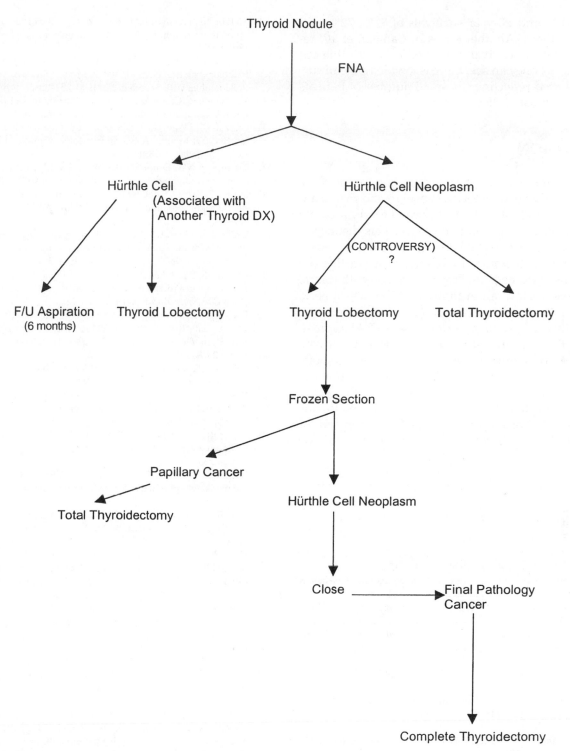

**Figure 14–4.** Hürthle cell nodule.

cer. It tends to be more multifocal and bilateral and more frequently involves the lateral neck nodes than follicular carcinoma. It has the highest incidence of metastatic cancer among the differentiated cancers. Patients with Hürthle cell carcinoma present with metastatic disease 10–20% of the time and develop

metastatic disease 34% of the time.[21-24] The most common sites for metastatic disease are the lung, bone, and the central nervous system.[25]

Survival rates for Hürthle cell carcinoma are similar to or in many cases worse than follicular carcinoma. Ryan et al[26] reported in their series of Hürthle cell carcinoma 5-, 10-, and 20-year survivals of 92%, 72%, and 67%, respectively. Another series by Samaan et al[27] reported a 10-year survival rate of 65% for Hürthle cell carcinoma. As one can see, there is a wide range of survivals reported reflecting the small number of patients described in most of these papers.

## CONCLUSION

Hürthle cell neoplasms are an uncommon tumor of the thyroid. The distinction between benign and malignant is sometimes difficult to make but can be very accurate if done by an experienced pathologist. This distinction is similar to the difference between follicular adenoma and follicular carcinoma. Treatment for a Hürthle cell carcinoma should be a total thyroidectomy with central node dissection and an evaluation of the lateral neck. RAI is usually given to assess metastatic disease; however, Hürthle cell carcinomas only take up RAI approximately 10% of the time. Metastatic disease occurs in 34% of patients. Follow-up should include thyroid hormone and serum thyroglobulin levels. When thyroglobulin levels are elevated, RAI scans, CT scans, or PET scans should be done to assess extent of disease. If metastatic disease does not pick up RAI, surgical resection and/or external radiation therapy should be considered. The overall survival rate of Hürthle cell carcinoma is worse than the other well-differentiated cancers.

## References

1. McLeod MK, Thompson N. Hurthle Cell Neoplasms of the Thyroid. *Otol Clin North Am.* 1990;23(3):441–452.
2. Hurthle K. Beitrge sur Kenntiss der Secretionsvorgangs in der Schilddruse. *Arch Gesamte Physiol.* 1894;56:1–44.
3. Askanazy M. Pathologisch-anatomische Beitrage sur Kenntiss des Morbus Basedowii, Insbesondere uber die Dabei auftretende Muskelerkarankung. *Deutsches Arch F Klin Med.* 1898;61:118–186.
4. Langhans T. Uber die Epithelailan Forman der Malignen Struma. *Virchows Arch.* 1907;189:69.
5. Ewing J. *Neoplastic Disease.* 3rd ed. Philadelphia: WB Saunders; 1928.
6. Clark OH, Gerend PL. Thryotropin (TSH) receptor-adenylate cyclase system in Hurthle cell neoplasms. *J Clin Endocrinol Metab.* 1985;39:773–800.
7. Clark OH, Duk Q. *Textbook of Endocrine Surgery.* WB Saunders Co; Philadelphia: 1997:103.
8. McIvor NP, Freeman JL, Rosen I, et al. Value of fine needle aspiration in the diagnosis of Hurthle cell neoplasms. *Head Neck Surg.* 1993;15:335.
9. LiVolsi VA, Bennington JL. Hurthle cell lesions. Surgical Pathology of the Thyroid, Vol 22, *Major Problems in Pathology.* Philadelphia: W.B. Saunders Co. 1990. 281–286.
10. Vodanovic S, Crepinko I, Smoje J. Morphological diagnosis of Hurthle cell tumor of the thyroid gland. *Aeta Cytol.* 1993;37:17.
11. Gonzales JL, Wang HH, Ducatman BS. Fine needle aspiration to Hurthle cell lesions. A cytomorphologic approach to diagnosis. *Am J Clin Pathol.* 1993;100:231.
12. Thompson NW, Dunn EL, Batsakis JG, et al. Hurthle cell lesions of the thyroid gland. *Surg Gynecol Obstet.* 1974;139:555–560.
13. Grant CS, Barr D, Goellner JR, et al. Benign Hurthle cell tumors of the thyroid: a diagnosis to be trusted? *World J Surg.* 1988;12:488–495.
14. Grant CS. Operative and postoperative management of the patient with follicular and Hurthle cell carcinoma—do they differ? *Surg Clin North Am.* 1995;75(3):395–403.
15. Maxon HR, Smith HS. Radioiodine–131 in the diagnosis and treatment of metastatic well differentiated thyroid cancer. *Endocrinol Metab Clin North Am.* 1990;19:685.
16. Hundahl SA, Fleming ID, Fermgen AM, Menck HR. A National Cancer Data Base Report on 53,856 cases of thyroid carcinoma treated in the U.S., 1985–1995. *American Cancer Society:* 1998; 83(12):2638–2648.
17. Soh EY, Clark OH. Surgical consideration and approach to thyroid cancer. *Endocrinol Metab Clin North Am.* 1996;21:115.
18. Rossi RL, Cady B, Silverman ML, et al. Surgically incurable well-differentiated thyroid carcinoma prognostic factors and results of therapy. *Arch Surg.* 1988;123:569.
19. Young RL, Mazzaferri EL, Rabe AJ, et al. Pure follicular thyroid carcinoma: impact of therapy in 214 patients. *J Nucl Med.* 1980;21:733.
20. Barsano, CP, Skosey C, DeGroot JL, et al. Serum thyroglobulin in the management of patients with thyroid cancer. *Arch Intern Med.* 1982;142:763.
21. Har El G, Hardor T, Segal K, et al. Hurthle cell carcinoma of the thyroid gland. A tumor of moderate malignancy. *Cancer.* 1986;57: 1613.
22. Horn RC Jr. Hurthle cell tumors of the thyroid. *Cancer.* 1954;7:234.
23. Ruegemer JJ, Hay ID, Bergstralh EJ, et al. Distant metastases in differentiated thyroid carcinoma: a multivariate analysis of prognostic variable. *J Clin Endocrinol Metab.* 1988;67:501.
24. Watson RG, Brennan MD, Goellner Jr et al. Invasive Hurthle cell carcinoma of the thyroid: natural history and management. *Mayo Clin Proc.* 1986;59:851.
25. Carcangiu ML, Bianchi S, Savino D, et al. Follicular Hurthle cell tumors of the thyroid gland. *Cancer.* 1991;68:1944.
26. Ryan JJ, Hay ID, Grant CS, et al. Flow cytometric DNA measurement in benign and malignant Hurthle cell tumors of the thyroid. *World J Surg.* 1988;12:482.
27. Samaan NA, Schultz PA, Hickey RC, et al. The results of various modalities of treatment of well-differentiated thyroid carcinoma: a retrospective review of 1,599 patients. *J Clin Endocrinol Metab.* 1992;75:714.

# 15

# Medullary Carcinoma of the Thyroid

Gregory W. Randolph, M.D., F.A.C.S.
Anthony De la Cruz, M.D.
William C. Faquin, M.D., Ph.D.

Comprising less than 10% of all thyroid malignancies, medullary thyroid carcinoma (MTC) has a prognosis intermediate between well-differentiated thyroid carcinoma and anaplastic and is characterized by a propensity for early nodal metastasis. MTC arises from the thyroid's parafollicular C cells and not from the thyroid follicular parenchyma, as do most other thyroid malignancies. C cells secrete the polypeptide hormone calcitonin, which is normally involved in calcium homeostasis and has proven to be an invaluable marker in the diagnosis and follow-up of patients with MTC.[1] MTC may occur in both sporadic and inherited forms and can be associated with other tumors as part of the multiple endocrine neoplasia syndromes (MEN) types IIa and IIb. Hazard first described the pathologic findings of medullary thyroid carcinoma in 1952.[2] In 1968 Steiner found an association with hyperparathyroidism and pheochromocytoma as part of MEN II syndrome (now MEN IIa).[3] The familial form of MTC without other associated neoplasms was described by Famdon and associates in 1986.[4]

Medullary thyroid carcinoma is both a diagnostic and surgical challenge. The standard surgical treatment involves total thyroidectomy and central neck dissection. Recent work has demonstrated the importance of aggressive lateral neck surgery in patients with palpable thyroid lesions. Modem advances in calcitonin measurement, provocative calcitonin stimulation and RET oncogene testing, have become valuable tools in the management of patients at risk for this disease. The genetic advances associated with medullary carcinoma of the thyroid have provided us unique insight into the development of this inherited endocrine malignancy.

## INHERITED FORMS OF MTC

While the inherited forms of medullary thyroid carcinoma are often the first to come to a clinician's mind, approximately 75% represent sporadic, non-inherited lesions. For the 25% with inherited disease, different patterns of associated endocrinopathies, prognosis, and age at onset of disease characterize three separate clinically inherited entities (Table 15–1). All inherited forms of medullary thyroid carcinoma are autosomal dominant with incomplete penetrance and are associated with multifocal C cell hyperplasia and multifocal MTC. The multifocal nature of inherited MTC and the difficulty preoperatively in distinguishing sporadic from inherited forms have led to the recommendation of total thyroidectomy in all patients with MTC.

In MEN IIa, medullary is usually the first neoplasm to present. Also known as Sipple's syndrome, MEN IIa patients will develop pheochromocytoma in 50% and hyperparathyroidism in 10–30% of cases.[3] Medullary presents earlier in life in MEN IIa than in the sporadic form of MTC, typically, in the third decade of life (Table 15–2). In MEN IIa patients who develop pheochromocytoma or hyperparathyroidism these abnormalities typically occur after medullary presenta-

**Table 15–1.** The spectrum of MEN syndromes and hereditary MTC

| MEN Syndromes | | | Hereditary MTC |
|---|---|---|---|
| **MEN I** | **MEN 2a** | **MEN 2b** | **Familial MTC** |
| Werner's syndrome | Sipple's syndrome | MTC | MTC |
| • Pituitary adenomas | • MTC | Pheochromocytoma 50% | |
| • Pancreatic islet cell tumor | • Pheochromocytoma 50% | Marfanoid habitus | |
| • Adrenal cortical adenomas | • Hyperparathyroidism 10–30% | Multiple mucosal intestinal | |
| • Hyperparathyroidism | | ganglioneuromas 100% | |

MEN = multiple endocrine neoplasia

MTC = medullary carcinoma of the thyroid

From Randolph GW. Medullary Carcinoma of the Thyroid. *Curr Opin Otolaryngol Head Neck Surg.* 1997;5:55–68. Reprinted with permission.

tion. Two variant forms of MEN IIa have been described. The first is associated with a pruritic dermatologic condition called cutaneous lichen amyloidosis. The second form is associated with Hirschsprung's disease.[5] In MEN IIa, expressivity is variable and penetrance is age-related and incomplete with up to 30% of patients without clinical expression of disease by age 70.[6] Approximately 95% of gene carriers will demonstrate an elevation of calcitonin (through pentagastrin stimulation) by age 35, with average age of conversion to a positive test by 13 years.[5]

MEN IIb syndrome is characterized by MTC, marfanoid body habitus, pheochromocytoma, and multiple mucosal and intestinal neuromata. This syndrome becomes clinically evident as early as the first decade of life, typically through recognition of unique habitus or thyroid mass.

These patients have distinctive facial features such as thickened oral and labial mucosa, prominent corneal nerves, and a high, arched palate. As with MEN IIa, pheochromocytoma develops in approximately 50% of MEN IIb patients.[6,7] This subtype of MTC is believed to represent the most virulent form of MTC as compared to sporadic or other inherited types.[8]

Familial, non-MEN medullary thyroid carcinoma is also inherited as an autosomal dominant disease.[4] It typically presents in the fourth decade of life and has a relatively indolent course. These patients are free of other syndromic findings.

## CALCITONIN

Calcitonin is the major hormonal product of the parafollicular C cells. It is a 32 amino acid polypeptide hormone that acts to decrease serum calcium levels. Calcitonin has two main sites of action: bone and kidney.

Calcitonin inhibits osteoplastic activity, thereby decreasing bone reabsorption, and also acts to increase renal excretion of calcium. Calcitonin is elevated in all forms of MTC and may also be elevated in C cell hyperplasia. Calcitonin, therefore, represents an excellent marker for diagnosis of patients and family members at risk for MTC. Calcitonin levels may also be followed postoperatively to sensitively screen for recurrence of disease. Calcitonin levels can be increased postoperatively without clinical or radiographic correlates of disease.

In patients with inherited disease, C cell hyperplasia occurs multifocally throughout the gland prior to the development of frank MTC. As C cell hyperplasia develops and evolves into frank MTC, calcitonin levels rise. More than 30% of patients with C cell hyperplasia, or early MTC, have normal basal calcitonin levels.[9] In general, calcitonin levels correlate with tumor load. Patients with palpable neck disease may have serum levels greater than 1,000 pg/ml and patients with distant metastatic disease may have levels over 100,000.[10]

The physiologic importance of calcitonin in calcium homeostasis is slight. Even in patients with widely metastatic MTC and significant hypercalcitoninemia, calcium levels are typically within normal limits. Certainly after total thyroidectomy, patients typically do not have increased serum levels resulting from calcitonin deficiency. Calcitonin does have effects on the gastrointestinal track and can cause an increase in water and electrolyte secretion. This effect has been implicated in the chronic diarrhea that may occur in patients with high MTC loads and high calcitonin levels.

Calcium or pentagastrin infusion can provocatively stimulate calcitonin levels in patients with early MTC or C cell hyperplasia. Such provocative calcitonin stimulation has been used in early detection family screening programs to detect pre-clinical disease in relatives of patients with MTC. RET oncogene testing has, in

**Table 15–2.** Subtypes of MTC

| | Mode of Transmission | Family History | Age at Presentation Decade | Likelihood of Regional LN Involvement | Pheochromocytoma | Hyperparathyroidism | Mucosal Neuromata Marfanoid Habitus |
|---|---|---|---|---|---|---|---|
| Sporadic | — | Negative | 4th | High | No | No | No |
| MEN IIa | Autosomal dominant | Positive or negative | 3rd | High—with diagnostic mass<br><br>Low—with diagnostic screen | Yes | Yes | No |
| MEN IIb | Autosomal dominant | Usually negative | 1st or 2nd | High | Yes | No | Yes |
| FMTC | Autosomal dominant | Positive or negative | 4th | Low | No | No | No |

FMTC—familial nonmultiple endocrine neoplasia medullary carcinoma of the thyroid; MEN—mulitple endocrine neoplasia.

From Rancolpn GW. Medullary Carcinoma of the Thyroid *Curr Opin Otolaryngol Head Neck Surg.* 1997;5:55–68. Reprinted with permission.

large measure, replaced such biochemical screening programs. Approximately 95% of gene carriers will convert to a positive stimulated calcitonin biochemical test by the age of 35.[5,9]

## ONCOGENESIS

Although follicular parenchyma arises from the first and second pharyngeal pouches, C cells derive from neural crest, as does the adrenal medulla. In humans, C cells migrate not to a discreet ultimobranchial body, but to an intra-thyroidal position. C cells are mainly concentrated bilaterally in the upper two-thirds of the thyroid lateral lobes.

In hereditary forms of MTC, C cell hyperplasia occurs multifocally throughout the thyroid gland. This hyperplasia represents multiple sites of clonal C cell expansion as shown by glucose-6 phosphate dehydrogenase isoenzyme studies and does not occur in the sporadic form of MTC.[11] With time, the individual foci of C cell hyperplasia evolve into multiple foci of frank malignancy. Interestingly, the pheochromocytoma in MEN IIa and MEN IIb arise from a pre-existing bilateral diffuse nodular hyperplasia.[9]

The common neural crest origin of the adrenal medulla and parafollicular C cells led to speculation that MEN IIa and MEN IIb result from a fundamental genetic lesion, which results in proliferation of neural crest derived tissues. Knudsons "two hit" model of oncogenesis has been used to explain the sequence of events in oncogenesis in medullary carcinoma as for hereditary retinoblastoma.[12] According to this model, the germline autosomally dominant inherited genetic defect results in premalignant proliferation of certain neural crest derived tissues. The second and, perhaps inevitable, acquired genetic factor results in the development of frank malignancy from these proliferating tissues. Sporadic MTC would then require two acquired events consistent with the older age at onset of sporadic patients (Figure 15–1). The RET proto-oncogene has been recently identified in all forms of inherited MTC.[13,14] The exact role of RET in the development of C cell hyperplasia and ultimately MTC is not fully understood. It is not known if the RET oncogene alone is sufficient for the development of malignancy, although in in vitro assays, RET activation is associated with transforming potential.[6,15-19]

## GENETIC ADVANCES: RET PROTO-ONCOGENE

The RET proto-oncogene was identified during transformation assays in 1985 and has been completely cloned.[20] The RET gene codes for a transmembrane tyrosine kinase receptor whose natural ligand and nor-

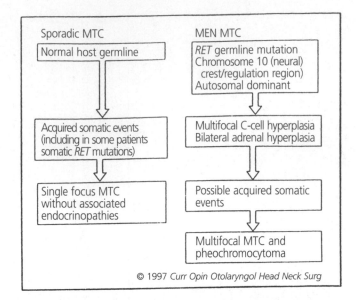

**Figure 15–1.** Oncogenesis in medullary carcinoma of the thyroid. MEN—multiple endocrine neoplasia; MTC—medullary carcinoma of the thyroid. (Reproduced from Randolph, GW. Medullary Carcinoma of the Thyroid, *Curr Opin Otolaryngol Head Neck Surg.* 1997;5:55–68. Reprinted with permission.)

mal physiologic function are poorly understood. The RET proto-oncogene is expressed in certain branchial arch and neural crest derived tissues and appears to have a role in neural crest/neuroendocrine tissue development and migration. RET expression has been found in several neural crest derived neoplasms, including neuroblastoma, as well as MTC and pheochromocytoma.[3,15,20] RET mutations have also been found in familial Hirschsprung's disease, an intestinal disorder associated with an absence or decrease in enteric ganglia.[5] Enteric ganglia abnormalities have been associated with a MEN IIa kindred. MEN IIb can be associated with intestinal ganglioneuromatosis and toxic megacolon similar to Hirschsprung's disease.[8] The RET oncogene has been mapped to the centromeric region of chromosome 10, a region implicated in neural crest and neuroendocrine tissue development and migration.

In 1993, missense point mutations in the RET proto-oncogene were identified in patients with MTC. Since that time the vast majority of patients with inherited forms of MTC have been found to have such RET point mutations.[13,21-24] These mutations are germline changes that are detectable in DNA from lymphocytes, obtained through peripheral blood samples. These mutations are not found as germline lesions in sporadic MTC patients. The RET mutations are thought to convert RET to a dominant transforming gene.[16,24,25] Ninety-seven percent of MEN IIa, 95% of MEN IIb, and 86% familial non-MEN medullary carcinoma have been found to have specific RET point mutations in a limited number of RET codons (Table 15–3).[6,26,27] In one surgi-

**Table 15–3.** Hereditary medullary carcinoma of the thyroid

| Syndrome | Cases with Known RET Mutations | Exon | Codons |
|---|---|---|---|
| MEN 2a | 97% | 10 | 609, 611, 618, 620 |
| | | 11 | 630, 634 |
| | | 13 | 768, 790 |
| MEN 2b | 95% | 15 | 883 |
| | | 16 | 918, 922 |
| FMTC | 86% | 10 | 609, 611, 618, 620 |
| | | 11 | 630, 634 |
| | | 13 | 768, 790, 791 |
| | | 14 | 804 |
| | | 15 | 891 |

Reproduced by permission from *Cancer Control: Journal of the Moffitt Cancer Center.*

cal series there have been no RET oncogene false positives.[28] The small fraction of inherited patients without known RET oncogene changes are believed to result from RET mutations which have not yet been discovered.

Identified RET mutations in inherited MTC are thought to lead to an increase in tyrosine kinase receptor activity and a change in tyrosine kinase substrate specificity.[15,19] Such increased tyrosine kinase activity may lead to changes in cell surface signaling and response to growth factors involved in neuroepidermal tissue differentiation and regulation.[5,15]

For patients with sporadic MTC, somatic (ie, tumor, not germline) RET mutations have been found in almost 70% of cases.[6,13,29] These RET changes at the somatic level are associated with sporadic tumor development. When present in sporadic tumors these RET changes have been associated with a poor prognosis[30] (Figure 15–1).

Eng has shown that there can be a relationship between a specific codon affected by RET oncogene mutation and the individual clinical disease manifestation (phenotype).[31] For example, with RET mutation at codon 634, the development of pheochromocytoma and hyperparathyroidism is likely, whereas these endocrinopathies do not occur when mutation occurs in codon 768 or 804. Further, mutation in codon 918 has only been associated with MEN IIb phenotype.[31,32]

## CLINICAL PRESENTATION

One must keep in mind that 75% of all medullary thyroid carcinoma is of the sporadic type. These patients typically present with a thyroid mass and will be diagnosed by fine needle aspiration. The cytology report, which describes malignant cells without further subtyping of the thyroid malignancy, should lead to con-

sideration for calcitonin immunohistochemical staining. We must also keep in mind during clinical assessment that these patients with palpable thyroid disease very frequently have regional nodal metastasis.[1,14] As it is often not possible preoperatively to separate sporadic MTC patients from inherited patients, all patients must be approached as possible inherited cases and have pheochromocytoma ruled out preoperatively with urine studies.

Sporadic MTC typically presents in the fourth decade usually as a thyroid mass. For sporadic patients, regional lymph nodes are involved in over 50% of cases with distant metastasis occurring in 10–20%[9,33] (Table 15–4).

MEN IIa presents usually in the third decade of life. If the diagnosis of MEN IIa is made through identification of a thyroid mass, regional lymph nodes are positive in nearly 50%.[34] If a patient is found to have MEN IIa by family screening methods, the incidence of lymph node metastasis at presentation drops to 14%.[35] Distant metastases are present in 20% of MEN IIa pa-

**Table 15–4.** MTC diagnostic workup

1. FNA, with calcitonin immunohistochemical staining
2. Calcitonin, CEA
3. Calcium, Albumin, Phosphate and intact PTH
4. 24-hour urine for catecholemines, VMA, metanephrines
5. Neck CT, ± thyroid ultrasound
6. Consider chest/abdominal imaging
7. Alert pathologist to check for multifocal MTC and C cell hyperplasia
8. RET oncogene assessment of patient and as appropriate, family screening

tients with clinically palpable MTC, but are not typically present in patients discovered through familial screening programs.[35] Although hyperparathyroidism and pheochromocytomas usually present clinically after MTC in patients diagnosed with MEN IIa, preoperative screening is essential.[35]

MEN IIb represents the most virulent subtype of medullary thyroid carcinoma. Such patients present through recognition of marfanoid habitus, mucosal ganglioneuromas, or thyroid mass. Regional lymph nodes are positive in 80% of patients with clinical disease and distant metastases at initial diagnosis are found in 20%.[9,33] Invasive MTC has been found at birth in children with MEN IIb. As these tumors are often fatal before reproductive age, many of these patients are thought to represent new mutations. Due to the poor prognosis at early age, families with MEN IIb are rare.

Familial (non-MEN) medullary thyroid carcinoma (FMTC) is the least virulent form of MTC. It typically presents in the fourth decade of life, similar to the sporadic form of disease. Its older age at onset and lack of associated endocrinopathy make it hard to differentiate from sporadic MTC. Regional lymph node disease is present in 10% and distant metastasis is uncommon at presentation.[4]

## PATHOLOGY

### Gross and Histologic Features

Gross examination of a resected medullary carcinoma typically shows a firm, circumscribed but rarely encapsulated tumor with a grey-white to red-brown cut surface (Figure 15–2).[36] Larger tumors may display central necrosis and hemorrhage as well as abundant amyloid deposition. These features are not typically seen in medullary microcarcinomas (less than 1 cm), which are more often seen with hereditary disease. Microcarcinomas are associated with C cell hyperplasia and have an excellent prognosis.[37]

Histologically, medullary carcinoma is known as a great mimicker because of the variability of its histologic and cytologic appearances, and its resemblance in histologic sections to a wide variety of other tumors, both primary in the thyroid and metastatic. This variable microscopic appearance includes a range of both architectural patterns as well as a varied array of cell types. Because of this histologic variability, the diagnosis of medullary carcinoma in metastatic sites may be particularly challenging.

The most frequently encountered histologic pattern is an arrangement of loosely cohesive sheets and clusters of polygonal to elongate cells set in a desmoplastic stroma and surrounded by delicate fibrovascular septa (Figure 15–3).[36] Individual cells are most often

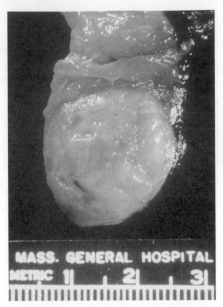

**Figure 15–2.** Gross appearance of a medullary carcinoma. The tumor is circumscribed but unencapsulated with an orange-tan cut surface.

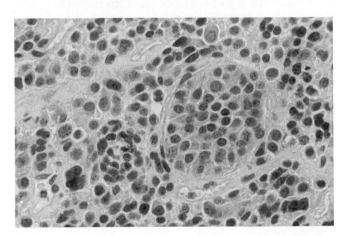

A

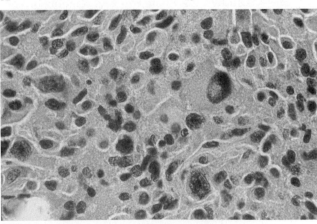

B

**Figure 15–3. A.** Histologic appearance of medullary carcinoma showing groups of plasmacytoid epithelial cells surrounded by fibrovascular septa. **B.** Medullary carcinoma showing loosely cohesive cells with focal atypia.

plasmacytoid with an eccentrically placed round to oval nucleus with stippled neuroendocrine-type chromatin. A moderate amount of finely granular eosinophilic cytoplasm is present, and up to 50% of cases may contain cytoplasmic mucin.[38] At least small amounts of amyloid are seen in the majority of cases as amorphous acellular globules and sheets of pink-staining stromal-associated material.[39] Especially in larger tumors, amyloid deposition may be extensive. Definitive identification of amyloid is based upon its reactivity using a Congo red stain and its characteristic apple-green birefringence when polarized (Figure 15–4). Other architectural patterns of medullary carcinoma include a follicular arrangement (mimicking a follicular thyroid neoplasm), a paraganglioma-like pattern, and a papillary pattern.[36] A number of cell types may be seen and include plasmacytoid, oncocytic (Hürthle cell-like), spindled, clear, pigmented, squamous, small cell, and giant cell (anaplastic) (Figure 15–5). In the head and neck, medullary carcinoma should be considered in the differential diagnosis of any oncocytic or spindled neoplasm in the thyroid or metastatic to cervical lymph nodes.

## Immunohistochemistry

Because medullary carcinomas may exhibit a variety of histologic patterns and cell types seen in other tumors, ancillary studies such as immunohistochemistry can be quite helpful in arriving at a definitive diagnosis. Among the more useful immunostains is calcitonin which is positive in the majority of medullary carcinomas (Figure 15–6).[40] Other immunohistochemical stains include carcinomembryonic antigen (CEA), chromogranin, and keratin.[36] Importantly, medullary carcinomas (except for the very rare mixed follicular and medullary carcinomas) are negative for thyroglobulin. In addition to immunhistochemistry, if material is obtained for electron microscopy, it will demonstrate the presence of 100–300 nm membrane-bound electron-dense cytoplasmic neurosecretory granules.[41]

## Fine Needle Aspiration (FNA)

In cytologic preparations, medullary carcinoma is characterized by a fairly uniform, predominantly dispersed population of neuroendocrine-type cells in a background of blood and scattered amorphous globules of amyloid (Figure 15–7).[41–43] The amyloid in alcohol-fixed cytology smears is indistinguishable from colloid. While some loose cell clusters, papillae, or even follicles may be present, the predominant cell pattern is one of single cells with occasional scattered enlarged atypical

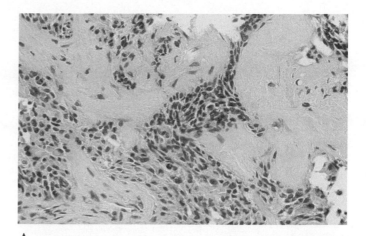

A

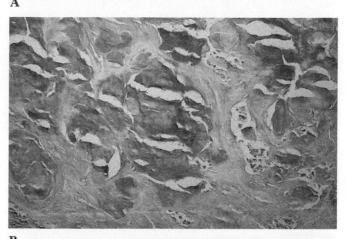

B

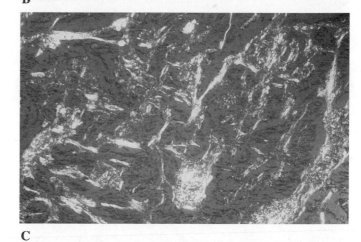

C

**Figure 15–4. A.** Medullary carcinoma with abundant stromal amyloid. **B.** The amyloid stains pale red using Congo red and **C.** exhibits apple-green birefringence when polarized.

cells and multinucleated cells. The nuclei in medullary carcinoma have a typical neuroendocrine "salt-and-pepper" chromatin texture with inconspicuous nucleoli and occasional intra-nuclear pseudoinclusions. A moderate to abundant amount of finely granular cytoplasm that may contain characteristic red cytoplasmic gran-

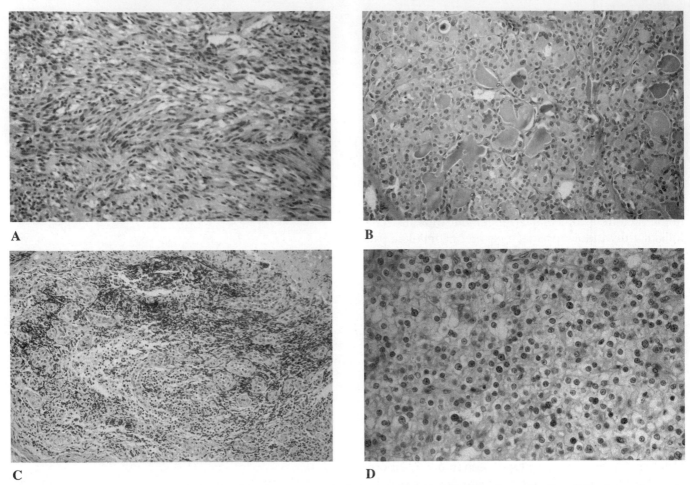

**Figure 15–5.** Histologic variants of medullary carcinoma include **A.** spindled, **B.** follicular, **C.** small cell, and **D.** clear cell.

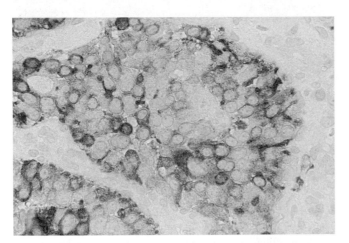

**Figure 15–6.** Positive immunocytochemical reactivity of medullary carcinoma for calcitonin. Immunoperoxidase method.

ules in air-dried preparations is present. As in histologic sections of this neoplasm, the cytologic features of medullary carcinoma are variable.[44] The cell types most often encountered in FNAs include plasmacytoid cells as well as spindled and oncocytic cells, the latter closely

mimicking a Hürthle cell neoplasm (Figure 15–7). The "salt-and-pepper" chromatin of medullary carcinoma helps to distinguish it from both papillary carcinoma with its pale "powdery" chromatin and from Hürthle cell neoplasms with their prominent nucleoli and hyperchromatic chromatin. In cases of medullary carcinoma with a predominant spindle cell pattern, anaplastic carcinoma may be considered in the differential diagnosis, but giant cells and marked nuclear atypia are usually absent.

## DIAGNOSTIC WORKUP

the initial evaluation in all patients suspected of having MTC should include a thorough personal and family history. Questions should be directed towards regional neck and thyroid symptoms, symptoms of hypercalcemia, pheochromocytoma, and hypercalcitoninemia (ie, diarrhea). All patients should have vocal cord mobility checked by mirror or fiberoptic laryngeal exam. As with all thyroid nodules, fine needle aspiration represents the central diagnostic tool. When initial cy-

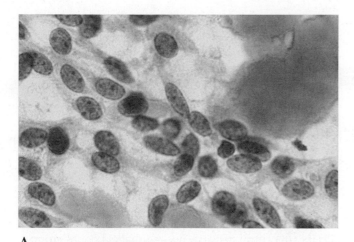

**A**

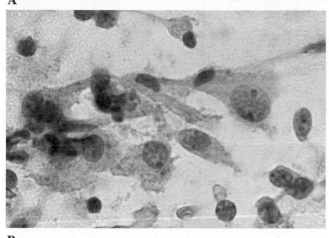

**B**

**Figure 15–7. A.** FNA of medullary carcinoma showing a dispersed population of neuroendocrine-type cells, many of which have a plasmacytoid appearance. Amorphous globules of amyloid are present in the background. **B.** FNA of a medullary carcinoma mimicking a Hürthle cell neoplasm. The neoplastic cells have abundant oncocytic cytoplasm.

topathologic diagnosis confirms malignancy, but cannot subtype that malignancy, thyroglobulin negative and calcitonin positive immunohistochemical staining makes the diagnosis of medullary carcinoma. In terms of regional radiographic evaluation, we prefer neck CT scanning and thyroid ultrasound. In terms of distant metastatic preoperative workup, we prefer chest CT scan (for lung metastasis), abdominal MRJ scan (for hepatic metastasis), and consideration for bone scanning.

All patients suspected of having MTC should have a basal calcitonin drawn. Keep in mind that only 60–70% of patients presenting will have elevation of basal calcitonin level.[9,45] If fine needle aspiration is suggestive of medullary provocative stimulation of calcitonin with pentagastrin, infusion can be performed. In general, the higher the calcitonin the greater the tumor burden and the lower the chance for cure.[46,47] CEA is a useful marker

to monitor disease status along with calcitonin postoperatively and should be drawn preoperatively.

All patients suspected of having MTC should have parathyroid function evaluated with calcium albumin, phosphate and intact PTH level. Similarly, a 24-hour urine for catecholamines, VMA and metanephrines must be obtained to rule out pheochromocytoma. If urine tests are positive, abdominal radiographic evaluation for pheochromocytoma should be aggressively pursued preoperatively.

Although sporadic and inherited forms of MTC seem to be discrete and perhaps easily distinguished entities, up to one-third of patients thought to have sporadic disease preoperatively are ultimately diagnosed with inherited forms. Thus, all patients need preoperative urine studies to rule out pheochromocytoma and total thyroidectomy. Family history may be unreliable. Inherited patients may represent new germline mutations or index cases of undiagnosed kindred. Patients with FMTC lack associated endocrinopathy. Associated endocrinopathy (ie, parathyroid or adrenal) typically presents after thyroid pathology in patients with MEN IIa.

RET oncogene testing is mandatory in all patients diagnosed with MTC and can be performed postoperatively as surgical approach would not be altered with this information. If a patient has an identified RET mutation, all family members should be tested for this mutation. This blood testing of family members represents an accurate, less costly, and less morbid form of screening than biochemical screening programs used in the past. Given the autosomal dominant inheritance and the age-related penetrance of inherited MTC, offspring of a patient within inherited MTC have a 35% chance of developing clinical disease in their lifetime.[15] Detection of provocatively elevated (through pentagastrin infusion) calcitonin elevation in gene carrier family members occurs in 95% of such gene carriers by the age of 35.[5,9] Such biochemical screening is unpleasant and may be associated with chest and abdominal pain, nausea, and flushing. This screening must be started by 1–3 years of age and continue every 6–12 months until the age of 35. Such biochemical testing is subject to both false positives and false negatives.[48,49] False positive estimates range between 1–10% of patients tested.[48–50] RET oncogene testing has not been associated with significant false positive or false negative results.[49,50] RET oncogene testing also allows surgical intervention at a stage before calcitonin provocative elevation is possible. If one waits until calcitonin elevation occurs, a greater percentage will have invasive disease, distant metastasis and postoperative calcitonin elevation. Wells and others have shown that surgery based on RET oncogene testing alone results in an increased percent of patients with C cell hyperplasia on pathology, a lower rate of frank MTC and a lower rate of metastasis.[51–53]

Although metastatic MTC has been documented in a patient as young as 6 years of age, some have suggested that there is little additional benefit to be realized by operating prior to provocative calcitonin elevation based on only RET oncogene informatiom.[5] It is interesting to note that between 1–5% of patients diagnosed with sporadic MTC, when undergoing RET oncogene analysis, postoperatively are found to have inherited disease.[17,54]

If a patient tests positive for RET oncogene mutation, but family members test negative for the same mutation (with testing confirmed twice) they can be reassured that no further evaluation or treatment is necessary. Those family members testing positive for the mutation can be appropriately evaluated and treated. In those patients with medullary thyroid carcinoma, testing negative for known RET oncogene mutations with negative parathyroid and adrenal workup, and surgical pathology that is interpreted as consistent with sporadic disease, sporadic MTC is the likely diagnosis. However, there is still a possibility that such a patient represents one of the 3–5% of patients with MEN IIa or 15% of patients with FMTC without known RET oncogene mutations. Eng has estimated that in such patients with current negative RET oncogene analysis there is still a 0.5% chance of MEN IIa and a 3% chance of FMTC. Family members of such a patient can be offered repetitive biochemical calcitonin screening.[31,54] All such genetic testing must be performed in the setting of fully informed patients and family, with an understanding for the potential for genetic discrimination as recommended by the Advisory Council for the U.S. Human Genome Research Project.[55] The advantage of early detection through RET oncogene analysis is understood when appreciating that the majority of patients with MEN who present with clinical (palpable thyroid) disease have elevated calcitonin levels posoperatively.[1,47,56]

## TREATMENT

The primary treatment modality for medullary carcinoma of the thyroid is surgery. The predilection towards multifocal thyroid disease, early regional nodal metastasis, coupled with the lack of T$_4$ suppressive or radioactive iodine therapeutic postoperative options emphasizes the need for adequate initial thyroid and nodal surgery. This is further appreciated when reviewing the high rate of postoperative regional cervical nodal recurrence and the postoperatively high rate of calcitonin elevations in patient with medullary carcinoma. Because of the high incidence of central neck nodal disease at presentation, central neck dissection is included in all patients undergoing total thyroidectomy for medullary carcinoma of the thyroid. Central neck nodes include prelaryngeal, pretracheal, paratracheal/tracheoesophageal groove/RLN chain and upper mediastinal nodes

extending to the innominate on the right and to an equivalent level beneath the clavicle on the left. Central neck dissection extends from the hyoid superiorly to the level of the innominate inferiorly and laterally to the bilateral internal jugular veins. Intraoperative frozen section of these nodes can be followed by lateral neck dissection if positive. Radical neck dissection has not been shown to improve prognosis and should be reserved for patients with gross jugular or sternocleidomastoid muscle involvement. An aggressive central neck dissection, including tracheoesophageal groove/RLN chain nodes and thymic resection places at risk the inferior parathyroids. Superior parathyroids generally can be preserved, as they are not commonly adjacent to significant central neck tracheoesophageal nodal groups. The aggressiveness of central neck dissection is controversial. The balance between aggressive nodal resection and inferior parathyroid preservation should favor nodal resection. After thorough resection in the tracheoesophageal groove/RLN chain and thymic regions, the resected specimen can be examined and the inferior parathyroid, if resected, can be identified, biopsied, and autotransplanted. In MEN IIa patients, all four parathyroid glands must be explored. Recurrence of hyperparathyroidism is rare if only enlarged glands are removed. Superior mediastinal dissection and thymic resection may be facilitated by sternothyroid muscle resection as has been suggested by Evans.[57] Sternotomy is not generally necessary unless significant mediastinal adenopathy is identified on preoperative radiographic studies.[58]

## The Importance of Addressing Lateral Neck Nodal Disease at Initial Surgery

Recent evidence suggests that it is of extreme importance to aggressively treat the lateral neck. Despite this, relatively recent recommendations have echoed past sentiment that lateral neck dissection should only be considered for patients with clinically palpable lateral neck nodal disease.[59,60] The inclusion of lateral neck lymphadenectomy in initial surgery for MTC, has been shown to improve biochemical cure rate by 20% with compartmental cervical lymphadenectomy being superior overall to selective lymphadenectomy.[61] Nodal groups in the lateral neck (not including central VI or mediastinal VII, which are very frequently involved) most frequently involved in order are: III, IV, II, V. Virtually all studies looking at modified radical neck dissection in patients with medullary carcinoma do not routinely dissect region I or extend into region V posterior to the XIth nerve.[62] Evans and co-authors, in reviewing eight studies, describe cervical lymph node recurrence rate in patients with medullary carcinoma as averaging 45%.[57] Recent work suggests that the treatment of recurrent gross nodal disease infrequently results in normalization of calcitonin level and is associated with a greater incidence of complications, especially permanent hyperparathyroidism.[58] Moley found in patients with palpable unilateral intra-thyroidal primaries (including both sporadic and familial cases) lymph node metastasis were found in 81% of central neck dissection specimens, 81% of ipsilateral lateral neck dissection specimens (ipsilateral regions II–V), and even in 44% of contralateral neck dissection specimens (contralateral neck regions II–V).[63] Contralateral nodal involvement occurred in up to 22% of patients, even when thyroid lesions were less than 1 cm. He found that intraoperative palpation was poor (sensitivity 64%, specificity 71%) in the detection of metastatic nodal involvement.[63] Another recent series also describes a rate of over 40% of positive nodal disease in the contralateral neck, with sporadic unilateral thyroid primaries.[58] We believe, therefore, that all patients with palpable thyroid primaries should have ipsilateral neck dissection and be considered for contralateral neck dissection. All patients presenting with palpable lymph node metastasis should undergo bilateral lateral neck dissection (Figure 15–8).

## Course and Prognosis

MTC metastasizes early on to regional nodes in the central and lateral neck and the superior mediastinum. Eventually distant hematogenous metastasis may occur to the liver, lung and bone.[9] Approximately one-third of MTC will clinically recur after initial surgery and approximately 50% of patients will have postoperative calcitonin elevations.[9,64] Metastatic disease can often be indolent and show little change over the course of several years, despite calcitonin elevation.[64]

For all types of MTC the five-year survival rate is between 78–92% and ten-year survival is between 61–75%.[9,33] The most important prognostic factor is disease stage at presentation (Table 15–5). Sporadic and MEN IIa, corrected for stage, have similar long-term prognoses. FMTC has the best prognosis of all subtypes of MTC. The most virulent form of MTC is MEN IIb. Stage and initial presentation is a significant prognostic factor. In turn, the method of diagnosis relates to stage at presentation. Patients diagnosed through family calcitonin or RET oncogene screening programs have earlier stage disease than patients presenting clinically. Block found that only 17% of patients diagnosed with palpable disease had normal calcitonin levels postoperatively.[1] vanHeerden found that patients with greater than three positive lymph nodes at initial surgery had an increased risk of recurrent disease.[64] Saad found that provocatively stimulated calcitonin levels were postoperatively elevated in 70% of patients with intra-thyroidal disease and 94% of patients with positive nodal disease or local invasion at first surgery.[9] Wells and colleagues have shown that when preoperative stimulated calcitonin levels are less than 1,000 pg/ml, only 4% of patients will have positive lymph nodes at surgery, none will have distant metastasis and only 4% will have persistent postoperative hypercalcitoninemia. When preoperative levels of calcitonin are greater than 10,000 pg/ml, regional and distant metastasis increases to 57% and 17%, respectively, and 61% have elevated calcitonin levels postoperatively.[56]

The incidence of regional nodal disease increases with age at presentation. Thus, age is a negative prognostic factor. Other factors that have been associated with poor outcome include male gender, nondiploid DNA tumor ploidy, and decreased calcitonin immunoreactivity.

## POSTOPERATIVE TREATMENT AND FOLLOW-UP

A variety of chemotherapeutic agents, including doxorubicin, dacarbazine, cyclophosphamide, bleomycin, cisplatin, fluorouracil and vincristine have shown re-

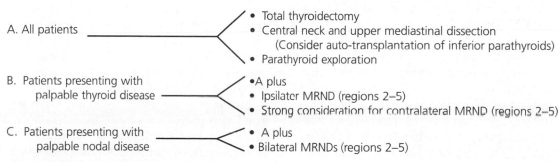

**Figure 15–8.** Surgical treatment of MTC.

**Table 15–5.** American Joint Committee on Cancer Staging for Papillary, Follicular, and Medullary Thyroid Carcinoma

| | **Papillary or Follicular:** Age <45 yrs | **Age 45 or Older** |
|---|---|---|
| Stage I | Any T, any N, M0 | Any T1, N0, M0 |
| Stage II | Any T, any N, M1 | T2 or 3, N0, M0 |
| Stage III | | T4, N0, M0, or any T, N1, M0 |
| Stage IV | | Any T, any N, M1 |
| | **Medullary:** | |
| Stage I | T1, N0, M0 | |
| Stage II | T2-4, N0, M0 | |
| Stage III | Any T, N1, M0 | |
| Stage IV | Any T, any N, M1 | |
| | **Undifferentiated:** | |
| Stage IV (all cases) | Any T, any N, any M | |

**Definition of TNM:**

| | | |
|---|---|---|
| Primary Tumor (T) | T0 = No evidence of primary tumor | |
| | T1 = Tumor I cm or less in greatest dimension limited to the thyroid | |
| | T2 = Tumor more than 1 cm but not more than 4 cm in greatest dimension limited to the thyroid | |
| | T3 = Tumor more than 4 cm in greatest dimension limited to the thyroid | |
| | T4 = Tumor of any size extending beyond the thyroid capsule | |
| Regional Lymph Nodes (N) | N0 = No regional lymph node metastasis | |
| | N1 = Regional lymph node metastasis<br>N1 a = Metastasis in ipsilateral cervical lymph node(s)<br>N1b = Metastasis in bilateral, midline, or contralateral cervical or mediastinal lymph node(s) | |
| Distant Metastasis (M) | M0 = No distant metastasis | |
| | M1 = Distant metastasis | |

Used with the permission of the American Joint Committee on Cancer (AJCC), Chicago Ill. The original source for this material is the *AJCC Cancer Staging Handbook,* 5th ed (1997), published by Lippincott-Raven Publishers, Philadelphia, Pa.

sponse rates of between 15–30%.[65,66] Radioiodinated meta-iodo-benzyl guanidine (MIBG) and somatostatin analogues have met with limited success.[67,68] Octreotide therapy can be considered for patients with metastatic disease or retractory diarrhea.[67] I[131] labeled anti-CEA antibodies have been investigated and show limited anti-tumor effect.[69]

External beam radiation therapy is generally recommended for palliation of bony metastasis.[70] Some investigators have suggested that postoperative radiation therapy may be helpful in terms of regional control.[71] Brierley has recently shown that in patients with microscopic residual disease, nodal involvement, or extraglandular invasion, postoperative external beam radiation therapy reduced locoregional recurrence rate from 48% to 14%.[72] Clearly, with extensive regional disease

after adequate surgery, external radiation beam therapy should be considered.

Calcitonin levels should be checked no sooner than two months postoperatively. Normal basal and stimulated calcitonin levels are excellent indications that the resection has been curative.[34] In inherited cases postoperatively, Zalcium, PTH and adrenal urine studies should be monitored intermittently. Calcitonin and CEA levels should be followed postoperatively to help identify those patients who are at risk for recurrence or the development of metastasis.[9,70] Should calcitonin levels become elevated, assuming the head and neck exam is negative for obvious disease, a regional and distant metastatic search is warranted. A regional search should include neck and mediastinal CT, MRI and sonography. Distant metastatic search should include chest CT scan, abdominal MRI scan, and bone scanning. A variety of scans have been used, including technetium-99Tc-DMSA (dimercaptosuccinic acid), thallium chloride, I[131]-MIBG, I[131] labeled CEA or anti-calcitonin antibodies, technetium sestamibi, and octreotide scans. All of these scans are generally poor in detecting small volume microscopic disease, especially in the liver.[57]

Hepatic metastasis may occur early in the course of MTC and may elude detection on MRI or CT scanning. Tung has reviewed the usefulness of laparoscopic detection of MTC hepatic metastasis.[73] This evaluation only identifies surface metastasis. Recent series suggest laparoscopic hepatic examination yield is low.[58] Selective venous catheterization is considered to be the most sensitive method for detecting hepatic metastasis.[74]

In a patient with elevated calcitonin with a negative head and neck examination and a metastatic search that is negative, indolent cervical disease has been presumed. In such a patient with elevated calcitonin and without obvious metastatic disease, the specific clinical course cannot be predicted.[75] Tisell, Buhr, and Moley have recommend an aggressive microsurgical neck dissection.[76–78] Controversy exists as to whether in patients with elevated calcitonin and no obvious distant metastasis, the extirpation of cervical nodal disease is a worthwhile goal. Some studies have shown that patients with indolent MTC may have regional nodal disease without distant metastasis.[76] Others suggest that regional nodal involvement is more likely a marker of systemic disease and that lymphadenectomy should not have an impact on survival.[79] In fact, increased survival has not been demonstrated through aggressive neck reoperation. vanHeerden noted good long-term survival in patients without evidence of regional or metastatic disease, despite elevated calcitonin levels with an 86% 15-year survival rate.[64] The most recent work by Moley and colleagues suggest that up to 38% of patients may have normal stimulated calcitonin levels after neck reoperative surgery. Most studies suggest that approximately one-third of patients may be cured by aggressive neck reoperation with the remaining two-thirds showing either no change or decreased, but still elevated, calcitonin levels postoperatively. Gimm and Drale found that 28% of patients undergoing reoperative neck surgery for MTC, subject to random lung biopsy, showed pulmonary micrometastasis.[80] Patients who had first surgery had disease extending beyond the thyroid capsule or lymph node capsule typically fail aggressive cervical reoperative attempts.[76,77] Fleming found that in patients undergoing reoperative neck surgery for elevated calcitonin levels a preoperative calcitonin of greater than 835 pg/ml, the presence of nodal metastasis, the presence of extranodal extension of tumor and time greater than two years from first surgery, all decrease the chance of a normal calcitonin after revision surgery.[58] In patients without obvious metastatic disease with postoperative elevated calcitonin who initially presented with intra-thyroidal disease, aggressive neck reoperation should be considered.

## References

1. Block MA. Clinical characteristics distinguishing hereditary from sporadic MTC. *Arch Surg.* 1980;115:142–148.
2. Hazard JB, Hwk WA, Crile G Jr. Medullary (solid) carcinoma of the thyroid: a clinicopathologic entity. *J Clin Endocrinol Metab.* 1959;19:152–161.
3. Steiner AL, Goodman AD, Powers SR. Study of kindred with pheochromocytomas, medullary carcinoma of the thyroid, hyperparathyroidism and Cushing's disease: MEN type II. *Medicine,* 1968;47:371–409.
4. Farndon JR, Leight GS, Dilley WG, et al. Familial medullary thyroid carcinoma without associated endocrinopathies: a distinct clinical entity. *Brit J Surg.* 1986;73:278–281
5. Gagel RF, Cote G. Decision making in MEN type II. In: Mazzaferri EL, Bar RS, Kriesberg RA (eds) *Advances in Endocrinology and Metabolism.* St. Louis: Mosby; 1994;1–23.
6. Eng C. The RET proto-oncogene in MEN II and Hirschsprung's disease. *New Engl J Med.* 1996;335:943–951.
7. Chong GC, Beahrs OH, Sizemore GW, Woolner L. Medullary carcinoma of the thyroid. *Cancer.* 1975;35:695–704.
8. O'Riordain D, O'Brien T, Crotty T, et al. Multiple endocrine neoplasia type IIb: more than an endocrine disorder. *Surgery* 1995; 118:936–942.
9. Saad MF, OrdonezNG, Rashid RK, et al. Medullary thyroid carcinoma: a study of the clinical features and prognostic factors in 161 patients. *Medicine.* 1984;63:319–342.
10. Dunn JM, Farndon JR. Medullary thyroid carcinoma. *Brit J Surg.* 1993;80:6–9.
11. Baylin SB, Hsu SH, Gann DS, Smallridge RC, Wells SA, Jr. Inherited MTC: a final monoclonal mutation in multiple clones of susceptible cells. *Science.* 1978; 199:429–431.
12. Knudson AG, Jr, Strong LC, Andeson DE. Heredity and cancer in man. *Medicine.* 1973;9:133–158.
13. Eng C, Mulligan L, Smith D, et al. Mutation of the RET proto-oncogene in sporadic medullary thyroid carcinoma. *Genes Chromo Cancer.* 1995;12:209–212.
14. Gagel RF, Cote G, Martins BM, et al. Clinical use of molecular information in the management of multiple endocrine neoplasia type IIa. *J Intern Med.* 1995;238:333–341.
15. Mulligan LM, Ponder BAJ. Genetic basis of endocrine disease in MEN type 11. *J Clin Endocrinol Metab.* 1995;80:1989–1995.
16. Santoro M, Carlomagno, F, Romano A, et al. Activation of RET as a dominant transforming gene by germline mutations of MEN IIa and MEN IIb. *Science.* 1995;267:381–383.
17. Komminoth P, Kunz E, Matias-guiu X, et al. Analysis of RET oncogene point mutations distinguishes heritable from non-heritable medullary thyroid carcinoma. *Cancer.* 1995;76:479–489.
18. vanHeyningen V. One gene: four syndromes. *Nature.* 1994;367: 319–320.
19. Marsh DJ, Andrew SD, Eng C. Germline and somatic mutations in an oncogene: RET mutations in inherited MTC. *Cancer Res.* 1996;56:124-1243.
20. Pasini B, Horstra R, Yin L. The physical map of the human RET proto-oncogene. *Oncogene.* 1995;11:1737–1743.
21. Mulligan LM, Kwok JBJ, Healey CS, et al. Germline mutations of the RET proto-oncogene in multiple endocrine neoplasia type II. *Nature.* 1993;363:458.
22. Donis-Keller H, Dou S, Chi D, et al. Mutations in the RET proto-oncogene in MEN IIa and FMTC. *Hum Mol Genet.* 1993;2:851–856.

23. Eng C, Smith DP, Mulligan LM, et al. Point mutation within the tyrosine kinase domain of the RET proto-oncogene in MEN type IIb, and related sporadic tumors. *Hum J Mol Genet.* 1994;3:237–241.

24. Lloyd RV. RET proto-oncogene mutation and rearrangements in endocrine disease. *Am J Pathol.* 1995;147:1539–1544.

25. Takahashi L. Oncogenic activity of the RET proto-oncogene in thyroid cancer. *Crit Rev Oncol.* 1995;61(1):35–46.

26. Landstratr RM, Jansen RP, Hofstra RM, et al. Mutation analysis of the RET proto-oncogene in Dutch families with MEN IIa, MEN IIb and FMTC. Two novel mutations and one de novo, mutation for MEN IIa. *Hum Genet.* 1996;97:11–14.

27. Frilling A, Dralle H, Eng C. Presymptomatic DNA screening in families with multiple endocrine neoplasia Type II and FMTC. *Surgery.* 1994; 1 18:1099–1104.

28. Decker RA, Peacock ML, Borst MJ, Sweet J, Thompson N. Progress in genetic screening on MEN type IIa: is calcitonin testing obsolete? *Surgery.* 1995; 118:257–264.

29. Eng C, Smith D, Mulligan LK, et al. A novel point mutation in the tyrosine kinase domain of the RET proto-oncogene in sporadic MTC and in a family with FMTC. *Oncogene.* 1995;10:509–513.

30. Zedenius J, Larsson C, Bergholm U, et al. Mutation of the codon 918—the RET proto-oncogene correlates to poor prognosis in sporadic MTC. *J Clin Endocrinol Metab.* 1995;80:3088–3090.

31. Eng C, Clayton D, Schuffenecker I, et al. The relationship between specific RET proto-oncogene mutations and the disease phenotype in MEN II: international RET mutation consortium analysis. *JAMA.* 1996;276:1575–1579.

32. Frank-Raue K, Hoppener W, Frilling A, et al. Mutations of the RET proto-oncogene in German multiple endocrine neoplasia families: relationship between genotype and phenotype. *J Clin Endocrinol Metab.* 1996;81:1780–1783.

33. Kkudo, K. Carney JR, Sizemore GW. Medullary carcinoma of the thyroid: biologic behavior of the sporadic and familial neoplasm. *Cancer.* 1985;55:2818–2821.

34. Cance WG, Wells SA. MEN type IIa. *Curr Prob Surg.* 1985;22:7–56.

35. Bergholm. U, Adami HO, Bergstrom R. Clinical characteristics in sporadic and familial medullary thyroid carcinoma. *Cancer.* 1989;63:1196–1204.

36. Rosai J, Carcangiu M, DeLellis R. *Atlas of Tumor Pathology: Tumors of the Thyroid Gland.* Washington, DC: Armed Forces Institute of Pathology; 1992.

37. Gallagher LA, Pilch BZ, Gaz RD, Randolph GW, Faquin MTC. Histologic and clinicopathologic features of 31 medullary microcarcinomas and their precursors. *Mod Pathol.* 2001;14:76A.

38. Zaatari GC, Saigo PE, Huvos AG. Mucin production in medullary carcinoma of the thyroid. *Arch Pathol Lab Med.* 1987;107:70–74.

39. Albores-Saavedra J, Livolsi VA, Williams Ed. Medullary carcinoma. *Semin Diagnos Pathol.* 1985;2:137–146.

40. Krisch K, Krisch I, Howat G, et al. The value of immunohistochemistry in medullary thyroid carcinoma. A systematic study of 30 cases. *Histopathology.* 1985;9:1077–1089.

41. Bose S, Kapila K, Verma K. Medullary carcinoma of the thyroid: a cytological, immunocytochemical and ultrastructural study. *Diagnos Cytopathol.* 1992;8:28–32.

42. Kini SR, Miller JM, Hamburger JI, Smith MJ. Cytopathologic features of medullary carcinoma of the thyroid. *Arch Pathol Lab Med.* 1984;108:156–59.

43. Faquin MTC. Cytopathology of the thyroid gland. In BZ Pilch, ed, *Head and Neck Surgical Pathology.* Philadelphia: Lippincott Williams & Wilkins; 2000.

44. Das A, Gupta SK, Banerjee AK, et al. Atypical cytologic features of medullary carcinoma of the thyroid. A review of 12 cases. *Acta Cytol.* 1992;36:137–141.

45. Samaan N, Hickey R. Medullary carcinoma of the thyroid: differentiating the types and current management. *Oncology.* 1987,1:21–28.

46. Olson JE, Hughes J, Alpern H. Family members of patients with sporadic medullary thyroid carcinoma must be screened for hereditary disease. *Surgery.* 1992;112:1074–1079.

47. Wells SA, Baylin SB, Leight GS, Dale JK, Dilley WG. The importance of early diagnosis in patients with hereditary medullary thyroid carcinoma. *Ann Surg.* 1982;195:595–599.

48. Marsh DJ, McDowall D, Valentine J, et al. The identification of false positive responses to the pentagastrin stimulation test in RET mutation negative members of MEN IIa families. *Clin Endocrin.* 1996;44:213–220.

49. Lips CJ, Landvater RM, Hoopener JW, et al. Clinical screening as compared with DNA analysis in families with MEN type IIa. *New Engl J Med.* 1994;331:828–835.

50. Pacini F, Romei C, Miccoli P, et al. Early treatment of hereditary medullary thyroid carcinoma after attribution on MEN type II gene carrier status by screening for RET gene mutation. *Surgery.* 1995;118:1031–1035.

51. Wells SA, Chi D, Toshima K, et al. Predictive DNA testing in prophylactic thyroidectomy in patients at risk for multiple endocrine neoplasia type 11. *Ann Surg.* 1994;220:237–250.

52. Lips CJ, Landsvater RM, Hoppener JW, et al. From medical history and biomedical tests to presymptomatic treatment in a large MEN IIa family. *J Intern Med.* 1995;238:347–356.

53. O'Riordain D, O'Brien T, Weaver A, Hay I. Medullary thyroid carcinoma in multiple endocrine neoplasia. Type IIa and IIb. *Surgery.* 1994; 116:1017–1023.

54. Eng C, Mulligan LM, Smith DP. Low frequency of germline mutation with RET proto oncogene in patients with apparently sporadic medullary thyroid carcinoma. *Clin Endocrin.* 1995;43:123–127.

55. National Advisory Council for Human Genome Research. Statement on the use of DNA testing for presymptomatic identification of cancer risk. *JAMA.* 1994;27:785.

56. Wells SA, Baylin SB, Gann DS, et al. Medullary thyroid carcinoma relationship of method of diagnosis to pathologic staging. *Ann Surg.* 1990;188:377–383.

57. Evans DB, Fleming JB, Lee JE, Cote G, Gagel RF. The surgical treatment of medullary thyroid carcinoma. *Semin Surg Oncol.* 1999; 16:50–63.

58. Fleming JB, Lee JE, Bouvent M, et al. Surgical strategy for the treatment of medullary thyroid carcinoma. *Ann Surg.* 1999;230:697–707.

59. Shaha AR. Thyroid cancer: extent of thyroidectomy. *Cancer Control.* 2000;7:240–245.

60. Shaha AR, Byer RM, Terz JJ. Thyroid cancer surgical practice guidelines. In: *Practice Guidelines for Major Cancer Sites.* Arlington Heights, IL; Society of Surgical Oncology; 1997.

61. Dralle H, Scheumann G, Proye C. The value of lymph node dissection in hereditary MTC: a retrospective European multicenter study. *J Intern Med* 1995;238:357–361.

62. Ellenhorn J, Shah J, Brennan M. Impact of therapeutic regional lymph node dissection for MTC. *Surgery.* 1993;114:1078–1082.

63. Moley JF, DeBenedetti MK. Patterns of nodal metastases in palpable medullary thyroid carcinoma. *Ann Surg.* 1999;6:880–888.

64. vanHeerden JA, Grant CS, Gharib H, Hay 1, Ilstrup DM. Long-term course of patients with persistent hypercalcitoninemia after apparent curative primary surgery for MTC. *Ann Surg.* 1990;212:395–400.

65. Gravier A, Rave F, Gagel RF. Changing concepts in the management of hereditary and sporadic medullary thyroid carcinoma. *Endocrinol Metab Clin North Am.* 1990;19:613–635.

66. Wu LT, Averbuch SD, Ball DW. Treatment of advanced MTC with combination of cyclophosphamide, vincristine and decarbonize. *Cancer.* 1994;73:432.

67. Modigliani E, Cohen R, Joannidis S, et al. Results of long-term continuous subcutaneous octreotide administration in 14 patients with MTC. *Clin Endocrinol.* 1992;36:183.

68. Hoefnagel CA, Delprat CC, Valdeo Olmoo. Role of I[131] MIBG therapy in MTC. *J Nucl Biol Med.* 1991;35:334–336.

69. Juweid M, Sharkey R, Behr T, Swayne LC, Rubin AD, Hanley D. Targeting an initial radioimmunotherapy of MTC with I[131] labeled monoclonal antibodies to carcinoembryonic antigen. *Cancer Res* (suppl). 1995;55:5945–5951.

70. Brunt LM, Wells SA. Advances in the diagnosis and treatment of medullary thyroid carcinoma. *Surg Clin North Am*. 1987;67:263–279.

71. Rougier P, Parmentier A, Planche A, Lafevre M, Travogli JP. MTC: prognostic factors in treatment. *Int J Radiat Oncol Biol Phys*. 1983;9(2):161–169.

72. Brierley J, Tsang R, Simpson WJ, et al. Medullary thyroid cancer: analysis of survival and prognostic factors and the role of radiation therapy in local control. *Thyroid*. 1996;6:305–310.

73. Tung W, Vessely T, Moley J. Laparoscopic detection of hepatic metastasis in patients with residual recurrent medullary thyroid carcinoma. *Surgery*. 1995;118:1024–1030.

74. Gautvik KM, Talle K, Hager B. Early liver metastasis in patients with medullary carcinoma of the thyroid gland. *Cancer*. 1989; 63:174–180.

75. Tisell LE, Dilley WG, Wells SA. Progression of postoperative residual MTC as monitored by plasma calcitonin levels. *Surgery*. 1996;199:34–39.

76. Tisell HE, Hansson G, Jansson S. Reoperation in the treatment of the asymptomatic metastasizing medullary thyroid carcinoma. *J Surg*. 1986;99:60–69

77. Buhr H, Kallinowski R, Rave F, Herfaith C. Microsurgical neck dissection of occultly metastasizing medullary thyroid carcinoma. *Cancer*. 1993;72:3685–3693.

78. Moley JF, Wells SA, Dilley WG. Reoperation for recurrent or persistent MTC. *Surgery*. 1993;114:1090–1096.

79. Cady B. In discussion of: Gimm O, Dralle H: Reoperation in metastatic medullary thyroid carcinoma: is a tumor stage oriented approach justified? *Surgery*. 1997;122:1130–1131.

80. Gimm O, Dralle H. Reopeartion in metastasizing medullary thyroid carcinoma: is a tumor stage oriented approach justified? *Surgery*. 1997;122:1124–1131.

# 16

# Anaplastic Thyroid Carcinoma

## Diane Hershock, M.D., Ph.D. and Randal Weber, M.D.

## INTRODUCTION

Anaplastic thyroid cancers comprise 5–14% of primary malignant thyroid neoplasms and are lethal.[1,2] Patients usually present with rapidly progressive local disease or distant metastasis with an abysmal overall five-year survival of 3.6% and a median survival of four months.[3–5] Reports of combined modality treatment may increase survival only to one year.[6] This type of thyroid cancer is noted for its rapid growth either from a pre-existing thyroid cancer or on initial presentation. This tumor type generally affects older women with a peak incidence in the seventh decade of life.[2]

Twenty percent of patients have had a prior history of a well-differentiated carcinoma of the thyroid. In goiter endemic regions of the world, anaplastic cancers are twice as common in those with prior histories of long-standing goiter.[7] Some investigators have also suggested that prior radiation exposure or use of iodine 131 may lead to transformation of differentiated to anaplastic thyroid cancer, but this has not been substantiated by the literature.[8–9] In a study at the Mayo Clinic, 11% of 71 patients evaluated had received therapeutic radiation in the region of the thyroid.[4] Radiation doses were, however, poorly defined in some cases, with some patients having had low doses for benign conditions and others having had high doses for the therapy of another malignant neoplasm in the neck region. No definite conclusions were made as to the etiologic role of irradiation in these patients. As has been documented with papillary thyroid carcinoma, a remarkably high incidence of a previous malignant lesion was noted, the two most common being breast and skin.[10]

The first report of the coexistence of two histologic types of thyroid cancer was reported in 1957.[11] It was suggested that prolonged stimulation of papillary or follicular carcinoma by thyroid-stimulating hormone (TSH) could transform low-grade tumors into highly malignant anaplastic carcinoma. The incidence of coexistence of tumors varies in the literature from 10–89%.[1] In a Mayo Clinic study, 5% of patients had co-existent papillary cancers with 17% having a dual follicular cancer as well.[4] Follicular carcinoma, as opposed to papillary carcinoma, has demonstrated a greater asssociation with anaplastic transformation.

## CLINICAL PRESENTATION

In general, anaplastic thyroid cancers present as a rapidly growing, painful, low anterior neck mass which is often firm and fixed to underlying structures. It is not uncommon to have areas of tumor necrosis, producing fluctuant areas within the mass. Enlargement of metastatic lymph nodes in the cervical region may occur early. The growth rate of thyroid masses was evaluated at Mayo Clinic several years ago in 71 patients, 56 of whom had rapid growth.[4] The duration of the mass varied as well; 32 patients reported a mass within 12 weeks, 17 had been aware of the mass for more than 2 years, and 5 did not know they had a nodule until examined by a physician.

The second most common finding was dyspnea which was frequently associated with either hoarseness (35 patients) or irritable cough (25 patients).[4] Pain from the neck mass or in the neck itself was also noted. Dysphagia and weight loss are common findings as well. None of the patients in the Mayo study were suspected of having hyper- or hypothyroidism. Other presenting symptoms may include those suggestive of metastatic pulmonary disease, superior vena cava syndrome, signs of asphyxiation, or exsanguination caused by massive erosion.

Physical findings are commonly documented as multiple nodules, bilateral neck involvement, tumor size of greater than 5 cm, fixed lesions, enlarged lymph nodes or vocal cord paralysis.[4] Other physical findings may include symptoms of recurrent laryngeal nerve paralysis and Horner's syndrome.

## PATHOLOGY

The pathology of this tumor can be quite varied with an extensive variety of histologic patterns. Three distinct histologic types have been designated as spindle cell, giant cell or squamoid.[12] In general, there appears to be no difference in biologic behavior, although recognition of these growth patterns may have some diagnostic importance. What is characteristic microscopically for all anaplastic thyroid cancers is a high mitotic index, marked cellular pleomorphism, extensive necrosis, tumor emboli and vascular invasion.[13] As mentioned, coexistence of a well-differentiated carcinoma can exist.[1,12,13] In addition, anaplastic cells do not produce thyroglobulin nor are they able to transport iodine. They do not have thyrotropin receptors on their cell surfaces. There is a consensus among pathologists that in almost all cases of anaplastic thyroid cancer, coexistent papillary, follicular or Hürthle cell malignancy may be identified.

With the advent of electron microscopy and immunohistochemical staining, it is possible to distinguish anaplastic spindle cell thyroid carcinomas from sarcomas, melanomas and lymphomas.[12] Leukocyte common antigen is negative and is helpful for differentiating anaplastic thyroid carcinoma from lymphomas. The identification of epithelial cell features such as desmosomes and tight junctions can distinguish sarcomas from anaplastic features.

## PROGNOSTIC FEATURES

Tumor staging is based upon the extent of disease. Stage I tumors are confined to the region of the gland; stage II tumors palpable regional lymphadenopathy; stage III extensively invade the soft tissues of the neck; and stage IV is the presence of distant metastases. Survival is adversely influenced by increasing extent of disease. Patients with regional or distant metastatic disease do not survive longer than three years. Those patients with tumors less than 5 cm which are unilateral with no invasion of adjacent tissue and absence of nodal involvement have the best survival advantage.[4]

Only 3% of patients with lesions greater than 6 cm are alive at five years. Patients with small cell histology have the best survival advantage while patients having both spindle and giant cell pattern experience the worst survival. Patients with rapid growth in a preexisting goiter also have a poorer prognosis.[4]

## THERAPEUTIC MODALITIES

With five year survival rates of about 3%, treatment for anaplastic thyroid cancer is usually considered palliative at best. Generally, anaplastic thyroid carcinoma is resistant to most forms of therapy and is considered one of the most aggressive and lethal human cancers. Generally, symptom management is the rule in this disease. If patients present with symptoms of airway compromise, emergent tracheotomy may be required. The majority of patients die within a few months usually from invasion of tumor into the aerodigestive tract or complications from pulmonary metastases.

Surgery, radiotherapy or chemotherapy as single modality treatment is not adequate to control disease; however, a combination of these modalities may improve local control. Each treatment entity will be subsequently discussed below, both as single modality therapy and in combination.

### Role of Surgery

Surgical management of anaplastic thyroid cancer centers around airway management and resection of the primary tumor with or without regional lymph node dissection. Patients with rapid tumor growth are at risk for airway obstruction by one of three mechanisms: external compression of the trachea, intraluminal tumor extension or bilateral vocal cord paralysis. With anaplastic thyroid cancer, the most common cause for airway impairment and indication for tracheotomy is external tracheal compression. Airway management may be elective or emergent depending upon the patient's presentation. Patients with either stridor or rapid tumor growth should be considered for tracheotomy since further airway degradation can be expected. Preoperative CT scanning should be obtained to determine the extent of airway compromise and the presence of intraluminal tumor.

For tracheotomy, the patient is taken to the operating room for secure airway management. Preoperative sedation should be avoided. A rigid bronchoscope should be available in all instances should the airway be lost acutely. The patient is intubated under direct vision or fiberoptically. In the absence of intraluminal tumor this may be safely accomplished. Once the airway is secured, the tracheotomy is performed under more controlled conditions. A generous low collar incision is made and the neck flap is elevated to the level of the thyroid notch. Because the laryngotracheal complex is frequently deviated and the trachea may be deep to massive tumor bulk, the thyroid notch serves as a useful landmark for identifying the airway. The tumor is debulked from superior to inferior directly over the airway until the cricoid cartilage is identified. The first and second tracheal rings are subsequently exposed and the airway entered. Sufficient tumor debulking will usually permit placement of a standard or extended length tracheotomy tube. In rare instances an endotracheal tube may be necessary until a custom-made tracheotomy tube is available. The wound is closed laterally with the central portion remaining open to provide wound drainage.

The second potential indication for surgery is management of the primary thyroid tumor and regional metastases. Unfortunately, patients often present at a very advanced stage making surgical resection not feasible. Radical surgery, even when combined with postoperative radiotherapy, does not provide long term disease control because of the high risk for distant metastasis and local recurrence. When diagnosed early, surgical extirpation of limited disease is possible and should be combined with postoperative radiotherapy. The incidence of regional metastasis is high and neck dissection should be performed for clinically evident cervical metastasis. Prior to surgery, a complete metastatic work-up should include a CT of the chest and abdomen. Contraindications to surgical resection are carotid encasement, fixation to the prevertebral fascia and distant metastasis. Surgical resection of the larynx, hypopharynx and cervical esophagus for advanced disease are of minimal therapeutic benefit because of a very high incidence of distant metastasis. More recently surgery has been combined with chemotherapy and external beam radiation for patients who obtain a significant response to cytoreductive therapy.

Surgical resection in anaplastic thyroid cancer has been recommended for those patients with small foci of disease or those detected at an earlier stage.[6,14-17] The number of these cases is usually small however. In several case reports, complete resection or extended operations have been reported to have good outcomes.[15-16] In 21 cases of anaplastic carcinoma, it was reported that patients treated with complete resection for tumors with extrathyroidal extension and mean tumor sizes greater than 5 cm had a median survival of 131 months.[17] In those patients who underwent incomplete resections, the median survival was 4.2 months with 0% alive at two years.

A recent publication reviewed the survival rates of a total of 46 patients treated with or without surgical intervention with the intended question being: is there any benefit in performing surgery for the purpose of influencing survival?[18] Patients in this study had either locally advanced disease or distant metastasis at presentation. Fifteen of 20 patients with locally advanced disease underwent surgery; 13 in the distant metastasis group also received surgical therapy. For the locally advanced group, the mean survival was 12.8 months versus 8.6 months in the non-surgical arm (p= 0.46). Those with distant metastasis after surgery had a mean survival of 3.5 months versus 2.8 months in the non-surgical arm (p=0.72). These data suggested no surgical advantage in terms of overall survival. Thus, surgery as a single modality in these patients does not appear to be a viable treatment option.

## Radiation Therapy

Conventional radical radiotherapy is generally administered in 5–6 week courses with a partial or complete response noted in less than 45% of patients with anaplastic carcinoma of the thyroid. Since almost 75% of these patients die from local progression with airway and/or esophageal obstruction, treatment with radiation often fails to control disease locally.[3,19-21] In addition to demonstrating little impact on overall survival, most patients undergoing treatment with radiation spend a significant portion of their remaining survival coping with the long-term morbidity of radiotherapy.

Retrospective data analyzing fifty-one patients treated from 1970–1986 treated with external beam radiation was published focusing on overall survival, local control and patterns of metastasis.[21] External beam radiation was given to all 51 patients. Fifty-seven percent of these patients were irradiated to a dose of more than 30 Gy; 9 patients received less than 15 Gy because of early death. A median dose of 35 Gy (range 1–60 Gy) was delivered to a target volume encompassing the primary tumor and both sides of the neck, as well as the superior mediastinum. The interval between diagnosis and the start of radiation was 31–175 days. Overall survival of these patients was poor; 94% were dead in the first year. Cause of death was residual tumor or local relapse with or without distant metastasis in 32 patients. Pulmonary metastasis and/or other metastases without local tumor was found in 10 others. Patients with metastatic disease but who were locally free of tumor experienced a median survival of 7.5 months. Those with local-regional residual disease after therapy had a 100% mortality at eight months and a median survival of 1.6 months.

As an attempt to improve local control, several investigators have tried other means, such as hyperfractionated radiotherapy or chemotherapy or both.[6,14,22-25]

Moderate responses were observed with hyperfractionated therapy but with greater toxicity, especially if combined with chemotherapy. Based on the oncophysiologic theory that anaplastic carcinoma, particularily high-grade, has a short doubling time, it is postulated that accelerated radiotherapy may be of benefit.[26] An intial pilot study was encouraging, leading to a Phase II evaluation.[27–28] Seventeen patients received twice daily radiation (1.8 Gy in a.m. and 2.0 Gy in p.m.) in 16 fractions over 10–12 days for two cycles to a total of 30.4 Gy each cycle. Endpoints were outcome and treatment toxicity. Three patients had a complete response and seven patients achieved a partial response with five having stable disease. Two died prior to completion of therapy. Most deaths were caused by metastatic disease. The major problem was acute toxicities, particularly grade III/IV esophagitis which developed 2–3 weeks into treatment and persisted for several weeks after the completion of therapy. Thus, it was concluded from this study that a high response rate was achieved with local symptom control at the expense of great toxicity. Other treatment approaches appeared necessary, such as 3-D conformal planning, the introduction of gaps in treatment, dose reduction or the addition of chemotherapy.

## Chemotherapy

In the 1970s–1980s, chemotherapy as single modality treatment was given to patients with advanced thyroid cancers.[29–30] Several active agents were identified; more recently combined multiple agent chemotherapy for patients with thyroid cancer in general has been documented.[31–33] It has been difficult to do a randomized trial based on the rarity of anaplastic thyroid carcinoma. In 1985, the Eastern Cooperative Oncology Group (ECOG) initiated a group wide study comparing the therapeutic indications and toxicities of combination doxorubicin (ADR) and cisplatin (CDDP) with doxorubicin alone in both medullary and anaplastic thyroid cancer.[23]

Ninety-two patients were entered in the study; 84 were evaluable.[23] Selected patients had histologically diagnosed thyroid cancer, 39 of whom had anaplastic, 35 with differentiated and 10 with medullary thyroid cancers. There were two treatment arms: single agent ADR 60 mg/m$^2$ every three weeks versus CDDP 40 mg/m$^2$ with ADR 60 mg/m$^2$ every three weeks. Patients received at least three cycles. Forty-one patients received single agent ADR with seven patients having a partial response (PR). Forty-three patients received combined therapy, 5 with a complete response (CR) and 6 with a PR. Four of 5 who had a CR lived more than 2 years. Of those having anaplastic thyroid cancer, 0 had a CR and 5% had a PR in the ADR arm

versus 17% CR and 17% PR in the ADR/CDDP arm. Increased hematologic and gastrointestinal toxicities were noted with the combination, but this was not statistically significant. Thus, with both CDDP and ADR there was a combined 35% response rate as compared to 5% with ADR alone in anaplastic thyroid cancer. However, most patients with anaplastic thyroid cancer were not alive at 6.7 months.

## Concurrent Strategies—Chemoradiation

The rationale for combining radiotherapy and chemotherapy is based on the fact that since the toxicities of these modalities are not entirely overlapping, enhanced tumoricidal effect might be accomplished.[34] The first promising results of combined radiotherapy and chemotherapy were published in 1973.[35] In 1974, another study suggested that the combination of dactinomycin and radiotherapy given in 6 patients had a 50% overall survival benefit at two years, with no survivors at four years.[1,36]

From 1971–1985 consecutive groups of patients were treated at Radiumhemmet in Sweden utilizing various combinations of radiotherapy, chemotherapy and surgery.[17] Eight patients were initially treated with a combination of methotrexate (MTX) and radiation. The dose of MTX was 5 mg IV/PO daily with 30–40 Gy (one fraction/day) radiation for 3–4 weeks. Of the eight patients, tumor reduction by more than 50% was noted in 7. Remission was temporary in 5 patients. The mean survival time was 9 months (6/8 patients died between 6–12 months after diagnosis). All patients, however, experienced grade III/IV hematologic or gastrointestinal toxicities. Despite the degree of toxicity, this study served as an encouraging basis for utilizing combined modality therapy as a means to improve response and local control.

A second trial evolved from the above, this involving 9 patients treated with a 3 drug regimen given concurrently with radiation. This included Bleomycin 5 mg/d; cyclophosphamide 200 mg/d; and 5-fluorouracil, 500 mg every second day (BCF). Radiotherapy included 30–40 Gy over 3–4 weeks, one fraction per day, with large portals including the cervical nodes and upper mediastinum. Treatment related toxicity was experienced by all patients but was less severe than the above noted study. An objective response was had by 7/9 patients; however, the response was short-lived with a median survival of 3 months. Since BCF provided a transient remission, surgery was planned during remission. Long-term survivorship (12 years) was documented in the only patient who then underwent surgery subsequent to completion of combined chemoradiotherapy.

Based on this study, surgery was then considered for all patients. A third Radiumhemmet study thus evolved where 20 patients received pre- (30 Gy) and postoperative (16 Gy) radiation. Radiation was given in two fractions per day, with BCF administered concurrently. All patients subsequently underwent surgery. The results of this study demonstrated 15/20 patients showing objective responses with grade III/IV toxicity, mostly gastrointestinal, noted in 9. Of the initial 25 patients, 2 were alive and disease free 3.5 and 11 years after treatment. Thus, this appeared to be encouraging but limiting in terms of toxicities and number of patients.

As suggested by the ECOG doxorubicin versus doxorubicin/cisplatin study, doxorubicin was found to be the most effective single cytostatic agent against thyroid cancers in general.[37-39] The combination of ADR and radiation in mammalian tumor cells is synergistic when a low dose of this cytostatic agent (less than 0.15mg/kg) is used.[40] The mechanism is postulated to be as a radiosensitizer. Low dose adriamycin plus hyperfractionated radiation intially gave a 30–45% response rate with few remissions.[41] Hyperfractionated radiotherapy can reduce the early reaction in normal tissues.[42-43] Since anaplastic cancers are rapidly dividing, it was postulated that it might be important to decrease treatment time by accelerating the fractionation of the radiation time, reducing the chance for tumor cells to repopulate during treatment. Additionally, debulking surgery can remove any residual necrotic tumor mass which may improve the efficacy of other treatment modalities.[44-45]

Two studies served as the basis of a combined modality treatment involving surgery, radiation and chemotherapy. Radiotherapy (3000 rads given in 2.5 weeks in two fractions per day, 5 days per week) and weekly adriamycin, 20 mg IV, demonstrated less toxicity but essentially no response.[46] Another study at Radiumhemmet where low dose weekly adriamycin (ADR), superfractionated radiation (30 plus 16 Gy) resulted in a median survival of 5 months in two patients.[41] This study led to 33 patients treated at Radiumhemmet with 20 mg IV ADR weekly, radiotherapy of 30 Gy/30 fractions or 30 Gy/23 fractions for 3 weeks preoperatively and 16 Gy in either 16 or 12 fractions 1.5 weeks after surgery administered daily.[41] Debulking surgery was done after preoperative chemoradiation was completed. Maintenance ADR was then given weekly at 20 mg IV to a maximum dose of 750 mg/m². Median survival in these cohorts was 3.5 versus 4.5 months, respectively. Forty-eight percent of all patients had no evidence of local recurrence, however er 24% died because of local failure. Toxicity was mainly non-hematologic, including skin reactions and mucositis. The conclusion offered from this study was improved local control with minimal toxicity. However, there was no improvement in overall survival.

## CONCLUSIONS

Surgery, radiotherapy or chemotherapy as single modality therapy does not appear adequate to control anaplastic thyroid disease. Accelerated radiotherapy alone has an impressive response rate but considerable long-term toxicity. Combined chemotherapy (ADR/CDDP) has a poor response rate with associated toxicity. There is modest improvement with combined modality treatment including radiation/chemotherapy/and debulking surgery with evidence of local control as well as a minimal survival benefit. The combination of adriamycin and radiation appears synergistic. Thus, the currently accepted standard of care includes the combination of adriamycin with or without cisplatin and hyperfractionated radiation.[47] In Europe and some areas in the United States, the combination of adriamycin and concurrent radiation is followed by debulking surgery.[41] Despite these efforts, the majority of patients die within a few months from tumor invasion into the aerodigestive system or from complications of pulmonary metastasis. However, the advent of new agents such as anti-angiogenesis inhibitors and other biological substances used as single agents or in combination with radiation may improve local control and overall survival.

## References

1. Aldinger KA, Samaan NA, Ibanez ML, et al. Anaplastic carcinoma of the thyroid: a review of 84 cases of spindle and giant cell carcinoma of the thyroid. *Cancer*. 1978;41:2267–2275.
2. Venkatesh YS, Ordonez NG, Schultz PN, et al. Anaplastic carcinoma of the thyroid. *Cancer*. 1990;66:321–330.
3. Harmer CL. Multidisciplinary management of thyroid neoplasms. In: Preece PE, Rosin RD, Mann AGD, eds. *Head and Neck Oncology for the General Surgeon*. London: W.B. Saunders; 1991:55–90.
4. Nel CJC, van Heerden JA, Goellner JR, et al. Anaplastic carcinom of the thyroid: a clinicopathologic study of 82 cases. *Mayo Clinic Review*. 1985;60:51–58.
5. Schoumacher P, Metz R, Bey P, Chesneau AM. Anaplastic carcinoma of the thyroid gland. *Br. J. Cancer*. 1977;13:383–383.
6. Kim J, Leeper R. Treatment of locally advanced thyroid carcinoma with combination of doxorubicin and radiation therapy. *Cancer*. 1987;60(10) 2372-5.
7. Hofstadter F. Frequency and morphology of malignant tumors of the thyroid before and after the introduction of iodine prophylaxis. *Virchows Arch*. 1980;385:263–274.
8. Kapp D, Livolsi V, Sanders M. Anaplastic carcinoma. well differentiated thyroid cancer. *Yale J. Biol. Med*. 1982;55:521.
9. Maheshwari Y, Hill C, Haynie T, et al. I-131 therapy of differentiated cacinoma. *Cancer*. 1981;47:664–71.

10. McConahey WM, Hay ID, Woolner LB, van Heerder JA, Taylor WF. Papillary thyroid cancer treated at the Mayo Clinic, 1946 through 1970: initial manifestations, pathologic findings, theory + outcome. *Mayo Clin Proc.* 1986;61(12):978–96.

11. Crile G Jr. The endocrine dependency of certain thyroid cancers and the danger that hypothyroidism may stimulate their growth. *Cancer.* 1957;10:119–1137.

12. Samaan NA, Ordonez NG. Uncommon types of thyroid cancer. *Endocrinol Metab Clin North Am.* 1990;19:637–648.

13. Carcangiu ML, Steeper T, Zampi G, et al. Anaplastic thyroid carcinoma: a study of 70 cases. *Am. J. Clin. Pathol.* 1985;83:135–158.

14. Werner B, Abele J, Alveryd A, et al. Multimodal therapy in anaplastic giant cell thyroid carcinoma. *World J Surg.* 1984;8:64–70.

15. Kobayashi T, Asakawa H, Umeshita K, et al. Treatment of 37 patients with anaplastic carcinoma of the thyroid. *Head Neck.* 1996;18:36–41.

16. Tan RK, Finley RK III, Driscoll D, et al. Anaplastic carcinoma of the thyroid: a 24 year experience. *Head Neck.* 1995;17:41–48.

17. Tallroth E, Wallin G, Lundell G, et al. Multimodality treatment in anaplastic thyroid carcinoma. *Cancer.* 1987;60:1428–1431.

18. Lu WT, Lin JD, Huang HS, Chao TC. Does surgery improve the survival of patients with advanced anaplastic thyroid carcinoma? *Otoloaryngol Head Neck Surg.* 1998;118:728–731.

19. Jebeb B, Sternsward J, Lowhagen T. Anaplastic giant-cell carcinoma of the thyroid. a study of treatment and prognosis. *Cancer.* 1975;35:1293–1295.

20. Junor EJ, Paul J, Reed NS. Dyspnoea: a major prognostic indicator in anaplastic thyroid carcinoma. *Clin. Oncol.* 1991;3:299.

21. Levendag, PC, DePorre PMZR, van Putten WLJ. Anaplastic carcinoma of the thyroid gland treated by radiation therapy. *Int. J. Rad. Oncol. Biol. Phys.* 1993;26:125–128.

22. Schlumberger M, Parmentier C, Delisle MJ, Coette JE, Sarrazin D. Combination therapy for anaplastic giant cell thyroid carcinoma. *Cancer.* 1991;67:564–566.

23. Shimaoka K, Schoenfeld DA, DeWys WD, Creech RH, DeConti R. A randomized trial of doxorubicin versus doxorubicin plus cisplatin in patients with advanced thyroid carcinoma. *Cancer.* 1985;56:2155–2160.

24. Simpson JW. Anaplastic thyroid carcinoma: a new approach. *Canc. Surg.* 1980;23:25–27.

25. Tallroth E, Wallin G, Lundell G, Lowhagen T, Einhorn J. Multimodality treatment in anaplastic giant cell thyroid carcinoma. *Cancer.* 1987;60:1428–1431.

26. Thames HD, Peters LJ, Withers HR, Fletcher GH. Accelerated radiofractionation: rationales for several treatments per day. *Int. J. Rad. Oncol. Biol. Phys.* 1981;9:127–138.

27. Huddart RA, Hoskin P, Rhys-Evans P, Harmer CL. High grade thyroid cancer treated by accelerated radiotherapy. *Clin. Oncol.* 1993;5:329.

28. Mitchel G, Huddart R, Harmer C. Phase II evaluation of high dose accelerated radiotherapy for anaplastic thyroid carcinoma. *Radiotherapy Oncol.* 1999;50:33–38.

29. Shimaoka K, Reyes J. Chemotherapy of thyroid carcinoma. In: Robbins J, Braverman LE, eds. *Thyroid Research 1975.* Oxford: Elsevier Publishing Co; 1976:586–589

30. Leeper RD, Shimaoka K. Treatment of metastatic thyroid cancer. In: Abe K, ed. *Endocrinology and Cancer: clinics in Endocrinology and Metablism, vol 9.* Philadelphia: W.B. Saunders; 1980:383–404.

31. Alexieva-Figusch J, VanGilse HA, Treurniet RE. Chemotherapy in carcinoma of the thyroid: retrospective and prospective. *Ann. Radiol.* 1977;20:810–813.

32. Benker G, Hackenberg K, Hoff HG, et al. Zytostatische kombinationshehandlung metastasierender schilddrusen karzinome mit doxorubicin und bleomycin. *Dtsch Med Wochenschr.* 1977;102:1908–1913.

33. Sokal MM, Harmer CL. Chemotherapy for anaplastic carcinoma of the thyroid. *Clin. Oncol.* 1978;4:3–10.

34. Wendt TG, Chucholowski M, Hartensein R, Rohloff R, Willich N. Sequential chemo-radiotherapy in locally advanced squamous cell carcinoma of the head and neck. *Int. J. Radiat. Oncol. Biol. Phys.* 1985;12:397–399.

35. Wallgren A, Norin T. Combined chemotherapy and radiation therapy in spindle and giant cell carcinoma of the thyroid gland: report of a case. *Acta Radiol. Ther. Phys. Biol.* 1973;12:17–20.

36. Rogers JD, Lindberg RD, Hill CS Jr, Gehan EG. Spindle and giant cell carcinoma of the thyroid: a different therapeutic approach. *Cancer.* 1974;34:1328–1332.

37. Poster DS, Bruno S, Penta K, Catane R. Current status of chemotherapy in the treatment of advanced carcinoma of the thyroid gland. *Cancer Clin. Trials.* 1981;4:301–307.

38. Benker G, Reinwein R, Windeck HG, Seber S. Experiences with chemotherapy in 52 patients with thyroid tumors. *Acta Endocrinol.* 1983;102:77.

39. Tallroth EE, Lundell G, Tennvall J, Wallin G. Chemotherapy and multimodality treatment in thyroid carcinoma. *Otolaryngologic Clin. North Am.* 1990;233:523–527.

40. Byfield JE, Lynch M, Kulhanian F, Chan PYM. Cellular effects of combined adriamycin and X-irradiation in human tumor cells. *Int J Cancer.* 1977;19:194–204.

41. Tennvall J, Lundell G, Hallquist A, Wahlberg P, Wallin G, Tibblin S and the Swedish Anaplastic Thyroid Cancer Group. Combined doxorubicin, hyperfractionated radiotherapy, and surgery in anaplastic thyroid carcinoma. *Cancer.* 1994;74:1348–1354.

42. Thames HD, Peters LJ, Rodney WH, Fletcher GH. Accelerated fractionation vs hyperfractionation: rationales for several treatments per day. *Int. J. Radiat. Oncl. Biol. Phys.* 1982;9:127–138.

43. Withers HR. Biologic basis for altered fractionation schemes. *Cancer.* 1985;55:2086–2095.

44. Schlumberger M, Parmentier C, Delisle MJ, Couette JE, Droz JP. Combination therapy for anaplastic giant cell thyroid carcinoma. *Cancer.* 1991;67:564–566.

45. Tennvall J, Andersson T, Biorklund A, Ingemansson S, Landberg T, Akerman M. Undifferentiated giant and spindle cell carcinoma of the thyroid: report on two combined treatment modalities. *Acta Radiol. Oncol.* 1979;18:408–416.

46. Kim JH, Leeper RD. Treatment of locally advanced thyroid carcinoma with combination doxorubicin and radiation therapy. *Cancer.* 1987;60:2372–2375.

47. Tennvall J, Lundell G, Hallquist A, et al. Anaplastic thyroid carcinoma. *Acta Oncol.* 1990;29:1025–1029.

# 17

# Thyroid Carcinocma in Children and Adolescents

## Thomas V. McCaffrey, M.D.

Thyroid cancer in children is rare, with only 0.4 to 1.5 reported cases per million, but it has become a topic of particular interest as a result of the observed increase in incidence of this neoplasm in children exposed to radioactive fallout in the regions surrounding the Chernobyl nuclear reactor accident in 1986.[1]

The characteristics of childhood thyroid cancer differ distinctly from adult cases in presentation and response to treatment. The evaluation and management of these tumors should be based on the unique characteristics of thyroid cancer in this age group. The relative rarity of thyroid cancer in children has limited the amount of information available on the clinical behavior of these tumors. There are few institutional studies with large numbers of patients, and as diagnostic techniques and clinical practices have evolved over the time intervals evaluated, it is difficult to draw definitive conclusions on the optimal treatment for these patients.

## CLINICAL FEATURES OF THYROID CANCER IN CHILDREN

### Papillary and Follicular Carcinoma

The incidence of thyroid cancer in children is between 0.4 and 1.5 cases per million and is two to three times more frequent in girls than in boys.[1] Between 80% and 90% of differentiated thyroid cancers in childhood are papillary or the follicular variant of papillary carcinoma.[2] The most frequent presenting sign for thyroid cancer in children is a palpable cervical lymph node or thyroid mass.

Although papillary thyroid cancer in children tends to present at a more advanced stage than in adults, the overall prognosis and survival is quite good.[3] The clinical features of thyroid cancer in children have been compared to adult patients. In a study reported from the Mayo Clinic in Rochester, Minnesota, the characteristics of 58 patients 17 years of age and younger with the diagnosis of papillary thyroid cancer were compared to 981 adult patients treated during the same period.[4] This study showed that children presented with larger tumors (3.1 cm vs. 2.1 cm), more frequent neck node involvement (90% vs. 35%), and more frequent distant metastases (7% vs. 2%) than adults. Although papillary thyroid cancer in children was more often metastatic to neck nodes and lungs before initial surgery and more often recurrent in neck lymph nodes postoperatively, it was less often fatal than in adults.

There is evidence that there has been some change in the extent of disease at the time of diagnosis when comparing older cohorts of patients with more recent series. A study reported from the University of Michigan compared cases seen between 1936 and 1970 with those seen between 1971 and 1990.[2] The cases seen in the later time interval had less advanced disease on presentation. The rate of cervical adenopathy fell from 63% to 36%, local infiltration of the primary from 31% to 6%, and initial pulmonary metastases from 19% to 6%. However, cervical node metastases were present in 88% of both groups.

It is known that thyroid carcinoma is two to three times more frequent in girls than in boys, but this ratio is

189

not constant with age. At puberty the incidence of thyroid cancer is 14 times higher in females, but before and after puberty the ratio is close to two to one.[5] This excess of thyroid cancer in females was present only for papillary thyroid carcinoma and not follicular thyroid carcinoma. This finding suggests that sex hormones have a role in the pathogenesis of papillary thyroid cancer.

Pulmonary metastases are more common in children with thyroid cancer than adults. Pulmonary metastases occur more frequently in males.[5] Most often pulmonary metastases have a micronodular pattern and in some cases are not visible on chest X-ray.[6] Although pulmonary metastases at the time of diagnosis would generally be considered a poor prognostic finding, the survival reported for children is no worse than for older patients with less advanced disease.

Papillary carcinoma is the predominant differentiated thyroid carcinoma in children representing approximately 80% of childhood thyroid cancers. Papillary carcinoma presents in children as a more aggressive tumor than follicular thyroid carcinoma. Papillary carcinoma is associated with a significantly higher frequency of advanced disease (35% vs. 8%), lymph node involvement (58% vs. 28%), and distant metastases (30% vs. 8%) compared with follicular thyroid carcinoma.[5]

## Medullary Carcinoma

Most medullary carcinoma seen in children is a component of a familial multiple endocrine neoplasia syndrome type 2 (MEN II). When very young patients are diagnosed with medullary thyroid carcinoma, it is the result of calcitonin or genetic screening prompted by having a relative diagnosed with MEN II. Because the results for surgery for medullary thyroid carcinoma depend on the extent of extrathyroidal disease, early diagnosis is essential. Genetic screening can identify the specific mutations of the *ret* oncogene.[7] Because this leads to earlier diagnosis, total thyroidectomy can be performed at a much earlier age than if serum calcitonin is used to identify C-cell hyperplasia or early carcinoma.[8] Genetic testing should be performed at birth in children at risk for MEN IIb and no later than one year for those at risk of MEN IIa. If *ret* oncogene mutations are noted, total thyroidectomy should be performed before 5 years of age in MEN IIa and during the first 6 months in MEN IIb. Only in this way can uncontrollable dissemination of the disease be avoided.

## Radiation Related Thyroid Cancer

Radiation exposure, including radiation exposure for medical treatment and environmental exposure has been implicated in thyroid malignancy. Between 1920 and 1960 radiation was used to treat a variety of benign conditions in children. This led to an observed increase in thyroid cancers with a lag time of five to 20 years.[9] Radiation doses as low as 6.5 cGy have been implicated in thyroid cancer. There is a linear increase in the risk of thyroid cancer with a radiation exposure from 20 to 1125 cGy, but there is a reduced risk at doses over 3000 cGy.[10] Subsequent studies have also shown that there is an inverse linear relation between relative risk of thyroid cancer and age up to the age of five years when the risk abruptly decreases.[11] In addition to the increased risk of thyroid malignancy, the risk of benign thyroid abnormalities is also greatly increased in patients receiving radiation to the thyroid gland during infancy.[10]

Beginning in 1990 a dramatic increase in thyroid cancer was noted in children in Belarus and the Ukraine.[12] This increase was confined to the Gomel region of Belarus and the Ukraine that lie immediately to the north of Chernobyl. This region received a high level of radioactivity as fallout after the breakdown of Chernobyl reactor number four on April 26, 1986. The fallout contained large amounts of I[131] and significant amounts of short-lived radioactive isotopes of iodine.

The histologic type of these radiation-induced thyroid cancers has been almost exclusively papillary. In addition, the primary increase in thyroid cancers has been in children. This follows the observed pattern of radiation-induced thyroid malignancy from the medical uses of external radiation.

This event has produced distinctly different effects than the previously observed effects of radiation on thyroid cancer in children. The most notable difference is related to the short interval of four years between the exposure to radiation and the onset of the tumors. A review of environmental exposure to radiation and thyroid cancer shows a clearly linear dose response curve with the largest number of cases occurring in patients in areas receiving radiation doses of greater than 50 cGy.[13] The risk of developing thyroid carcinoma is inversely related to age at exposure and the tumor most commonly caused by radiation is papillary thyroid carcinoma. The natural history of radiation-induced carcinoma may differ from naturally occurring sporadic cases of thyroid carcinoma. The carcinomas affected younger children, were less influenced by gender, and appeared to be more aggressive at presentation.[12]

Because of the high incidence of thyroid malignancy in children with known radiation exposure, whether environmental or medical, a more aggressive approach should be taken for thyroid abnormalities in this population. This population must be closely observed for palpable thyroid abnormalities, and any identified nodules should be biopsied. Total thyroidectomy should be performed for biopsy-proven malignancy. Some have advocated thyroidectomy for any palpable thyroid abnormality in patients with a history of childhood radiation exposure.[10]

## PROGNOSIS OF THYROID CANCER IN CHILDREN

In spite of the more advanced stage of thyroid cancer in children at the time of diagnosis as well as the relatively conservative management of these tumors, the survival rate observed in several large series has been equivalent or better than the outcome in adults. The study from the Mayo Clinic of 58 papillary thyroid cancers showed that survival for both children and adults were no different from expected survival rates for age-matched controls.[4] Only adults older than 40 years at the time of diagnosis had a significantly higher mortality than expected. Although papillary thyroid carcinoma in children was more often metastatic to neck nodes and lungs before initial surgery and more often recurrent in neck lymph nodes postoperatively, it tended to be less often fatal than in adults.

A series of 89 children and adolescents with thyroid carcinoma followed at the University of Michigan between 1936 and 1990 had a long-term mortality of only 2.2%. This was in spite of advanced stage of disease on presentation, with 51% having a palpable thyroid nodule, 53% cervical adenopathy, 21% local infiltration of tumor and 15% pulmonary metastases.[2]

In adults, follicular thyroid cancer is thought to have a poorer prognosis than papillary thyroid cancer. However, in children the opposite appears to be the case. La Quaglia from Memorial Sloan-Kettering Cancer Center reported a lower rate of recurrence in children with follicular thyroid cancer compared to papillary thyroid cancer.[14] Schlumberger also reported a lower recurrence rate for follicular thyroid cancer compared to papillary thyroid cancer in a series of 72 children with differentiated thyroid cancer.[6]

## TREATMENT OF THYROID CANCER IN CHILDREN

Because thyroid cancer in children is rare, and final evaluation of the effectiveness of treatment requires many years follow-up, optimal treatment protocols have not been established. Treatment recommendations have been made largely on retrospective analysis of outcomes in relatively small groups of patients.

As with adults, thyroid cancer fine needle aspiration biopsy of suspicious thyroid nodules is an important tool for evaluation. The incidence of malignancy in clinically solitary thyroid nodules is higher in children (14% to 40%) than in adults (10% to 15%), so all palpable thyroid nodules in children should be biopsied.[15] In children fine needle biopsy has a reported diagnostic accuracy of 87% and a high degree of safety.[16]

Because of the high reported incidence of nodal and distant metastases in children, these sites need to be assessed preoperatively. Many children will have palpable cervical lymph nodes on presentation. Those without can be assessed with ultrasonography or CT scanning. Pulmonary metastases can be evaluated by chest X-ray or may require total body radioactive iodine scanning postoperatively to detect unidentified pulmonary metastases.

Because of the frequent advanced stage of disease on presentation many early series included aggressive surgery consisting of total thyroidectomy and often radical or modified radical neck dissection or cervical metastases. These series have shown an excellent survival rate but a relatively high incidence of complications, including vocal cord paralysis, hypoparathyroidism, and spinal accessory nerve paralysis.[6,14] It appears that the positive outcome of treatment of advanced thyroid carcinoma in children may be a result of the indolent nature of the disease rather than the aggressiveness of treatment. Other studies have noted good results with total or near total thyroidectomy to minimize postoperative hypoparathyroidism.[4] The advantages of total thyroidectomy include treatment of potentially multifocal disease in the case of papillary carcinoma, more efficient postoperative radioactive iodine scanning for distant metastases, and the reduced need for central compartment re-exploration for recurrent disease and its known risks.

The available information in the literature would tend to favor total thyroidectomy with central compartment node dissection when it can be performed without injury to the parathyroid glands, with lateral selective neck dissection for clinically positive nodal disease.[2,4,6,15,17] Some cases of recurrent laryngeal nerve involvement will be identified. In these cases extensive tumor involvement will require sacrifice of the nerve intentionally. Some authors have advocated shaving tumor from the nerve when involvement is not extensive to preserve laryngeal function.[15]

The most powerful factor influencing the risk for distant metastases is advanced stage of the tumor.[5] Because of the high risk of pulmonary metastases in the pediatric patient and the observation that over one-half of patients with normal chest X-rays will have pulmonary metastases, postoperative whole body I[131] scanning should be performed.[18] It can be expected that pulmonary metastases will respond to I[131].[6,18]

## RELAPSE

Recurrence of thyroid cancer in children is more common than in adults. Most often the recurrence is in cervical lymphatics.[4] Factors related to recurrence are papillary histology and younger age of the patient.[14] In spite of recurrence in the neck or lungs the tumors remain responsive to treatment in most cases.[2] Regional lymph node recurrence can be surgically excised. Pulmonary recurrence is treated with I[131].[18]

Radioactive iodine is effective in clearing radiographic abnormities on chest X-ray. Although the chest X-ray may clear, radioactive iodine uptake in the lungs may remain abnormal despite repeated doses of radioactive iodine.[18] In these cases the clinical response has lasted up to 10 years in most patients.

Thyroid cancer in childhood remains a rare event except in exceptional cases of medical or environmental radiation exposure. The characteristics of childhood cancer are distinct from adult thyroid cancer. Despite an apparently aggressive initial presentation, most childhood cancers respond favorably to treatment. The preferred management is total thyroidectomy and lymphadenectomy of involved nodes with aggressive use of postoperative I[131] for treatment of pulmonary metastases. Because recurrences are frequent, close follow-up is essential. Medullary thyroid cancer in children is primarily the result of *ret* oncogene mutations in MEN II kindreds. Effective management of this disease depends on early genetic detection and total thyroidectomy in affected individuals.

# References

1. Storm HH, Plesko I. Survival of children with thyroid cancer in Europe 1978—1989. *Eur J Cancer.* 2001;37(6):775–779.
2. Harness JK, Thompson NW, McLeod MK, Pasieka J, Fukuuchi A. Differentiated thyroid carcinoma in children and adolesents. *World J. Surg.* 1992;16:547–554.
3. Zohar Y, Strauss M, Laurian N. Adolescent versus adult thyroid carcinoma. *Laryngoscope.* 1986;96(5):555–559.
4. Zimmerman D, Hay ID, Gough IR, et al. Papillary thyroid carcinoma in children and adults: long-term follow-up of 1039 patients conservatively treated at one institution during three decades. *Surgery.* 1988;104(6):1157–1166.
5. Farahati J, Bucsky P, Parlowsky T, Mader U, Reiners C. Characteristics of differentiated thyroid carcinoma in children and adolescents with respect to age, gender, and histology. *Cancer.* 1997;80(11):2156–2162.
6. Schlumberger M, De Vathaire F, Travagli JP, et al. Differentiated thyroid carcinoma in childhood: long term follow-up of 72 patients. *J Clin Endocrinol Metab.* 1987;65(6):1088–1094.
7. Brandi ML, Gagel RF, Angeli A, et al. Guidelines for diagnosis and therapy of MEN type 1 and type 2. *J Clin Endocrinol Metab.* 2001;86(12):5658–5671.
8. Skinner MA, DeBenedetti MK, Moley JF, Norton JA, Wells SA, Jr. Medullary thyroid carcinoma in children with multiple endocrine neoplasia types 2A and 2B. *J Pediatr Surg.* 1996;31(1):177–181; discussion 181–172.
9. Fraker DL. Radiation exposure and other factors that predispose to human thyroid neoplasia. *Surg Clin North Am.* 1995;75:365–375.
10. Witt TR, Meng RL, Economou SG, Southwick HW. The approch to the irradiated thyroid. *Surgical Clinics of North America.* 1979;59(1):45–63.
11. Ron E, Kleinerman RA, Boice JD, Jr., LiVolsi VA, Flannery JT, Fraumeni JF, Jr. A population-based case-control study of thyroid cancer. *J Natl Cancer Inst.* Jul 1987;79(1):1–12.
12. Leenhardt L, Aurengo A. Post-Chernobyl thyroid carcinoma in children. *Baillieres Best Pract Res Clin Endocrinol Metab.* 2000; 14(4):667–677.
13. Tronko MD, Bogdanova TI, Komissarenko IV, et al. Thyroid carcinoma in children and adolescents in Ukraine after the Chernobyl nuclear accident: statistical data and clinicomorphologic characteristics. *Cancer.* 1999;86(1):149–156.
14. La Quaglia MP, Corbally MT, Heller G, Exelby PR, Brennan MF. Recurrence and morbidity in differentiated thyroid carcinoma in children. *Surgery.* 1988;104(6):1149–1156.
15. Stael AP, Plukker JT, Piers DA, Rouwe CW, Vermey A. Total thyroidectomy in the treatment of thyroid carcinoma in childhood. *Br J Surg.* 1995;82(8):1083–1085.
16. Al-Shaikh A, Ngan B, Daneman A, Daneman D. Fine-needle aspiration biopsy in the management of thyroid nodules in children and adolescents. *J Pediatr.* 2001;138(1):140–142.
17. Segal K, Arad-Cohen A, Mechlis S, Lubin E, Feinmesser R. Cancer of the thyroid in children and adolescents. *Clin Otolaryngol.* 1997;22(6):525–528.
18. Vassiopoulou-Sellin R, Klein MJ, Smith TH, et al. Pulmonary metastases in children and young adults with differentiated thyroid cancer. *Cancer.* 1993;71(4):1348–1351.

# 18

# Management of the Neck in Thyroid Malignancy

## K. Thomas Robbins, M.D. and Sandeep Samant, M.S., F.R.C.S.

The biology of thyroid gland cancer varies significantly from conventional models of tumor behavior applicable to most other neoplastic processes. Thus, much controversy surrounds almost every aspect of this disease. The difficulty in understanding the behavior of these cancers also relates to their unique epidemiologic characteristics. Not only are these cancers relatively uncommon, but a majority of patients with differentiated thyroid cancer will do well regardless of the nature of treatment provided. Recurrence and death from this cancer continues to occur as late as 20 or even 30 years after initial diagnosis. This delayed and infrequent occurrence of disease-related mortality, the usual endpoint for measuring efficacy in cancer treatment, makes design of clinical trials nearly impossible. Hence, recurrence of disease is often used as an alternate, surrogate endpoint, but recurrence does not necessarily portend diminished survival.

Lymphatic metastasis in differentiated thyroid cancer occurs frequently, yet as with other aspects of this disease, controversy surrounds the question of its prognostic implication and treatment. In this chapter, we attempt to analyze the existing knowledge about the anatomic basis, prognostic value, and surgical management of lymphatic metastasis from thyroid cancer. Management of the neck in differentiated thyroid cancers and medullary cancer is discussed separately.

## PATTERNS OF LYMPHATIC METASTASIS IN DIFFERENTIATED THYROID CANCER

From a study of the thyroid gland in dog and man, Reinhoff, in 1931, described its lymphatic drainage as being initiated in a rich intraglandular plexus, located throughout the gland in the interfollicular space, and emptying into an extraglandular plexus on the surface of the gland.[1] From this external plexus, lymphatic trunks emanate in superior and lateral directions, and travel along superior thyroid vessels to drain into the jugular group of lymph nodes. Another set of lymphatics courses inferiorly, forming a pretracheal reticulum, to drain into the mediastinum.

Patterns of metastatic lymph node involvement reported in patients with thyroid cancer also contribute to our understanding of the lymphatic drainage of this gland. The majority of nodal metastases occur in the central compartment of the neck and in the mid and lower jugular nodes.[2] In a report on 586 patients with differentiated thyroid cancer, of whom 415 underwent neck dissections, Ozaki et al found metastatic disease in the central nodes (prelaryngeal, pretracheal, paratracheal and parathyroidal) in 72.3% and in the jugular nodes in 67% of patients whose necks were dissected.[3] Among the jugular group of lymph nodes, the mid and lower jugular groups are involved more commonly than upper jugular lymph nodes.[4] Involvement of other areas of the neck (spinal accessory, submandibular and submental) is relatively uncommon.

Thyroid cancer metastasis occurs much more commonly on the side of neck ipsilateral to the primary tumor. This was evident in the 546 patients with differentiated thyroid cancer reported from Institut Gustav-Roussy, France by Tubiana et al, in whom neck metastases were unilateral in 176 and bilateral in 48, resulting in a 41% (224/546) overall incidence of positive cervical lymph nodes.[5] Bilateral metastases can be particularly significant in individuals with tumors involving both lobes, tumors located in the isthmus and in those with recurrent tumors.[6]

## INCIDENCE OF LYMPHATIC METASTASES IN DIFFERENTIATED THYROID CANCER

Cervical lymphatic metastases have been reported to occur in 11% to 82% of patients with differentiated cancers.[3,7-14] For the most part, this variability can be explained on the basis of the difference in the way nodal metastasis is diagnosed in various institutions. It is apparent from the literature that the reported incidence relates directly to the diligence for which metastases have been looked. For instance, upon reviewing the records of 792 patients treated at the Lahey Clinic Foundation over a 40-year period, Cady et al acknowledged that the incidence of nodal metastasis—11%, 28%, 35% and 27% in the four decades—correlated roughly with the number of nodal resections performed.[7] Nodal dissections, performed only in 21% of all cases in the 1930s, increased to 47% in the 1950s, and fell again to 38% in the latter part of the 1960s. Also, while 92% of resections were radical neck dissections in the 1950s, only 43% of the resections were radical neck dissections in the latter part of 1960s—limited perithyroidal nodal excisions (41%) or modified neck dissections (16%) were more commonly utilized during this time.

Approach to diagnosis and treatment of nodal disease varies widely between institutions. While some recommend surgery only for palpable lymphadenopathy, others perform lymph node sampling to look for occult disease, completing a formal neck dissection if this is found. Less common is the routine use of elective modified radical neck dissections. Studies employing this last approach should provide the most accurate estimate of the incidence of cervical metastases in thyroid cancer. Sato et al performed a modified radical neck dissection in all 139 patients with differentiated thyroid cancer reported in their series.[14] They found cervical lymphatic metastases in 102 patients (73%). Similarly, Ozaki et al found the incidence of histologic metastases to be 81.7% in a group of 415 cases of differentiated thyroid cancer who had either a modified neck dissection or local dissection performed along with thyroid surgery. The rate of positive disease ranged from 60.4% for the local dissection group to 83.6% for the ipsilateral modified neck dissection group and 89.8% for the bilateral modified neck dissection group. Likewise, other studies where the majority of patients were subjected to a neck dissection report the rate of cervical metastasis to be around 65% or higher.[13,15]

## FACTORS INFLUENCING THE INCIDENCE OF CERVICAL METASTASES IN DIFFERENTIATED THYROID CANCER

Cady et al from the Lahey Clinic Foundation showed that lymphatic metastases were more frequent and more numerous in younger patients.[7] Although a similar trend was noted in a study by Harwood et al from the Veterans Hospital at San Francisco, California, closer inspection of the data presented shows no significant correlation of age with incidence of positive nodes.[16] In yet another study, McHenry et al from the University of Toronto School of Medicine found that patients with lymph node metastases did not differ from those without nodal metastases in terms of mean age (42 years versus 42 years).[12] Similarly, no difference in the incidence of nodal metastases was noted in patients above and below 50 years of age in a report on 212 differentiated thyroid cancers from Birmingham, Alabama.[17]

Nodal metastases show no clear predilection for gender. In Harwood's report, there were 31 women and 19 men in the group with lymph node metastases, and 36 women and 14 men among those without nodal metastases.[16] On the other hand, a study in Sweden found the incidence of node positivity to be higher in men (70%) than in women (45%).[18]

By contrast, tumor histology does seem to have an influence on the likelihood of finding cervical metastases. Although there are occasional reports suggesting no such influence,[15] the weight of the evidence in the literature supports the view that papillary thyroid cancers metastasize more readily to cervical nodes than follicular or Hurthle cell cancers. In a report on 1578 differentiated thyroid cancers, Simpson et al found the incidence of cervical metastases to be 27% and 12% for papillary and follicular thyroid cancers, respectively.[10] McHenry et al found positive cervical nodes in 38% of papillary, 14% of follicular, and in none of the 19 Hürthle cell cancers in their study.[12]

The size of the primary tumor in the thyroid gland and extension of disease outside the gland capsule also have a bearing on the likelihood of lymphatic metastases; however, this association is not as clear as it is in mucosal epithelial malignancies of the head and neck. Tisell et al found that in those with metastatic nodal disease, there was a positive correlation between the size of the primary tumor and the number of involved nodes in the neck.[18] It is not clear from their report, however, whether there was an increase in the incidence of cervical metastatic disease with increasing size of the primary tumor. Ozaki et al, on the other hand, warned that nodal metastases develop as often with smaller primary tumors as with the advanced ones. They classified their patients on the basis of a staging system where patients with T3 (larger than 5 cm, or involving both lobes) and T4 tumors (extraglandular extension) were included in the advanced category and those with Tis (less than 1 cm), T1 (1cm to 2 cm, confined to one lobe or isthmus), and T2 tumors (2 cm to 5cm in size, or extending into the isthmus) were in the nonadvanced category. Neck dissections were carried out in 138 of 185 advanced cases and in 277 of 401 nonadvanced cases. Lymph node metastases were discovered in the central nodes in 68.6% and in the jugular nodes in 62.1% of the nonadvanced cases; by comparison, these figures were 79.7% and 76.8%, respectively, for the patients in the advanced category.[3] In contrast, Cody and Shah selected 32 patients with locally invasive thyroid cancer treated at Memorial Sloan-Kettering Cancer Center over a 22–year period. Clinically overt nodal disease was present in 18 patients. In addition, 6 other patients underwent elective neck dissection; 5 of these were found to have occult metastases. Furthermore, 4 of 8 patients with clinically negative necks that were simply observed developed cervical metastases later. The authors therefore suggested that locally aggressive thyroid cancers have a higher than usual incidence of clinically positive and occult cervical nodal metastases.[19]

To conclude this point, while papillary histology, advanced primary tumor, particularly that showing extrathyroidal extension, and possibly younger age increase the likelihood of metastatic neck disease, nodal involvement is not at all unusual even with follicular cancers, smaller primaries, and older age.

## PROGNOSTIC SIGNIFICANCE OF NODAL METASTASIS IN DIFFERENTIATED THYROID CANCER

How does the presence of palpable cervical adenopathy affect the outlook of a patient with differentiated thyroid cancer? Also, if no clinically obvious lymphadenopathy exists at the time of presentation, how should the neck be treated? As is typical for the literature on thyroid cancer, answers to these questions remain buried in controversy. Confusion has arisen from the discrepancy between the high incidence of cervical metastases when neck dissections are routinely performed and the relatively low incidence of recurrences when necks are not dissected. Hence, the biologic behavior of lymphatic metastases remains unclear. While there is no doubt that palpable metastases must be excised, there is some disagreement on how to handle the clinically negative neck. Suffice it to say, lymphatic metastases probably do have some negative impact on survival, although there are some studies suggesting otherwise. They clearly increase the likelihood of neck recurrence. Finally, it is possible that certain groups of patients may benefit from elective neck dissection. In this section, we will examine the evidence which supports these conclusions.

First, in assessing the evidence supporting the notion that lymph nodes do not affect survival adversely, Cady et al in analyzing 792 patients with differentiated thyroid cancers inferred the opposite: that lymph node metastases exert a protective effect.[7] However, this was not a multivariate analysis, nor had any attempt been made to control for such variables as age of the patient and the size of the primary tumor. In this study, lymph node metastases were more frequent and more numerous in the younger patients. Hence, the strong positive influence of age should have been adequately accounted for. The authors also stated that the protective effect of nodes was directly related to the number of lymph node metastases present such that no deaths occurred in those patients who had more than 10 node metastases. However, the authors again failed to note that not a single patient older than 51 years of age (the high risk group) happened to fall in the category of those with more than 10 positive nodes.

Sato et al were unable to demonstrate any adverse impact of lymph node metastases in their study of 139 differentiated thyroid cancers. They, however, conceded that their study did suffer from the limitations of a small number of patients, a relatively short follow-up of 7 years, and the absence of a multivariate life-curve analysis.[14]

In a matched-pair analysis published from Memorial Sloan-Kettering Cancer Center, Hughes et al put forward a strong argument against lymphatic metastases having any detrimental effect on survival.[20] From a database of 931 cases of differentiated thyroid cancers treated at that hospital between 1930 and 1980, 100 node-positive patients were selected and compared to corresponding N0 patients matched for age, tumor size, histology, and intrathyroidal extent. No difference in survival could be demonstrated between the two groups. However, there was a trend for a lower survival in the node-positive patients over 45 years of age in comparison to their node-negative counterparts. Recurrences were significantly higher in the N1 patients over 45 years of age than in the N0 patients.

In contrast, a number of studies have demonstrated a detrimental effect of lymph node metastases in differentiated thyroid cancer. Harwood et al compared 50 consecutive patients with differentiated thyroid cancer having nodal metastases treated at the University of California, San Francisco, with 50 consecutive patients without nodal metastases.[16] They found the groups to be evenly matched for age, sex, histology, pathologic findings, and extent of nodal involvement. Tumor recurred in 32% of those with lymphatic metastases compared to 14% of those without. Twenty-four percent of the patients with nodal disease died of thyroid cancer, whereas only 8% of those without nodal metastases died of their cancer. This difference in cancer related mortality was much more striking in patients older than 40 years of age: nine patients (41%) with nodal metastases died, while only four (15%) without nodal disease died. Although this study addresses the effect of confounding variables such as age, sex, and histologic features, it does suffer from the limitations of small sampling and a lack of determinate survival calculations (survival is expressed only as percentage of tumor-related deaths in each category).

In 1984, Tubiana et al from Institut Gustav-Roussy, France, published their results on 546 patients with differentiated thyroid cancer.[5] No patient had distant metastasis at the time of presentation. Follow-up ranged from 8 to 40 years. All patients with palpable adenopathy underwent a modified radical neck dissection. In patients with no palpable nodes, an intraoperative biopsy was performed by excising the paratracheal, lower jugular and supraclavicular nodes; a neck dissection was later completed if histology showed cancer in the excised lymph nodes. Postoperative radiation was administered to 203 patients for suspected or frank invasion of tumor into the neighboring tissues. Radioiodine ablation was performed in 100 patients. The authors calculated survival by the actuarial method. Cox's regression model was used for multivariate analysis to study the relative effect of four parameters: age, sex, histologic type and presence of involved nodes. Lymphatic metastases were shown to be associated with a lower survival (relative risk 1.4) and a higher recurrence rate (relative risk 1.85). The strongest influence on survival, however, was exerted by age.

In a Canadian survey of 1074 papillary thyroid cancers and 504 follicular thyroid cancers, Simpson et al performed a multivariate analysis on 12 possible prognostic variables.[10] They found that, in descending order of influence, age, extrathyroidal invasion, and differentiation were significant for cause-specific survival with papillary cancers and extrathyroidal invasion, distant metastasis, tumor size, lymph node metastasis, age, and postoperative gross status were significant, in that rank order, for cause-specific survival in follicular cancers. When the two histologies were considered together, there was no significant difference in survival between node-positive and node-negative patients; however, poorer survival was noted specifically in the subgroup of patients with extrathyroidal extension— those having positive nodes demonstrating worse survival compared to those with negative nodal status.

McHenry et al studied 227 consecutive patients with differentiated thyroid carcinoma treated at the University of Toronto School of Medicine.[12] All patients were subjected to an intraoperative sampling of middle and lower cervical lymph nodes, and a modified radical neck dissection was performed when metastases were detected. Additionally, most patients with cervical metastases were subjected to radioactive iodine thera-

py. Patients with nodal disease were similar in age, sex, and tumor size to those without nodal involvement. Only four patients died of their disease; hence, no survival difference could be demonstrated statistically. However, all four patients who died had cervical nodal metastases. There were a disproportionate number of patients with extrathyroidal extension (41% versus 8%) and distant metastases (6% versus 0.1%) in the group with cervical metastases. Thirteen of 15 patients with distant metastases had cervical metastases. The authors, therefore, argued that the presence of cervical metastases was a marker for a more aggressive tumor behavior. As with other studies, recurrences were higher in the node-positive group (19% versus 2%). The influence of treatment with radioactive iodine on the outcome was suggested in this study: patients with positive nodes, who were administered radioactive iodine, recurred less frequently (16%) compared to those who were not (42%).

This theme of increased recurrence, association with distant metastases, and a prospect of diminished survival has been echoed in many other studies.[15,17,21] Finally, a recent study by Noguchi et al has produced strong evidence favoring a negative prognostic impact of nodal metastases on survival based on a multivariate analysis performed on a very large number of patients.[13] Two thousand nine hundred and sixty-six patients were treated over a 45-year period with a mean follow-up of 15.6 years. A modified radical neck dissection was performed in 72.1% of patients, while a limited node excision was carried out in 8.5%. Two thousand and five patients (67.6%) had histologically confirmed metastases; 39.1% had gross nodal disease. The study demonstrated that sex, age, tumor size, extrathyroidal invasion, and lymphatic metastases were significant risk factors affecting survival. The study also showed that performing a neck dissection resulted in improved survival (p=.02) among patients having extrathyroidal invasion by the tumor and in women older than 60 years. However, it was not clearly stated how many of these patients had an elective versus therapeutic neck dissection.

Thus, the evidence for lymphatic metastases having an adverse prognostic impact is more compelling than the opposite effect. While this impact appears insignificant in younger individuals and in those with favorable disease (small, intrathyroidal tumors), it achieves significance in older patients and those in whom tumors extend beyond the confines of the gland.

## SURGICAL MANAGEMENT OF THE NECK IN THYROID CANCER SURGERY

Our approach to the neck is based upon the premise that a neck dissection should be performed when there is clinical evidence of lymphadenopathy, or when abnormal nodes are identified intraoperatively. While the Japanese studies suggest that an elective neck dissection for patients who are elderly or have extrathyroidal extension may be beneficial, at the present time, this is not the standard of practice.

A standard thyroidectomy incision can be enlarged when a neck dissection is to be performed, curving it from the lateral end, and directing it up along the lateral border of the sternomastoid muscle to stop a little below the level of mandibular angle. Elevating and retracting the skin beyond the superior edge of this incision will afford adequate clearance of level II nodes, while still avoiding a long and unsightly incision.

We do not believe in the strategy of lymph node sampling from central compartment and lower jugular nodes to be used as a guide to perform neck dissection in patients with N0 necks. The decision to perform a neck dissection should instead be based upon the presence or absence of enlarged or abnormal appearing lymph nodes. Given the high incidence of occult metastatic disease, if lymph node sampling were used to select patients for neck dissection, a large proportion (about 50%) would end up having a neck dissection on the ipsilateral side of the neck, and a substantial number (probably close to 20%) would have to have surgery on both sides. We believe that this approach would be overly aggressive for the majority of patients in whom the course of this disease is mostly benign and seems to be unaffected by the presence of microscopic tumor in cervical nodes.

The extent of nodal resection is similar in clinically N0 or N+ necks. This should be a selective compartmental neck dissection including levels II–VI nodes (upper, middle and lower jugular, posterior triangle, and central compartment nodes). As mentioned before, the likelihood of involvement of level I nodes (submandibular and submental nodes) is negligible. Thus, level I should be dissected only when there is clinically positive disease in this region or extensive nodal disease in adjacent nodal groups. Central compartment dissection should include a transcervical clearance of paratracheal nodes down to the level of the innominate artery. More thorough clearance below this region requires a median sternotomy, which should only be considered if enlarged mediastinal nodes have been demonstrated radiographically.

Caution should be exercised in removing the paratracheal and perithyroidal nodes to avoid devascularizing the parathyroid glands or injuring the recurrent laryngeal nerves. If it is necessary to thoroughly dissect the paratracheal region on one side, a more conservative dissection is recommended on the opposite side. A gland with compromised blood supply may be autotransplanted after confirming its parathyroid nature on frozen sections. Permanent hypoparathyroidism is a real complication of thyroid cancer surgery, occurring in 2.8% to 33% of cases.[15,22-24] The likelihood of developing this complication increases with the extent of surgery in this area, with the combination of total thyroidectomy and neck dissection resulting in the highest incidence.[15,25] Attie and Khafif reported continued reduction in the incidence of hypoparathyroidism with increasing surgical experience in their series.[24] This underscores the fact that surgery for thyroid cancer should not be performed by the occasional thyroid surgeon.

Before the concept of modified radical and selective neck dissections became popular, many authors promoted the use of conservative lymph node excision ("berry picking") as an alternative to the much more morbid radical neck dissection. They quoted somewhat similar disease control and lower complication rates as reasons for preferring the former approach.[8,26] No direct comparison of the two approaches is available in the literature, although some reports have quoted a higher recurrence rate with conservative nodal excisions.[27] We subscribe to the view that a carefully performed modified radical neck dissection, preserving the accessory nerve, internal jugular vein, and sternocleidomastoid muscle, is the treatment of choice for both N0 (when indicated) and N+ disease, as it maximizes disease control in the neck without any significant increase in morbidity. Occasionally, a radical neck dissection is necessary for patients who have massive adenopathy in which the disease has extended through the capsule and invaded non-lymphatic structures such as the internal jugular vein, sternocleidomastoid muscle, and the spinal accessory nerve. Interestingly, the presence of extracapsular spread associated with differentiated thyroid cancer, does not appear to adversely affect survival.[28]

## MANAGEMENT OF THE NECK IN MEDULLARY THYROID CANCER

Medullary carcinoma arises from the C cells in the thyroid gland and occurs in hereditary and sporadic forms. Lymph node metastasis is common, occurring in as many as 81% of cases.[29] Both the central compartment as well as the lateral compartments of the neck can be the site of metastatic disease. While clearance of the central compartment and ipsilateral neck dissection is recommended, it has been argued that bilateral neck dissections may be necessary in order to maximize regional control, as metastatic disease has been noted to occur in as many as 44% of contralateral neck dissections.[29] The risk of bilateral metastasis is particularly significant in familial cancers as well as in sporadic cancers involving both lobes of the thyroid gland. Others have followed the policy of dissecting only in cases with clinically or radiologically demonstrable lymphadenopathy.[30] Neck dissection should include the jugular chain nodes (levels II through IV), the posterior triangle nodes (level V), the central compartment nodes (level VI), and those lymph nodes of the superior mediastinum, which can be removed transcervically. As medullary thyroid cancer has a greater tendancy to extend into the perinodal connective tissue, care should be taken to remove the disease with adequate margins. For this reason, radical neck dissection may be required in a higher percentage of cases. Based on this biologic behavior, Dralle et al recommended the use of microscopic dissection of each compartment involved by tumor. This thorough systematic approach to neck dissection was reported to be superior to more limited lymph node dissections based on improved survival, lower recurrence, and a higher rate of normalization of calcitonin level with the former method.[31]

The argument for adopting the more radical approach of performing bilateral neck dissection is supported by the fact that persistent hypercalcitoninemia after initial surgery is thought to be caused by microscopic disease in the neck in many instances. Tisell et al found metastatic disease in the neck in all 11 patients operated for elevated calcitonin levels persisting after initial thyroidectomy and central neck dissection.[32] Reduction in calcitonin levels has been achieved by performing modified radical neck dissections in a number of patients who remain biochemically positive after initial thyroid surgery.[32,33] Moley et al achieved normalization of calcitonin levels in 28% of patients and a decrease in calcitonin levels by 40% or more in another 42% of patients.[34] However, localization of residual disease with the aid of CT and MR imaging of neck, chest and abdomen and radionuclide studies should always be undertaken before planning the surgery in order to rule out wider dissemination of disease.

## CONCLUSION

Cervical lymphatic metastasis occurs very frequently in patients with cancers of the thyroid gland. For differentiated thyroid cancer, neck dissection is indicated in patients with clinically positive disease (cN+). For patients with clinically negative disease (cN-), only those who are found to have evidence of abormal nodes intraoperatively should have an elective neck dissection. Otherwise, there is no compelling evidence to perform an elective neck dissection even among patients with poor prognosis disease. For medullary thyroid cancer, surgical treatment of the cervical nodes is very important and should include the central compartment and both the ipsilateral and contralateral neck when indicated. Unlike papillary and follicular thyroid carcinoma,

elective neck dissection is recommended for patients with medullary thyroid cancer who have clinically N0 nodal disease. The extent of nodal dissection in thyroid cancer should include the nodes in the central compartment (level VI); the jugular chain (level II-IV), and the posterior triangle (level V). Nodes in the superior mediastinum and level I should be removed whenever there is clinical evidence of disease in these subzones.

## References

1. Strong EW, Evaluation and surgical treatment of papillary and follicullar carcinoma. In: SA Falk, ed. *Thyroid Disease*. Lippincott-Raven: Rochester, NY: 1997; 565–586.
2. Rossi RL, Nieroda C, Cady B, et al. Malignancies of the thyroid gland. The Lahey Clinic experience. *Surg Clin North Am.* 1985; 65(2): 211–230.
3. Ozaki O, Ito K, Kobayashi K, et al. Modified neck dissection for patients with nonadvanced, differentiated carcinoma of the thyroid. *World J Surg.* 1988; 12(6): 825–829.
4. Sako K, Marchetta FC, Razack MS, et al. Modified radical neck dissection for metastatic carcinoma of the thyroid. A reappraisal. *Am J Surg.* 1985; 150(4): 500–502.
5. Tubiana M, Schlumberger M, Rougier P, et al. Long-term results and prognostic factors in patients with differentiated thyroid carcinoma. *Cancer.* 1985; 55(4): 794–804.
6. Noguchi M, Kinami S, Kinoshita K, et al. Risk of bilateral cervical lymph node metastases in papillary thyroid cancer. *J Surg Oncol.* 1993; 52(3): 155–599.
7. Cady B, Sedgwick CE, Meissner WA, et al. Changing clinical, pathologic, therapeutic, and survival patterns in differentiated thyroid carcinoma. *Ann Surg.* 1976; 184(5): 541–553.
8. Mazzaferri EL, Young RL. Papillary thyroid carcinoma: a 10 year follow-up report of the impact of therapy in 576 patients. *Am J Med.* 1981; 70(3): 511–518.
9. Rossi RL, Cady B, Silverman ML, et al. Current results of conservative surgery for differentiated thyroid carcinoma. *World J Surg.* 1986; 10(4): 612–622.
10. Simpson WJ, McKinney SE, Carruthers JS, et al. Papillary and follicular thyroid cancer. Prognostic factors in 1,578 patients. *Am J Med.* 1987; 83(3): 479–488.
11. Attie JN. Modified neck dissection in treatment of thyroid cancer: a safe procedure. *Eur J Cancer Clin Oncol.* 1988; 24(2): 315–324.
12. McHenry CR, Rosen IB, Walfish PG. Prospective management of nodal metastases in differentiated thyroid cancer. *Am J Surg.* 1991; 162(4): 353–356.
13. Noguchi S, Murakami N, Yamashita H, et al. Papillary thyroid carcinoma: modified radical neck dissection improves prognosis. *Arch Surg.* 1998; 133(3): 276–280.
14. Sato N, Oyamatsu M, Koyama Y, et al. Do the level of nodal disease according to the TNM classification and the number of involved cervical nodes reflect prognosis in patients with differentiated carcinoma of the thyroid gland? *J Surg Oncol.* 1998; 69(3): 151–155.
15. Simon D, Goretzki PE, Witte J, et al. Incidence of regional recurrence guiding radicality in differentiated thyroid carcinoma. *World J Surg.* 1996; 20(7): 860–866; discussion 866.
16. Harwood J, Clark OH, Dunphy JE. Significance of lymph node metastasis in differentiated thyroid cancer. *Am J Surg.* 1978; 136(1): 107–112.
17. Sellers M, Beenken S, Blankenship A, et al. Prognostic significance of cervical lymph node metastases in differentiated thyroid cancer. *Am J Surg.* 1992; 164(6): 578–581.

18. Tisell LE, Nilsson B, Molne J, et al. Improved survival of patients with papillary thyroid cancer after surgical microdissection. *World J Surg.* 1996; 20(7): 854–859.

19. Cody HSD, Shah JP. Locally invasive, well-differentiated thyroid cancer. 22 years' experience at Memorial Sloan-Kettering Cancer Center. *Am J Surg.* 1981; 142(4): 480–483.

20. Hughes CJ, Shaha AR, Shah JP, et al. Impact of lymph node metastasis in differentiated carcinoma of the thyroid: a matched-pair analysis. *Head Neck.* 1996; 18(2): 127–132.

21. Scheumann GF, Gimm O, Wegener G, et al. Prognostic significance and surgical management of locoregional lymph node metastases in papillary thyroid cancer. *World J Surg.* 1994; 18(4): 559–567; discussion 567–568.

22. McKenzie AD. The natural history of thyroid cancer. A report of 102 cases analysed 10 to 15 years after diagnosis. *Arch Surg.* 1971; 102(4): 274–277.

23. Harrold CC, Wright J. Management of surgical hypoparathyroidism. *Am J Surg.* 1966; 112(4): 482–487.

24. Attie JN, Khafif RA. Preservation of parathyroid glands during total thyroidectomy. Improved technic utilizing microsurgery. *Am J Surg.* 1975; 130(4): 399–404.

25. Wingert DJ, Friesen SR, Iliopoulos JI, et al. Post-thyroidectomy hypocalcemia. Incidence and risk factors. *Am J Surg.* 1986; 152(6): 606–610.

26. Hamming JF, van de Velde CJ, Fleuren GJ, et al. Differentiated thyroid cancer: a stage adapted approach to the treatment of regional lymph node metastases. *Eur J Cancer Clin Oncol.* 1988; 24(2): 325–330.

27. McGregor GI, Luoma A, Jackson SM. Lymph node metastases from well-differentiated thyroid cancer. A clinical review. *Am J Surg.* 1985; 149(5): 610–612.

28. Spires J, Robbins KT, Luna M, Byers RM. Metastatic papillary thyroid carcinoma: the significance of extranodal extension. 1989; *Head Neck Surg.* 11:242.

29. Moley JF, DeBenedetti MK. Patterns of nodal metastases in palpable medullary thyroid carcinoma: recommendations for extent of node dissection. *Ann Surg.* 1999; 229(6): 880–887; discussion 887–888.

30. Ellenhorn JD, Shah JP, Brennan MF. Impact of therapeutic regional lymph node dissection for medullary carcinoma of the thyroid gland. *Surgery.* 1993; 114(6): 1078–1081; discussion 1081–1082.

31. Dralle H, Damm I, Scheumann GF, et al. Compartment-oriented microdissection of regional lymph nodes in medullary thyroid carcinoma. *Surg Today.* 1994; 24(2): 112–121.

32. Tisell LE, Hansson G, Jansson S, et al. Reoperation in the treatment of asymptomatic metastasizing medullary thyroid carcinoma. *Surgery.* 1986; 99(1): 60–66.

33. Fleming JB, Lee JE, Bouvet M, et al. Surgical strategy for the treatment of medullary thyroid carcinoma. *Ann Surg.* 1999; 230(5): 697–707.

34. Moley JF, Wells SA, Dilley WG, et al. Reoperation for recurrent or persistent medullary thyroid cancer. *Surgery.* 1993; 114(6): 1090–1095; discussion 1095–1096.

# 19

# Radio-Iodine Treatment in Differentiated Thyroid Malignancy

Ana O. Hoff, M.D.

Steven I. Sherman, M.D.

Robert F. Gagel, M.D.

## INTRODUCTION

The concept of destroying thyroid tissue by using a radioactive iodine compound emerged in 1936 when physicists from the Massachusetts Institute of Technology lectured to a group of Harvard University faculty that included members of the Thyroid Unit of Massachusetts General Hospital.[1] Following this lecture, these groups started to investigate the potential role of radio-iodine in the diagnosis and treatment of thyroid disease. Within a few years, radioactive iodine ($^{131}$I) became an established treatment for hyperthyroidism and thyroid cancer.[1] The utility of $^{131}$I for diagnosis and treatment of thyroid diseases is the unique and specific ability of the thyroid cell to take up iodine. This chapter will discuss the use of $^{131}$I as a tool for diagnosis, treatment and follow-up of well-differentiated thyroid cancer.

Differentiated thyroid cancer comprises papillary and follicular thyroid carcinomas. Most patients with differentiated thyroid cancer are potentially cured after an appropriate primary treatment, but a few remain at risk of recurrence or cancer-related death.[2-4] The risk of recurrence or death is determined by several prognostic factors[5] that can be identified at the time of diagnosis (Table 19–1) and by the extent of initial treatment. Surgery is the mainstay of primary treatment for thyroid cancer. Although the extent of initial surgery is still controversial, most advocate near-total or total thy-

roidectomy for tumors larger than 1 cm as this surgery is associated with fewer cancer recurrences and tumor-related deaths.[4,6-8] Most patients with differentiated thyroid cancer undergo radio-iodine treatment after surgery for ablation of residual thyroid tissue and destruction of adjacent microscopic cancer cells. After the initial surgery and radio-iodine ablation, patients are followed with radio-iodine whole-body scans to determine whether residual or recurrent foci of disease are present. In most circumstances, local (cervical) metastatic disease is treated with node dissection followed by radio-iodine therapy. In the case of distant metastases which can involve the lungs, bone, and, less commonly, the brain, radio-iodine therapy becomes the mainstay of therapy as many of these tumors tend to maintain their ability to take up iodine.

The indications, dosage and the potential complications for radio-iodine treatment for differentiated thyroid cancer will be reviewed in further detail in the subsequent sections of this chapter.

## ADJUVANT RADIO-IODINE ABLATION OF POSTSURGICAL THYROID REMNANTS

Most retrospective studies have shown that adjuvant radio-iodine ablation lowers the recurrence rate and the disease-specific mortality rate in patients with differentiated thyroid cancer.[2-4] Most series demonstrate a clear

**Table 19–1.** Prognostic factors at time of diagnosis

---

### Differentiated Thyroid Carcinomas

---

Large tumor size

Age > 40 years

Male gender

Tumor multicentricity

Extra-thyroidal invasion

Vascular invasion

Cervical lymph node metastases

Distant metastases

Poorly differentiated histologic subtypes (eg, tall-cell and diffuse sclerosing variants of papillary thyroid carcinoma, Hürthle cell carcinoma)

---

benefit of radio-iodine ablation in patients with invasive and metastatic disease.[2,3] However, the role of postsurgical [131]I therapy in patients with low-risk disease (tumors < 1.5 cm, age ≤ 40 years, no soft tissue invasion, and no distant metastases) remains controversial. These patients have an excellent prognosis (96–98% survival rate at 15-year follow-up and less than 10% chance of recurrence),[6,9] and it has not been determined whether the benefits of [131]I therapy outweigh the potential risks in this group. The lack of consensus about which patients should receive postsurgical [131]I ablation also occurs because of other issues. First, there are no large randomized, prospective trials with long-term follow-up on the value of [131]I ablation in patients with low-risk disease. Second, the presence of distant metastasis may not be apparent at the time of initial treatment.

However, although the benefits of adjuvant radio-iodine ablation have not been proven in prospective clinical trials, there are still compelling arguments for its use. One rationale for postsurgical ablation of residual normal thyroid tissue is to increase the sensitivity of tests (whole-body scans and serum thyroglobulin measurements) used during long-term follow-up. Lack of normal thyroid tissue increases relative radio-iodine uptake by tumor cells, resulting in better detection of recurrent or metastatic disease and higher specificity of serial serum thyroglobulin measurements as a tumor marker. An additional benefit of postsurgical radio-iodine ablation is the destruction of any microscopic foci of disease that is adjacent to or intermixed with normal thyroid tissue being ablated, reducing the risk of recurrence.[6,7,10,11]

In general, radio-iodine ablation is given to patients with any of the following presentations: tumor larger than 1.5 cm, evidence of extra-thyroidal disease, or age of at least 40 years at diagnosis. Patients with low-risk disease who have multifocal disease or a history of irradiation may also benefit from radio-iodine ablation.[6,7]

One critical determinant of the efficacy of the RAI dose administered is the amount of residual thyroid tissue; it has been suggested that larger residues require larger [131]I doses for complete ablation.[12] Other critical determinants of the success of radio-iodine ablation are the thyroid-stimulating hormone (TSH) level at the time of ablation and the size of the body's iodine stores. The TSH concentration should be elevated to at least 30 mμ/L to optimize [131]I uptake. This level usually requires a period of thyroid hormone withdrawal of at least 4 weeks. One approach is to suspend thyroid hormone replacement for 4 to 6 weeks after the patient undergoes the thyroidectomy. Another approach is to give a short-acting form of thyroid hormone (T$_3$) for 2 weeks after thyroidectomy followed for a period of 2 to 3 weeks of total hormone withdrawal. The latter approach can spare the patient the symptoms of hypothyroidism. To optimize radio-iodine uptake, patients should follow a low-iodine diet.[13] Patients should avoid computed tomography with iodine-containing contrast for at least 6 to 8 weeks prior to any radio-iodine scan, although older patients and those with compromised renal function may require an even longer period of iodine restriction. A common procedure that we follow is to perform a 24-hour urine collection for iodine in patients whose scans are negative so that excessive endogenous iodine stores can be excluded as a cause for the lack of uptake. Another strategy that can be used to optimize the radio-iodine uptake is a short course of lithium therapy.[14] Lithium augments radio-iodine retention by thyroid cells, so administration of lithium before radio-iodine treatment can enhance the absorbed radiation dose delivered to the thyroid tissue. Pretreatment with lithium is particularly helpful for tumors that are not iodine avid, including less well differentiated papillary and follicular thyroid cancer, Hürthle cell carcinoma, the tall-cell variant of papillary thyroid carcinoma, and thyroid tumors in older patients

A diagnostic radio-iodine whole-body scan is frequently done prior to the ablation therapy; this scan is useful for the localization of uptake (Figures 19–1, 19–2). The activity of radio-iodine administered ranges from 2 to 5 mCi. Areas of uptake can be demonstrated more effectively with higher doses; however, higher doses are not recommended as they can lead to a decreased capacity of the thyroid cells to take up the subsequent therapeutic radio-iodine dose, a phenomenon called "stunning."[15-17] A way to permit higher radio-iodine doses without the risk of stunning is to use [123]I instead of [131]I as [123]I delivers a minimal radiation dose.

No consensus has been reached as to the optimal required dose of radio-iodine for the ablation of residual thyroid tissue. The doses of [131]I used for ablation of remnant thyroid tissue range from 30 mCi to 150 mCi.[17] At our institution, a typical dose used to ablate residual thyroid tissue in the thyroid bed area is 100 mCi (Figure 19–1). Some physicians have used a 29-mCi dose, the major benefit of which is that it can be administered on an outpatient basis. The 29-mCi dose is believed to result in successful ablation when the radio-iodine uptake is less than 5%;[7,17-19] however, larger studies are needed to establish the long-term efficacy of this dose. Maxon et al found that 56% of patients who received [131]I activities of up to 30 mCi and 86% of patients who received at least 100 mCi had successful ablation after the first treatment.[20] Another critical factor in achieving a successful ablation is the amount of residual thyroid tissue. Arad et al showed that 28% of patients with large thyroid remnants (patients who had undergone hemithyroidectomy) and 80% of patients with small thyroid remnants had

successful ablation after a mean single dose of 141 mCi of [131]I.[21] Therefore, patients in whom ablation is indicated should have a near-total thyroidectomy. Another benefit of a smaller thyroid remnant is the lower frequency of post-treatment radiation thyroiditis, a common complication seen in patients with large remnants.

## USE OF RADIO-IODINE WHOLE-BODY SCANS FOR LONG-TERM FOLLOW-UP

In addition to lowering the recurrence rate, another value of radio-iodine ablation of postsurgical thyroid remnants is that this procedure clearly improves the value of the follow-up radio-iodine whole-body scan, and makes serial serum thyroglobulin measurements useful.[16,22] After radio-iodine ablation, patients with differentiated thyroid cancer are started on thyroid suppression therapy with levothyroxine, and are followed with serum thyroglobulin measurements, thyroid function tests, sonography of the neck, and chest roentgenography. For the first 2 years the follow-up visits are performed every 3 to 6 months depending on the severity of the case. The first follow-up [131]I whole-body scan is performed 6 to 12 months after the ablation therapy. Afterwards, [131]I whole-body scans may be repeated annually until at least two negative scans have been obtained. A recent study of the predictive value of annual scanning showed that the 10-year recurrence-free survival rate was greater than 95% in patients with two consecutive negative scans and only 90% in patients with one negative scan.[23]

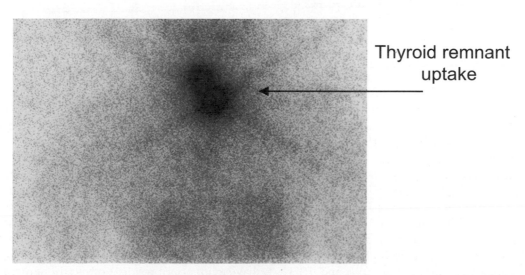

Thyroid remnant uptake

**Figure 19–1.** A 20-year-old patient with papillary thyroid carcinoma who presented to our institution after undergoing a near total thyroidectomy. The pathology revealed a 2.8-cm, multifocal papillary thyroid carcinoma. This figure shows a post-thyroidectomy diagnostic [131]I scan revealing a significant amount of thyroid tissue in the thyroid bed area. This patient received 100 mCI of [131]I for ablation of thyroid remnant.

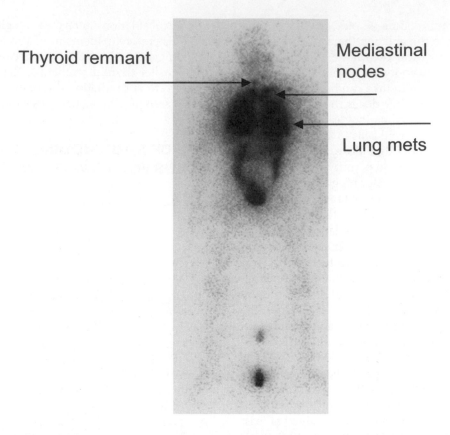

Thyroid remnant

Mediastinal nodes

Lung mets

**Figure 19–2.** A 30-year-old male who presented with a 6-year history of a neck mass. The fine needle aspiration biopsy was consistent with papillary thyroid carcinoma. The patient underwent a total thyroidectomy and bilateral cervical and mediastinal lymph node dissection. The [131]I diagnostic scan revealed faint uptake in the thyroid bed area and significant uptake in the mediastinum and both lungs. The preoperative chest roentgenography revealed a 0.7-cm nodule in the left upper lung and computed tomography of the chest (performed without iodinated contrast) revealed bilateral micronodular metastatic disease. This patient was treated with 200 mCI of [131]I.

Similar to the case for patients undergoing whole-body scanning prior to radio-iodine ablation, patients undergoing follow-up whole-body scanning need to have a TSH level of more than 30 mμ/ml. This can be accomplished by thyroid hormone withdrawal or by administration of recombinant human TSH (rhTSH).[24] Most patients, especially those with no evidence of recurrent or residual disease and with serum thyroglobulin levels of less than 5 ng/ml during levothyroxine therapy, can be prepared with rhTSH injections.[25,26] Recombinant human TSH is given at a dose of 0.9 mg intramuscularly for 2 days. On the third day, [131]I is given at a dose of 2 to 5 mCi. The whole-body scan is performed 48 hours later. Serum thyroglobulin and TSH levels are measured on the same day of the whole-body scan.[25,26] Patients with positive uptake on a rhTSH-stimulated radio-iodine scan should undergo thyroid hormone withdrawal before radio-iodine therapy be

cause the efficacy of rhTSH compared with thyroid hormone withdrawal in preparation for treatment of residual thyroid cancer has not yet been established.[25] At our institution, the doses of [131]I given for treatment of residual or recurrent disease are as follows: thyroid bed uptake, 100–150 mCi; uptake in cervical lymph nodes or lungs, 150 mCi; and bone metastases, 200 mCi.

The significant benefit of rhTSH is that it spares patients from symptoms of hypothyroidism. However, [131]I scans performed after rhTSH stimulation are somewhat less sensitive than those obtained after thyroid hormone withdrawal.[27,28] Therefore, patients who are expected to require radio-iodine therapy, patients who have evidence of residual or recurrent disease detected by other imaging modalities, and patients with a serum thyroglobulin level greater than 5 ng/ml should be prepared with thyroid hormone withdrawal rather than with rhTSH stimulation.[27]

## RADIO-IODINE TREATMENT OF METASTATIC DISEASE

The frequency of distant metastases in patients with differentiated thyroid cancer is reported to be between 7% and 23%.[2-4] The most common sites of metastatic disease are the lungs, bone, and brain. Lung involvement is more frequent in papillary thyroid carcinoma, while bone involvement is more common in follicular thyroid carcinoma.[28] Patients with distant metastases have a high risk of disease-related morbidity and mortality.

Treatment of distant metastases in patients with differentiated thyroid cancer usually involves different modalities, including surgical resection, radio-iodine treatment, thyroid hormone suppression, external radiotherapy, and, less commonly, systemic chemotherapy.[29] Radio-iodine treatment of distant metastases has been proven to reduce morbidity and prolong survival. However, the efficacy of therapy depends on the size and location of the metastatic lesions and on their ability to take up iodine. Important prognostic indicators of outcome include not only the radio-iodine uptake by the metastases but also the patient's age at diagnosis of distant metastases, the extent of tumor involvement (involvement of single vs. multiple organ sites) and, in the case of lung metastases, the pattern of lung involvement.[29-32] The chance for cure is greatest in the case of micronodular diffuse lung metastases revealed only by the [131]I whole-body scan and not by chest roentgenography or computed tomography. However, the reported cure rates for these lesions range from 15% to 80%.[28,31,33-35] One possible explanation for the poor cure rates is that lesions not detected by computed tomography are usually smaller than 3 mm, and lesions that small are unable to concentrate the radio-iodine long enough to be destroyed. Children with diffuse, micronodular lung involvement tend to have a very good prognosis.[36]

In the case of bone metastases from follicular thyroid carcinoma, radio-iodine therapy is rarely curative but can provide significant pain relief and can result in significant reduction of serum thyroglobulin levels (Figure 19–3). Cure is seen in fewer than 10% of treated patients, and partial remission is seen in just 35%.[33] The poor prognosis of patients with bone metastases is most

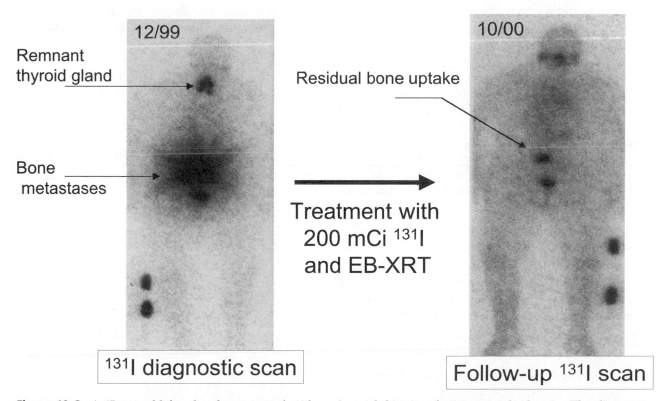

**Figure 19–3.** A-65-year-old female who presented with an 8-month history of progressive back pain. The diagnostic workup revealed a large lumbar-sacral lesion and a 7-cm neck mass. Fine needle aspiration biopsies of both lesions were consistent with follicular thyroid carcinoma. After total thyroidectomy, the [131]I scan revealed uptake in the thyroid bed area and at the lumbar-sacral spine. The patient received 200 mCI of [131]I and external radiotherapy to the lumbar-sacral lesion resulting in almost complete resolution of the back pain. Ten months later, a follow-up [131]I scan revealed residual uptake in the lumbar-sacral region and the patient received a second treatment with 200 mCI of [131]I.

likely related to the large size of the lesions and the heterogeneity of the cancer cells in terms of iodine avidity.

Few trials have attempted to determine the optimal radio-iodine dose for treatment of distant metastases; therefore, the most commonly used radio-iodine doses in patients with distant metastases from differentiated thyroid cancer are derived mainly from the available experience. Common doses used for distant metastatic disease range between 150 mCi (for pulmonary metastases) and 200 mCi (for bone metastases) (Figures 19–2, 19–3). An alternative method is to deliver the largest tolerable dose, which is based on dosimetric analysis of a tracer dose.[37] This approach is expensive, cumbersome, and of unclear long-term benefit and is used in only a few centers. The dose given ranges from 200 to 500 mCi and is intended to deliver no more than 200 cGy to the red marrow with 80 to 120 mCi of whole-body retention.

## TREATMENT OF SCAN-NEGATIVE, THYROGLOBULIN-POSITIVE METASTATIC THYROID CANCER

Approximately 15% to 20% of patients with differentiated thyroid cancer have an elevated serum thyroglobulin level but no uptake detected by [131]I whole-body scan.[6,29] One option for these patients is empirical treatment with high doses (100–300 mCi) of [131]I. A significant percentage of patients treated this way have metastatic foci revealed by the post-treatment whole-body scan. Several authors have reported that this approach not only increases the sensitivity of whole-body scans for the detection of previously unrecognized metastases but also may have a therapeutic effect, reflected by a reduction in serum thyroglobulin level and decreased radio-iodine uptake on subsequent scans.[38-41] However, the validity of this form of therapy is still questionable. The available studies have shown its potential short-term benefits, but this therapy exposes patients to significant radiation, and it is still unclear how beneficial the therapy will be in decreasing morbidity and improving long-term survival.[10,29]

## ARTIFACTS IN RADIO-IODINE SCANS

Radio-iodine scans are quite specific to the thyroid tissue which is able to concentrate, organify, and store [131]I. However, in rare cases, [131]I scans reveal nonthyroid foci of uptake. This topic was recently reviewed by Shapiro et al.[42] In this review, the authors discuss the various artifacts, anatomic and physiologic variants, and nonthyroidal diseases that can lead to a false-positive result on a whole-body scan (Table 19–2). Common nonthyroidal areas of uptake (physiologic variants) include tissues that concentrate [131]I but do not retain it in the organic form (eg, salivary glands, nasopharynx, stomach, and choroid plexus). Other organs typically seen on whole-body scans are the kidneys, liver, gut, and bladder, which are part of the excretion pathway for [131]I. Other

**Table 19–2.** Reported artifacts in radio-iodine scans

---

**Ectopic normal thyroid tissue** (lingual thyroid, high cervical thyroid, paracardiac thyroid [struma cordis], thyroglossal duct, esophageal and intratracheal thyroid, ovarian thyroid [struma ovarii], intrahepatic thyroid tissue).

**Nonthyroidal physiologic uptakes** (salivary gland; nasal, gastric, and bowel mucosa; choroid plexus; urinary tract; heart and great vessels; nonlactating and lactating breast tissue; liver and gallbladder; lacrimal gland).

**Contamination by body secretions** (urine, saliva, nasal and respiratory secretions, sweat, vomit, breast milk, tears).

**Uptake by ectopic gastric mucosa** (Meckel's diverticulum, hiatus hernia, gastric pull-through, Barrett's esophagus, gastric duplication cysts).

**Other gastrointestinal abnormalities** (Zenker's diverticulum, stricture of esophagus, achalasia, poorly dissolved [131]I capsule with esophageal retention, gastroesophageal reflux, constipation).

**Urinary tract abnormalities** (hydronephrosis, renal cysts, urinary tract fistula, atonic bladder, ectopic or transplanted kidney).

**Mammary abnormalities** (unilateral mammary hypertrophy, supernumerary breast, asymmetric lactation, lactational duct cyst).

**Uptake in serous cavities and cysts** (pericardial effusion, scrotal hydrocele, lymphoepithelial cysts, ovarian cysts, pleuropericardial cysts).

**Uptake in sites of inflammation or infection** (pericarditis, skin burn, pulmonary bronchiectasis, pulmonary fungal infection, sinusitis, psoriatic plaques, folliculitis, infected sebaceous cysts, sialoadenitis, recent myocardial infarction).

**Uptake by nonthyroidal neoplasms** (meningioma, gastric adenocarcinoma, salivary adenocarcinoma, ovarian adenocarcinoma, ovarian cystadenoma, ovarian teratoma, uterine fibromyoma, abdominal neurilemoma, lung cancer)

---

Modified from Shapiro et al.[42]

potential and misleading artifacts can arise from contamination by secretions such as saliva, urine, nasal secretions, sweat, vomit, and breast milk. Therefore, patients should always be imaged dressed in a clean gown, and in the case of suspected contamination, the whole-body scan should be repeated after an attempt has been made to clean the potential contamination site.

## ACUTE AND LONG-TERM COMPLICATIONS OF RADIO-IODINE THERAPY

The most common complication of [131]I treatment is acute radiation thyroiditis. The thyroiditis varies from transient, mild neck tenderness to prolonged, severe neck pain requiring treatment with nonsteroidal anti-inflammatory drugs. The severity and frequency depend mostly on the size of the thyroid remnant (see second section). Sialoadenitis is another frequent acute complication of [131]I therapy that occurs in 8% to 33% of cases.[43-45] It is caused by irradiation of the salivary glands, which results in tissue inflammation, obstruction of the salivary flow, and a change in the composition of the saliva. A significant percentage of patients with sialoadenitis develop chronic impairment of salivary gland function, and a few can develop complete xerostomia.[43] One simple measure to protect salivary function is to have patients suck on sour candies during the immediate post-therapy period, which increases salivary flow and thus has the potential to decrease the duration of iodine retention. Amifostine, an organic thiophosphate, is a cytoprotective agent that accumulates in the salivary glands following intravenous administration. Because of its properties, it has been studied in patients with differentiated thyroid cancer who undergo radio-iodine treatment.[46,47] In one study, 50 patients with differentiated thyroid cancer were assessed by quantitative salivary gland scintigraphy, before and 3 months after therapy.[47] Twenty-five patients received amifostine, and 25 received saline and served as controls. Amifostine-treated patients maintained normal salivary function, while saline-treated patients had a significant reduction in salivary function (40%). The data are promising, but larger trials with longer follow-up will be necessary to confirm the benefits of amifostine. In addition, concerns about the effect of amifostine on iodine uptake by thyroid cancer cells will need to be addressed.

Other common and transient symptoms of radio-iodine therapy related to radiation sickness include nausea, vomiting, headache, and malaise. Leukopenia and thrombocytopenia can occur in up to 10% of patients and can last up to 1 year.[48] Oligospermia or azoospermia can occur in up to 70% of patients; this condition is transient but can last up to 4 years.[45,49,50] Transient ovarian failure in women has also been reported.[51] Other more serious complications include a slight but real increase in the risk of developing other malignancies such as leukemia, breast cancer, and bladder cancer.[52,53] The risk is higher in patients who receive larger cumulative doses of [131]I (usually higher than 600 mCi).[52] In patients treated repeatedly for diffuse pulmonary metastases, another possible complication of [131]I therapy is radiation-induced pulmonary fibrosis.[54] Therefore, patients with known iodine-avid pulmonary metastases should always have a pretreatment pulmonary function test. Significantly decreased pulmonary function should be considered a contraindication to further [131]I therapy.

## References

1. Becker DV, Sawin CT. Radioiodine and thyroid disease: the beginning. *Semin Nucl Med.* 1995;26:155–164.
2. Mazzaferri EL, Jhiang SM. Long-term impact of initial surgical and medical therapy on papillary and follicular thyroid cancer. *Am J Med.* 1994;97:418–428.
3. Samaan NA, Schultz PM, Hickey RC, Goepfert H, Haynie TP, Johnston DA. The results of various modalities of treatment of well-differentiated thyroid carcinoma: a retrospective review of 1599 patients. *J Clin Endocrinol Metab.* 1992;75:714–720.
4. DeGroot LJ, Kaplan EL, McCormick M, Straus FH. Natural history, treatment, and course of papillary thyroid carcinoma. *J Clin Endocrinol Metab.* 1990;71:414–424.
5. Treseler PA, Clark OH. Prognostic factors in thyroid carcinoma. *Surg Oncol Clin North Am.* 1997;6:555–598.
6. Pacini F, DeGroot LJ. Thyroid neoplasia. In: DeGroot LJ, Jameson JL, eds. *Endocrinology.* Philadelphia, PA: WB Saunders Company; 2001:1541–1566.
7. Sherman SI, Gillenwater AM, Goepfert H. Advances in the management of cancer of the thyroid gland. *Adv Otolaryngol Head Neck Surg.* 2000;14:75–105.
8. Bi J, Lu B. Advances in the diagnosis and management of thyroid neoplasms. *Curr Opin Oncol.* 2000;12:54–59.
9. Krausz Y, Uziely B, Karger H, Isacson R, Catane R, Glaser B. Recurrence-associated mortality in patients with differentiated thyroid carcinoma. *J Surg Oncol.* 1993;52:164–168.
10. Wartofsky L, Sherman SI, Gopal J, Schlumberger M, Hay ID. Therapeutic controversy. The use of radioactive iodine in patients with papillary and follicular thyroid cancer. *J Clin Endocrinol Metab.* 1998;83:4195–4199.
11. Schlumberger M. Medical progress: papillary and follicular thyroid carcinoma. *N Engl J Med.* 1998;338:297–306.
12. Vermiglio F, Violi MA, Finocchiaro MD, et al. Short-term effectiveness of low-dose radioiodine ablative treatment of thyroid remnants after thyroidectomy for differentiated thyroid cancer. *Thyroid.* 1999;9: 387–391.
13. Lakshmanan M, Schaffer A, Robbins J, et al. A simplified low iodine diet in I-131 scanning and therapy of thyroid cancer. *Clin Nucl Med.* 1988;13: 866–868.
14. Koong SS, Reynolds JC, Movius EG, et al. Lithium as a potential adjuvant to 131 I therapy of metastatic, well-differentiated thyroid carcinoma. *J Clin Endocrinol Metab.* 1999;84:912–916.
15. Muratet JP, Daver A, Minier JF, et al. Influence of scanning doses of iodine-131 on subsequent first ablative treatment outcome in

patients operated on for differentiated thyroid carcinoma. *J Nucl Med.* 1988;39:1546–1550.

16. Sherman SI, Tielens ET, Sostre S, Wharam MD, Ladenson PW. Clinical utility of posttreatment radioiodine scans in the management of patients with thyroid carcinoma. *J Clin Endocrinol Metab.* 1994;78:629–634.

17. Park HM, Park YH, Zhou XH. Detection of thyroid remnant/metastasis without stunning: an ongoing dilemma. *Thyroid.* 1997;7:277–280.

18. Bal C, Padhy AK, Jana S, et al. Prospective randomized clinical trial to evaluate the optimal dose of 131 I for remnant ablation in patients with differentiated thyroid carcinoma. *Cancer.* 1996;77:2574–2580.

19. Samuel AM, Rajashekharrao B. Radioiodine therapy for well-differentiated thyroid cancer: a quantitative dosimetric evaluation for remnant thyroid ablation after Surgery. *J Nucl Med.* 1994;35:1944–1950.

20. Maxon, HR, Englaro EE, Thomas SR, et al. Radioiodine-131 therapy for well-differentiated thyroid cancer—a quantitative radiation dosimetric approach: outcome and validation in 85 patients. *J Nucl Med.* 1992;33:1132–1136.

21. Arad E, O'Mara RR, Wilson GA. Ablation of remaining functioning thyroid lobe with radioidine after hemithyroidectomy for carcinoma. *Clin Nucl Med.* 1993;18:662–663.

22. Roelants V, De Nayer P, Bouckaert A, Beckers C. The predictive value of serum thyroglobulin in the follow-up of differentiated thyroid cancer. *Eur J Nucl Med.* 1997;24:722–727.

23. Grigsby PW, Baglan K, Siegel BA. Surveillance of patients to detect recurrent thyroid carcinoma. *Cancer.* 1999;85:945–951.

24. Meier CA, Braverman LE, Ebner SA, et al. Diagnostic use of recombinant human thyrotropin in patients with thyroid carcinoma (phase I/II study). *J Clin Endocrinol Metab.* 1994;78:188–196.

25. Ladenson PW. Recombinant human thyrotropin symposium. Strategies for thyrotropin use to monitor patients with treated thyroid carcinoma. *Thyroid.* 1999;9:429–433.

26. Mazzaferri EL. Recombinant human thyrotropin symposium. An overview of the management of papillary and follicular thyroid carcinoma. *Thyroid.* 1999;9:421–427.

27. Haugen BR, Pacini F, Reiners C, et al. A comparison of recombinant human thyrotropin and thyroid hormone withdrawal for the detection of thyroid remnant or cancer. *J Clin Endocrinol Metab.* 1999;84:3877–3885.

28. Ladenson PW, Braverman LE, Mazzaferri EL, et al. Comparison of administration of recombinant human thyrotropin with withdrawal of thyroid hormone for radioactive iodine scanning in patients with thyroid carcinoma. *N Engl J Med.* 1997;337:888–896.

29. Ruegemer JJ, Hay ID, Bergstralh EJ, Ryan J J, Offord KP, Gorman CA. Distant metastases in differentiated thyroid carcinoma: a multivariate analysis of prognostic variables. *J Clin Endocrinol Metab.* 1988;67:501–508.

30. Sherman SI. The management of metastatic differentiated thyroid carcinoma. *Reviews in Endocrine & Metabolic Disorders.* 2000;1:165–171.

31. Schlumberger M, Tubiana M, De Vathaire F, et al. Long-term results of treatment of 283 patients with lung and bone metastases from differentiated thyroid carcinoma. *J Clin Endocrinol Metab.* 1986;63:960–967.

32. Massin J-P, Savoie J-C, Garnier H, Guiraudon G, Leger FA, Bacourt F. Pulmonary metastases in differentiated thyroid carcinoma. Study of 58 cases with implications for the primary tumor treatment. *Cancer.* 1984;53:982–992.

33. Hoie J, Stenwig AE, Kullmann G, Lindegaard M. Distant metastases in papillary thyroid cancer. A review of 91 patients. *Cancer.* 1988;61:1–6.

34. Vassilopoulou-Sellin R, Delpassand E S. Follicular thyroid cancer: clinical outcome and impact of radioiodine therapy in patients with distant metastases. *Int J Oncol.* 1996;8:969–976.

35. Sisson JC, Giordano TJ, Jamadar DA, et al. 131-I treatment of micronodular pulmonary metastases from papillary thyroid carcinoma. *Cancer.* 1996;78:2184–2192.

36. Samaan NA, Schultz PN, Haynie TP, Ordonez NO. Pulmonary metastasis of differentiated thyroid carcinoma: treatment results in 101 patients. *J Clin Endocrinol Metab.* 1985;65:376–380.

37. Maxon HR, Thomas SR, Samaratunga RC. Dosimetric considerations in the radioiodine treatment of macrometastases and micrometastases from differentiated thyroid cancer. *Thyroid.* 1997;7:183–187.

38. Pacini F, Lippi F, Formica N, et al. Therapeutic doses of iodine-131 reveal undiagnosed metastases in thyroid cancer patients with detectable serum thyrogobulin levels. *J Nucl Med.* 1987;28:1888–1891.

39. Pineda JD, Lee T, Ain K, Reynolds JC, Robbins J. Iodine-131 therapy for thyroid cancer patients with elevated thyroglobulin and negative diagnostic scan. *J Clin Endocrinol Metab.* 1995;80:1488–1492.

40. Schlumberger M, Arcangioli O, Piekarski JD, Tubiana M, Permentier C. Detection and treatment of lung metastases of differentiated thyroid carcinoma in patients with normal chest x-rays. *J Nucl Med.* 1988;29:1790–1794.

41. Fatourechi V, Hay ID. Treating the patient with differentiated thyroid cancer with thyroglobulin-positive iodine-131 diagnostic scan-negative metastases: including comments on the role of serum thyroglobulin monitoring in tumor surveillance. *Semin Nucl Med.* 2000;30:107–114.

42. Shapiro B, Rufini V, Jarwan A, et al. Artifacts, anatomical and physiological variants, and unrelated diseases that might cause false-positive whole-body 131-I scans in patients with thyroid cancer. *Semin Nucl Med.* 2000;2:115–132.

43. DiRusso G, Kern KA. Comparative analysis of complications from I-131 radioablation for well-differentiated thyroid cancer. *Surgery.* 1994;116:1024–1030.

44. Alexander C, Bader JB, Schaefer A, Finke C, Kirsch CM. Intermediate and long-term side effects of high-dose radioiodine therapy for thyroid carcinoma. *J Nucl Med.* 1998;39:1551–1554.

45. Maxon HR III. The role of 131 I in the treatment of thyroid cancer. *Thyroid Today.* 1993;16:1–9.

46. Bohuslavizki KH, Brenner W, Klutmann S, et al. Radioprotection of salivary glands by amifostine in high-dose radioiodine therapy. *J Nucl Med.* 1998;39:1237–1242.

47. Bohuslavizki KH, BrennerW, Klutmann S, Mester J, Henze E, Clausen M. Salivary gland protection by amifostine in high-dose radioiodine treatment: results of a double-blind placebo-controlled study. *J Clin Oncol.* 1998;16:3542–3549.

48. Keldsen N, Mortensen BT, Hansen HS. Haematological effects from radioiodine treatment of thyroid carcinoma. *Acta Oncol.* 1990;29:1035–1039.

49. Ahmed SR, Shalet SM. Gonadal damage due to radioactive iodine (131 I) treatment for thyroid carcinoma. *Postgrad Med J.* 1985;61:361–362.

50. Pacini F, Gasperi M, Fugazzolam L, et al. Testicular function in patients with differentiated thyroid cancer treated with radioactive iodine *J Nucl Med.* 1994;35:1418.

51. Raymond JP, Izembart M, Marliac V, et al. Temporary ovarian failure in thyroid cancer patients after thyroid remnant ablation with radioactive iodine. *J Clin Endocrinol Metab.* 1989;69:186–190.

52. Edmonds CJ, Smith T. The long-term harzards of the treatment of thyroid cancer with radioiodine. *Br J Radiol.* 1986;59:45.

53. Vassilopoulou-Sellin R, Palmer L, Taylor S, et al. Incidence of breast carcinoma in women with thyroid carcinoma. *Cancer.* 1999;85:696–705.

54. Rall JE, Alpers JB, Lewalleu CG, et al. Radiation pneumonitis and fibrosis: a complication of radioiodine treatment of pulmonary metastases from cancer of the thyroid. *J Clin Endocrinol Metab.* 1957;17:1263.

# 20

# Management of Locally Invasive Thyroid Carcinoma

## Michael Friedman, M.D.

## INTRODUCTION

The relatively benign nature of well-differentiated thyroid carcinoma has led to the misconception that incomplete resection of the tumor may be adequate treatment if complete resection would be difficult or require violation of a nearby vital structure. Of patients who eventually die of thyroid carcinoma, local recurrence with invasion of vital structures constitutes the major cause of death and is the most common postmortem finding.[1] Laryngotracheal invasion by well-differentiated thyroid carcinoma is rare, with the reported incidence ranging from 1 to 13%.[2-6] Treatment of laryngotracheal invasion in well-differentiated thyroid cancer is of great importance because of the tumor's great responsiveness to surgical therapy with possible long-term survival. We frequently treat well-differentiated thyroid carcinoma even in patients with known metastatic disease because most patients die from their local disease, and effective treatment of metastatic disease with radioiodine is more effective after eradication of the local tumor and all normal functioning thyroid tissue.

Selection of surgical procedure depends on several variables, including age of patient, cell type of tumor, extent of disease, and input from the informed patient. Procedures for eradicating thyroid carcinoma with invasion of the larynx and/or trachea include total or partial laryngectomy, circumferential tracheal resection with end-to-end anastomosis, or partial tracheal resection and reconstruction.

Shaving off the segment of involved cartilage has been associated with a high recurrence rate, and should not be performed. On the other hand, total laryngectomy is not necessary in most cases unless there is extensive laryngeal involvement.[7] Conservative or partial laryngeal and/or tracheal resection should be performed whenever possible. Conservative resection, which requires intimate knowledge of the anatomy of the larynx, involves excision of the segment of larynx or trachea that has been invaded by cancer. Friedman et al clarified the concept of subglottic laryngectomy for thyroid carcinoma and showed that up to 15 to 25% of the anterolateral cricoid cartilage can be resected without appreciable airway compromise.[7] More extensive cricoid cartilage resection requires reconstruction. In 1986, Friedman et al[8] described the sternocleidomastoid myoperiosteal flap for reconstruction of subglottic or tracheal defects. The flap incorporates clavicular periosteum. The periosteum, which receives its vascular supply from the sternocleidomastoid muscle pedicle, is used to close the tracheal defect over a stent, providing an airtight seal and eventually forming bone to provide a rigid, stable airway.

This chapter reviews our experience with the surgical treatment of thyroid carcinoma invading the trachea and/or larynx, and the application of the sternocleidomastoid myoperiosteal flap is described for reconstruction of laryngeal, subglottic, or tracheal defects after thyroid tumor resection. Long-term follow-up of these patients adds insight into the natural history of this disease process.

## PREOPERATIVE ASSESSMENT

Patients with thyroid carcinoma invading the airway present difficult diagnostic and therapeutic problems to the thyroid surgeon. Extent of disease is an important factor influencing the mode of therapy. Patients with thyroid carcinoma invading the airway may present with hemoptysis, stridor, or dyspnea, which occurs only very late in the disease. Computed tomography (CT) and magnetic resonance imaging (MRI) are extremely helpful in evaluating the extent of tumor invasion because most patients are asymptomatic.

Computed tomography scan is helpful because of its ability to define thyroid gland, tumor, and tissue planes; to identify areas of cartilage invasion without intraluminal extension; and to localize vascular structures.[9] MRI has the advantage of readily providing images in the coronal plane that provide a large-field view and demonstrate the neck, cervicothoracic junction, and mediastinum in one or two images.[10] Furthermore, MRI can identify vascular structures without the need for intravenous contrast.[11] Whenever possible, radiologic studies that require the administration of contrast should be avoided since the iodine in the contrast will prevent postoperative scanning from detecting residual or metastatic disease. When imaging the thyroid gland and the region of the thoracic inlet, shoulder artifact is not a problem with MRI as it is with CT. We feel that either CT or MRI can provide the information needed for preoperative diagnostic evaluation of thyroid tumors with tracheal invasion and postoperative follow-up.

Three basic principles of thyroid surgery are: 1) all gross tumor should be removed; 2) wide margins are not necessary; and 3) normal structures should not be sacrificed.[7] In observing these principles, the treatment of thyroid carcinoma with airway invasion proposes a surgical dilemma. A common site of airway invasion is the subglottic space, where no standard form of partial laryngectomy is applicable.[7]

In cases of obvious intraluminal involvement of the subglottic space, the surgeon has the option of performing a total laryngectomy or preserving phonation by utilizing a more conservative resection. We do not consider shaving the tumor of the trachea or larynx when there is evidence of cartilage invasion. Friedman et al showed that after shave excision there was a high recurrence rate of thyroid carcinoma that was invading the airway.[11] Most studies report the use of total laryngectomy when there is any evidence of laryngeal involvement. In 1958, Frazell et al performed total laryngectomies on 4 patients of a total of 393 cases of papillary thyroid cancer.[2] No conservation procedures were performed. Clark et al treated 218 patients, 5 of whom underwent total laryngectomy.[12] He believed that if the larynx or trachea were involved, these structures should be removed. Schindel performed total laryngectomy in 8 of 225 patients with thyroid carcino-

ma.[3] In a review of 2,000 cases, Djalilian et al noted that 7 patients underwent total laryngectomy, while only 2 patients underwent partial laryngectomy.[4] Conversely, Lawson et al believed that conservation surgery should be performed whenever possible.[13] He reported on 6 patients with airway invasion, 5 of whom had local control with conservation surgery. Most of these studies do not provide criteria for the extent of resection and the method of reconstruction.

In our series, only one patient underwent total laryngectomy.[7, 8] Subglottic invasion does not necessarily dictate that a total laryngectomy be performed rather than a subtotal subglottic resection. However, when more than 15% of the cricoid cartilage was resected, reconstruction was important to provide a stable airway.[7, 8] The goals of partial subglottic laryngectomy include complete tumor excision with clear margins, minimal functional alteration, and few complications.[7]

Patients with extensive cricoid or tracheal involvement (greater than 60% of the circumference) may require extensive resection, and primary thyrotracheal anastomosis is the preferred treatment.[7] Gerwat and Bryce[14] and Pearson et al[15] described the technique of thyrotracheal anastomosis. The larynx is stabilized, and the recurrent laryngeal nerves are protected by preserving the cricothyroid joints (if they are not invaded by tumor). If necessary, the ipsilateral recurrent laryngeal nerve can be sacrificed with minimal functional deficit. In our series, no cases required extensive resection with primary thyrotracheal anastomosis.

Tracheal invasion by thyroid carcinoma can be treated by circumferential tracheal resection with end-to-end anastomosis, partial tracheal resection, or tracheotomy for palliation. Ishihara et al treated 24 patients with thyroid carcinoma that invaded the trachea.[16] They commented on the difficulty in preserving the recurrent laryngeal nerves, and the problem of tracheal stenosis that occurred in 7 patients. Nakao et al performed tracheal resections on 12 patients with thyroid carcinoma, with two patients developing tracheal stenosis at the anastomotic site.[17] Fujimoto et al performed aggressive radical resections on 18 of 21 patients with locally invasive papillary carcinoma of the thyroid.[18] They found that patients with extensive tracheal invasion by thyroid carcinoma frequently had esophageal or mediastinal involvement. Circumferential tracheal resection with end-to-end anastomosis is difficult and requires extensive dissection of the larynx and trachea to permit a reasonable closure without tension. There is a high risk of recurrent laryngeal nerve damage, along with tracheal stenosis at the anastomotic site.

When thyroid cancer invades the trachea, it tends to grow along the trachea more readily than actually invading into the lumen. Therefore, thyroid carcinoma can advance along the trachea, invading numerous tracheal rings, along with the pharynx, esophagus, and both recurrent laryngeal nerves.[17] Esophageal invasion is extremely rare but occurs. In cases with minimal invasion, the tumor can be resected and the defect closed primarily. If there is moderate invasion, the defect can be reconstructed with a myocutaneous flap. The resectability of an invasive thyroid tumor is primarily based on the surgeon's technical ability to remove the tumor and reconstruct the defect. Patient input after discussion about the quality of life is an important consideration. Age is usually not considered a factor. Major contraindications to thyroid tumor resection include 1) massive tracheal or esophageal invasion beyond reconstructive capacity; 2) innominate artery invasion; and 3) deep invasion into the mediastinum. Carotid artery invasion is not considered a contraindication because the vessel can be ligated and resected in selected cases after appropriate preoperative assessment.

## EXTENT OF RESECTION AND METHODS OF RECONSTRUCTION

Friedman et al have previously described the sternocleidomastoid myoperiosteal flap for reconstruction of the subglottis and trachea.[8,19] The surgical technique is reviewed in Figures 20–1 and 20–2. We have used this method of reconstruction to close defects encountered after resecting thyroid carcinoma with airway invasion. At the time of thyroidectomy, the extent of laryngeal or tracheal invasion was assessed. Airway invasion of thyroid carcinoma tends to extend over the surface of the cricoid or tracheal cartilages without extending through the cartilage. In these cases we performed full-thickness excision of the involved cartilage, ensuring clear margins by frozen section histopathology whenever possible.

The different degrees of tumor invasion are demonstrated in Figure 20–3. The method of reconstruction is discussed for each case. Minimal tumor invasion of the thyroid cartilage (Figure 20–3A) required full-thickness resection of the involved cartilage but no reconstruction. When tumor invasion required resection of less than 15% of the circumference of the cricoid cartilage (Figure 20–3B), no reconstruction was necessary. If tumor invasion required resection of 15 to 35% of the cricoid cartilage (Figure 20–3C), a sternocleidomastoid myoperiosteal flap without a stent is used to reconstruct the defect. If 35 to 70% of the cricoid cartilage is resected (Figure 20–3D), a sternocleidomastoid myoperiosteal flap is used with a stent. When tumor invaded less than 30% of the circumference of the first tracheal ring, as shown in Figure 20–3E, the defect is reconstructed with a sternocleidomastoid myoperiosteal flap without a stent. Defects of the first tracheal ring are treated in a

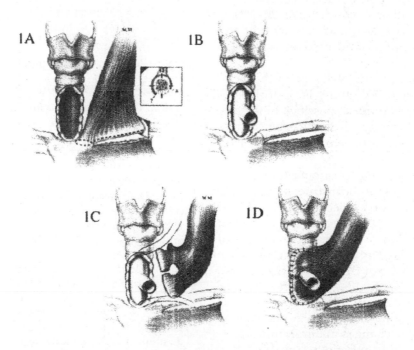

**Figure 20–1.** Sternocleidomastoid myoperiosteal flap for reconstruction of large tracheal defects. **A.** Elevation of the myoperiosteal flap off the clavicle after making incision at about the 4 o'clock position. Flap is elevated to the 7 o'clock position (see inset). **B.** A T-tube is inserted into the defect to act as an airway and a stent. **C.** The flap is fashioned to fit over the T-tube and to close the defect. **D.** Closure of the defect.

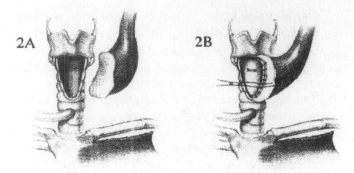

**Figure 20–2. A.** Subglottic and tracheal defect demonstrated. (Note the resection of the cricoid.) The myoperiosteal flap has been elevated. **B.** A myoperiosteal flap is fashioned to fit the defect with the stent in place.

fashion similar to cricoid defects. With anterior midline invasion of less than 30% of the circumference of the second and third tracheal rings (Figure 20–3F), the involved cartilage is excised and a tracheotomy tube is inserted into the defect. These patients are managed as any other patients with a tracheotomy, except they were decannulated in 3 to 5 days. In these cases, no flap is required for reconstruction.

When the defect is greater than 30% of the circumference of the airway but less than 6 cm in length (Figure 20–3G), a stent is used with a sternocleidomastoid myoperiosteal flap to close the defect. With tracheal defects longer than 6 cm (Figure 20–3H), a Montgomery T-tube serves as a tracheotomy tube and stent for the sternocleidomastoid myoperiosteal flap (Figure 20–1A–D).

When there is extensive involvement of the hemilarynx, a vertical hemilaryngectomy is performed to conserve as much of the larynx as possible. In the case of extensive laryngeal or subglottic invasion (greater than 50% of the laryngeal architecture), total laryngectomy is performed.

In our experience, the sternocleidomastoid myoperiosteal flap has been ideal for reconstruction of defects encountered after conservative resection of thyroid carcinoma invading the airway. The sternocleidomastoid myoperiosteal flap requires minimal dissection and provides fibrous, vascular, and autogenous periosteum that conforms to the shape of the airway (over a stent or T-tube if necessary) with tension-free closure. The periosteum has been demonstrated to form bone, which provides the rigidity necessary to maintain an adequate airway, despite changes in intraluminal pressure.[7,20] This added rigidity permits reconstruction of large defects, earlier decannulation, and superior long-term results. The myoperiosteal flap allows the surgeon to actually mold a new anterior wall out of the subglottic airway, which will resume its previous circular conformation.

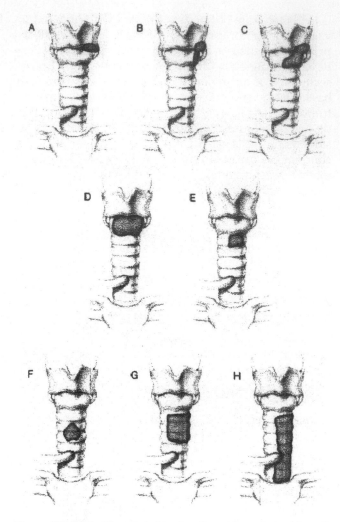

**Figure 20–3. A.** Diagram showing thyroid carcinoma invading the thyroid cartilage. A full-thickness resection of involved cartilage is performed. No reconstruction is necessary. **B.** Thyroid carcinoma invading the thyroid cartilage and less than 15% circumference of the cricoid cartilage. After resection of the involved cartilage, no reconstruction is necessary. **C.** Invasion of 15–35% of the circumference of the cricoid cartilage. After cartilage resection, a sternocleidomastoid myoperiosteal flap is used to reconstruct the defect without a stent. **D.** Invasion of 35–70% of the circumference of the cricoid cartilage. A sternocleidomastoid myoperiosteal flap with a stent is used for reconstruction. **E.** Thyroid carcinoma invading less than 30% of the circumference of the first tracheal ring. A myoperiosteal flap without a stent is used for reconstruction. The first tracheal ring is treated like the cricoid cartilage. **F.** Anterior midline invasion (less than 30% of the circumference) of the second and third tracheal rings. No flap is required for reconstruction. A tracheotomy tube is placed through the defect for 3 to 5 days. The patient is decannulated as a typical tracheotomy patient. **G.** Invasion of more than 30% of the circumference of several tracheal rings. A sternocleidomastoid myoperiosteal flap and a stent are used for reconstruction of the defect. **H.** Invasion of a segment of trachea greater than 6 cm in length. With these large defects, a T-tube is used to support the myoperiosteal flap and to provide an airway.

The only complication associated with the use of the sternocleidomastoid myoperiosteal flap is granulation tissue formation around the stent, which resolves after the stent is removed. The relative ease and effectiveness of this procedure makes it an attractive option in airway reconstruction after resection of thyroid cancer with laryngotracheal invasion.

## CONCLUSION

1. Thyroid carcinoma invading the airway can be treated in most cases by partial laryngectomy and/or partial tracheal resection.
2. Total laryngectomy or circumferential tracheal resection may be required in cases with extensive disease.
3. Full-thickness cartilage resection is necessary in cases of cartilage invasion, even when there is no evidence of intraluminal involvement.
4. The sternocleidomastoid myoperiosteal flap is a relatively simple, single-stage procedure for airtight closure of subglottic and tracheal defects.
5. The sternocleidomastoid myoperiosteal flap provides long-term airway stability with a low complication rate.
6. Conservative resection of thyroid carcinoma with airway invasion can be performed without compromising margins of resection, yielding good functional results with a low local recurrence rate.

## References

1. Silverberg S, Hutter R, Foote FW. Fatal carcinoma of the thyroid: histology, metastasis, and causes of death. *Cancer.* 1970;25:792-802.
2. Frazell E, Foote FW. Papillary cancer of the thyroid: a review of 25 years of experience. *Cancer.* 1958;11:895–921.
3. Schindel J. Surgery of malignant tumors of the thyroid gland: a review of 15 years' experience with 225 cases. *Ann Otol Rhinol Laryngol.* 1971;80:61–66.
4. Djalilian M, Beahrs O, Devine K, et al. Intraluminal involvement of the larynx and trachea by thyroid cancer. *Am J Surg.* 1974;128:500–504.
5. Breaux E, Guillamondegui O. Treatment of locally invasive carcinoma of the thyroid: how radical? *Am J Surg.* 1980;140:514–517.
6. Cody H, Shah J. Locally invasive, well-differentiated thyroid carcinoma: 22 years' experience at Memorial Sloan-Kettering Cancer Center. *Am J Surg.* 1981;142:480–483.
7. Friedman M, Shelton VK, Skolnik EM, et al. Laryngotracheal invasion by thyroid carcinoma. *Ann Otol Rhinol Laryngol.* 1982;91:363–369.
8. Friedman M, Grybauskas V, Toriumi DM, et al. Reconstruction of the subglottic larynx with a myoperiosteal flap: clinical and experimental study. *Head Neck Surg.* 1986;8:287–295.
9. Kikuchi T, Kawamura M, Nakayama M, et al. Computed tomography in thyroid carcinoma infiltrating the trachea. *Kyobu-Geka.* 1987;40:450–454.
10. Higgins CB, McNamara MT, Fisher MR, Clark OH. MR imaging of the thyroid. *Am J Radiol.* 1986;147:1255–1261.
11. Friedman M, Skolnik E, Baim H, et al. Thyroid carcinoma. *Laryngoscope.* 1980;90:1991–2003.
12. Clark RL, Ibanez M, White E. What constitutes an adequate operation for carcinoma of the thyroid? *Arch Surg.* 1966;92:23–26.
13. Lawson W, Som ML, Biller HF. Papillary adenocarcinoma of the thyroid invading the upper air passages. *Ann Otol Rhinol Laryngol.* 1977;86:751–755.
14. Gerwat J, Bryce DP. The management of subglottic laryngeal stenosis by resection and direct anastomosis. *Laryngoscope.* 1974;84:940–947.
15. Pearson FG, Cooper JD, Nelems JM, Van Nostand AWP. Primary tracheal anastomosis after resection of cricoid cartilage with preservation of the recurrent laryngeal nerves. *J Thorac Cardiovasc Surg.* 1975;70:806–816.
16. Ishihara T, Yamazaki S, Kobayashi K, et al. Resection of the trachea infiltrated by thyroid carcinoma. *Ann Surg.* 1982;195:496–500.
17. Nakow K, Miyata M, Izukura M, et al. Radical operation for thyroid carcinoma invading the trachea. *Arch Surg.* 1984;119:1046–1049.
18. Fujimoto Y, Obara T, Ito Y, et al. Aggressive surgical approach for locally invasive papillary carcinoma of the thyroid in patients over forty-five years of age. *Surgery.* 1986;100:1098–1106.
19. Friedman M, Toriumi DT, Owens R, Grybauskas VT. Experience with the sternocleidomastoid myoperiosteal flap for reconstruction of subglottic and tracheal defects: modifications of technique and report of long-term results. *Laryngoscope.* 1988;98:1003–1011.
20. Friedman M, Grybauskas V, Skolnik E, et al. The sternomastoid myoperiosteal flap for reconstruction of the subglottic larynx. *Ann Otol Rhinol Laryngol.* 1987;96:163–168.

# 21

# Lymphoma and Other Unusual Thyroid Neoplasms

Chul S. Ha, M.D.

Fernando Cabanillas, M.D.

Phillip K. Pellitteri, D.O., F.A.C.S.

## PRESENTATION AND EPIDEMIOLOGY

Lymphoma of the thyroid gland is very uncommon. Although Hodgkin's disease of the thyroid gland has been reported,[1,2] most of the lymphomas arising from the thyroid gland are non-Hodgkin's lymphoma.[3-6] It constitutes less than 2 to 3 % of non-Hodgkin's lymphoma and 2 to 8 % of all malignancies of the thyroid gland.[4-7] It occurs predominantly in females with a male:female ratio ranging from 1:14 to 1:2.[2,5,8-12] The median age at diagnosis is about 60 years with most of the diagnoses made after the 6th decade of life.[2,9,13,14] However, it has been reported in pediatric patients.[15] The most characteristic presentation is a rapidly enlarging anterior neck mass. This is often accompanied by cervical lymphadenopathy helping to raise the suspicion of malignant lymphoma. Some patients present with hoarseness, difficulty with breathing, cough and dysphagia.[1,2,7] Clinical or sub-clinical hypothyroidism is observed in 30 to 40% of the patients although hyperthyroidism has been reported.[14,16,17] Presence of Hashimoto's thyroiditis has been documented usually in association with hypothyroidism even before biopsy of the thyroid, and careful pathologic examination has documented background thyroiditis in up to 100% of the patients.[2,14,16] Anti-thyroglobulin or anti-microsomal antibodies have been detected in 30 to 100% of the patients, suggesting a relationship between autoimmune process and development of thyroid lymphoma.[14,16,18,19] Although an association of Epstein-Barr virus to the development of thyroid lymphoma has been suggested, it has not been firmly established.[20,21] Of interest, patients with Hashimoto's thyroiditis were found to have up to 67–80 fold increased risk of developing non-Hodgkin's lymphoma of the thyroid compared to the general population.[22,23]

Different definitions of primary non-Hodgkin's lymphoma of the thyroid gland have been used by different authors. Dawson proposed criteria for diagnosis of extranodal lymphoma stipulating that patients had to present with the main manifestation of their disease at an extranodal site. Lymphadenopathy, if present, could only be regional.[24] This would essentially limit the application of the terminology "primary non-Hodgkin's lymphoma of the thyroid gland" to stage I or II disease. However, some authors have included patients with stage III or IV disease as long as the patients presented with symptoms or signs associated with the thyroid gland.[10,12,25,26] In this chapter we will limit the discussion to stages I and II disease because of the concern that the lymphoma of the thyroid in stages III or IV presentations are very likely from metastatic involvement of the gland from other more common primary sites.

## DIAGNOSIS AND STAGING WORKUP

Although the majority of enlarged thyroid glands are benign and malignant lymphoma is still uncommon even among the malignant thyroid neoplasms, it should be kept in mind during evaluation of the enlarged thyroid gland to minimize misdiagnosis and to avoid unnecessary operative procedures.[5,4,18] A rapidly enlarging neck mass in the presence of Hashimoto's thyroiditis should raise a very strong suspicion for thyroid lymphoma.[27] As the majority of the thyroid neoplasms are carcinoma, an attempt at a diagnosis using a fine needle aspiration (FNA) is a reasonable initial approach in most cases, although some patients may need an emergency tracheostomy first to establish an airway. The FNA can be guided by palpation or ultrasound.[28] Although up to 80% accuracy in diagnosing lymphoma by FNA has been reported,[16] differentiation from other conditions such as thyroiditis and anaplastic carcinoma can occasionally be difficult from the limited sample obtainable from FNA.[29-31] Of note, this problem has decreased with the use of immunocytochemistry. Unless a firm diagnosis of a specific lymphoma can be established from FNA, a surgical biopsy, at least core needle biopsy or incisional biopsy, is recommended to have sufficient tissue to evaluate the growth pattern and to do immunohistochemical studies for lymphoma.[16] Once diagnosis of lymphoma is established, staging evaluation is done to define the extent of the disease. This includes history, physical examination, complete blood counts, urinalysis, electrolytes, biochemical survey including serum lactate dehydrogenase (LDH) and $\beta_2$-microglobulin, bilateral bone marrow biopsy and aspiration, chest films, computed tomography (CT) scans of abdomen and pelvis and gallium or positron emission tomography (PET) scan. Thyroid lymphoma does not take up [123]I-iodine used for thyroid scan. However, this finding is very non-specific.[16] Although ultrasound can be used to visualize the thyroid nodules and there are reports of asymmetric pseudocystic patterns found by ultrasound in more than 90% of patients with thyroid lymphoma compared with only 11% of patients with Hashimoto's thyroiditis,[16] CT scan or magnetic resonance imaging (MRI) of the neck is preferred because of certain limitations of the ultrasound such as difficulty in assessing the tumor invasion of the blood vessels, esophagus, and lymph nodes.[16,28,32,33] CT or MRI scan is also preferred to ultrasound for radiation therapy planning. The most commonly used staging system for lymphoma is Ann Arbor system, which is based on the extent of lymphatic chain involvement on each side of the diaphragm.[34] Briefly, stage I is involvement of a single lymph node region on the same side of the diaphragm, stage II is involvement of two or more lymph node regions on the same of the diaphragm, stage III is lymph node involvement on both sides of the diaphragm (and localized continuous involvement of up to one extra-lymphatic organ), and stage IV is disseminated (multi-focal) involvement of one or more

than one extra-lymphatic organ or isolated extra-lymphatic organ involvement with non-regional nodal involvement. The Ann Arbor staging system was initially developed for Hodgkin's disease and its usefulness in non-Hodgkin's lymphoma was limited because of more diffuse patterns of presentation and occurrence of extranodal non-Hodgkin's lymphoma. In the latter cases, disease arising from a primary extranodal site is considered stage I, and disease arising from regional lymph nodes involvement is considered stage II. The M.D. Anderson Cancer Center tumor score[35] and International Prognostic Index[36] for malignant lymphoma have been developed to better group the patients with intermediate and high-grade lymphoma according to prognostic categories and to develop treatment strategies accordingly. The M.D. Anderson Cancer Center tumor score assigns one point for any bulky site $\geq 7.0$ cm, Ann Arbor stage III or IV, B-symptoms, LDH $\geq 110\%$ of the upper normal limit, and $\beta_2$-microglobulin $\geq 150\%$ of the upper normal limit. This modeling has yielded two prognostic groupings. Patients in the low risk group (tumor score 0, 1, or 2) are expected to have a 3-year freedom from treatment failure of 83% compared to 24% for those in the high risk group (tumor score $\geq 3$). The tumor score has been used to stratify the patients for clinical trials at M.D. Anderson Cancer Center. The International Prognostic Index for malignant lymphoma assigns a score based on age > 60 years, Ann Arbor stage III or IV, Eastern Cooperative Oncology Group (ECOG) performance status 2, LDH > upper normal limit, and more than 1 extranodal site of involvement. This modeling yields four prognostic groupings with decreasing five-year survival with increasing IPI.

## PATHOLOGY

Grossly the cut-surface of thyroid lymphoma is usually white and smooth with relatively homogeneous appearance.[16] Microscopically the most common pathology of thyroid lymphomas per the Working Formulation, now considered obsolete by some, is diffuse large cell lymphoma (DLCL), usually accounting for more than 50% of thyroid lymphomas.[26,27] Other pathologies are follicular, diffuse small cleaved or non-cleaved, immunoblastic, and small lymphocytic lymphoma.[27] In general, most lymphomas of the thyroid gland tend to be of intermediate or high grade.[9,10,16] When the newer Revised European American Lymphoma (REAL) classification is applied, DLCL of B cell origin still appears to be the most common histologic entity.[37] Most thyroid lymphomas are of B cell origin though T cell lymphoma has been reported.[38] Isaacson et al suggested that the majority of thyroid lymphomas arise from a low-grade

MALT (mucosa associated lymphoid tissue) lymphoma only to transform into a more aggressive higher grade pathology such as DLCL during the course of the disease.[14,37,39] MALT lymphoma was first described by Isaacson et al in 1983 to describe the histologic features of low-grade B cell lymphoma of extranodal origin such as stomach, salivary gland, and thyroid.[40,41] The features are thought to recapitulate those of normal MALT tissue. These are characterized by the presence of B cell follicles, infiltration of the thyroid epithelium by B cells (so called lymphoepithelium) and plasma cell differentiation. The lymphoid tissue is thought to have accumulated through chronic antigen stimulation leading to an inflammatory process (Hashimoto's thyroiditis in case of thyroid lymphoma). It is often difficult to differentiate a lymphomatous process from the background lym-

phoid cells, which occur in chronic thyroiditis, although sometimes invasion of the wall of the blood vessels and extension outside the thyroid gland can help establish the diagnosis of lymphoma.[14] Immunohistochemistry can also help differentiate monoclonal malignant process from polyclonal reactive proliferation.[14] MALT lymphoma has been subclassified into high grade and low grade by some investigators depending on the proportion of large cell components. However, it has been proposed, for the next lymphoma classification, which will be the World Health Organization (WHO) classification, to classify primary large cell lymphoma of MALT sites as "DLCL" instead of "high grade MALT lymphoma." The term MALT lymphoma will be reserved exclusively for the low-grade lymphoma types.[42,43] Figure 21–1 demonstrates a typical DLCL of

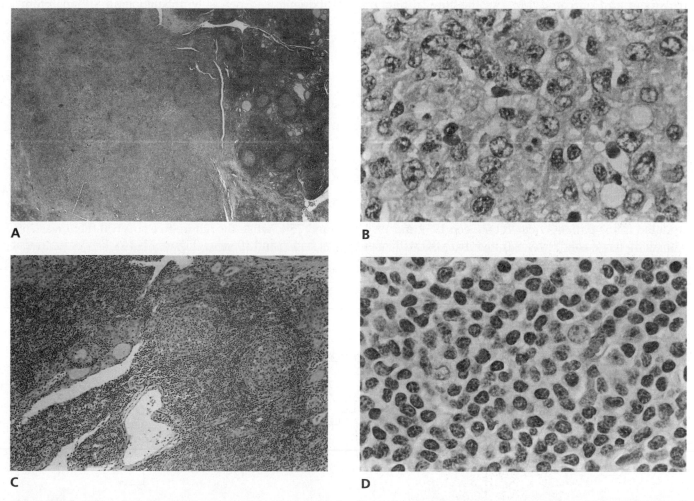

**A**   **B**   **C**   **D**

**Figure 21–1.** Diffuse large B cell lymphoma arising in thyroid gland, associated with Hashimoto's thyroiditis and low-grade B cell lymphoma of mucosa associated lymphoid tissue (MALT). **A.** Low power figure of diffuse large B cell lymphoma (left) and thyroid gland with Hashimoto's thyroiditis (right). **B.** High power figure of diffuse large B cell lymphoma. The neoplastic cells are large and noncleaved with vesicular nuclear chromatin. **C.** Low power figure of low-grade B cell lymphoma of MALT. The neoplastic cells surround reactive germinal centers in field. **D.** High power figure of low-grade MALT lymphoma. The neoplastic cells are small with round nuclei and abundant pale cytoplasm. (A, 20X; B, 400X; C, 200X; D, 400X) (Photo courtesy of L. Jeffrey Medeiros, M.D.)

the thyroid arising from the background of Hashimoto's thyroiditis and MALT lymphoma. One of the major morphologic differential diagnoses of thyroid lymphoma is small cell and anaplastic carcinoma.[14] Although anaplastic carcinoma has marked cellular pleomorphism compared to lymphoma, it is essential to run immunohistochemical studies using a battery of lymphoid markers to make the diagnosis of lymphoma and further classify it to tailor the treatment accordingly.

## TREATMENT AND PROGNOSIS

The treatment decision should be based on the pathology and prognostic factors. As most non-Hodgkin's lymphomas of the thyroid gland are DLCL, and as other types are very uncommon, most reports tend to combine all the pathologies together to present the data on treatment and outcome. Most of the clinical data on thyroid lymphoma are from retrospective analyses, making direct comparisons of the treatment modalities or prognostic factors difficult because of the inherent patient selection biases and evolving treatment philosophy. The treatments and their outcomes by different pathologies are summarized below.

### Intermediate Grade Lymphoma

The treatment outcome of Ann Arbor stage I and II thyroid lymphoma treated at M.D. Anderson cancer Center was previously reported[44] and has been recently updated for 51 patients treated between 1959 and 1994. The median age was 59 years (range 16 to 84) with male to female ratio of 18:33. The Ann Arbor stages were: I—21 patients, II—30 patients. International Prognostic Index (IPI) was known for 43 patients (0—16 patients, ≥ 1—27 patients). Fifteen patients had mediastinal involvement.

Forty seven (92%) of the 51 patients had intermediate or high grade lymphomas per the Working Formulation. Diffuse large cell lymphoma (n=35, 69%) was most common. Other pathologies were follicular and diffuse large cell (n=4), diffuse small noncleaved cell (n=2), and follicular large cell (n=2) lymphomas. One of each of the following pathologies was also identified: small lymphocytic, diffuse mixed, lymphoblastic, immunoblastic, follicular small cleaved, follicular mixed, and large cell (not otherwise specified) lymphoma. One patient's slides were not available for reclassification. Forty-one patients (80%) had the abdomen evaluated by computed tomography of the abdomen and pelvis, lymphangiogram or laparotomy. The treatments were: thyroidectomy alone—4, radiation therapy alone (XRT)—18, chemotherapy alone—5, combined modality therapy (CMT) with chemotherapy and radiation therapy—24. A doxorubicin-containing regimen was used in 26 of the 29 patients with a median of 7 cycles. Radiation therapy was either modified mantle or involved field at a median dose of 42 Gy in 21 fractions.

At a median follow-up of 10 years (range 1 month–26 years), the overall survival (OS) of the entire patient population was 64% at 5 years and 49% at 10 years, with the corresponding cause-specific survival (excluding death unrelated to lymphoma) rates of 75% and 75%, while the failure-free survival (FFS) was 76% at both 5 and 10 years (Figure 21–2A). FFS by treatment

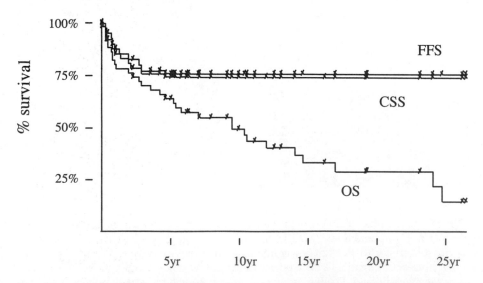

**Figure 21–2A.** Overall survival (OS), failure-free survival (FFS), and cause-specific survival (CSS) for the entire patient population.

regimen were: 76% for XRT, 50% for chemotherapy and 91% for CMT at both 5 and 10 years (p=0.15) (Figure 21–2 B).

Among the five variables (treatment modality, gender, IPI, Ann Arbor stage, and mediastinal involvement) analyzed for significance in terms of OS, IPI was the only factor statistically significant. The 5-year OS was 86% and 50% for IPI of 0 and ≥ 1, respectively (p=0.022). None of the 5 variables analyzed for significance in terms of FFS was statistically significant, although the 5-year FFS was 93% and 68% for IPI of 0 and ≥ 1, respectively (p= 0.08). Eleven patients failed treatment. Of the ten patients whose details of relapse are known, nine had a component of distant failure across the diaphragm, mainly in the abdomino-pelvic cavity. Only two patients were salvaged with additional treatments with chemotherapy with or without radiation therapy. It also appears from the literature that the gastrointestinal tract is a common site of failure for thyroid lymphoma[14] although there are data indicating otherwise.[8] Table 21–1 summarizes the major findings of the studies on thyroid lymphoma reported in the literature since 1985 which contained more than 30 patients. Although there have been reports favoring the role of debulking surgery, especially for the patients who have disease limited to the thyroid, surgical resection alone is not recommended in the management of intermediate or high grade lymphoma because of the propensity to fail in distant sites.[7,31,45] There may be a subgroup of patients who do well with radiation therapy alone. These are probably the patients with localized disease without any adverse prognostic factors such as high IPI. However, doxorubicin based combination chemotherapy with or without radiation therapy is considered a standard treatment for the management of DLCL in

general. It is also possible in patients with favorable presentations to use only three courses of cyclophosphamide, doxorubicin, vincristine, and prednisone (CHOP) chemotherapy and then consolidative radiation therapy.[46] The role of involved field radiation therapy for patients treated with combination chemotherapy has been well established by two prospective randomized clinical trials by the Southwest Oncology Group[46] and Eastern Cooperative Oncology Group[47] in terms of improved OS and FFS.

## Lymphomas with Background Evidence of MALT

Laing et al reported 45 patients with stage I and II non-Hodgkin's lymphoma of the thyroid gland.[48] Thirty-one patients had evidence of tumor origin from MALT and 14 did not. The overall cause-specific survival at 5 and 10 years in patients with evidence of tumor origin from MALT was 90% compared with 55% in 5 years for patients without such evidence (p=0.003). The complete response rate among 39 patients who were treated with radiation therapy alone initially was 97% with disease-free survival rate at 5 years of 67%. There was a trend for a more favorable relapse-free survival in patients with tumor with evidence of MALT lymphoma. Although there are a very limited number of reports on MALT lymphoma without evidence of DLCL of the thyroid gland, each with a very small number of patients, it appears that patients with MALT lymphoma can be managed well with loco-regional therapy alone such as thyroidectomy or radiation therapy.[37,49] However, given the concern about microscopic residual disease and surgical complications from thyroidectomy

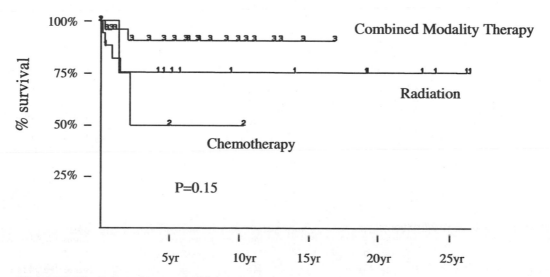

**Figure 21–2B.** Failure-free survival by treatment regimen.

**Table 21–1.** Summary of studies on thyroid lymphoma

| Author | Patients | Treatments | Outcomes |
|---|---|---|---|
| Laing[48] (1968–1990) pub. 1994 British National Lymphoma Investigation and Royal Marsden Hospital, UK | 45 Patients 37 Stage 1 8 Stage 2 | XRT 39 CMT 4 Chemo 1 Surgery 1 | 5 yr CCS 79% (31 patients with evidence of tumor origin from MALT— 5 yr CSS 90% 14 patients without evidence of tumor origin form MALT— 5 yr CSS 55%) |
| Logue[11] (1965–1983) pub. 1992 Christie Hospital and Holt Radium Institute, UK | 70 Patients 32 Stage 1 38 Stage 2 | XRT 68 CMT 2 | 5 yr survival corrected for death from intercurrent dz—49% (Stage 1 68% Stage 2 36%) |
| Pedersen[19] (1983–1991) pub. 1996 Odense University Hospital, Denmark | 38 Patients. 26 Stage 1 12 Stage 2 | not reported | 5 yr CCS: Stage 1 – 57% Stage 2 – 50% |
| Tupchong[2] (1948–1980) pub.1986 Royal Marsden Hospital, UK | 46 Patients. 24 Stage 1 22 Stage 2 | XRT 40 Surgery 2 CMT 4 | 5 yr OS 40% |
| Blair[26] (1965–1979) pub. 1985 Mayo Clinic, Rochester, USA | 38 Patients 20 Stage 1 14 Stage 2 1 Stage 3 1 Stage 4 2 Unstaged | XRT 31 CMT 7 | 5 yr OS—57% 5 yr DFS—59% for all 38 patients |
| Tsang[25] (1978–1986) pub. 1993 Princess Margaret Hospital, Canada | 52 Patients 16 Stage 1 28 Stage 2 8 Stage 3 or 4 | 5 patients treated as anaplastic CA of thyroid and excluded. Among 39 stage 1 & 2 XRT 18 CMT 18 Chemo 3 | 5 yr OS—64% 5 yr RFS—66% for 39 patients with stage 1 and 2 dz |
| Pledge[10] (1973–1992) pub. 1996 Nottinghamshire Lymphoma Registry, UK | 39 Patients 20 stage 1 19 stage 2 4 Stage 3 or 4 | XRT 22 CMT 10 Chemo 11 | 5 yr OS—39% 5 yr CSS—60% for 35 patients with intermediate or high grade dz |
| Aozasa[12] (1963–1984) pub. 1986 Osaka University Medical School, Japan | 70 Patients 47 Stage 1 23 Stage 2 6 Stage 3 or 4 3 No data on staging | XRT 56 Chemo 2 CMT 19 None 2 | 5 yr OS low grade—92% intermediate grade—79% high grade—13% for all 79 patients |
| Pyke[31] (1965–1989) pub. 1992 Mayo Clinic, Rochester, USA | 50 Patients 34 Stage 1 16 Stage 2 | XRT—39 CMT—4 Chemo—4 Surgery only—3 | 5 yr OS Stage 1 (confined to capsule)— 80% Stage 1E (extra-thyroidal invasion)—58% Stage 2E—50% 2 yr. OS |
| Junor[9] (1962–1988) pub. 1992 Beatson Oncology Center, Scotland | 87 patients 48 Stage 1 31 Stage 2 8 Stage 3 or 4 | XRT as a component of treatment—78 Chemo with XRT or surgery— 10 Chemo—3 | 5 yr OS Stage 1—56% 2 yr OS Stage 1—64% Stage 2—30% |

*(continued)*

**Table 21–1.** *(continued)*

| Author | Patients | Treatments | Outcomes |
|---|---|---|---|
| Matsuzuka[16] (1963–1990) pub. 1993 Kuma Hospital, Kobe, Japan | 119 patients (stages not given) | XRT—31 CMT—88 | 8 yr OS—100% for 16 patients treated with XRT + CHOPx6 and 75% for 21 patients treated with XRT+ CHOP or MOPPx1or 2 |

Abbreviations: pub = published; yr = year; dz = disease; CA = cancer; chemo = chemotherapy; RFS = relapse-free survival; DFS = disease-free survival; CCS = cause-specific survival)
Refer to the text for other abbreviations.

such as damage to the recurrent laryngeal nerve, radiation therapy is the preferred choice of treatment. It appears that patients with intermediate or high grade lymphoma arising from MALT lymphoma have worse prognosis, and these patients need to be treated more aggressively with combined modality therapy as discussed above. When the diagnosis of MALT lymphoma of the thyroid gland is made, we recommend esophagogastroduodenoscopy to rule out involvement of the upper gastrointestinal tract.[50] The yield of colonoscopy and small bowel series is less well defined even though there are reports of bowel involvement by thyroid lymphoma at presentation.[51] A prospective trial has been activated at the M.D. Anderson Cancer Center for treatment of stages I and II MALT lymphoma. Every patient is to have esophagogastroduodenoscopy, small bowel series, and colonoscopy to prospectively study the yield of these tests.

## Low-Grade Lymphoma Other Than MALT Lymphoma

This is a less common entity among non-Hodgkin's lymphomas of the thyroid. When the diagnosis of low-grade follicular lymphoma is made, the possibility of MALT lymphoma or invasion of the thyroid gland by adjacent primary nodal lymphoma needs to be ruled out. The treatment options for low-grade follicular lymphoma range from watchful waiting to intensive chemotherapy or radiation therapy.[52-54] At M.D. Anderson Cancer Center, there is an ongoing prospective randomized clinical trial for Ann Arbor stages I, II, and III follicular low-grade lymphoma. This protocol compares intensive 12-cycle chemotherapy regimen with central lymphatic irradiation (CLI). The preliminary results of the CLI arm have been published.[55] While the clinical data from CLI essentially reproduced previously published experiences,[56-58] the molecular biologic correlation appears very interesting. The patients with low IPI had a significantly better chance of achieving a molecular response as determined by the disappearance of the bcl-2 oncogene measured by the polymerase chain reaction technique compared with patients with high IPI, suggesting the possibility of potential cure for these patients.[59] Another option for these patients is combined modality therapy with ten cycles of CHOP or cyclophosphamide, doxorubicin and vincristine (COP) with involved field radiation therapy. This approach has been shown to achieve 60% relapse-free survival at 15 years for stages I and II disease.[60]

## High-Grade Lymphoma

Burkitt's lymphoma, or diffuse small non-cleaved cell lymphoma of the thyroid gland, has been reported. This entity has been treated with 3 sequential chemotherapy combinations and intrathecal prophylaxis with methotrexate and cytarabine at M.D. Anderson Cancer Center yielding 95% 5-year freedom from tumor mortality.[61] These results refer to Burkitt's lymphoma arising mainly from sites other than the thyroid.

## UNUSUAL NEOPLASMS OF THE THYROID GLAND

### Squamous Cell Carcinoma

Pure squamous cell carcinoma of the thyroid gland, as defined by obvious squamous differentiation and cytologic atypia, is rare.[62] These neoplasms are most often found in elderly patients who may have a history of goiter. The tumors exhibit rapid growth with aggressive and extensive local invasiveness involving adjacent cervical and aerodigestive structures. Some patients exhibit a marked inflammatory response manifested by fever, leukocytosis and hypercalcemia, which is postulated to be mediated by the release of interluekin-1.[63] These tumors demonstrate a wide range of differentiation from well-differentiated cancers to undifferentiated lesions appearing similar to anaplastic carcinoma. It is not uncommon to demonstrate foci of differentiated thyroid cancer within the main tumor mass, lending credence to the theory that these tumors may develop from metaplastic foci of differentiated thyroid cancer, usually papillary thyroid carcinoma.

Primary squamous cell carcinoma of the thyroid must be distinguished from those squamous cancers that may metastasize from other regions, particularly as a result of local extension from primary lesions of aerodigestive tract origin (larynx, trachea and esophagus).

The treatment for these tumors is generally palliative because of the early aggressive behavior exhibited and the propensity to extend into adjacent critical structures within the neck and mediastinum, making complete surgical resection unlikely and highly morbid. Surgery and adjuvant radiation therapy are the main modalities utilized, with tracheotomy often required for airway support because of tracheal resection or sacrifice of the recurrent laryngeal nerves. Combined chemoradiotherapy for lesions judged to be unresectable may be implemented in a palliative setting. Interestingly, this modality has not demonstrated the degree of effectiveness as has been seen when used for primary squamous cancers of the upper aerodigestive tract. The prognosis in patients with this tumor is uniformly poor, with the majority dying as a result of the effects of local invasion.

## Plasmacytoma

Plasma cell tumors of the thyroid gland may arise primarily or as an extramedullary focus of multiple myeloma. Primary tumors arising within the gland usually occur in the elderly and in the background of chronic lymphocytic thyroiditis.[64] These lesions should be distinguished from MALT lymphoma and medullary thyroid carcinoma, both of which demonstrate cytologic characteristics similar to plasmacytoma. Treatment is that which is usually administered for this lesion occurring in any other organ or region. When restricted to the thyroid gland, primary resection via total thyroidectomy represents adequate treatment. The presence of multifocal disease should be excluded, and when present, may be treated with external beam radiotherapy.

## Mesenchymal Tumors

Benign mesenchymal tumors and sarcomas may arise within the thyroid gland. Benign lesions include hemangioma, lymphangioma, leiomyoma, neurilemmoma (schwannoma) and lipoma. Treatment is almost exclusively surgical with the extensiveness of resection based on the degree of thyroid and surrounding cervical involvement. Large lymphangiomatous lesions involving the thyroid primarily or secondarily as a result of extension from a larger cervical/aerodigestive process may be conservatively followed for regression, particularly in younger children, provided the airway is not compromised.[65]

Sarcomas, malignant tumors of mesenchymal origin, have been variously described as primary thyroid malignancies, although they constitute a very small portion of thyroid cancers.[66] Their demographic characteristics and biologic behavior is similar to that of undifferentiated carcinoma in that they occur in older patients, exhibit rapid unrelenting growth with local invasion and usually result in death from local disease. The most common of these malignant tumors is an angiosarcoma occurring generally in the seventh decade of life with a slight male predominance. These lesions are usually quite large, replace most if not all the thyroid gland and frequently extend grossly to involve lateral cervical soft tissues. Angiosarcomas may commonly be hemorrhagic with necrotic degeneration into blood-filled cystic loculations. As with most of the unusual malignant neoplasms occurring in thyroid tissue, the differential diagnosis of primary sarcoma includes undifferentiated carcinoma and is usually distinguished by special ultrastructural and immunohistochemical techniques. Prognosis for patients with these tumors is extremely poor. Treatment is usually surgery with radiotherapy in a palliative setting. Chemotherapy is rarely effective for these tumors.

## Thymic and Thymic-Like Neoplasms

Thymomas may arise primarily within the thyroid gland. They most commonly occur in middle-aged women, probably as a result of intra-thyroidal thymic remnants. Most behave as benign neoplasms requiring lobectomy for cure. Malignant thymomas do occur and may be confused with undifferentiated carcinoma or malignant lymphoma, both of which can be distinguished from thymoma by cytologic and immunohistochemical characteristics. Treatment for malignant thymoma is similar to that for lymphoma.

An unusual tumor of the thyroid that has recently been described as occurring in late adolescence is the spindle epithelial tumor with thymus-like differentiation or SETTLE tumor.[67] These tumors exhibit spindle cell cytologic characteristics fusing with epithelial type cells and forming cords and tubules. Although these tumors usually behave in a benign fashion responding to partial thyroidectomy, they may develop late metastasis years after surgery. Carcinomas with thymus-like differentiation have also been described.[68] These tu mors, in contrast to the SETTLE tumors, usually occur in middle-aged patients and demonstrate nodal metastasis in up to 50% of patients. Primary resection with or without neck dissection is the treatment with satisfactory long-term survival.

## Teratoma

Teratomas occur in the thyroid gland usually as a consequence of direct extension from the central neck in which they arise from embryonic tissue remnants containing all three germ cell lines. They have been reported in both neonates and adults, more commonly in the former in which they generally pursue a more benign course. In contrast, these tumors in adults may behave quite aggressively with a very malignant clinical course. The treatment in both instances is primarily surgical with radiotherapy reserved for adults with tumors exhibiting local extension, regional metastasis or subtotal resectability.

## Mucoepidermoid Carcinoma

Mucoepidermoid carcinomas may rarely arise within the thyroid gland, most often in older adults although they have been reported across a broad age range.[69] Within the thyroid gland they demonstrate a similar combination of squamous and mucous cells arranged in a solid or cystic pattern as is seen in the salivary entity. In contrast to the salivary variety, mucoepidermoid carcinomas of the thyroid gland demonstrate a more indolent clinical behavior with a tendency to metastasize to cervical nodes in a pattern similar to that of papillary carcinoma. Foci of mucoepidermoid carcinoma within a follicular variant of papillary carcinoma has been reported.[70] These findings suggest a genetic link between mucoepidermoid carcinoma and papillary carcinoma. Treatment of these tumors is primarily surgical, with thyroidectomy and lymph node dissection for metastasis.

## Paraganglioma

Paragangliomas of the thyroid gland are extremely rare. Most tumors probably arise from ganglial elements associated with the thyroid capsule.[71] Tumors generally do not attain a large size and some may be grossly quite small. Histologically, these tumors are composed of chief cells, which perform a neurosecretory function, and sustentacular cells, which are the supporting cellular elements. Prognosis is uniformly good with conservative thyroidectomy. There does not appear to be any supporting evidence linking this entity with multiple endocrine neoplasia (MEN).

## Metastatic Tumors

Metastatic disease to the thyroid may occur as a consequence of direct extension from upper aerodigestive malignancies, ie, squamous cell carcinoma, or by hematogenous spread. Evidence at autopsy has demonstrated up to 20% of patients exhibiting distant metastasis to the thyroid gland from breast, lung, kidney and melanoma skin most commonly.[72,73] The appearance of distant metastasis to the thyroid gland from a remote primary site may be quite delayed (greater than eight years) and, thus, any thyroid mass presenting in a patient with known history of malignancy should be considered as a potential metastatic focus. Treatment generally involves surgical resection of the metastatic focus within the thyroid, together with appropriate management of the primary process.

## SUMMARY

Non-Hodgkin's lymphoma of the thyroid gland is a disease seen mostly in patients over 55 years of age but can also be seen in younger patients. A significant number appear to arise from MALT lymphoma in the background of Hashimoto's thyroiditis. However, diffuse large cell lymphoma with or without MALT background remains the most common pathology among thyroid lymphomas. Procurement of adequate biopsy specimen to study the architecture of the lymphoma and to perform immunophenotyping is recommended through incisional or at least core needle biopsy. Standard lymphoma staging evaluation needs to be done once diagnosis of lymphoma of the thyroid gland is made, which would also include esophagogastroduodenoscopy in case of MALT lymphoma. The treatment of choice is combined modality therapy with a combination of chemotherapy and involved field radiation therapy for intermediate and selected high-grade lymphoma. Radiation therapy alone is probably an adequate treatment for localized MALT lymphoma. The overall five-year disease-free survival for stages I and II disease is higher than 70% and perhaps somewhat higher for MALT lymphoma.

Unusual tumors of the thyroid gland may arise as a result of a primary process or by secondary extension or distant metastasis. These may include tumors which may be difficult to distinguish from undifferentiated carcinoma, ie, squamous cell carcinoma and sarcoma, and which characteristically carry a poor prognosis. The presence of a thyroid mass occurring in a patient with a prior history of malignancy must be suspected as being a metastatic focus, even if the interval since primary treatment seems long. In most instances, treatment for these peculiar thyroid tumors remains surgical excision, with or without radiotherapy depending on biologic aggressiveness and resectability.

# References

1. Kapadia SB, Dekker A, Cheng VS, Desai U, Watson CG. Malignant lymphoma of the thyroid gland: a clinicopathologic study. *Head & Neck Surg*. 1982;4:270–280.

2. Tupchong L, Hughes F, Harmer CL. Primary lymphoma of the thyroid: clinical features, prognostic factors, and results of treatment. *Int J Rad Oncol Biol Phys*. 1986;12:1813–1821.

3. Isaacson PG. Lymphoma of the thyroid gland. *Curr Topics in Path*. 1997;91:1–14.

4. Pasieka JL. Anaplastic cancer, lymphoma, and metastases of the thyroid gland. *Surg Oncol Clin North Am*. 1998;7:707–720.

5. Austin JR, el-Naggar AK, Goepfert H. Thyroid cancers. II. Medullary, anaplastic, lymphoma, sarcoma, squamous cell. *Otol Clin North Am*. 1996;29:611–627.

6. Ansell SM, Grant CS, Habermann TM. Primary thyroid lymphoma. *Seminars in Oncology*. 1999;26:316–323.

7. Skarsgard ED, Connors JM, Robins RE. A current analysis of primary lymphoma of the thyroid. *Arch Surg*. 1991;126:1199–203; discussion 1203–1204.

8. Compagno J, Oertel JE. Malignant lymphoma and other lymphoproliferative disorders of the thyroid gland. A clinicopathologic study of 245 cases. *Am J Clin Path*. 1980;74:1–11.

9. Junor EJ, Paul J, Reed NS. Primary non-Hodgkin's lymphoma of the thyroid. *Euro J Surg Oncol*. 1992;18:313–321.

10. Pledge S, Bessell EM, Leach IH, et al. Non-Hodgkin's lymphoma of the thyroid: a retrospective review of all patients diagnosed in Nottinghamshire from 1973 to 1992. *Clin Oncol*. (Royal College of Radiologists). 1996;8:371–375.

11. Logue JP, Hale RJ, Stewart AL, Duthie MB, Banerjee SS. Primary malignant lymphoma of the thyroid: a clinicopathological analysis. *Int J Rad Oncol Biol Phys*. 1992;22:929–933.

12. Aozasa K, Inoue A, Tajima K, Miyauchi A, Matsuzuka F, Kuma K. Malignant lymphomas of the thyroid gland. Analysis of 79 patients with emphasis on histologic prognostic factors. *Cancer*. 1986;58:100–104.

13. Makepeace AR, Fermont DC, Bennett MH. Non-Hodgkin's lymphoma of the thyroid. *Clin Radiol*. 1987;38:277–281.

14. Anscombe AM, Wright DH. Primary malignant lymphoma of the thyroid—a tumour of mucosa-associated lymphoid tissue: review of seventy-six cases. *Histopathol*. 1985;9:81–97.

15. Marwaha RK, Pritchard J. Primary thyroid lymphoma in childhood: treatment with chemotherapy alone [published erratum appears in Pediatr Hematol Oncol 1991 Apr-Jun;8(2):201]. *Ped Hematol & Oncol*. 1990;7:383–388.

16. Matsuzuka F, Miyauchi A, Katayama S, et al,. Clinical aspects of primary thyroid lymphoma: diagnosis and treatment based on our experience of 119 cases. *Thyroid*. 1993;3:93–99.

17. Aozasa K, Ueda T, Katagiri S, Matsuzuka F, Kuma K, Yonezawa T. Immunologic and immunohistologic analysis of 27 cases with thyroid lymphomas. *Cancer*. 1987;60:969–973.

18. Burman KD, Ringel MD, Wartofsky L. Unusual types of thyroid neoplasms. *Endocrinol Metab Clin North Am*. 1996;25:49–68.

19. Pedersen RK, Pedersen NT. Primary non-Hodgkin's lymphoma of the thyroid gland: a population based study. *Histopathol*. 1996;28:25–32.

20. Takahashi K, Kashima K, Daa T, Yokoyama S, Nakayama I, Noguchi S. Contribution of Epstein-Barr virus to development of malignant lymphoma of the thyroid. *Pathology International*. 1995;45:366–374.

21. Tomita Y, Ohsawa M, Kanno H, Matsuzuka F, Kuma K, Aozasa K. Sporadic activation of Epstein-Barr virus in thyroid lymphoma. *Leukemia & Lymphoma*. 1995;19:129–134.

22. Holm LE, Blomgren H, Lowhagen T. Cancer risks in patients with chronic lymphocytic thyroiditis. *N Engl J Med*. 1985;312:601–604.

23. Aozasa K. Hashimoto's thyroiditis as a risk factor of thyroid lymphoma. *Acta Pathologica Japonica*. 1990;40:459–468.

24. Dawson I, Cornes J, Morson B. Primary malignant lymphoid tumours of the intestinal tract. *Br J Surg*. 1961;49:80–89.

25. Tsang RW, Gospodarowicz MK, Sutcliffe SB, Sturgeon JF, Panzarella T, Patterson BJ. Non-Hodgkin's lymphoma of the thyroid gland: prognostic factors and treatment outcome. The Princess Margaret Hospital Lymphoma Group. *Int J Rad Oncol Biol Phys*. 1993;27:599–604.

26. Blair TJ, Evans RG, Buskirk SJ, Banks PM, Earle JD. Radiotherapeutic management of primary thyroid lymphoma. *Int J Rad Oncol Biol Phys*. 1985;11:365–370.

27. Wolf BC, Sheahan K, DeCoste D, Variakojis D, Alpern HD, Haselow RE. Immunohistochemical analysis of small cell tumors of the thyroid gland: an Eastern Cooperative Oncology Group study. *Human Pathol*. 1992;23:1252–1261.

28. Takashima S, Nomura N, Noguchi Y, Matsuzuka F, Inoue T. Primary thyroid lymphoma: evaluation with US, CT, and MRI. *J Comp Assist Tomog*. 1995;19:282–288.

29. Matsuda M, Sone H, Koyama H, Ishiguro S. Fine-needle aspiration cytology of malignant lymphoma of the thyroid. *Diag Cytopathol*. 1987;3:244–249.

30. Tani E, Skoog L. Fine needle aspiration cytology and immunocytochemistry in the diagnosis of lymphoid lesions of the thyroid gland. *Acta Cytolog*. 1989;33:48–52.

31. Pyke CM, Grant CS, Habermann TM, et al. Non-Hodgkin's lymphoma of the thyroid: is more than biopsy necessary? *World J Surg*. 1992;16:604–609; discussion 609–610.

32. Shibata T, Noma S, Nakano Y, Konishi J. Primary thyroid lymphoma: MR appearance. *J Comp Assist Tomog*. 1991;15:629–633.

33. Takashima S, Ikezoe J, Morimoto S, et al. Primary thyroid lymphoma: evaluation with CT. *Radiology*. 1988;168:765–768.

34. Hodgkin's Disease. In: Fleming I, Cooper J, Henson D, et al, eds. *AJCC Cancer Staging Manual*. 5th ed. Philadelphia: Lippincott-Raven; 1997:285–287.

35. Rodriguez J, Cabanillas F, McLaughlin P, et al. A proposal for a simple staging system for intermediate grade lymphoma and immunoblastic lymphoma based on the "tumor score." *Ann Oncol*. 1992;3:711–717.

36. Shipp M, Harrington D, Anderson J. A predictive model for aggressive non-Hodgkin's lymphoma. *N Engl J Med*. 1993;329:987–994.

37. Burke JS. Are there site-specific differences among the MALT lymphomas—morphologic, clinical? *Am J Clin Pathol*. 1999;111 (Suppl. 1):S133–S143.

38. Coltrera MD. Primary T-cell lymphoma of the thyroid. *Head & Neck*. 1999;21:160–163.

39. Hyjek E, Isaacson PG. Primary B cell lymphoma of the thyroid and its relationship to Hashimoto's thyroiditis. *Hum Pathol*. 1988;19:1315–1326.

40. Isaacson P, Wright D. Malignant lymphoma of mucosa-associated lymphoid tissue: a distinctive type of B-cell lymphoma. *Cancer*. 1983;52:1410–1416.

41. Isaacson P, Wright DH. Extranodal malignant lymphoma arising from mucosa-associated lymphoid tissue. *Cancer*. 1984;53:2515–2524.

42. Harris NL, Jaffe ES, Diebold J, Flandrin G, Muller-Hermelink HK, Vardiman J. Lymphoma classification—from controversy to consensus: the R.E.A.L. and WHO Classification of lymphoid neoplasms. *Ann Oncol*. 2000;11(Suppl. 1):3–10.

43. Harris NL, Jaffe ES, Diebold J, et al. The World Health Organization classification of neoplastic diseases of the haematopoietic and lymphoid tissues: Report of the Clinical Advisory Committee Meeting, Airlie House, Virginia, November 1997. *Histopathology.* 2000;36:69–86.

44. Vigliotti A, Kong JS, Fuller LM, Velasquez WS. Thyroid lymphomas stages IE and IIE: comparative results for radiotherapy only, combination chemotherapy only, and multimodality treatment. *Int J Rad Oncol Biol Phys.* 1986;12:1807–1812.

45. Friedberg MH, Coburn MC, Monchik JM. Role of surgery in stage IE non-Hodgkin's lymphoma of the thyroid. *Surgery.* 1994;116: 1061–1066; discussion 1066–1067.

46. Miller TP, Dahlberg S, Cassady JR, et al. Chemotherapy alone compared with chemotherapy plus radiotherapy for localized intermediate- and high-grade non-Hodgkin's lymphoma [see comments]. *N Engl J Med.* 1998;339:21–26.

47. Glick J, Kim K, Earle J, O'Connell M. An ECOG randomized phase III trial of CHOP vs. CHOP+radiothcrapy (XRT) for intermediate grade early stage non-Hodgkin's lymphoma (NHL). *Proc Amer Soc Clin Oncol.* 1995;14:391.

48. Laing RW, Hoskin P, Hudson BV, et al. The significance of MALT histology in thyroid lymphoma: a review of patients from the BNLI and Royal Marsden Hospital. *Clin Oncol.* (Royal College of Radiologists). 1994;6:300–304.

49. Zinzani PL, Magagnoli M, Galieni P, et al. Nongastrointestinal low-grade mucosa-associated lymphoid tissue lymphoma: analysis of 75 Patients. *J Clin Oncol.* 1999;17:1254–1258.

50. Liao Z, Ha C, McLaughlin P, et al. MALT (Mucosa Associated Lymphoid Tissue) lymphoma with initial supradiaphragmatic presentation: natural history and patterns of failure. in press. *Int J Rad Oncol Biol Phys.*

51. Stone CW, Slease RB, Brubaker D, Fabian C, Grozea PN. Thyroid lymphoma with gastrointestinal involvement: report of three cases. *Am J Hematol.* 1986;21:357–365.

52. Mendenhall N, Lynch JW. The low-grade lymphomas. *Seminars in Radiation Oncology.* 1995;5:254–266.

53. Young R, Longo D, Glatstein E, Ihde D, Jaffe E, DeVita VT. The treatment of indolent lymphomas: watchful waiting vs. aggressive combined modality treatment. *Seminars in Hematology.* 1988; 25:11–16.

54. Longo DL. What's the deal with follicular lymphomas? [editorial; comment] [see comments]. *J Clin Oncol.* 1993;11:202–208.

55. Ha C, Cabanillas F, Lee M, Besa P, Mclaughlin P, Cox J. Serial determination of the bcl-2 gene in the bone marrow and peripheral blood after central lymphatic irradiation for stages I-III follicular lymphoma: a preliminary report. *Clin Cancer Res.* 1997;3:215–219.

56. Jacobs J, Murray K, Schultz C, et al. Central lymphatic irradiation for Stage III nodular malignant lymphoma: long-term results. *J Clin Oncol.* 1993;11:233–238.

57. De Los Santos JF, Mendenhall NP, Lynch JW, Jr. Is comprehensive lymphatic irradiation for low-grade non-Hodgkin's lymphoma curative therapy? Long-term experience at a single institution [see comments]. *Int J Rad Oncol Biol Phys.* 1997;38:3–8.

58. Paryani S, Hoppe R, Cox R, Colby T, Kaplan H. The role of radiation therapy in the management of Stage III follicular lymphomas. *J Clin Oncol.* 1984;2:841–848.

59. Ha C, Tucker S, Lee M, Cabanillas F, McLaughlin P, Cox J. The significance of molecular response rate of follicular lymphoma to central lymphatic irradiation (CLI) as measured by polymerase chain reaction (PCR) for t(14;18)(q32;q21). *Int J Rad Oncol Biol Phys.* 1999;45(3):218.

60. Besa P, McLaughlin P, Cox J, Fuller L. Long term assessment of patterns of treatment failure and survival in patients with stage I or II follicular lymphoma. *Cancer.* 1995;75:2361–2367.

61. Lopez TM, Hagemeister FB, McLaughlin P, et al. Small noncleaved cell lymphoma in adults: superior results for stages I-III disease [published erratum appears in *J Clin Oncol* 1994 Mar; 12(3):646]. *J Clin Oncol.* 1990;8:615–622.

62. Simpson WJ, Carruthers J. Squamous cell carcinoma of the thyroid gland. *Am J Surg.* 1988;156:44–46.

63. Saito K, Fujii Y, Ono M. Production of interleukin-1 alpha like factor and colony stimulating factor by a squamous cell carcinoma of the thyroid ($T_3$ M-5) derived from a patient with hypercalcemia and leukocytosis. *Cancer Res* 1987;47:6474–6480.

64. Aozasa K, Inone A, Yashimura A. Plasmacytoma of the thyroid gland. *Cancer.* 1986;58:105–110.

65. Rosai J, Carcanqui M, Delellis R. Tumors of the thyroid gland. Atlas of tumor pathology. Washington, DC: Armed Forces Institute of Pathology, 1992:259–265.

66. Kennedy, T. (Personal Communication).

67. Chan J, Rosai J. Tumors of the neck showing thymic or related branchial pouch differentiation, a unifying concept. *Hum Pathol.* 1991;22:349–367.

68. Rosai J, Saxen E, Woolner L. Undifferentiated and poorly differentiated carcinoma. *Semin Diagn Pathol.* 1985;2:123–136.

69. Wenig B, Adair C, Heffess C. Primary mucoepidermoid carcinoma of the thyroid gland: a report of six cases and a review of the literature. *Hum Pathol.* 1995;26:1099–1108.

70. Miranda RN, Myint MA, Gnepp DR. Composite follicular variant of papillary carcinoma and mucoepidermoid carcinoma of the thyroid. *Am J Surg Pathol.* 1995;19:1209–1215.

71. Buss DH, Marshall RB, Baird FG, Myers RT. Paraganglioma of the thyroid gland. *Am J Surg Pathol.* 1980;4:589–593.

72. Ivy HK. Cancer metastatic to the thyroid. A diagnostic problem. *Mayo Clin Proc.* 1984;59:856–859.

73. Nakhjauani M, Gitarib H, Goellner JR, Van Hesrden JA. Metastasis to the thyroid gland. A report of 43 cases. *Cancer.* 1997;79: 574–578.

# 22

# Suppression and Long-Term Surveillance in Thyroid Malignancy

## R. Michael Tuttle, M.D.

Since the 10 year disease specific mortality rate is less than 7% in papillary thyroid cancer, and less than 15% in follicular thyroid cancer, the majority of patients diagnosed with differentiated thyroid cancer will become long term survivors.[1,2] While death from thyroid cancer is a relatively uncommon event, as many as 30% of patients will develop a recurrence if followed for 20–30 years after diagnosis.[2-4] Two thirds of these recurrences will develop in the first 10 years following diagnosis, but the remaining third will present clinically more than 10 years after initial diagnosis and therapy.[2]

While the majority of recurrences are detected in cervical lymph nodes or thyroid bed remnants and are readily treated with additional surgery or radioactive iodine, more serious recurrences develop outside the neck in approximately 20% of the cases (usually pulmonary metastases).[2] Recurrences are clinically significant events. Up to 15% of patients will die of thyroid cancer following a recurrence, and an additional 30% will live with persistent disease that cannot be eradicated.

Any effective follow-up strategy begins with an assessment of the likelihood of recurrence or death from thyroid cancer. Many investigators have identified important characteristics of the patient and the tumor at diagnosis that are independent predictors of these important clinical endpoints.[2,3,5-8] Furthermore, since the risk of recurrence and death from thyroid cancer decreases with longer periods of disease free survival, the intensity of testing for disease detection should also decrease in long term survivors. Widely differing approaches to the follow-up of thyroid cancer patients was reported following a survey of thyroid cancer "experts" in the American Thyroid Association.[9] An appropriate level of follow-up may vary from an annual physical examination on levothyroxine therapy in low risk patients to yearly whole body radioactive iodine scanning for selected high risk patients.[5,10,11]

This chapter will focus on the use of levothyroxine suppression to decrease long term recurrence rates and current management recommendations regarding appropriate testing to detect local and distant recurrences developing years after initial diagnosis and therapy.

## LEVOTHYROXINE SUPPRESSIVE THERAPY

The use of levothyroxine as adjuvant therapy to thyroidectomy has been shown to decrease recurrence rates and disease specific mortality.[2,12,13] In a retrospective French study of 141 thyroid cancer patients, improved relapse free survival was noted in patients with a TSH constantly suppressed to less than 0.05 microU/ml compared to patients with TSH values consistently greater than 1 microU/ml.[14] In this study, TSH suppression was an independent predictor of relapse free survival in a multi-variate analysis that included age, gender, histology and stage of disease at diagnosis. However, a prospective U.S. study of 617 thyroid cancer patients did not find the degree of TSH suppression to be an independent predictor of disease progression.[15]

Since TSH is known to be a growth factor for both normal and malignant thyroid cells, it has become routine clinical practice to place thyroid cancer patients on levothyroxine suppressive therapy.[16] Recent data demonstrating an increased risk of atrial fibrillation[17] and osteoporosis[18-20] in thyrotoxic patients has caused us to re-examine the risk/benefit ratio of levothyroxine suppressive therapy, particularly in low risk, long term survivors.

While there is little data to provide guidance regarding the optimal magnitude of TSH suppression, it has become common clinical practice to suppress TSH values to less than 0.1 microU/ml for the first several years after initial therapy. In low risk patients who are disease free for several years, it is quite reasonable to decrease the levothyroxine suppression so that a TSH just below the normal reference range is achieved. However, patients with persistent disease are likely to benefit from continued levothyroxine suppression at the minimal levothyroxine dose necessary to maintain the TSH less than 0.1 microU/ml.[16]

## PRIMARY TESTING MODALITIES FOR DETECTION OF RECURRENT/PERSISTENT DISEASE

### Serum Thyroglobulin

Thyroglobulin is synthesized by thyroid cells as a key substrate in the production and storage of thyroid hormones.[21,22] Since thyroglobulin production is restricted to thyroid cells, its presence in the peripheral circulation serves as a valuable tumor marker for most differentiated thyroid cancers. In recent years, serum thyroglobulin has developed as the simplest, readily available testing modality for the detection of recurrent disease.

Reliable, accurate serum thyroglobulin measurements are now commercially available from many laboratories. Lower levels of detection of 0.5–1.5 ng/ml are common in immuno-metric assays. Because of the lack of an international thyroglobulin standard, measurements of thyroglobulin vary considerably between manufacturers. Therefore, a direct comparison between thyroglobulin measurements performed by different laboratories is difficult at best.[23] Maximal sensitivity for detection of recurrent disease is obtained when a patient has serial thyroglobulin values measured in the same laboratory over time.[24]

Furthermore, the presence of anti-thyroglobulin antibodies in up to 20% of thyroid cancer patients makes the standard thyroglobulin measurement unreliable.[25,26] Depending on the individual characteristics of the assay, either falsely elevated or falsely suppressed thyroglobulin determinations are possible. Therefore, thyroglobulin values can only be reliably interpreted in the absence of anti-thyroglobulin antibodies. Newer generations of thyroglobulin measurements based on recovery assays are currently available which may provide a reliable thyroglobulin measurement in the face of many anti-thyroglobulin antibodies. The validity of these recovery assays is still the source of considerable controversy.[25,27]

Serum thyroglobulin is a sensitive and specific marker of persistent/recurrent disease only after total or near total thyroidectomy followed by radioactive iodine ablation.[28] Normal thyroid tissue as well as autonomous functioning thyroid tissue is a rich source of thyroglobulin which cannot be differentiated from thyroid cancer.

However, most patients treated with lobectomy alone will have thyroglobulin values less than 5 ng/ml on levothyroxine suppression. Often the thyroglobulin is undetectable in this situation. Therefore, a significant elevation of serum thyroglobulin should always prompt an evaluation for recurrent/persistent thyroid cancer. However, the specificity of an elevated thyroglobulin is much less in patients with remaining normal thyroid tissue than in those treated with appropriate surgery and radioactive iodine ablation.

Since thyroglobulin synthesis and release is stimulated by TSH, it is not surprising that measurement of serum thyroglobulin is most sensitive for disease detection when measured in the presence of an elevated TSH (thyroid hormone withdrawal, or stimulation with recombinant human TSH).[27,29-33] Therefore, most authorities recommend measurement of thyroglobulin during TSH stimulation as part of the routine follow-up algorithm.

### Radioactive Iodine Whole Body Scanning

While all normal thyroid follicular cells have the ability to concentrate radioactive iodine, only 75% of thyroid cancers retain this property. Whole body radioactive iodine scanning has long been used to detect and localize radioactive iodine avid thyroid cancers. Since the maximal uptake of radioactive iodine requires TSH stimulation, whole body radioactive iodine scans have traditionally been performed following levothyroxine withdrawal (TSH > 30 microU/ml). Discontinuation of levothyroxine results in a marked rise in pituitary synthesis and secretion of TSH but also is associated with significant symptoms of clinical hypothyroidism.

Recently, the advent of recombinant human TSH has allowed an alternative method for TSH stimulation that does not require discontinuation of thyroid hormone.[34,35] Several recent studies have demonstrated that rhTSH stimulated whole body scanning has similar sensitivity and specificity to standard hypothyroid levothyroxine withdrawal scanning.[35,36]

While whole body scanning is an excellent test for detection and localization of recurrent/persistent thyroid cancer, it is less sensitive than serum thyroglobulin measurements and cannot be used in pregnant women.[37,38] Perhaps the most problematic issue with diagnostic whole body radioactive iodine scanning is the potential for small scanning doses of I[131] (3–5mCi) to interfere with the subsequent uptake of therapeutic doses of radioactive iodine (30–200 mCi).[39-41] This interference, commonly referred to as "stunning," may be more common than previously recognized. Some investigators are now using I[123] instead of I[131] while others are foregoing the diagnostic scan prior to definitive radioactive iodine therapy altogether. Further studies are needed to better define the prevalence and, more importantly, the clinical significance of stunning.

## STAGES OF FOLLOW-UP

Management issues in thyroid cancer therapy can be readily divided into three arbitrary phases (see Figure 22–1).[5] Phase 1 begins immediately following the initial surgical management of the thyroid cancer. Phase 1 includes all other testing used to determine the extent of disease at diagnosis (including radioactive iodine scans if indicated). After all evidence of disease is eliminated, either with surgical intervention or radioactive iodine therapy, the patient enters Phase 2 of follow-up (usually 6–12 months following initial therapy). Phase 2 covers the period during which recurrence of thyroid cancer is most likely to be detected: the first several years after this initial therapeutic intervention. After patients have been free of disease for several years, it is quite likely that the patient is "cured" of disease and he may transition into Phase 3 surveillance. However, it is important to remember that clinically significant recurrences continue to develop in a small number of patients during Phase 3 of follow-up. Patients in Phase 3 require life-long, but less aggressive, follow-up.

If recurrent disease is detected at any phase, the management approach returns to the Phase 1 strategy of determining the extent of disease and undertaking appropriate therapeutic interventions. If the patient can be rendered free of disease, he then enters Phase 2 once again and is followed closely for a second recurrence using the same strategies as normally employed in Phase 2 follow-up.

## Determination of Extent of Disease at Diagnosis (Phase 1)

Low risk patients (less than 45 years old) with low risk tumor characteristics (small intra-thyroidal tumors) are often treated with less than a total thyroidectomy. The presence of significant amounts of normal thyroid tissue makes radioactive iodine scanning so insensitive that it is not routinely used in this setting. Therefore, determination of extent of disease at diagnosis requires a careful physical examination, review of intra-operative findings, judicious use of cervical ultrasound,[42] and chest radiographs in selected patients. In general, the risk of recurrence or death in these selected patients is considered to be so low that highly sensitive disease detection techniques are not required.

Moderate to high risk patients are often treated with total or near total thyroidectomy and radioactive iodine ablation of any normal thyroid remnants. Because these patients have a higher risk of spread of the thyroid cancer outside the thyroid gland at the time of initial diagnosis, more sensitive detection methods are employed (see Table 22–1). Therefore, Phase 1 extent of disease determination in these higher risk patients often includes a whole body radioactive iodine scan. This whole body scan can be done with a small tracer dose of radioactive iodine (2–5 mCi) before radioactive iodine ablation or can be done following a standard radioactive iodine ablation dose (30–100mCi) if there is concern for stunning.

Thyroglobulin values in the months following thyroidectomy and radioactive iodine ablation need to be

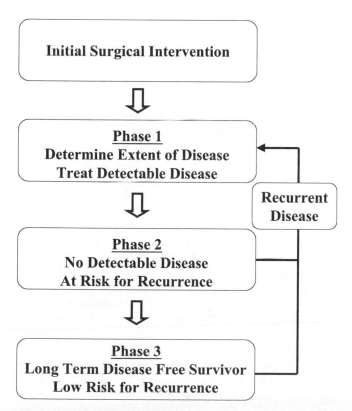

**Figure 22–1.** The three phases of thyroid therapy. (Adapted from Mazzaferri, EL. An overview of the management of papillary and follicular carcinoma. *Thyroid.* 1999;421–427.)

**Table 22–1.** Detection methods during phases 1, 2, and 3

| Diagnostic Testing | Phase 1 | Phase 2 | Phase 3 |
|---|---|---|---|
| Physical Examination | Every 3–4 months | Every 3–6 months for 2 years, then every 6–12 months | Annually |
| Serum Tg on Suppression | — | Every 6–12 months | With each examination |
| Serum Tg with TSH stimulation* | 4–6 weeks post-op | 12 months after initial therapy, then yearly until 2 consecutive negative studies** | At infrequent intervals in high risk patients*** |
| Serum TSH | 4–6 weeks post-op | Every 6–12 months | With each examination |
| Whole Body RAI scan* | 4–6 weeks post-op | Yearly until 2 consecutive negative studies** | At infrequent intervals in high risk patients*** |
| Chest X-ray | Pre-op | Consider at infrequent intervals*** | Consider at infrequent intervals*** |
| Neck Ultrasound | Not routine | Consider for selected patients at high risk for cervical recurrence | Consider for selected patients at high risk for cervical recurrence |

*Only in patients treated with near total or total thyroidectomy.

** A negative study means that the whole body scan has no non-physiologic foci of radioactivity and that the stimulated Tg does not rise to higher than approximately 2 ng/ml.

***Infrequent intervals may be every 3–5 years depending on the individual risk factors for recurrence and death from thyroid cancer.

Abbreviations: Tg = thyroglobulin, RAI = radioactive iodine

interpreted with caution. In fact, 3–12 months may elapse following radioactive iodine ablation before the serum thyroglobulin becomes undetectable.[27,29,30] However, thyroglobulin values greater than 30 ng/dl are quite suspicious for persistent thyroid cancer either local/regionally or at distant metastatic sites even in the early months following initial therapy. Serial determinations of the serum thyroglobulin can be used to judge the adequacy of the initial therapy.

Many other imaging techniques can be used to determine the extent of disease in selected clinical situations. These include cervical ultrasound and fluorine-18 fluorodeoxyglucose positron emission tomography in patients with elevated thyroglobulin but no radioactive iodine avid disease on whole body scanning.[43,44] Spiral CT scans are quite useful in defining the extent of disease in patients with an abnormal chest X-ray. Occasionally, other nuclear medicine scans such as thallium, sestamibi, gallium, tetrafosmin, furifosmin and/or somatostatin analogs may be useful in detecting thyroid cancer that does not concentrate radioactive iodine. However, each of these scanning agents suffers from poor sensitivity and specificity in the detection of thyroid cancer, which makes the clinical utility quite limited.

## Detection of Early Recurrences (Phase 2)

Patients free of clinically evident disease 6–12 months after initial therapy enter Phase 2 of follow up. The method of disease detection during Phase 2 is in large part dependent on the initial therapeutic management approach. If normal thyroid tissue is still present in the thyroid bed, then surveillance for recurrent disease will rely largely on physical exam and judicious use of non-radioactive iodine imaging of the neck and chest. Since the majority of recurrences in these low risk patients present as enlarged cervical lymph nodes, a careful physical examination and cervical ultrasound can be used to detect recurrent disease. Obviously, these techniques are less sensitive for disease detection than radioactive iodine scanning.

When radioactive iodine ablation of remnant normal thyroid tissue is used as part of the initial therapeutic strategy, very sensitive methods of detection of recurrent disease can be employed. Destruction of functional normal thyroid tissue allows the use of radioactive iodine whole body scanning and serum thyroglobulin measurements to be used with maximal sensitivity.

In general, Phase 2 detection of disease includes a careful physical examination of the neck for recurrence of disease and thyroglobulin determinations every 3–6 months for the first 2 years. Even in the presence of a normal thyroid lobe, serum thyroglobulin measurements should be low and should not rise on serial evaluations. In patients who did not receive ablation of thyroid remnants, a rising thyroglobulin level is likely to represent recurrent disease, but could also represent development of benign autonomous thyroid function (benign nodules, autoimmune thyroid disease).[45] However, an increasing thyroglobulin level certainly deserves a careful evaluation for recurrent thyroid cancer with a careful physical examination, cervical ultrasound and imaging of the lungs.

Individual thyroglobulin measurements are more meaningful in patients previously treated with radioactive iodine ablation. In this setting, an elevated thyroglobulin level almost certainly indicates recurrent thyroid cancer since it is quite unlikely for benign thyroid disease to arise following aggressive thyroid surgery and radioactive iodine ablation.

Maximal sensitivity for detection of recurrent disease is achieved when the thyroglobulin is measured at a time of TSH stimulation.[27,29] A significant increase in thyroglobulin is seen in approximately 20% of patients whose thyroglobulin is undetectable on levothyroxine suppression.[27,29-33] Previously, measurement of a TSH stimulated thyroglobulin required discontinuation of levothyroxine for several weeks (usually in preparation for whole body radioactive iodine scanning). The FDA recently approved a biosynthetic form of injectable TSH (recombinant human TSH, *Thyrogen*, Genzyme Corporation) as an alternative method for TSH stimulation prior to whole body scanning.[34,35] This recombinant human TSH now gives us the option of obtaining a stimulated thyroglobulin without having to discontinue the levothyroxine suppressive therapy. Trials are ongoing to evaluate the sensitivity and specificity of using just the TSH stimulated thyroglobulin value (without whole body radioactive iodine scanning) in the detection of recurrent thyroid cancer.

Until these studies are complete, it seems wise to continue to perform both whole body scans and stimulated thyroglobulin determinations together in order to achieve maximal sensitivity for disease detection.[35,36] However, it does seem likely that the TSH stimulated thyroglobulin measurement will likely be used alone in patients who have previously undergone 1–2 TSH stimulated whole body radioactive iodine scans that showed no evidence of disease. Ongoing studies will clarify the exact role of whole body scanning and stimulated thyroglobulin measurements in the follow-up of Phase 2 and Phase 3 thyroid cancer patients.

## Detection of Late Recurrences (Phase 3)

By the time the patient enters Phase 3, several years have passed since the initial diagnosis and therapy. Many of these patients will have had 2 or more negative whole body radioactive iodine scans. Therefore, the risk of recurrence or death from thyroid cancer in these patients is quite low.

In general, patients in Phase 3 are followed annually with physical examination and thyroglobulin measurements on levothyroxine therapy. Because thyroid cancer can recur up to 30 years or longer after diagno-

sis, lifelong follow-up is required. However, whole body radioactive iodine scanning is generally not needed, except in patients at very high risk for disease recurrence (older than 45 years at diagnosis, very high risk tumor features).

As in Phase 2, any increase in serum thyroglobulin needs to be appropriately evaluated in an attempt to identify recurrent thyroid cancer. Recurrent disease is often treated with surgical removal, followed by radioactive iodine therapy. Evaluation of recurrent disease would proceed as described for Phase 1 patients above.

While a small number of Phase 3 patients will show recurrence, subjecting all patients to the clinical hypothyroidism necessary for whole body scanning does not seem reasonable. However, the advent of rhTSH does allow whole body scanning and stimulated thyroglobulin measurements to be made with minimal clinical impact. Therefore, the role of rhTSH stimulated thyroglobulin measurements is being reassessed in these Phase 3 patients. More studies are needed before wide-spread screening for recurrent thyroid cancer can be advocated in these low risk patients. While there is little doubt that rhTSH stimulated thyroglobulin determinations will identify recurrent disease in some of these Phase 3 patients, it is less clear that the identification of very small recurrences will have a significant clinical impact on these long term survivors.

## NATIONAL COMPREHENSIVE CANCER NETWORK (NCCN) GUIDELINES

A panel of thyroid cancer experts was convened in 1998–1999 to discuss diagnostic and treatment approaches and to arrive at a consensus practice guideline for the management of thyroid nodules and thyroid cancers.[46] The guidelines assume that most patients will be treated with total or near total thyroidectomy and radioactive iodine ablation, and are therefore heavily weighted toward the use of serum thyroglobulin and whole body radioactive iodine scanning for the detection of recurrent disease. These guidelines call for periodic examinations, as well as serum thyroglobulin measurements and whole body radioactive iodine scans during several phases of follow-up. The combination of physical examination with these two testing modalities detects clinically significant residual/recurrent disease in nearly all patients who have undergone total thyroidectomy and radioactive iodine ablation.

The NCCN guidelines call for a physical examination every 3–6 months for 2 years, then annually if the patient is disease free. A TSH stimulated thyroglobulin is measured at 6 and 12 months post-operatively, then annually if disease free. Whole body radioactive iodine scans are recommended annually until 2 negative scans are obtained in patients treated with total thyroidectomy and radioactive iodine (RAI) ablation during Phase 1. Periodic neck ultrasound and chest X-ray should also be considered at infrequent intervals.

## SUMMARY OF RECOMMENDED FOLLOW-UP STUDIES

Table 22–1 presents a general outline of diagnostic studies recommended by the author for the usual thyroid cancer patient who easily passes through Phase 1 and is thought to be disease free a year after initial therapy. The first 2–3 years of Phase 2 represent the most intensive diagnostic approaches to detection of recurrent disease with serum thyroglobulin (Tg) levels measured on suppression at 6 and 12 months, and annual TSH stimulated Tg measurements and whole body scans until at least 2 negative consecutive studies are obtained. For the next several years, these patients are followed with clinical examination and thyroglobulin measurements on levothyroxine suppression.

Low risk patients with low risk tumor characteristics can then transition into Phase 3 surveillance within 3–5 years of diagnosis. However, high or moderate risk patients may continue for 5–10 years in Phase 2 with more frequent monitoring of TSH stimulated thyroglobulin values (probably with rhTSH stimulation), periodic neck ultrasound evaluation, and infrequent chest X-rays.

Phase 3 surveillance relies on yearly physical examinations and measurement of Tg on levothyroxine suppression. More data are needed to determine the proper role for whole body radioactive iodine scanning and rhTSH stimulated Tg values in these long term survivors who had high risk characteristics at initial diagnosis.

If recurrent thyroid cancer is detected in any Phase of follow-up, then the patient is considered Phase 1 once again. As with patients entering Phase 1 for the first time, a vigorous search for thyroid cancer is warranted to define the extent of disease. Appropriate therapy can then be offered based on an understanding of the extent of disease, radioactive iodine avidity of the tumor, and underlying health of the patient.

## References

1. Hundahl SA, Fleming ID, Fremgen AM, Menck HR. A National Cancer Data Base report on 53,856 cases of thyroid carcinoma treated in the U.S., 1985–1995 *Cancer*. 1998;83:2638–48.
2. Mazzaferri EL, Jhiang SM. Long-term impact of initial surgical and medical therapy on papillary and follicular thyroid cancer (published erratum appears in *Am J Med* 1995 Feb;98(2):215). *Am J Med*. 1994;97:418–28.
3. McConahey WM, Hay ID, Woolner LB, van Heerden JA, Taylor WF. Papillary thyroid cancer treated at the Mayo Clinic, 1946 through 1970: initial manifestations, pathologic findings, therapy, and outcome. *Mayo Clin Proc*. 1986;61:978–96.
4. Ruiz de Almodovar JM, Ruiz-Garcia J, Olea N, Villalobos M, Pedraza V. Analysis of risk of death from differentiated thyroid cancer. *Radiother Oncol*. 1994;31:207–12.
5. Mazzaferri EL. An overview of the management of papillary and follicular thyroid carcinoma. *Thyroid*. 1999;9:421–7.
6. Shaha AR, Loree TR, Shah JP. Prognostic factors and risk group analysis in follicular carcinoma of the thyroid. *Surgery*. 1995;118:1131–6; discussion 1136–8.
7. Tubiana M, Schlumberger M, Rougier P et al. Long-term results and prognostic factors in patients with differentiated thyroid carcinoma. *Cancer*. 1985;55:794–804.
8. Hay ID, Bergstralh EJ, Goellner JR, Ebersold JR, Grant CS. Predicting outcome in papillary thyroid carcinoma: development of a reliable prognostic scoring system in a cohort of 1,779 patients surgically treated at one institution during 1940 through 1989. *Surgery*. 1993;114:1050–7; discussion 1057–8.
9. Solomon BL, Wartofsky L, Burman KD. Current trends in the management of well differentiated papillary thyroid carcinoma. *J Clin Endocrinol Metab*. 1996;81:333–9.
10. Mazzaferri EL, Kloos RT. Using recombinant human TSH in the management of well-differentiated thyroid cancer: current strategies and future directions. *Thyroid*. 2000;10:767–78.
11. Singer PA, Cooper DS, Daniels GH et al. Treatment guidelines for patients with thyroid nodules and well-differentiated thyroid cancer. American Thyroid Association. *Arch Intern Med*. 1996;156:2165–72.
12. Simpson WJ, Panzarella T, Carruthers JS, Gospodarowicz MK, Sutcliffe SB. Papillary and follicular thyroid cancer: impact of treatment in 1,578 patients. *Int J Radiat Oncol Biol Phys*. 1988;14:1063–75.
13. Cady B, Sedgwick CE, Meissner WA, Bookwalter JR, Romagosa V, Werber J. Changing clinical, pathologic, therapeutic, and survival patterns in differentiated thyroid carcinoma. *Ann Surg*. 1976;184:541–53.
14. Pujol P, Daures JP, Nsakala N, Baldet L, Bringer J, Jaffiol C. Degree of thyrotropin suppression as a prognostic determinant in differentiated thyroid cancer. *J Clin Endocrinol Metab*. 1996;81:4318–23.
15. Cooper DS, Specker B, Ho M et al. Thyrotropin suppression and disease progression in patients with differentiated thyroid cancer: results from the National Thyroid Cancer Treatment Cooperative Registry. *Thyroid*. 1998;8:737–44.
16. Dulgeroff AJ, Hershman JM. Medical therapy for differentiated thyroid carcinoma. *Endocr Rev*. 1994;15:500–15.
17. Sawin CT, Geller A, Wolf PA et al. Low serum thyrotropin concentrations as a risk factor for atrial fibrillation in older persons. *N Engl J Med*. 1994;331:1249–52.
18. Ross DS, Neer RM, Ridgway EC, Daniels GH. Subclinical hyperthyroidism and reduced bone density as a possible result of prolonged suppression of the pituitary-thyroid axis with L-thyroxine. *Am J Med*. 1987;82:1167–70.
19. Stall GM, Harris S, Sokoll LJ, Dawson-Hughes B. Accelerated bone loss in hypothyroid patients overtreated with L-thyroxine. *Ann Intern Med*. 1990;113:265–9.
20. Diamond T, Nery L, Hales I. A therapeutic dilemma: suppressive doses of thyroxine significantly reduce bone mineral measurements in both pre-menopausal and post-menopausal women with thyroid carcinoma. *J Clin Endocrinol Metab*. 1991;72:1184–8.
21. Van Herle AJ, Vassart G, Dumont JE. Control of thyroglobulin synthesis and secretion. (First of two parts). *N Engl J Med*. 1979;301:239–49.
22. Van Herle AJ, Vassart G, Dumont JE. Control of thyroglobulin synthesis and secretion (Second of two parts). *N Engl J Med*. 1979;

23. Spencer CA, Takeuchi M, Kazarosyan M. Current status and performance goals for serum thyroglobulin assays. *Clin Chem*. 1996; 42:164–73.
24. Black EG, Sheppard MC, Hoffenberg R. Serial serum thyroglobulin measurements in the management of differentiated thyroid carcinoma. *Clin Endocrinol (Oxf)*. 1987;27:115–20.
25. Spencer CA, Takeuchi M, Kazarosyan M et al. Serum thyroglobulin autoantibodies: prevalence, influence on serum thyroglobulin measurement, and prognostic significance in patients with differentiated thyroid carcinoma. *J Clin Endocrinol Metab*. 1998;83:1121–7.
26. Mariotti S, Barbesino G, Caturegli P et al. Assay of thyroglobulin in serum with thyroglobulin autoantibodies: an unobtainable goal? *J Clin Endocrinol Metab*. 1995;80:468–72.
27. Schlumberger MJ. Diagnostic follow-up of well-differentiated thyroid carcinoma: historical perspective and current status. *J Endocrinol Invest*. 1999;22:3–7.
28. Spencer CA, Wang CC. Thyroglobulin measurement. Techniques, clinical benefits, and pitfalls. *Endocrinol Metab Clin North Am*. 1995;24:841–63.
29. Pacini F, Lippi F. Clinical experience with recombinant human thyroid-stimulating hormone (rhTSH): serum thyroglobulin measurement. *J Endocrinol Invest*. 1999;22:25–9.
30. Ozata M, Suzuki S, Miyamoto T, Liu RT, Fierro-Renoy F, DeGroot LJ. Serum thyroglobulin in the follow-up of patients with treated differentiated thyroid cancer. *J Clin Endocrinol Metab*. 1994;79: 98–105.
31. Lo Gerfo P, Colacchio TA, Colacchio DA, Feind CR. Effect of TSH stimulation on serum thyroglobulin in metastatic thyroid cancer. *J Surg Oncol*. 1980;14:195–200.
32. Pacini F, Lari R, Mazzeo S, Grasso L, Taddei D, Pinchera A. Diagnostic value of a single serum thyroglobulin determination on and off thyroid suppressive therapy in the follow-up of patients with differentiated thyroid cancer. *Clin Endocrinol (Oxf)*. 1985;23:405–11.
33. Muller-Gartner HW, Schneider C. Clinical evaluation of tumor characteristics predisposing serum thyroglobulin to be undetectable in patients with differentiated thyroid cancer. *Cancer*. 1988;61:976–81.
34. Ladenson PW, Braverman LE, Mazzaferri EL et al. Comparison of administration of recombinant human thyrotropin with withdrawal of thyroid hormone for radioactive iodine scanning in patients with thyroid carcinoma. *N Engl J Med*. 1997;337:888–96.
35. Haugen BR, Pacini F, Reiners C et al. A comparison of recombinant human thyrotropin and thyroid hormone withdrawal for the detection of thyroid remnant or cancer. *J Clin Endocrinol Metab*. 1999;84:3877–85.
36. Robbins R, Tuttle R, Sharaf R et al. The use of rhTSH in the detection of persistent thyroid cancer. *JCEM*. 2001;Februrary, in press.
37. Ashcraft MW, Van Herle AJ. The comparative value of serum thyroglobulin measurements and iodine-131 total body scans in the follow-up study of patients with treated differentiated thyroid cancer. *Am J Med*. 1981;71:806–14.
38. Ronga G, Fiorentino A, Fragasso G, Fringuelli FM, Todino V. Complementary role of whole body scan and serum thyroglobulin determination in the follow-up of differentiated thyroid carcinoma. *Ital J Surg Sci*. 1986;16:11–15.
39. Park HM, Perkins OW, Edmondson JW, Schnute RB, Manatunga A. Influence of diagnostic radioiodines on the uptake of ablative dose of iodine-131. *Thyroid*. 1994;4:49–54.
40. Leger FA, Izembart M, Dagousset F et al. Decreased uptake of therapeutic doses of iodine-131 after 185-MBq iodine-131 diagnostic imaging for thyroid remnants in differentiated thyroid carcinoma. *Eur J Nucl Med*. 1998;25:242–6.
41. Muratet JP, Daver A, Minier JF, Larra F. Influence of scanning doses of iodine-131 on subsequent first ablative treatment outcome in patients operated on for differentiated thyroid carcinoma. *J Nucl Med*. 1998;39:1546–50.
42. Antonelli A, Miccoli P, Ferdeghini M et al. Role of neck ultrasonography in the follow-up of patients operated on for thyroid cancer. *Thyroid*. 1995;5:25–8.
43. Wang W, Larson SM, Fazzari M et al. Prognostic value of [18F]-fluoro-deoxy-glucose positron emission tomographic scanning in patients with thyroid cancer. *J Clin Endocrinol Metab*. 2000;85: 1107–13.
44. Wang W, Macapinlac H, Larson SM et al. [18F]-2-fluoro-2-deoxy-D-glucose positron emission tomography localizes residual thyroid cancer in patients with negative diagnostic (131)-I whole body scans and elevated serum thyroglobulin levels. *J Clin Endocrinol Metab*. 1999;84:2291–302.
45. Torrens J, Burch H. Clinical application of serum thyroglobulin testing. *The Endocrinologist*. 1996;6:125–144.
46. Mazzaferri EL. NCCN thyroid carcinoma practice guidelines. *Oncology*. 1999;13:391–412.

# 23

# Hyperthyroidism: Medical and Surgical Management

## Douglas L. Fraker, M.D.

Hyperthyroidism is a common functional abnormality of the thyroid that produces a recognizable symptom complex that can be readily confirmed by diagnostic blood tests. Hyperthyroidism and thyrotoxicosis are terms that although often used interchangeably have different implications. Thyrotoxicosis is the condition caused by excess thyroid hormone due to any etiology including exogenous ingestion of thyroid hormones or release of preformed thyroid hormones by various causes of thyroiditis.[1] Hyperthyroidism specifically refers to excess thyroid hormone produced by overactive function of the thyroid gland. Therefore, hyperthyroidism is a subset of the larger group of diseases that cause thyrotoxicosis. Hyperthyroidism may be caused by a relatively uniform overactivity throughout the entire thyroid gland referred to as diffuse toxic goiter or Graves' disease, or it may be caused by hyperfunction in specific nodules in the thyroid gland. Hyperthyroidism in nodular thyroid disease may be from multiple functional nodules throughout the thyroid referred to as a multinodular toxic goiter or Plummer's disease, or it may be a single hyperfunctioning nodule or toxic adenoma called Goetsch's disease. Graves' disease or diffuse toxic goiter account for the vast majority of cases of hyperthyroidism with only 4–10% of patients in most series having other etiologies as the cause of their increased thyroid function.[1,2]

The combination of cardiac palpitations and an enlarged thyroid gland was described as a discrete syndrome in 1835 by the Irish physician, Dr. Robert James Graves,[3] although the English physician, Caleb Parry, had described a single incidence of a patient with "an enlarged heart and an enlarged thyroid gland" ten years earlier. The association between hyperthyroidism and proptosis of the eyes was first described by Carl von Basedow in 1840 who felt that the ocular symptoms were the most relevant component of this disease. Many areas in Eastern Europe still refer to diffuse toxic goiter as Basedow's disease instead of Graves' disease. The initial treatment developed for Graves' disease was surgical resection of the thyroid as described by Kocher in the 1880s. Prior to that time, the intraoperative and perioperative mortality for thyroid resection primarily caused by hemorrhage was prohibitive. Kocher's initial series of 100 patients undergoing thyroidectomy reported a mortality of only 12.8%, a remarkable improvement at that time which was recognized by the Nobel Prize for Medicine in 1909.[4] The second category of treatment for hyperthyroidism was the use of radioactive iodine compounds to ablate the thyroid tissue. Advances in the understanding of radioactivity at the end of the 19th century coupled with the knowledge that the thyroid gland concentrates iodine made this treatment possible. Moeblin reported the first series of radioactive iodine ablation for hyperthyroidism in 1911.[5] The medical or drug therapy of hyperthyroidism was made possible by the surreptitious observation in 1941 from two groups studying the administration of thioamide compounds to rats.[6,7] One group was evaluating the anti-microbial effects of these compounds on gut flora and one group was observing the reaction to a bitter taste stimuli. Both groups noted that in animals taking these compounds, there was the development of significant thyroid hyperplasia. Astwood recognized the potential use of these drugs to ablate thyroid tissue and coined the term anti-thyroid drugs.[8] He reported the development of both propylthiouracil in 1946 and methimazole in 1949, the two drugs which are the mainstays of medical therapy now four decades later.[6] Key points in the history of Graves' disease and its treatment are documented in Table 23–1.

This chapter will deal with the medical and surgical management of Graves' disease and nodular causes of hyperthyroidism. The treatment strategies are similar for both types of hyperthyroidism as are the clinical signs and symptoms, with the exception of specific extra-thyroidal autoimmune manifestations such as ophthalmopathy that is only seen in Graves' disease.

## EPIDEMIOLOGY AND INCIDENCE

Graves' disease in virtually all series is overwhelmingly the most common etiology of hyperthyroidism. Most institutions report their experience with either Graves' disease or report nodular thyroid disease so it is difficult to obtain accurate data regarding the relative proportion of hyperthyroidism caused by these two broad categories of disease. The largest although somewhat outdated collection of patients that addresses this issue comes from data from the Cooperative Thyrotoxicosis Therapy Study Group which registered 35,609 patients in the United States and Great Britain between 1946 and 1964.[2] In this large series, 91% of the patients had Graves' disease, 8% had toxic nodular thyroid disease, and 1% had undefined hyperthyroidism. A more recent study from Tokyo evaluating patients with hyperthyroidism between 1981 and 1994 reported that in 607 consecutive patients, 579 (95.4%) had Graves' disease and 28 (4.6%) had toxic nodular disease.[9] In general, between 90–95% of cases of hyperthyroidism will be caused by Graves' disease.[1]

As with other autoimmune disorders, Graves' disease has a marked female predominance with incidence being between four-fold and ten-fold greater in women than in men in most series.[6] The prevalence of Graves' disease has been estimated to be 2% in females and 0.2% in males in the United States, with an overall prevalence in the general population of approximately 1%. Since hyperthyroidism is essentially a non-lethal disease, the annual incidence is much lower and has been estimated to be between 13 and 20 patients per 100,000 population.[6] The high prevalence rate occurs as the majority of patients with Graves' disease are young to middle age and patients will live for several decades after obtaining this diagnosis. However, this disease may be diagnosed anywhere from childhood up to the eighth decade of life.[10] In patients with hyperthyroidism over the age of 60, multinodular disease is more common with one series reporting 57% of new cases in this age range caused by nodular disease.[2] The predilection for females is still present in toxic nodule thyroid disease, with ratios of approximately 5:1 favoring females.

In patients with toxic nodular goiter, the distribution of patients with multinodular disease versus a single toxic adenoma depends to some degree on the geographic area of the patient population. In Europe, the majority of patients have multinodular goiter or Plummer's disease, whereas in the United States, the majority of patients have single toxic adenomas. In the recent series from Japan in which 28 patients were identified over a 15 year period with toxic nodular thyroid disease, 22 patients had a single adenoma (79%) versus 6 patients with multinodular disease (21%).[9]

## ETIOLOGY

Graves' disease is now clearly defined as an autoimmune disease characterized by antibodies produced against the thyroid stimulating hormone (TSH) or thyrotropin receptor. These autoantibodies act as agonists and simulate ligand binding, which leads to overproduction of thyroid hormone responding to signal transduction pathways from the stimulated thyrotropin re-

**Table 23–1.** Key historical points in the understanding and treatment of Graves' disease

| | |
|---|---|
| 1825 | Caleb Parry describes five cases of "enlargement of the heart and enlargement of the thyroid" in Bath in England. |
| 1835 | Robert James Graves describes three cases of "violent palpitations and . . . enlargement of the thyroid" in Ireland. |
| 1840 | Carl A. von Basedow describes exophthalmos in Germany. |
| 1880 | Ludwig Rehn performs the first thyroidectomy for diffuse toxic goiter in Germany. |
| 1943 | Astwood describes thioamides as antithyroid drugs and uses them clinically in Baltimore. |
| 1946 | Radioactive iodine treatments developed in Boston and Berkeley. |
| 1956 | Adams describes long-acting thyroid stimulation and Graves' disease is understood to be an autoimmune disease. |

ceptor. The circulating factor that caused overstimulation of the thyroid was first identified in 1956 as long-acting thyroid stimulator (LATS). As this antibody against the thyrotropin receptor has been better characterized and can be measured in a specific immunoassay, it has been referred to as thyroid stimulating immunoglobulin (TSI) or more specifically as TSH receptor antibodies (TRAb).[11]

Like most autoimmune diseases, the precise etiology or the cause of the breakdown in tolerance to self-antigen is unknown but is likely to be a combination of genetic and environmental factors. Twin studies have reported a concordance of hyperthyroidism between 30% and 76% in monozygotic or identical twins and of 11% in dizygotic or fraternal twins. The lack of complete concordance in identical twins as well as the incidence that is significantly higher than the general population in fraternal twins indicates the importance of environmental factors. Certain HLA alleles have been associated with a high incidence of Graves' disease specifically HLA-B8 and HLA-DR3. Linkage analysis has demonstrated an association of isotypes of CTLA-4 gene with Graves' disease.[1] In terms of environmental factors, there has been a report of association of *Yersinia enterocolitica* with Graves' disease. Other investigators have linked stress or stressful events to an onset of Graves' disease. There is an increased incidence of Graves' disease with cigarette smoking with a hazard ratio of 1.9 in smokers compared to non-smokers that is not found in other causes of hyperthyroidism or other thyroid disorders.[12]

A second component of Graves' disease is ophthalmopathy. The clinical manifestations of this ocular disorder will be described below. Since ophthalmopathy is limited only to patients with Graves' disease and does not occur in toxic nodular hyperthyroidism or other causes of thyrotoxicosis, these symptoms are clearly related to the autoimmune etiology of Graves' disease. The pathology of Graves' ophthalmopathy is caused by infiltration of the retro-orbital fat and ocular muscles with glycosaminoglycans and a large lymphocytic infiltration.[13] It is believed that an immune reaction occurs against antigens expressed on fibroblasts located in the retro-orbital area. Although initially theorized that there may be a cross-reactive antigen expressed on these fibroblast cells which shares an immunoreactive epitope with the TSH receptor, recent data suggest a second subset of immune effector cells against specific fibroblast targets that may be related to TSH epitopes.[14] The 5–10% of patients who have symptoms of ophthalmopathy without overt hyperthyroidism would argue that this interpretation is correct. Also, a similar immune reaction against dermal fibroblasts may explain the skin changes seen in the small subset of patients with Graves' disease described as pretibial myxedema or pretibial dermopathy.

The etiology of toxic nodular hyperthyroidism is less well understood. For patients with single toxic nodules, molecular genetics has indicated that alterations or mutations may occur in various components of the TSH receptor. These mutations may result in the TSH receptor being in the "on" position as if there was a ligand-binding. These lesions have been seen in the minority of nodules and the majority of toxic nodules, and patients with multinodular disease have less clear etiologies.

## CLINICAL MANIFESTATIONS OF HYPERTHYROIDISM

Virtually all the clinical signs and symptoms of hyperthyroidism of any etiology relate to excess $T_4$ and $T_3$ acting via their specific receptors on essentially all tissues of the body. The one major exception to this general rule regarding symptoms of hyperthyroidism is the effect of thyrotropin receptor antibodies, which cause the ophthalmopathy and dermopathy described above associated only with Graves' disease.

The most common symptoms of thyroid hormone excess experienced by the patient are palpitations, intolerance to heat, and neuropsychiatric symptoms of fatigue and inability to concentrate.[15] Other symptoms such as tremor, weight loss despite adequate appetite, diaphoresis, and diarrhea may be present. The list of common signs and symptoms of hyperthyroidism is presented in Table 23–2.[15,16] There have been a variety of attempts to create grading scales for the severity of hyperthyroidism in the literature.[17]

The most common clinical signs identified on physical examination in patients with hyperthyroidism include an increased resting heart rate, lid lag on eye exam, and increased deep tendon reflexes. Examination of the neck generally shows either general or focal enlargement of the thyroid gland. In a large series of patients with Graves' disease, over 97% of patients have been documented to have a diffuse but soft enlargement of the thyroid that can be detected on physical examination. For patients with a single toxic adenoma as the cause of hyperthyroidism, there is generally a focal enlargement of a thyroid nodule that moves with swallowing and can be palpated on physical examination. The majority of toxic adenomas are >2.5 cm in diameter and thus within the size range of lesions that can be palpated. For patients with multinodular toxic goiter it would be generally bilateral nodular involvement of the thyroid that would be difficult to distinguish from Graves' disease, although the character of the gland may be more firm with distinctly palpable nodules.

Approximately 40% to 50% of patients with Graves' disease have clinical evidence of ophthalmopathy which is pathognomonic for this disorder (Table 23–3).[18] No other cause of hyperthyroidism is associat-

**Table 23–2.** Signs and symptoms of hyperthyroidism

| Organ System | Symptoms | Signs |
|---|---|---|
| Cardiovascular | Palpitations<br>Dyspnea | Resting tachycardia<br>Accelerated heart sound<br>Atrial fibrillation |
| Gastrointestinal | Increased appetite<br>Diarrhea | Weight loss |
| Neuropsychiatric | Insomnia<br>Irritability<br>Nervousness | Fine distal tremor<br>Brisk deep tendon reflexes<br>Clonus<br>Lid lag |
| Skin/General | Heat intolerance<br>Sweating<br>Pruritus | Moist skin<br>Palmar erythema |
| Musculoskeletal | Weakness<br>Fatigability | Muscle wasting<br>Decreased bone density |
| Hematopoietic | | Leukopenia<br>Lymphocytosis |
| Reproductive System | Oligomenorrhea/Amenorrhea<br>Infertility<br>Impotence<br>Decreased libido | Gynecomastia (male) |

**Table 23–3.** Signs and symptoms of autoimmune and dermopathy of Graves' disease

| | Signs | Symptoms |
|---|---|---|
| Ophthalmopathy | Gritty feeling in eyes<br>Photophobia<br>Excess tearing<br>Diplopia<br>Deep pain/pressure in eye | Proptosis<br>Chemosis or erythema of conjunctiva<br>Eyelid edema<br>Ophthalmoplegia |
| Dermopathy | Swollen thickened skin of calf<br>  (pretibial myxedema)<br>Swelling of distal phalanx aria<br>  of toes and finger (thyroid<br>  acropathy) | Non-pitting edema of pretibial skin<br>Red/brown discoloration<br>peau d'orange |

ed with these ocular changes, and they are so distinctive that they generally can secure the diagnosis on physical examination prior to laboratory confirmation.[13] The patients complain of symptoms in mild cases of excess tearing, photophobia, and a feeling of grittiness in their eyes. With more advanced disease, they will complain of the bulging of the eyes or proptosis that would be visible on self-examination, double vision, pressure in the eye, and occasionally decreased visual acuity.[19] On examination of the eyes, there is often obvious proptosis, chemosis, or conjunctival injection, periorbital and eyelid edema, and in severe cases there may be ophthalmoplegia.[20] Even in the 50–60% of patients who do not have overt complaints of ophthal-

mopathy with Graves' disease, if they are examined by CT scan or MRI this will confirm excess tissue in the retro-orbital fat and muscle tissues.[21]

A second manifestation of autoimmune effect against tissue fibroblasts in Graves' disease is pretibial myxedema or pretibial dermopathy (Table 23–1). Clinically, this is a finding of brawny, non-pitting edema or swelling of the anterior lower legs. Microscopically this is caused by a deposition of hyaluronic acid within the subcutaneous tissues. This may be seen in only 5–10% of patients with Graves' disease. An extremely rare finding in Graves' disease is thyroid acropathy which is a diffuse enlargement of the soft tissues surrounding the distal digits of the hands and feet.[22]

In patients who present with the complete classic triad of palpitations, a diffusely enlarged thyroid gland, and proptosis, the diagnosis of Graves' disease can be easily made on clinical evaluation. In patients who present without ophthalmopathy the diagnosis may be more subtle, particularly in the elderly population.[23] Older patients may present with predominantly neuropsychiatric symptoms and the treatable disorder of hyperthyroidism may be attributed to depression or even senile dementia. Atrial fibrillation is a very common finding for patients with hyperthyroidism in the elderly population, but associated enlargement of the thyroid, ophthalmopathy, and other signs may not be present and a high level of suspicion and screening with thyroid function tests is indicated in these clinical situations.

## LABORATORY DIAGNOSIS AND DIFFERENTIAL DIAGNOSIS OF HYPERTHYROIDISM

For patients who are felt to have hyperthyroidism on clinical grounds, these suspicions may be confirmed and the specific cause of hyperthyroidism ascertained by a combination of laboratory tests and a radioactive iodine uptake scan (RAIU) of the thyroid. The single most appropriate screening test to diagnose or to rule out hyperthyroidism is measurement of serum thyrotropin with a second generation sensitive assay (Figure 23–1). For most patients with hyperthyroidism, TSH is undetectable in the serum by this sensitive assay. The second generation TSH assay has a level of sensitivity which detects TSH >0.05 mIu/L.[1,24] The result of an undetectable TSH may be confirmed by utilizing the ultrasensitive or third generation TSH assay which has a sensitivity of <0.005 mIu/L. An exception to the rule that TSH is undetectable in clinically relevant hyperthyroidism is in the very rare cases of hyperthyroidism caused by a pituitary tumor which secretes TSH[25] or a condition with a mutated TSH receptor.[26] For patients with an undetectable TSH, hyperthyroidism may be confirmed by measurement of free thyroxin ($FT_4$). If $FT_4$ is within normal range with a suppressed TSH, then measurement of free triiodothyronine may identify $T_3$ thyrotoxicosis. Patients who are biochemically hyperthyroid with an undetectable TSH and clinical signs of ophthalmopathy may be diagnosed with Graves' dis-

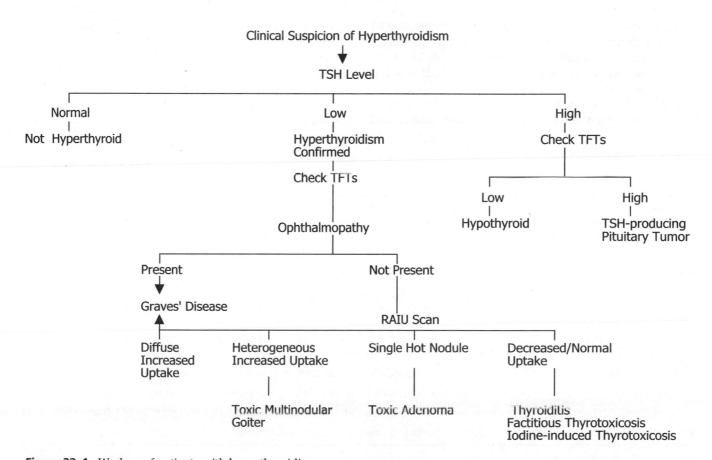

**Figure 23–1.** Workup of patients with hyperthyroidism.

ease without any further testing. Confirmatory measurements of thyrotropin related antibodies is available but not necessary and does not alter therapy.

In patients with no ophthalmopathy, the next study to obtain is a radioactive iodine uptake nuclear medicine scan. Two types of information can be obtained from RAIU scans. First, the proportion of administered iodine that is taken up and retained in the thyroid gland has both an early time point of 4–6 hours and a late time point of 20–24 hours which can be measured. Second, the distribution of iodine uptake throughout both lobes of the thyroid can be seen on an imaging scan. Patients with Graves' disease have uniformly diffuse uptake that is significantly elevated compared to the normal ranges of 6–14% at 6 hours and 15–25% at 24 hours after injection. Increased uptake with a diffuse pattern across both lobes of the thyroid will confirm Graves' disease in the setting of biochemical hyperthyroidism. Patients with iodine uptake in a single dominant nodule with suppression of the surrounding or remaining thyroid is indicative of a toxic adenoma. Multinodular toxic goiter will result in a heterogeneous uptake in both lobes of the thyroid that is overall greater than the normal range of uptake.

If patients have a normal to low iodine uptake on RAIU, an alternative diagnosis of thyrotoxicosis other than hyperthyroidism can be made (Table 23–4). Potential causes of low iodine uptake in the setting of elevated thyroid hormones levels include thyroiditis, factitious thyrotoxicosis, and iodine-induced thyrotoxicosis. A variety of causes of thyroiditis including subacute, silent, and post-partum thyroiditis are characterized by release of preformed thyroid hormone caused by inflammation of the thyroid gland which also results in a low uptake of iodine.[27] Factitious thyrotoxicosis due to an ingestion of exogenous thyroxin will cause suppression of TSH and generalized suppression of iodine uptake.[28] A third category of thyrotoxicosis with low iodine uptake is Jod-Basedow disease, or iodine-induced thyrotoxicosis.[29] Oral intake of high levels of iodine may in some situations lead to hyperthyroidism that is generally characterized by thyroid stunning and low iodine uptake on RAIU. The most common etiology currently is related to the use of amiodarone which is a widely used anti-arrhythmic drug.[30] Amiodarone by molecular weight is composed of 37% iodine. Patients treated with amiodarone develop thyrotoxicosis at a rate of 1–2%, and a recent series of patients from the Mayo Clinic demonstrated a low iodine uptake (4%) at 24 hours in this patient population. Alternative causes of iodine induced thyrotoxicosis include excessive intake of iodine based radiocontrast agents.

An unusual cause of thyrotoxicosis that may be identified on radioactive iodine scan is struma ovarii.[31] This very rare condition is ectopic production of thyroid hormone from tissues located within the substance of the ovaries. This excess production suppresses iodine uptake in the thyroid and, if the pelvis is imaged on RAIU, it will show a focus of iodine uptake in that ectopic location securing the diagnosis.

A second benefit of the RAIU scan is the ability to detect a cold or hypofunctional nodule within the setting of diffuse increased uptake in patients with Graves' disease. A cold nodule in a patient with Graves' disease has the same implications for malignancy as similar lesions in patients who are euthyroid. The recommended evaluation would be fine needle aspiration, and if there is any indication from this study that a patient may have a neoplastic or frankly malignant lesion appropriate sur-

**Table 23–4.** Etiologies of thyrotoxicosis and the key diagnostic criteria

| *Disease* | *Key Diagnostic Criteria* |
| --- | --- |
| Diffuse Toxic Goiter (Graves' disease) | Diffuse increased uptake on RAIU scan; ophthalmopathy; elevated thyrotropin receptor antibodies |
| Nodular Toxic Goiter (Plummer's Disease) | Heterogeneous increased uptake on RAIU scan |
| Toxic Adenoma (Goetsch's Disease) | Single hot nodules on RAIU scan with suppression of uptake in remaining thyroid |
| Iodine-induced Thyrotoxicosis (Jod-Basedow's Disease) | Decreased uptake on RAIU scans; often thyroid enlargement; history of amiodarone use or iodine based contrast dye use |
| Factitious Thyrotoxicosis | Decreased iodine uptake on RAIU scans; normal sized thyroid; no autoantibodies |
| Thyroiditis | Decreased iodine uptake on RAIU scan; elevated thyroid peroxidase and thyroglobulin antibodies |
| TSH-producing Pituitary Adenoma | Increased iodine uptake on RAIU scan; elevated TSH; pituitary lesion on MRI scan |
| Stoma Ovarii | RAIU scan positive in ovary; decreased or absent uptake in thyroid |

RAIU—Radioactive iodine uptake scan

gical resection is indicated. This information may influence therapeutic decisions regarding treatment of Graves' disease as described below. In a recent series, concurrent malignancies have been diagnosed in patients undergoing thyroidectomy for Graves' disease at levels of 5.9% and 7%.[32] Because of heterogeneity and iodine uptake, it is harder to detect cold areas in patients with diffuse toxic multinodular goiter.

Other studies which may be relevant for the differential diagnosis of thyrotoxicosis include measurements of thyroid peroxidase antibodies and anti-thyroglobulin antibodies that confirm a diagnosis of thyroiditis. A history of taking excess thyroid hormone, amiodarone, or iodine based contrast agents may also contribute to the differential diagnosis. Additional diagnostic studies that are appropriate for patients with hyperthyroidism and ophthalmopathy would be a CT scan or MRI of the orbits. These studies would be helpful in documenting the degree of abnormality causing the ophthalmopathy and may be helpful in treatment planning.

## THERAPY OF GRAVES' DISEASE

There are three general categories of treatment for Graves' disease: medical therapy with thioamide drugs, ablation of thyroid tissue with radioactive io-

dine, and surgical resection of the thyroid gland.[1,33,34] In the United States, medical therapy is not viewed as a definitive treatment and is typically combined or used as an initial treatment prior to radioactive iodine or surgical resection.[6] For most patients, radio-iodine ablation is the recommended definitive treatment and surgical resection is used for specific clinical situations. In Europe and Asia, there is a greater tendency for utilizing long-term medical therapy as a definitive treatment and less use of radioactive iodine ablation.[35,36]

## Medical Therapy with Anti-Thyroid Medications

The primary drugs that are utilized for treatment of Graves' disease are thioamides but other types of agents may play a role in therapy in specific situations (Table 23–5). For each of these drugs, their mechanisms of action in terms of hyperthyroidism will be described and then the overall strategies to apply these agents to patients with hyperthyroidism will be discussed.[8]

The thioamide drugs have been used for the treatment of Graves' disease for over 50 years since they were developed by Astwood in the 1940s.[8] In the United States, propylthiouracil and methimazole are the two available agents. In Europe, carbimazole is uti-

**Table 23–5.** Description of medications useful in treating hyperthyroidism

| Category of Drug | Specific Drugs | Characteristics | Clinical Utility |
|---|---|---|---|
| Thioamides | Methimazole | Longer T$\frac{1}{2}$, fewer side effects than PTU | Drug of choice for initial treatment of hyperthyroidism in US |
| | Carbimazole | Converted to methimazole | Drug of choice in Europe |
| | Propylthiouracil | Less release in breast milk; does not cross placenta as well; blocks peripheral conversion of T$_4$ → T$_3$ | Useful in pregnancy, in lactating females; Useful in thyroid storm |
| Inorganic Iodide | Lugol's Solution (5% sodium iodine and 10% potassium iodide) Supersaturated solution of Potassium iodide (SSKI) | Blocks uptake of iodine into thyroid cells and blocks organification of tyrosine Decreased thyroid blood flow | Used 7–10 days prior to surgical removal of thyroid |
| β-Blockers | Multiple | Blocks peripheral effects of excess thyroid hormone | Use to control initial symptoms of hyperthyroidism and thyroid storm; Primary agent to treat thyroiditis |
| Glucocorticoids | Hydrocortisone Prednisone | Blocks peripheral conversion of T$_4$ → T$_3$. Blocks effects of hyperthyroidism | Useful in thyroid storm |

T$\frac{1}{2}$ = half-life

lized instead of methimazole and it may be considered an equivalent agent as it is converted with near 100% efficiency to methimazole after ingestion.[6]

Thioamides act by blocking the production of thyroid hormone by inhibiting the organification of iodine and by blocking the coupling of iodotyrosines[8] (Figure 23–2). PTU has the additional effect of blocking peripheral conversion of $T_4$ to $T_3$. Methimazole has a longer half-life than PTU allowing daily dosing schedule, and it has slightly lower risks of significant adverse drug reactions making it the preferable agent for most cases of patients with Graves' disease. The half-life of methimazole is 4–5 hours in the circulation compared to 1–2 hours for PTU. However, both of these agents are concentrated in the thyroid and the effective half-lives are greater than the serum half-life. PTU crosses the placenta to a lesser degree than methimazole and is utilized as the principal agent for pregnant patients with Graves' disease.[37,38] Also, the ability of PTU to block the peripheral conversion of $T_4$ to $T_3$ makes it a preferred agent for acute therapy in thyroid storm.

A second category of drugs that plays a role in treatment of hyperthyroidism is beta-blockers (Table 23–5).[39] These drugs do not directly act against the thyroid gland or any step in the production and signal transduction pathways of thyroxine. Beta-blockers have the ability to decrease or partially control several of the symptoms patients feel with hyperthyroidism including palpitations and tremors (Figure 23–2). These agents are used in combination with thioamides to control symptoms at the time of initial diagnosis when patients are still biochemically hyperthyroid, but the beta-blockers should be discontinued when patients become euthyroid. Beta-blockers are the drugs of choice for treating symptoms of hyperthyroidism associated with thyroiditis as thioamides are ineffective for these diseases that are caused by release of preformed hormone. Beta-blockers are contraindicated in patients with asthma, COPD, or congestive heart failure.

There are two types of non-organic iodides which are utilized primarily in preparation for surgical resection of the thyroid in patients with Graves' disease. Lugol's solution, which is a combination of 5% sodium iodine and 10% potassium iodide, and supersaturated potassium iodide (SSKI) both provide very high content of non-organic iodide.[8] Administration of these agents has a "stunning effect" on the thyroid gland and decreases release of the thyroid hormone and also decreases vascular flow to the gland for a period of a few weeks.[40] After this initial effect, the thyroid returns to

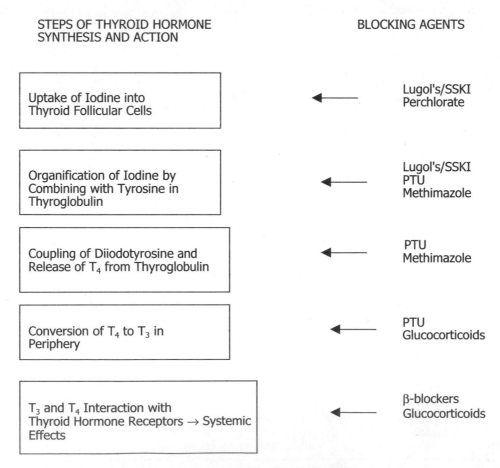

**Figure 23–2.** Mechanisms of action of anti-thyroid medications.

baseline function and that is why these agents are only used immediately prior to surgical resection.

Other agents that are useful for medical therapy of hyperthyroidism include high iodine content radiocontrast agents such as iopanoic acid as well as lithium chloride. These agents both block production of thyroid hormone or block action of thyroid hormone in the periphery. For thyroid storm, high-dose steroids may have beneficial effect in managing the symptoms by ameliorating some of the activity of the thyroid hormone in the periphery.

The general strategy employed for patients presenting with Graves' disease is to treat them with thioamide at a high initial dose to make the patients euthyroid and when they are biochemically corrected to decrease the dose to a maintenance level to maintain the euthyroid state for between 6 and 24 months (Figure 23–3).[1,33] At that point in time, the thioamide is withdrawn to determine whether the patient has gone into a spontaneous remission. Generally, the initial dose of thioamide is 30 mg qd for methimazole or 100 mg tid for PTU. Patients may be decreased to 5–10 mg of methimazole or 30–50 mg of PTU three times daily during the maintenance phase.[41]

If patients have significant symptoms at the time of initial presentation, the addition of a beta blocker may be beneficial to control these symptoms.[39] Again, as beta-blockers do not directly alter thyroid hormone metabolism once the patient's biochemical levels of thyroxine normalize, these agents should be discontinued.[1,6,42] While patients are being treated with thioamides, they need to be monitored for side effects. The most common side effects are a rash or pruritus which may require halting these drugs if significant and switching to an alternative treatment strategy. The most serious side effects are agranulocytosis which occurs in 0.3% of patients.[8] A baseline white blood cell count should be obtained and patients should be counseled that if they develop any infectious disease or fever they should be immediately evaluated and screened for agranulocytosis. A second major side effect is hepatic necrosis for PTU and cholestatic jaundice for methimazole, but these toxicities are so rare that routine screening of liver function tests is not indicated.

In most series when thyroid medications are withdrawn after a maintenance phase of between 6 and 24 months, 50–70% of patients will go into remission similar to other autoimmune disorders. Patients need to be followed closely after that withdrawal as between 50–80% of this group of patients in remission will eventually develop a relapse of Graves' disease. Seventy percent of these relapses will occur within the first six months but relapse may occur up to several years later.

An alternative strategy to the above plan of initial blocking and maintenance is a "block-replace" strategy[43] that was popularized in the 1980s (Figure 23–3). With

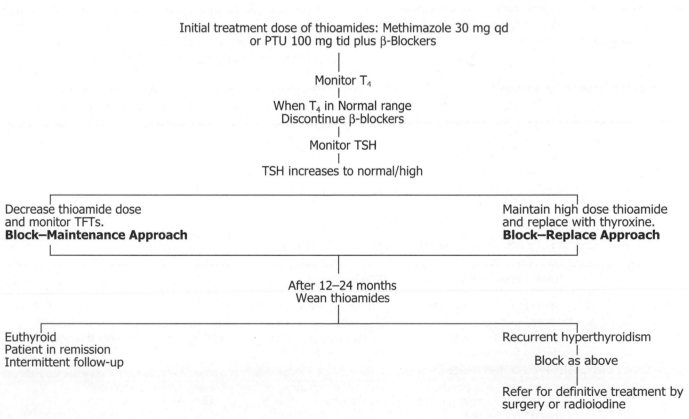

Initial treatment dose of thioamides: Methimazole 30 mg qd
or PTU 100 mg tid plus β-Blockers

Monitor T₄

When T₄ in Normal range
Discontinue β-blockers

Monitor TSH

TSH increases to normal/high

Decrease thioamide dose and monitor TFTs.
**Block–Maintenance Approach**

Maintain high dose thioamide and replace with thyroxine.
**Block–Replace Approach**

After 12–24 months
Wean thioamides

Euthyroid
Patient in remission
Intermittent follow-up

Recurrent hyperthyroidism

Block as above

Refer for definitive treatment by surgery or radioiodine

**Figure 23–3.** Algorithm for the initial management of patients with Graves' disease.

this approach, patients are maintained on very high levels of thioamides throughout the treatment phase and when they become hypothyroid they are given replacement thyroxin.[44] An initial report from Japan indicated that with this block-replace strategy the incidence of short-term relapse decreased from 37% to 1.4%. These investigators hypothesized that the high-dose thioamides had an immunosuppressive effect and would be beneficial in preventing recurrences of Graves' disease.[43] However, subsequent confirmatory studies did not show any benefit in terms of the relapse rate with a block-replace strategy compared to a block–maintenance approach.[41] Current recommendations would be to follow a standard block and maintenance program for one to two years and then withdraw the thioamide while following thyroid function tests closely.[6]

If patients' symptoms recur after an initial remission or if they recur during withdrawal of thioamide they should be counseled to have a definitive ablation by either radioactive iodine or surgery. The chance of a second durable spontaneous remission after an initial recurrence is negligible. Some investigators believe for patients in the older age range >50 years that after initial control of hyperthyroidism they should be ablated without any attempt at withdrawal of thioamides. The reasoning behind this strategy is that it is more cost-effective in an older patient population to definitively treat the disease with radioactive iodine, than to commit a patient to very close follow-up for several years hoping for a permanent euthyroid state with an unlikely spontaneous remission.

## Radio-Iodine Ablation

The two types of definitive ablative therapy for Graves' disease are radioactive iodine ablation or surgical resection (Table 23–6).[1,33,34] With both types of these ablative techniques, the overall goal is to reduce the amount of mass of hyperfunctional thyroid tissue. Radioactive iodine with [131]I decreases thyroid mass by cell death after thyroid tissue concentrates this isotope which has a relatively low energy beta-emission within the thyroid gland.[45] Surgical resection obviously is a direct instantaneous ablation of thyroid tissue depending upon the amounts of thyroid removed. For both radioactive iodine and surgical resection, there is a balance between the risk of recurrent hyperthyroidism versus the risk of long-term hypothyroidism. The greater the dose of iodine or the more thyroid tissue resected, the greater the chance of long-term hypothyroidism. On the other hand, with decreased radioactive iodine doses or subtotal thyroidectomies leaving larger remnants, the greater risk of recurrent hyperthyroidism. The pros and cons of these two ablative therapies are shown in Table 23-6. For most patients in the United States, the optimal ablation technique is radioactive iodine. Certain clinical situations either mandate or suggest benefit from surgical resection.

Patients undergoing radioactive iodine ablation need to be well blocked with thioamide medications to normalize the thyroid hormone levels prior to receiving the radioactive iodine.[33,34] Blocking excess thyroid hormone prevents a radiation-induced thyrotoxicosis or possible thyroid storm. The thioamide drugs are stopped 3–5 days prior to receiving radioactive iodine[46] and then re-started after treatment with iodine in the next week (Figure 23–4). Patients need to continue on thioamide medications after receiving radioactive iodine as the antithyroid effect is not immediate and there is a slow decline in thyroid function over 2–6 months before patients may obtain a complete response.

The dosing schedule for radioactive iodine can be either based on a fixed dose of [131]I for all patients or on a calculated dose dependent upon gland size and degree of radioactive iodine uptake.[33,34] For clinicians using a fixed dose, it is generally recommended that the dose level is between 5–10 mCi of radioactive iodine [131]I.[45,47] The calculated dose of mCi [131]I is based on a formula of:

**Table 23–6.** Comparison of different treatment strategies for hyperthyroidism

|  | *Advantages* | *Disadvantages* |
| --- | --- | --- |
| Anti-Thyroid Drugs | Rapid control of symptoms | Side effects: rash, granulocytopenia, hepatic toxicity; not definitive therapy |
| Radioactive Iodine | Minimal toxicities; Avoid surgical procedure; Effective for normal to moderately enlarged gland | Long-term hypothyroidism 2%/year; ineffective against large glands; contraindicated in pregnant or lactating patients; possible teratogenic effects for 4–6 months |
| Surgical Resection | Effective for large glands; Safe in mid-trimester patients; No fertility effects | Surgical complications of hypocalcemia, recurrent laryngeal nerve paresis/palsy |

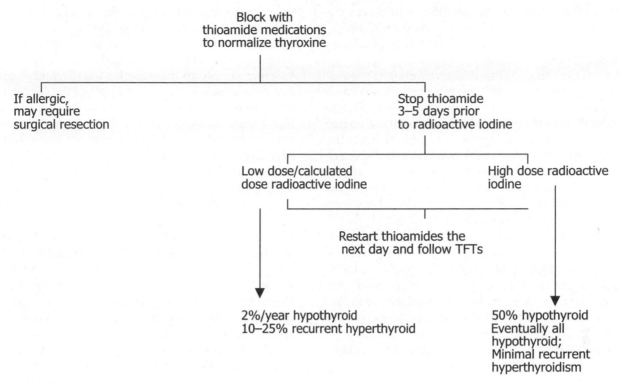

**Figure 23–4.** Algorithm for radioactive iodine treatment for hyperthyroidism.

$$mCi^{131}I =$$

$$\frac{\text{estimated thermal weight (grams)} \times \text{planned dose (Ci/g)}}{\text{fractional 24 RAIU uptake} \times 1000}$$

The planned dose is generally between 80 to 200 μCi/gm of tissue. Using this formula, a typical patient with an estimated thyroid mass of 50 gm and a 24-hour RAIU of 50% with a planned treatment dose of 100 mCi/gm of thyroid tissue produces a calculated dose of 10 mCi.[45]

After administration of radioactive iodine based on either of these techniques, the majority of patients will have normalized their thyroid hormone values within six months. With either technique, a certain proportion of patients will become hypothyroid. In general, 2–4% will become hypothyroid within the first six months and thereafter approximately 2% of patients per year are hypothyroid.[47] These rates translate into a 20% chance of hypothyroidism at ten years post-treatment and a 50% chance of hypothyroidism at 25 years post-treatment. Recurrence rates of hyperthyroidism generally are between 5–20% and depend on the gland size and iodine uptake. Patients with very large toxic goiters are often referred directly for surgical resection (see below) as it is felt that they may have too much thyroid mass to ablate with radioactive iodine. Patients with recurrent disease may be retreated with radioactive iodine at the same or higher dose after at least six

months after receiving the initial therapy, or they may undergo surgical resection.[48]

A third radioactive iodine dosing strategy is to give all patients a fixed high-dose of 15–20 mCi and accept a very high rate of postoperative hypothyroidism in return for virtually no chance of recurrent hyperthyroidism. With these very high doses, up to 50% of patients may be clinically hypothyroid by one year post-treatment and the vast majority of patients become hypothyroid within ten years. Again, this strategy accepts hypothyroidism not as a complication but as an acceptable result with relatively straightforward management with thyroid replacement.

There are few other complications to radioactive iodine except long-term hypothyroidism or treatment failure with recurrent hyperthyroidism.[49] Radioactive iodine may be teratogenic and, therefore, patients cannot become pregnant within six months of receiving a radioactive iodine treatment. The iodine also is transmitted in the breast milk and, therefore, lactating patients cannot be treated with radioactive iodine. There may be a very slight increase in cancer rates following radioactive iodine treatment. The hazard ratio in the large Cooperative Thyrotoxicosis Therapy Study Group had a ratio of 2.77 for development of thyroid cancer in the entire population.[21] Because of the low incidence of thyroid cancer this translated into approximately an additional 70–80 overall deaths in a population of greater than 35,000 patients. There is very slight increased risk of other cancers that may be developed in tissues exposed to the radioactive iodine including lung, breast, and kidney with hazard ratios of 1.11, 1.17, and 1.21, respectively.[2,49]

A final problem with radioactive iodine is a possibility that treatment in this manner may exacerbate ophthalmopathy.[50,51,52] Although prior retrospective studies suggested there was no difference in the degree or incidence of ophthalmopathy dependent upon the treatment type of Graves' disease, a recent prospective randomized study suggested that only 10% of patients who received thioamide drugs or surgical resection had worsened ophthalmopathy, whereas 33% of patients treated with [131]I ablation had worsened eye disease.[53] One criticism of this study is that the baseline incidence of ophthalmopathy in their entire patient population with Graves' disease was only 13%, which is almost three-fold lower than the typical rate. It is agreed that the worsened ophthalmopathy with radioactive iodine treatment is seen to a greater degree in patients who are cigarette smokers.[12] Further prospective studies with adequate follow-up will need to be performed to determine the degree of this problem.[50]

## Surgical Treatment of Graves' Disease

The classic operation popularized throughout the 20th century for surgical treatment of Graves' disease is a subtotal thyroidectomy.[4] With this operation on either one or both sides, a small crescent of thyroid tissue in the superior lateral margin of the thyroid where the recurrent laryngeal nerve enters the larynx is preserved by dividing across thyroid tissue at that location.[54] This operation also has the additional benefit of preserving vascular supply to the superior parathyroid gland on one or both sides. The general goal of the subtotal thyroidectomy is to leave between 3 and 6 grams of thyroid tissue with the overall results that patients become euthyroid on no medical replacement.[4,55] The amount of thyroid tissue left behind will have a direct impact on the recurrence rates of hyperthyroidism and the rates of long-term hypothyroidism.[56] For patients who have larger remnants left behind, there is an increased incidence of recurrent hyperthyroidism which can often be treated with radioactive iodine ablation as it generally involves a fairly small amount of residual tissue.[57,58,59] For patients with more complete thyroidectomies, it is virtually guaranteed there will be no recurrent hyperthyroidism but life-long hypothyroidism will be the outcome of the treatment (Figure 23–5).[60] These results with different surgical approach were demonstrated in a institutional report from Tokyo in which 436 patients with Graves' disease between 1981 and 1990 had operations that attempted to leave a 6-gram remnant of thyroid tissue. In the next 143 patients between 1991 and 1994, a 3-gram thyroid remnant was left.[9] For the patients with a larger remnant, there was an 8% rate of recurrent hyperthyroidism and a 10% rate of long-term clinical hypothyroidism. For patients who had a more significant resection, a lower recurrence rate of 3% was obtained but at a cost of having 51% of the patients be-

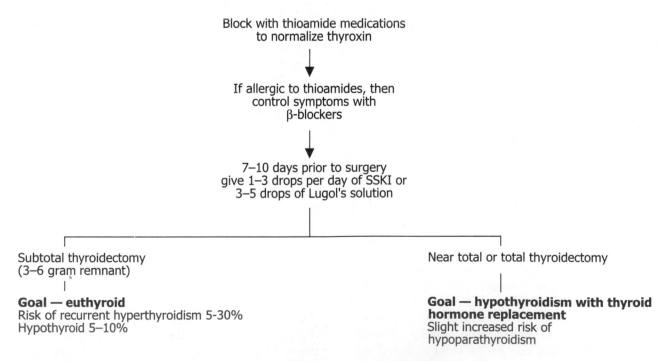

**Figure 23–5.** Algorithm for surgical approach to a patient with Graves' disease.

ing hypothyroid.[61] Some investigators have correlated the level of thyrotropin receptor antibodies with recurrence rate but the size of the thyroid remnant is much more important.[62]

As patients who are surgically rendered hypothyroid can be relatively inexpensively and easily managed with thyroid replacement, this is generally not viewed as a major complication to avoid more complete thyroidectomies in patients with Graves' disease.[63] Other arguments to perform subtotal thyroidectomy as opposed to near total thyroidectomy have been that there have been decreased complication rates by leaving remnants of thyroid tissue particularly in the superior lateral poles to avoid handling of the recurrent laryngeal nerve.[63] However, in experienced hands, the rate of permanent recurrent laryngeal nerve injury approaches zero as does the rate of long-term hypocalcemia.[64] In the report from Japan, there was a 4% transient hypocalcemic rate for patients with subtotal thyroidectomies leaving 6-gram remnants and 8% rate for patients with a near total thyroidectomy leaving 3-gram remnants, but no patient had permanent hypocalcemia caused by hypoparathyroidism.[9,65] The general trend now for patients who have strong indications for surgical therapy (see below) is a more aggressive subtotal or near total thyroidectomy performed with the bias towards preventing recurrent hyperthyroidism.[66,67]

Patients who have absolute indications for surgical treatment for their Graves' disease are those who have significant adverse reactions to thioamide drugs and cannot be appropriately blocked prior to radioactive iodine administration.[68] These would be patients with very severe skin reactions, hepatic damage, or patients with agranulocytosis. For these patients, they can be prepared for surgery using an alternative to thioamide drugs and surgical resection should be the treatment of choice in this small subgroup of patients. A second situation in which surgical resection is a preferred treatment is patients with very large goiters.[35] Patients who have estimated gland size over 75 grams will have very low success rate with radioactive iodine ablation because of the volume of thyroid tissue. In these patients, surgical resection should be the first ablative treatment. A third situation in which patients need surgical resection is when there is co-existent nodular disease that is known to be neoplastic or known to contain malignant tissue.[69] Patients who have cold nodules in the setting of diffuse toxic goiter should have those nodules sampled by fine needle aspiration. A finding of either follicular neoplasm or papillary cell features would require surgical resection and in patients with co-existing Graves' disease a near total thyroidectomy is indicated to treat both the hyperthyroidism and the neoplastic disease. The rate of incidental cancers in patients who had surgery for Graves' disease is 5 to 7%.[32] For all patients undergoing surgical resection for Graves' disease, they need their hyperthyroidism controlled from thioamide drugs or β-blockers for 7–10 days prior to surgery.[70] Patients are given inorganic iodide either as SSKI or Lugol's solution to decrease thyroid blood flow to simplify the surgical procedure (Figure 23–5).[40,71] This treatment will not only decrease the thyroid hormone production, but more importantly will decrease vascularity and blood flow through the thyroid gland making surgical resection easier with less blood loss.

Relative indications for surgical therapy are in young women of childbearing age.[72] As stated above, patients cannot become pregnant within six months of radioactive iodine ablation and patients who are lactating cannot receive radioactive iodine ablation. Young women of childbearing age who either want to attempt pregnancy or who are lactating and want to continue to do so must have surgical resection as a definitive thyroid ablation.[73,74] A second relative indication for surgery rather than radioactive iodine relates to the potential for worsening of ophthalmopathy with radioactive iodine ablation.[51,75,76] Patients with severe ocular symptoms particularly if they are cigarette smokers may opt for surgical resection as the data would indicate there would be no increased risk of worsening of ophthalmopathy with this choice of treatment.[77]

Patients need to be prepared for surgical resection so as not to induce thyrotoxicosis with general anesthesia and manipulation of the thyroid intraoperatively. The optimal management would include blocking of thyroid hormone production with thioamide drugs to achieve a euthyroid state. Addition of beta-blockers may be utilized to control other symptoms.[39] For patients who have significant adverse drug reactions to thioamide drugs, symptom control with beta-blockers alone is an appropriate alternative.

The major side effects from thyroidectomy besides hypothyroidism include development of a neck hematoma, permanent hypoparathyroidism, or recurrent laryngeal nerve injury or injury to the external branch of the superior laryngeal nerve. The incidence of neck hematoma should be <1–2%, and the incidence of permanent hypoparathyroidism should also be 1–2%.[64] There should be essentially zero risk of permanent injury to the recurrent laryngeal nerve for initial neck operations.[78]

## GRAVES' DISEASE IN PREGNANCY

For patients who are pregnant when diagnosed with Graves' disease, the initial treatment is with propylthiouracil as this drug does not cross the placenta to the degree of methimazole.[37,38] Patients can have their thyroid hormone levels decreased to a normal range with high-dose PTU and they should then go on a maintenance dose of PTU and should have their blood test followed closely.[73] Close follow-up is needed because patients in the last trimester of pregnancy may have a remission of their Graves' disease felt to be caused by immune tolerance.[79] Patients often can come off their thyroid medications during their final trimester, but they generally have to resume taking this medication post-partum.[37]

High-dose radioactive iodine is absolutely contraindicated during pregnancy and during times of breast-feeding. Definitive ablation with surgical resection may be performed during pregnancy but should be scheduled for the second trimester where risks of spontaneous abortion and induction of labor are more limited.[73] Indications for undergoing a relatively elective surgical procedure during pregnancy would be primarily adverse reactions to thioamide medications that did not allow them to be taken to control their symptoms of hyperthyroidism medically.

## TREATMENT OF NODULAR HYPERTHYROIDISM

The approach to treatment with medical therapy, radioactive iodine ablation, or surgical resection for toxic multinodular goiter or for a toxic adenoma is quite similar to treatment described above for Graves' disease. A few important differences exist that have an impact on therapy. First, patients with hyperfunctioning nodules never undergo spontaneous remission. Therefore, although thioamide drugs can be used to control the degree and symptoms of hyperthyroidism and prepare patients for radioiodine ablation or surgical resection, there are no plans to withdraw the thioamide medications and assess remission rates. All patients, once their hyperthyroidism is controlled by medical therapy, should be advised to plan and undergo definitive treatment. The definitive treatments for nodular hyperthyroidism include both radioactive iodine ablation and surgical resection with the third potential treatment for single functioning nodules of alcohol injection to ablate the lesion.

Radioactive iodine ablation is generally quite effective for toxic nodular thyroid disease.[80] In general, a higher dose of radioiodine is necessary because of less diffuse uptake and because of decreased degree of uptake. A typical radioactive iodine dose for nodular disease would be 15 mCi of [131]I. With this ablation technique, the majority of patients are cured of their hyperthyroidism. In patients who have a single nodule, there is a relatively low incidence of post-treatment hypothyroidism as the iodine uptake is only in the area of the abnormal nodule and there is incomplete exposure

to the entire thyroid gland.[81] For patients with bilobar multinodular toxic goiter, there is a greater incidence of post-treatment hypothyroidism. Contraindications to radioactive iodine are similar to that described for Graves' disease including young women who are lactating or are interested in becoming pregnant as well as patients with severe adverse drug reactions to thioamide medications.

Surgical resection for patients with a single toxic adenoma is more straightforward as only the lobe with the abnormal nodule needs to be removed leaving a normal contralateral lobe behind.[9] In general, these patients then have a recurrence of function and the incidence of hypothyroidism is quite low. The reported incidence of hypothyroidism after unilobar resection of a toxic adenoma is still 5%, probably based on some underlying thyroid pathology. For patients with multinodular toxic goiter, a near total thyroidectomy is necessary if patients opt for surgery over radioactive iodine. The surgical approach and complication rate is similar to that of diffuse toxic goiter.

A third choice of treatment is percutaneous injection of ethanol into the nodule.[82] Response rates with patients becoming euthyroid vary between 65% to 85% one year after therapy. In general, injections are repeated multiple times dependent on the size of the nodules and the clinical response.

It should be noted that virtually all nodules that are hyperfunctional in adult patients are benign and worries of malignancy in toxic adenomas should not influence therapy. These nodules do not need to undergo fine needle aspiration because the chance of malignancy is incredibly low. For patients with multinodular toxic goiter, again because of the heterogeneous iodine uptake, it may be very difficult to distinguish a cold nodule in this setting, and there have been malignancies reported that were surreptitiously uncovered after a surgical resection.

## IODINE-INDUCED THYROTOXICOSIS

Another setting for surgery in the treatment of hyperthyroidism is iodine-induced thyrotoxicosis. Far and away the most common etiology of this problem over the past decade has been use of the anti-arrhythmic drug amiodarone.[83,84] In this situation as with other occasions where iodine-induced thyrotoxicosis occurs there is a generalized low iodine uptake on radioactive scans.[85] A large series of patients at the Mayo Clinic with this diagnosis had only a 4% iodine uptake at 24 hours.[30] Therefore, radioiodine ablation is not an option for definitive treatment in this setting.

Amiodarone is retained in adipose tissue and often patients who have severe amiodarone-induced thyrotoxicosis may not have spontaneous resolution even with discontinuing the agent because of drug retained in the hepatic tissue. As iodine ablation is not effective, surgical resection is often needed. By definition, these patients have some type of cardiac history and may have an increased risk of operation, but a successful thyroidectomy is curative for this patient population.[86]

## THYROID STORM

The term thyroid storm refers to an acute exacerbation of either subclinical or baseline hyperthyroidism with constellation of symptoms that include high fever, severe tachycardia, and altered mental status. This condition generally results from an added event or insult such as an infection or surgical procedure that induces a marked release of thyroid hormone and this severe systemic response. Principles of management of this condition include removing the etiology of the thyroid storm (eg, performing an appendectomy for patients presenting with acute appendicitis in thyroid storm) and a series of measures to decrease the activity of thyroid hormone on the peripheral tissues.

In general, the treatment regimen for thyroid storm includes PTU as this not only blocks hormonal production but decreases the transition as a conversion of $T_4$ to $T_3$ in the peripheral tissues.[70] A second treatment agent would be radioiodine contrast agents as these block release of hormone from the thyroid and also block conversion of thyroxin in the periphery and any additional iodine uptake. Finally, high-dose steroids may be helpful in reducing the tissue response to high levels of thyroid hormones.[19]

## References

1. Woeber KA. Update on the management of hyperthyroidism and hypothyroidism. *Arch Int Med.* 2000;160(8):1067–1071.
2. Ron E, Doody MM, Becker DV, et al. Cancer mortality following treatment for adult hyperthyroidism. *JAMA.* 1998;280(4):347–355.
3. Stanbury JB, Ermans AE, Bourdoux P, et al. Iodine-induced hyperthyroidism: occurrence and epidemiology. *Thyroid.* 1998;8:83–100.
4. Mansberger AR. One hundred years of surgical management of hyperthyroidism. *Ann Surg.* 1988;207:724–729.
5. Sawin CT, Becker DV. Radioiodine and the treatment of hyperthyroidism: the early history. *Thyroid.* 1997;7:163–176.
6. Franklyn JA. The management of hyperthyroidism. *N Engl J Med.* 1994;330(24):1731–1738.
7. Astwood EB. Treatment of hyperthyroidism with thiourea and thiouracil. *JAMA.* 1943;122:78.
8. Cooper DS. Antithyroid drugs. *N Engl J Med.* 1984;311:1353–1362.
9. Okamoto T, Iihara M, Obara T. Management of hyperthyroidism due to Graves' and nodular diseases. *World J Surg.* 2000;24:957–961.
10. Witte J, Goretzki PE, Roher HD. Surgery for Graves' disease in childhood and adolescence. *Exper Clin Endocrin Diab.* 1997;4:58–60.
11. Costagliola S, Morgenthaler NG, Hoermann R, et al. Second generation assay for thyrotropin receptor antibodies has superior diagnostic sensitivity for Graves' disease. *J Clin Endocrinol Metab.* 1999;84:90–97.
12. Prummel MF, Wiersinga W. Smoking and risk of Graves' disease. *JAMA.* 1993;269(4):479–482.
13. Bahn RS, Heufelder AE. Pathogenesis of Graves' ophthalmopathy. *N Engl J Med.* 1193;329(20):1468–1474.
14. Utiger RD. Pathogenesis of Graves' ophthalmopathy. *N Engl J Med.* (Editorial) 1992;326(26):1772–1773.
15. Woeber KA. Thyrotoxicosis and the heart. *N Engl J Med.* 1992;327(2):94–98.
16. Wartofsky L. *Bone disease in thyrotoxicosis. Hospital Practice.* May 15, 1994; pp. 69–78
17. Klein I, Trzepacz PT, Roberts M, Levey GS. Symptom rating scale for assessing hyperthyroidism. *Arch Intern Med.* 1988;148:387–390.
18. Bartalena L, Pinchera A, Marcocci C. Management of Graves' ophthalmopathy: reality and perspectives. *Endocr Rev.* 2000;2:168–99.
19. Prummel MF, Mourits M, Berghout A, et al. Prednisone and cyclosporine in the treatment of severe Graves' ophthalmopathy. *N Engl J Med.* 1989;321(20): 1353–1358.
20. Burch HB, Wartofsky L. Graves' ophthalmopathy: current concepts regarding pathogenesis and management. *Endocr Rev.* 1993;14:747–793.
21. Tallstedt L. Surgical treatment of thyroid eye disease. *Thyroid.* 1998;8:447–52.
22. Fatourechi V, Fransway AF. Dermopathy of Graves' disease (pretibial myxedema). *Medicine.* 1994;73:1–7.
23. Wallace K, Hofmann MT. Thyroid dysfunction: how to manage overt and subclinical disease in older patients. *Geriatrics.* 1998;53:32–8.
24. Utiger RD. Subclinical hyperthyroidism—Just a low serum thyrotropin concentration, or something more? *N Engl J Med.* 1994;(Editorial) 331(19):1302–3.
25. Beck-Peccoz P, Brucker-Davis F, Persani L, et al. Thyrotropin-secreting pituitary tumors. *Endocr Rev.* 1996;16:610.
26. Kopp P, Van Sande J, Parma A, et al. Brief report: Congenital hyperthyroidism caused by a mutation in the thyrotropin-receptor gene. *N Engl J Med.* 1995;332(3):150–154.
27. Mariotti S, Caturegli P, Piccolo P, et al. Antithyroid peroxidase autoantibodies in thyroid diseases. *J Clin Endocrinol Metab.* 1990;71:661–669.
28. Mariotti S, Martino E, Cupini C, et al. Low serum thyroglobulin as a clue to the diagnosis of thyrotoxicosis factitia. *N Eng J Med.* 1982;307:410–412.
29. Stanbury JB, Ermans AE, Bourdoux P, et al. Iodine-induced hyperthyroidism: occurrence and epidemiology. *Thyroid.* 1998;8:83–100.
30. Meurisse M, Detroz B, Messens D, et al. The treatment of amiodarone-induced hyperthyroidism. Is there a place for surgery? *Acta Chirurgia Belgica.* 1994;94:36–41.
31. Ayhan A, Yanik F, Tuncer R, et al. Struma ovarii. *Int J Gynaecol. Obstet.* 1993;42:143–146.
32. Ozaki O, Ito K, Kobayashi K, Toshima K, Iwasaki H, Yashiro T. Thyroid carcinoma in Graves' disease. *World J Surg.* 1990;14:437–40.
33. Vanderpump MPJ, Ahlquist JAO, Franklyn JA, Clayton RN. Consensus statement for good practice and audit measures in the management of hypothyroidism and hyperthyroidism. *Br Med J.* 1996;313(7056):539–544.
34. Singer PA, Cooper DS, Legy EG, et al. Treatment guidelines for patients with hyperthyroidism and hypothyroidism. *JAMA.* 1995;273(10):808–812.
35. Weetman AP. The role of surgery in primary hyperthyroidism. *J Royal Soc Med.* 1998;33:7–11.

36. Wartofsky L, Glinoer D, Solomon B, Lagasse R. Differences and similarities in the treatment of diffuse goiter in Europe and the United States. *Exp Clin Endocrinol.* 1991;97:243–251.

37. Momotani N, Noh J, Oyanagi H, Ishikawa N, Ito Kunihiko. Antithyroid drug therapy for Graves' disease during pregnancy. *N Engl J Med.* 1986;315:24–8.

38. Marchant B, Brownlie BE, Hart DM, et al. The placental transfer of propylthiouracil, methimazole and carbimazole. *J Clin Endocrinol Metab.* 1977;45:1187–1193.

39. Adlerberth A, Stenstrom G, Hasselgren P. The selective $\beta_1$-blocking agent Metoprolol compared with antithyroid drug treatment of patients with hyperthyroidism. *Ann Surg.* 1987;205(2): 182–188.

40. Marigold JH, Morgan AK, Earle DJ, et al. Lugol's iodine: its effect on thyroid blood flow in patients with thyrotoxicosis. *Br J Surg.* 1985;72:45–47.

41. Gittoes NJ, Franklyn JA. Hyperthyroidism. Current treatment guidelines. *Drugs.* 1998;55:543–53.

42. Vitti P, Rago T, Chiovato L, et al. Clinical features of patients with Graves' disease undergoing remission after antithyroid drug treatment. *Thyroid.* 1997;7:369–375.

43. Hashizume K, Ichikawa K, Sakurai A, et al. Administration of thyroxine in treated Graves' disease. *N Engl J Med.* 1991; 324(14):947–953.

44. Ladenson PW. Treatments for Graves' disease. *N Engl J Med.* (Editorial) 1991;324(14):989–990.

45. Graham GD, Urman KD. Radioiodine treatment of Graves' disease. *Ann Int Med.* 1986;105:900–905.

46. Burch HB, Solomon BL, Wartofsky L, Burman KD. Discontinuing antithyroid drug therapy before ablation with radioiodine in Graves' disease. *Ann Intern Med.* 1994;121:553–559.

47. Sridama V, McCormick M, Kaplan EL, Fauchet R, DeGroot LJ. Long-term follow-up study of compensated low-dose $^{131}$I therapy for Graves' disease. *N Engl J Med.* 1984;311:426–32.

48. Hermann M, Roka R, Richter B, Koriska K, Gobl S, Freissmuth M. Reoperation as treatment of relapse after subtotal thyroidectomy in Graves' disease. *Surgery.* 1999;125:522–8.

49. Franklyn JA, Maisonneuve P, Sheppard MC, et al. Mortality after the treatment of hyperthyroidism with radioactive iodine. *N Engl J Med.* 1998;338:712–718.

50. Bartalena L, Marcocci C, Bogazzi F, Panicucci M, Lepri A, Pinchera A. Use of corticosteroids to prevent progression of Graves' ophthalmopathy after radioiodine therapy for hyperthyroidism. *N Engl J Med.* 1989;321:1349–52.

51. Fernandez Sanchez JR, Rosell Pradas J, Carazo Martinez O, et al. Graves' ophthalmopathy after subtotal thyroidectomy and radioiodine therapy. *Br J Surg.* 1993;80:1134–6.

52. Tallstedt L, Lundell G. Radioiodine treatment, ablation, and ophthalmopathy: a balanced perspective. *Thyroid.* 1997;7:241–5.

53. Tallstedt L, Lundell G, Torring O, et al. Thyroid Study Group. Occurrence of ophthalmopathy after treatment for Graves' hyperthyroidism. *N Engl J Med.* 1992;326(26):1733–1738.

54. Menegaux F, Ruprecht T, Chigot JP. The surgical treatment of Graves' disease. *Surgery, Gynecol Obstey.* 1993;176:277–82.

55. Sugino K, Mimura T, Toshima K, et al. Follow-up evaluation of patients with Graves' disease treated by subtotal thyroidectomy and risk factor analysis for post-operative thyroid dysfunction. *J Endocrin Invest.* 1993;16:195–9.

56. Sugino K, Mimura T, Ozaki O, et al. Management of recurrent hyperthyroidism in patients with Graves' disease treated by subtotal thyroidectomy. *J Endocrin Invest.* 1995;18:415–9.

57. Chou FF, Wang PW, Huang SC. Results of subtotal thyroidectomy for Graves' disease. *Thyroid.* 1999;9:253–7.

58. Sugino K, Mimura T, Ozaki O, et al. Early recurrence of hyperthyroidism in patients with Graves' disease treated by subtotal thyroidectomy. *World J Surg.* 1995;19:648–52.

59. Vestergaard H, Laurberg P. Radioiodine treatment of recurrent hyperthyoidism in patients previously treated for Graves' disease by subtotal thyroidectomy. *J Int Med.* 1992;231:13–7.

60. Razack MS, Lore JM, Lippes HA, Schaefer DP, Rassael H. Total thyroidectomy for Graves' disease. *Head & Neck.* 1997;19:378–83.

61. Ozaki O, Ito K, Mimura T, Sugino K, Ito K. Factors affecting thyroid function after subtotal thyroidectomy for Graves' disease: case control study by remnant-weight matched-pair analysis. *Thyroid.* 1997;7:555–9.

62. Sugino K, Mimura T, Ozaka O, et al. Preoperative change of thyroid stimulating hormone receptor antibody level: possible marker for predicting recurrent hyperthyroidism in patients with Graves' disease after subtotal thyroidectomy. *World J Surg.* 1996; 20:801–6.

63. Kuma K, Matsuzuka F, Kobayashi A, et al. Natural course of Graves' disease after subtotal thyroidectomy and management of patients with postoperative thyroid dysfunction. *Am J Med Sci.* 1991;302:8–12.

64. Yamashita H, Noguchi S, Tahara K, et al. Postoperative tetany in patients with Graves' disease: a risk factor. *Clin Endocrin.* 1997;47:71–7.

65. Noh SH, Soh EY, Park CS, Lee KS, Huh KB. Evaluation of thyroid function after bilateral subtotal thyroidectomy for Graves' disease—a long term follow up of 100 patients. *Yonsei Medical J.* 1994;35:177–83.

66. Winsa B, Rastad J, Larsson E, et al. Total thyroidectomy in therapy-resistant Graves' disease. *Surgery.* 1994;116:1068–74.

67. Miccoli P, Vitti P, Rago T, et al. Surgical treatment of Graves' disease. Subtotal or total thyroidectomy? *Surgery.* 1996;120:1020–1025.

68. Patwardhan NA, Moront M, Rao S, Rossi S, Braverman LE. Surgery still has a role in Graves' hyperthyroidism. *Surgery.* 1993;114:1108–12.

69. Zanella E, Rulli F, Muzi M, et al. Prevalence of thyroid cancer in hyperthyroid patients treated by surgery. *W J Surg.* 1998;22:473–7.

70. Hermann M, Richter B, Roka R, Freissmuth M. Thyroid surgery in untreated severe hyperthyroidism: perioperative kinetics of free thyroid hormones in the glandular venous effluent and peripheral blood. *Surgery.* 1994;240–5.

71. Chang DCS, Wheeler MH, Woodcock JP, et al. The effect of preoperative Lugol's iodine on thyroid blood flow in patients with Graves' hyperthyroidism. *Surgery.* 1987;102(6):1055–1061.

72. Sugino K, Ito K, Ozaki O, Mimura T, Iwasaki H, Wada N. Postoperative changes in thyrotropin-binding inhibitory immunoglobulin level in patients with Graves' disease: is subtotal thyroidectomy a suitable therapeutic option for patients of childbearing age with Graves' disease? *World J Surg.* 1999;23: 727–31.

73. Lazarus JH. Treatment of hyper- and hypothyroidism in pregnancy. *J Endocrinol Invest.* 1993;16:391–6.

74. Soreide JA, van Heerden JA, Lo CY, Grant SC, Zimmerman D, Ilstrup DM. Surgical treatment of Graves' disease in patients younger than 18 years. *World J Surg.* 1996;20:794–9.

75. Levitt MD, Edis AJ, Agnello R, McCormick CC. The effect of subtotal thyroidectomy on Graves' ophthalmopathy. *World J Surg.* 1988;12:593–597.

76. Winsa B, Rastad J, Akerstrom G, Johansson H, Westermark K, Karlsson FA. Retrospective evaluation of subtotal and total thyroidectomy in Graves' disease with and without endocrine ophthalmopathy. *Eur J Endocrin.* 1995;132:406–12.

77. Marcocci C, Bruno-Bossio G, Manetti L, et al. The course of Graves' ophthalmopathy is not influenced by near total thyroidectomy: a case control study. *Clin Endocrin.* 1999;51:503–8.

78. Andaker L, Johansson K, Smeds S, Lennquist S. Surgery for hyperthyroidism: hemithyroidectomy plus contralateral resection or bilateral resection? A prospective randomized study of post-

operative complications and long-term results. *World J Surg.* 1992;16:765–9.

79. Masiukiewicz US, Burrow GN. Hyperthyroidism in pregnancy: diagnosis and treatment. *Thyroid.* 1999;9:647–52.

80. Goldstein R, Hart IR. Follow-up of solitary autonomous thyroid nodules treated with [131]I. *N Eng J Med.* 1983;309:1473–6.

81. Ross DS, Ridgway EC, Daniels GH. Successful treatment of solitary toxic nodules with relatively low-dose [131]I with low prevalence of hypothyroidism. *Ann Intern Med.* 1984;101:488.

82. Martino E, Murtas ML, Loviselli A, et al. Percutaneous intranodular ethanol injection for treatment of autonomously functioning thyroid nodules. *Surgery.* 1992;112:1161–1165.

83. Dunn JT, Semigran MJ, Delange F. The prevention and management of iodine-induced hyperthyroidism and its cardiac features. *Thyroid.* 1998;8:101–6.

84. Martinoi E, Aghini-Lombardi F, Mariotti S, et al. Amiodarone: a common source of iodine-induced thyrotoxicosis. *Horm Res.* 1987;26:158.

85. Reichert LJ, de Rooy HA. Treatment of amiodarone induced hyperthyroidism with potassium perchlorate and methimazole during amiodarone treatment. *Br Med J.* 1989;298:547.

86. Bartalena L, Brogioni S, Grasso L, et al. Treatment of amiodarone-induced thyrotoxicosis, a difficult challenge: results of a prospective study. *J Clin Endocrinol Metab.* 1996;81:2930–2933.

# 24

# Surgical Evaluation and Management of Goiter

## Joseph A. Califano III, M.D. and Dennis H. Kraus, M.D.

Goiter is a term derived from the Latin appellation "tumidum gutter," translated as "swollen throat." In the intervening centuries since the origin of that nomenclature, the exact criteria by which goiter is described has only moderately improved in its precision and universal acceptance. The World Health Organization has described goiter as an enlargement of the lateral lobe of the thyroid gland that exceeds the dimensions of the terminal phalanx of the thumb.[1] Other definitions have included that of a gland greater than 40 grams in weight, or a volume twice that of a normal gland. Precise measurement of the *in situ* thyroid gland to determine goitrous enlargement may be accomplished by imaging techniques, with ultrasound being the most common modality used.

By even the most narrow definition, a plethora of underlying etiologies resulting in a diagnosis of goiter are recognized, each of which may range from insignificant, to annoying, to lethal. Varying definitions aside, appropriate evaluation and management of the thyroid goiter involve diagnosis of the nature and etiology of thyroid enlargement, its impact on thyroid function, and the risk for adverse sequelae related to the underlying disease process. This chapter will describe the evaluation of goiter as it relates to those processes which may be treated by appropriate surgical therapy. Information on the phenomenon of substernal goiter will not be explored in detail, as this is addressed in subsequent chapters in this volume.

## BACKGROUND AND CLASSIFICATION

Worldwide, goiter is most commonly caused by a deficiency in the dietary intake of iodine, a phenomenon termed "endemic goiter."[2,3] The prevalence of endemic goiter in populations that suffer from extreme iodine deficiency can approach 50%. In the United States, the routine practice of iodine supplementation in the food supply since the early part of the 20th century has resulted in dramatic decreases in the rate of endemic goiter. Consequently, endemic goiter is now seen only in a few geographic areas (Appalachia, eastern Kentucky) or in populations who have recently immigrated to the United States from areas where endemic goiter exists. However, thyroid goiter is still seen at a prevalence of approximately 5% in some populations despite effective iodine prophylaxis, and the annual incidence is 1% or less even in iodine-replete populations.[4,5]

As alluded to above, precise classification of goiter remains elusive, and remains almost synonymous with "thyroid enlargement." As such, "goiter" is a clinical term that may indicate the presence of several clinical entities, including a solitary thyroid nodule, multinodular thyroid enlargement, or diffuse thyroid enlargement. All these varieties may present with hyperfunction of the diseased thyroid nodule(s), resulting in the terms toxic adenoma and toxic multinodular goiter, or with diffuse hyperfunction of the thyroid gland from a variety of stimuli (see Table 24–1). At present, the only diagnostic terms which consistently use the word "goiter" are those of endemic goiter caused by iodine deficiency, and toxic and non-toxic multinodular goiter, referring to adenomatous hyperplasia of the thyroid gland with and without a hyperfunctioning thyroid adenoma, respectively. A presumption is made that at the conclusion of an appropriate diagnostic evaluation, an initial diagnosis of goiter may often be discarded in favor of a more precise diagnosis.

**Table 24–1.** Classification of thyroid enlargement

1. Nodular Goiter
   A. Non-toxic benign nodules
      1. Colloid nodule or colloid cyst
      2. Non-toxic multinodular goiter (adenomatous hyperplasia, colloid goiter)
      3. Follicular adenoma
      4. Hashimoto's thyroiditis with lymphoid follicles
   B. Hyperfunctioning nodules
      1. Toxic adenoma
      2. Toxic multinodular goiter
   C. Thyroid malignancy
      1. Carcinoma
         a. papillary carcinoma
         b. follicular carcinoma
         c. Hürthle cell carcinoma
         d. anaplastic carcinoma
         e. medullary carcinoma
      2. Lymphoma
      3. Metastasis and other
      4. Diffuse Goiter
   A. Endemic goiter caused by iodine deficiency
   B. Goitrogens
      1. Antithyroid medications
      2. Antithyroid foods or other ingested agents
   C. Autoimmune disease
      1. Graves' disease
      2. Toxic autoimmune thyroiditis
      3. Chronic lymphocytic thyroiditis
      4. Hashimoto's thyroiditis
   D. Acute bacterial thyroiditis
   E. Subacute thyroiditis
   F. Inherited enzymatic deficiency
   G. TSH-secreting pituitary adenoma
   H. Systemic and pituitary resistance to thyroid hormone

## GENERAL DIAGNOSTIC EVALUATION

Goiter is most commonly discovered on routine physical examination in an otherwise asymptomatic patient. A detailed clinical history should include a review of any symptoms of hypo- or hyperthyroidism. A history of prior therapeutic radiation exposure, a familial history of thyroid malignancy, or a history of immigration from an area where the entire population has been exposed to radioactive fallout (eg Chernobyl) will alert the examiner to the possibility of underlying malignancy. Those patients from an area where endemic goiter is common may well have underlying iodine deficiency.

A chronology of the rate at which the thyroid or thyroid mass has grown should be elicited. A recent history of sudden increase in the size of a particular nodule will increase the suspicion for the development of malignancy, although this may indicate hemorrhage into a benign cystic nodule. A sudden increase

in the size of the entire gland accompanied by pain and tenderness may be a symptom of a viral or acute lymphocytic thyroiditis. Symptoms of dysphagia and odynophagia are occasionally elicited, but must be carefully characterized to determine whether or not they may be attributable to the goiter itself. Airway symptoms including hoarseness, stridor, and dyspnea may be caused by compressive effects from a substernal goiter, or may be caused by recurrent laryngeal nerve involvement from a malignant process. Pain as a presenting symptom is rarely elicited, but may be caused by chronic or acute inflammation, or advanced malignancy.

The physical examination should include a complete head and neck examination with examination of the thyroid gland and cervical nodal beds, an ophthalmologic exam, a cranial nerve exam, and complete examination of the upper aerodigestive tract including an assessment of vocal cord function. A single, dominant, hard thyroid nodule that is adherent to the surrounding tissues suggests malignancy. The presence of cervical adenopathy accompanying a thyroid mass raises suspicion for metastatic thyroid cancer. Multiple nodules suggest a diagnosis of multinodular goiter, but does not exclude malignancy, as malignancy can arise in a background of multinodular adenomatous hyperplasia. Graves' disease often presents with a characteristic ophthalmopathy and/or dermopathy. Physical findings consistent with hyperthyroidism suggest the presence of early Graves' disease, an autonomously functioning adenoma, or toxic multinodular goiter. Symptoms and signs of thyrotoxicosis include anxiety, heat intolerance, weight loss despite adequate intake and appetite, heat intolerance, tremor, fatigue, muscle weakness, tachycardia, and heart failure. A diffusely tender, enlarged thyroid may be caused by autoimmune or viral thyroiditis. A diffusely firm, hard thyroid gland in a patient with symptoms and signs of hypothyroidism may be suffering from late stage Hashimoto's thyroiditis. As indicated, suspicion for malignancy rises with a solitary nodule, sudden increase in the size of a single nodule in a multinodular or normal gland, associated cervical adenopathy, a history of prior irradiation, large nodule size, fixation of the nodule to surrounding structures, or hard consistency to palpation.

## LABORATORY TESTING

Laboratory testing should include measurement of serum $T_3$, free $T_4$, and thyroid stimulating hormone (TSH). Many clinicians will also obtain a measurement of serum thyroid antibodies, including thyroglobulin antibodies (TgAb) and thyroperoxidase antibodies (TpAb) during initial assessment, since diffuse thyroid enlargement in iodine-sufficient areas is frequently caused by autoimmune thyroid disease. Some clinicians advocate only the measurement of TSH during initial evaluation, as newer generation TSH assays have a high degree of sensitivity in detection of hypo- and hyperthyroidism. Calcitonin and parathyroid hormone are not routinely measured during an initial evaluation, as the risk of medullary thyroid carcinoma and parathyroid adenoma are low in the setting of an initial diagnostic visit.

## FINE NEEDLE ASPIRATION BIOPSY

Fine needle aspiration biopsy (FNA) is a safe, inexpensive, and accurate modality for the evaluation of thyroid nodules. The primary utility of FNA is in diagnosis of a nodule as benign or malignant. It is the initial test of choice for a goiter caused by a solitary thyroid nodule, as its accuracy may be as high as 97% in that clinical context.[6] A review of series examining FNA in over 10,000 patients with single and multiple thyroid nodules showed a suspicious or malignant diagnosis in 16% of biopsied nodules.[7] Twenty-one percent of the surgically excised nodules were diagnosed as malignant on paraffin-embedded sections and 8% of the excised nodules were read as false negatives on FNA. The highest accuracy was noted in undifferentiated and medullary thyroid cancers, as well as papillary thyroid cancer. The ability of FNA to distinguish benign follicular lesions from follicular carcinoma is poor, however, since this distinction is primarily based on demonstration of invasion of capsular and vascular structures best revealed in tissue-block sections. Many benign conditions may yield an indeterminate or suspicious result from FNA, including Hashimoto's thyroiditis, benign goiter, follicular adenoma, and Hürthle cell adenoma. Even in medical centers with highly skilled clinicians, a 3% false-negative rate from FNA is seen in the evaluation of thyroid carcinoma. Therefore, FNA results need to be interpreted within a clinical context: a high suspicion for malignancy caused by progressive enlargement of a single or dominant thyroid nodule, fixation to adjacent structures, and/or a history of low-dose radiation exposure may mandate surgical intervention despite benign FNA result. In addition, a patient who has received a benign cytologic diagnosis by FNA still requires clinical surveillance.

Ultrasound guidance may be used to allow for the sampling of small nodules that may otherwise be difficult to access. Thyroid glands with multiple nodules may also be evaluated by ultrasound imaging. A solitary, enlarging nodule within that gland may be sampled individually. It should be noted that the same caveats regarding sampling error and risk of false negative cytology apply to these clinical scenarios, perhaps even more so.

## IMAGING

Ultrasonography is useful for a variety of clinical scenarios in the management of goiter. Its primary utility is based on its ability to measure the size and nature of multiple or single thyroid nodules. Nodules may be characterized as solid, cystic, or complex with a high degree of accuracy, and nodules less than 1 cm in size are routinely seen during thyroid ultrasound. Serial ultrasonography may be used to determine relative growth of specific nodules in a multinodular gland.

In the diagnosis of thyroid malignancy, ultrasound alone is of little or no utility.[8,9] It is highly sensitive in detection of nodules and may be used to detect multicentric disease in a gland already known to be involved with a papillary thyroid cancer. It may also be used to guide FNA of nodules that are small in size, inaccessible by palpation, or surrounded by other nodules in a multinodular goiter. The addition of ultrasound guidance in these scenarios will increase diagnostic accuracy. Ultrasound may also be used to monitor gland size and the increase in size of single nodules in a multinodular gland, in order to screen for suspicious lesions in a complex, multinodular goiter. It should be noted that the high sensitivity of ultrasound results in the diagnosis of nodules that are a few millimeters in size. In the absence of suspicion for thyroid malignancy in the remainder of the gland these are of little clinical importance, and may be observed as they are unlikely to represent occult malignancy.

## RADIONUCLIDE IMAGING

Iodine radionuclides are the most common of those used for thyroid imaging. They have limited use in the evaluation of goiter. Historically, this radiographic study was used to distinguish between a hypofunctioning and hyperfunctioning thyroid gland. Although this has been commonly used as an adjunctive test for determination of risk of malignancy for a particular thyroid nodule, it does not have an adequate sensitivity or specificity in determination of malignancy for thyroid nodules and has been largely supplanted by FNA.

## SUBTYPES OF THYROID GOITER: EVALUATION AND TREATMENT

Thyroid goiter may be classified on the basis of thyroid function and the presence and nature of nodularity in the involved gland. This information is obtained during the initial clinical evaluation from routine thyroid function tests, physical examination, and occasional ultrasonographic evaluation. Based on these results, goiter may be classified into those that are thyrotoxic versus non-toxic/hypo- and euthyroid. These may be further classified into those that are diffusely enlarged, uninodular, or multinodular. These entities will be examined separately in terms of further evaluation and treatment.

### Diffuse Toxic Goiter

The common etiologies of diffuse goiter with accompanying thyrotoxicosis include Graves' disease, subacute thyroiditis, chronic (lymphocytic) thyroiditis/Hashimoto's thyroiditis/autoimmune thyroiditis, and thyrotropin-induced thyrotoxicosis caused by a TSH-secreting pituitary tumor.

Graves' disease is the most common form of diffuse toxic goiter, and is the most common cause of hyperthyroidism in the United States.[10] Hyperthyroidism in this disease is thought to be caused by antibodies directed against the TSH receptors in thyroid tissue that directly stimulate these receptors. Affected patients are typically female, and present in the third and fourth decades of life. The classic triad of Graves' disease includes diffuse toxic goiter, infiltrative ophthalmopathy resulting in exophthalmos, and infiltrative dermopathy resulting in pretibial myxedema. Although initially presenting with thyrotoxicosis, Graves' disease is characterized by a waxing and waning clinical course, with spontaneous relapses and remissions. In addition, the disease is also characterized by production of antibodies that prevent stimulation of the TSH receptor, resulting in hypothyroidism.[11] Histologically, areas of lymphocytic infiltration may be present in the affected gland. A proportion of patients who present with thyrotoxicosis, infiltrative ophthalmopathy, and goiter may therefore have characteristics of both Hashimoto's thyroiditis and Graves' disease. Differentiation may only be possible after surgical removal of the gland, and determination of the unique histologic features of Graves' disease.

Radioactive iodine is the initial management of choice for Graves' disease in the United States. Long term results with this modality have been favorable with an incidence of recurrent hyperthyroidism of 6%. Radioactive iodine therapy is absolutely contraindicated in pregnant women, and is excreted in breast milk, preventing breast-feeding for several months after therapy. Radioactive iodine therapy is also contraindicated as first-line therapy for Graves' disease in children, but may be used in those who fail drug therapy and in those for whom surgery is contraindicated. Hypothyroidism after radioactive iodine therapy is not uncommon, and careful surveillance of thyroid status is warranted after treatment.

Drug therapy for Graves' disease is usually oral administration of propylthiouracil, or methimazole, and is usually reserved for younger patients and pregnant women, to avoid radiation exposure associated with radioactive iodine therapy. These agents block thyroid hormone formation by serving as a substrate for thyroid peroxidase, preventing organification of iodine. These agents are relatively safe, with a small risk of agranulocytosis and hepatitis. These agents are reported to result in permanent remission of hyperthyroidism on the order of 40%, with up to 60% recurrence of thyrotoxicosis within five years.[10,12]

Surgical therapy for thyrotoxic Graves' disease has traditionally consisted of subtotal thyroidectomy. It is primarily reserved for those who have failed to respond to radioactive iodine and thioamides, as well as pregnant women and children.[13] In a series of 321 patients treated surgically for Graves' disease, the incidence of recurrence of hyperthyroidism five years after subtotal thyroidectomy is 16%, with an incidence of hypothyroidism of approximately 10%.[14] Of note, a large thyroid remnant after subtotal thyroidectomy was found to be a risk factor for postoperative hyperthyroidism in this study. Postoperative hypothyroidism is easily treated, while persistent hyperthyroidism after subtotal thyroidectomy for Graves' disease may be very difficult to treat;[15] therefore appropriate surgical therapy should consist of an aggressive subtotal thyroidectomy with a minimal thyroid remnant.

The presence of nodularity found intraoperatively in a thyroid gland initially thought to be diffusely enlarged because of Graves' disease should immediately raise the suspicion for occult malignancy. Well differentiated thyroid cancer is greater than two-fold more prevalent in patients with Graves' disease when compared to the population-at-large.[16] Primary thyroid cancers occurring in a background of Graves' disease tend to have features that suggest that they are more aggressive, including larger size, and a higher incidence of both extrathyroidal extension and lymph node metastasis.[17] A palpable, non-functioning nodule found in a diffuse thyrotoxic goiter caused by Graves' disease has a greater than 40% chance of representing an occult malignancy, and a definitive diagnosis should be aggressively pursued in this clinical scenario.

Preoperative preparation for thyrotoxic Graves' disease includes control with thioamides or β-adrenergic blockade, either in combination or alone. Some authors advocate addition of iodine to β-adrenergic blockade in the belief that the requirement for β-blockade is reduced and the vascularity of the thyroid gland is reduced as well, but solid evidence for these views is lacking.

Subacute thyroiditis has also been termed pseudo-granulomatous thyroiditis, de Quervain's thyroiditis, or viral thyroiditis, although no clear viral etiology has been established. It presents with fever, myalgia, leukocytosis, and a painful and enlarged thyroid. Serum antithyroid antibodies are absent, differentiating this from other autoimmune causes of thyroiditis. The clinical course of this disease includes mild thyrotoxicosis during the acute phase for about one month, followed by a brief euthyroid state and subsequent hypothyroidism for several months. Finally a euthyroid state is reached. Medical therapy is directed at relieving associated symptoms, and surgical intervention is not indicated.

Hashimoto's thyroiditis is the most common form of thyroiditis, usually found in women from the fourth to sixth decade of life. It is an autoimmune thyroiditis that is often found in patients with other autoimmune conditions. Patients present with an asymptomatic goiter, with or without associated exophthalmos. They may be thyrotoxic, euthyroid, or hypothyroid. The thyroid gland is usually firm, and may be lobulated, giving the clinical impression of multiple nodules. Diagnosis is made on the basis of clinical presentation and anti-thyroglobulin, anti-TSH receptor, and other antibodies.

Hashimoto's thyroiditis is often clinically indistinguishable from Graves' disease, particularly when presenting with exophthalmos and thyrotoxicosis. Diagnosis is made by the characteristic lymphocytic infiltration of the thyroid tissue. However, it should be noted that these changes may often be mistaken for malignancy on FNA, and it is not uncommon for thyroidectomy to be performed on a benign thyroid gland involved by Hashimoto's thyroiditis to rule out malignancy. In addition, there is an approximately 70-fold increase in the risk of thyroid lymphoma in patients with Hashimoto's thyroiditis.[18] Therefore, nodules with a cytology consisting of lymphocytes in patients with Hashimoto's require definitive tissue diagnosis to exclude lymphoma as a diagnosis. In addition, a sudden increase in size of a nodule or sudden appearance of a nodule in a patient with this disease should raise the suspicion of lymphoma. At this time, it should be noted that there are no data indicating an increased risk of well differentiated thyroid carcinoma in these patients.

Acute suppurative thyroiditis is a bacterial infection usually caused by skin flora seeded by adjacent infection of the deep neck spaces, local trauma, or hematogenous spread from a distant site of infection. Mild thyrotoxicosis may occur caused by leakage of thyroid hormone from an inflamed gland. This syndrome occurs more often in children, and is characterized by erythema and cellulitis over the affected gland, fever, pain, and leukocytosis. Fluctuance may be difficult to palpate since the abscess is located deep to the musculature overlying the central compartment of the neck. Needle aspiration will obtain purulent material, which may be sent for culture. Appropriate incision and drainage with intravenous antibiotic therapy are required if abscess exists. Careful attention to preservation of vital structures, including the recurrent laryngeal nerves and parathyroid glands, is obviously maintained. An aggressive approach to drainage of abscesses is indicated, as the central compartment of the neck is in direct continuity with the mediastinum.

## Toxic Adenoma/Toxic Uninodular Goiter

A toxic adenoma is a solitary thyroid nodule that produces greater than normal amounts of $T_3$ or $T_4$, resulting in thyrotoxicosis sufficient to result in a reduction of TSH levels to a low or unmeasurable level. The term "autonomous nodule" refers to a functioning thyroid nodule that does not respond to low levels of serum TSH with an appropriate reduction in thyroid hormone production. By this definition, an autonomously functioning nodule does not necessarily imply that a state of thyrotoxicosis exists. Recently the pathogenesis of autonomously functioning thyroid nodules has been elucidated, including constitutively activating mutations of the alpha-subunit of the $G_s$ protein that is the downstream effector of TSH stimulation in the cyclic AMP cascade,[19] and constitutively activating mutations in the TSH receptor itself.[20]

The prevalence of toxic adenoma is variable in different populations, and is thought to be caused by variability in iodine supplementation. Studies of iodine-sufficient and iodine-deficient populations in Sicily found a significant difference in the prevalence of toxic nodular thyroid disease of 2.7% versus 4.4%, respectively.[21] Toxic adenomas are more prevalent in women than in men.

The largest series in the United States found a prevalence of autonomously functioning nodules of <1% in over 39,000 patients referred to an outpatient endocrinology clinic.[22] In this series of 349 patients with autonomously functioning nodules, those patients aged greater than 60 years were more likely to be thyrotoxic, and almost all thyrotoxic nodules were greater than 3 cm in size. In those patients with non-toxic, autonomously functioning nodules greater than 3 cm, only 20% developed toxicity over a 6 year period, and most nodules tended to remain unchanged in size. By these data, benign autonomously functioning nodules in euthyroid patients may be observed safely, with appropriate surveillance.

During clinical evaluation, it must be remembered that signs and symptoms of thyrotoxicosis may be subtle or absent. Autonomously functioning nodules typically grow slowly, and may be present for years before brought to the attention of a physician. As some nodules will secrete only $T_3$, the remainder of the normally functioning thyroid gland will respond to lack of stimulation, producing small amounts of $T_4$. Therefore, it is important to obtain TSH, $T_3$, and $T_4$ levels. Customary evaluation for a solitary thyroid nodule includes FNA, which is often performed simultaneously with measurement of thyroid function tests. If suspicion of a hyperfunctioning nodule is high because of clinical evaluation or prior measurement of a suppressed TSH, radionuclide imaging with $I^{123}$ will allow determination of an autonomously functioning nodule surrounded by a suppressed normal gland. In this clinical scenario, FNA may be deferred in favor of close surveillance, as the risk of malignancy in an autonomously

functioning nodule has been reported from 2–6%.[23,24] FNA will most likely show cytologic findings consistent with a follicular neoplasm with or without cellular atypia, resulting in an indeterminate interpretation at best, and may push the clinician to recommend unwarranted surgery.

Therapy for toxic adenoma includes radioactive iodine ablation, surgical excision, and percutaneous ethanol injection. Oral thioamide therapy is effective in controlling thyroid hormone levels and is often used to control thyrotoxicosis prior to surgical intervention. However, thioamides do not address the inherent autonomous function of the adenoma, and must be continued indefinitely to control thyrotoxicosis. Because of this inherent limitation, thioamides are rarely used as long term therapy for toxic adenoma.

First used approximately thirty years ago, $I^{131}$ is a relatively safe, non-invasive means of ablating toxic adenomas or controlling thyrotoxicosis. Contraindications include pregnancy and breast-feeding because of risk to the fetus and infant, respectively. Radioactive iodine therapy is particularly helpful in patients for whom surgery is contraindicated because of other medical comorbidities. A recent review of radioactive iodine therapy for solitary toxic adenomas reported variable, but generally favorable results. Thyrotoxicosis remained persistent or recurred in an average of 10% of patients, but series have reported varying rates of recurrence and persistence from 0% to 40%. Post-treatment hypothyroidism was reported 12% of the time, with series ranging from 0% to 58%.[25]

Ultrasound-guided percutaneous ethanol injection has been developed in Europe, and consists of multiple sterile ethanol injections directly into the nodule during ultrasonographic guidance. Several sessions are required, and the mechanism of action is caused by the direct toxic effect of the ethanol. Treatment success has been reported to be 59%, with 0% recurrence and minimal hypothyroidism at 5 year follow-up.[25] Drawbacks include transient dysphonia, thought to be caused by direct toxic effects on the recurrent laryngeal nerve.[26] This option remains less attractive because of its variable efficacy, requirement for repeat treatments, and possible side effects.

Surgery remains the preferred method of treating toxic adenoma in young patients and those with large adenomas, because of the variability of reported results with radioactive iodine therapy and ethanol injection. Thyroid lobectomy is the procedure of choice, although nodulectomy is acceptable as well. Recurrent hyperthyroidism occurs in less than 1% of cases in a review of surgical series, with a low incidence of postoperative complications.[25] The rate of hypothyroidism is noted to be less than 10%, although some smaller series have noted an increasing rate of hypothyroidism with extended follow-up. Preoperative preparation should include treatment with thioamides to ensure a euthyroid state at the time of surgery, with β-adrenergic blockade used to ensure intraoperative hemodynamic stability. Preoperative iodine should not be given, since the autonomously functioning nodule will not respond to changes in serum TSH, and exacerbation of thyrotoxicosis may result.

## Toxic Multinodular Goiter

Toxic multinodular goiter or "Plummer's disease" as it is eponymously known, is more prevalent in iodine-deficient regions, and is usually listed as one of the top two causes of thyrotoxicosis in various population studies internationally. As Plummer observed in his landmark article, multinodular goiter predates development of an autonomous nodule within the gland for years and sometimes decades.[27] Plummer's series noted an average interval of 17 years before the presence of goiter and the onset of thyrotoxicosis in patients with toxic multinodular goiter.

In iodine sufficient areas, toxic multinodular goiter may be caused by thyroid stimulating immunoglobulins,[28] or constitutively activating mutations in the TSH receptor in hyperfunctioning nodules.[29] In iodine-deficient areas, a consistent increase in the incidence of thyrotoxicosis associated with multinodular goiter is seen when widespread implementation of iodine supplementation is started. This transient increase occurs in the first year of supplementation and then decreases thereafter.

Therapy for multinodular goiter includes surgery, radioactive iodine ablation, or thioamide drug therapy. Thioamides must be used indefinitely if they are intended as long term therapy, since cessation of therapy almost invariably results in recurrence of thyrotoxicosis. These drugs are usually reserved as preparation for surgery, or for control of thyrotoxicosis in the interval before definitive treatment with surgery or radioactive iodine.

Surgery for toxic multinodular goiter is advocated for patients who are younger, for those in whom radioactive iodine is contraindicated, and when associated airway, swallowing, or cosmetic issues are present. As patients become more advanced in age, medical comorbidities are more prevalent, presenting a higher incidence of relative contraindications to surgery. Nevertheless, surgery is a rapid and effective means to treat thyrotoxicosis caused by multinodular goiter.

As in patients with toxic adenoma, preoperative preparation requires maintenance of a euthyroid state via thioamides and β-adrenergic blockade. Iodine is not given preoperatively, as this may exacerbate or precipi-

tate thyrotoxicosis in an analogous fashion. Subtotal thyroidectomy has been proposed as the operation of choice in the past, but, increasingly, authors are advocating total thyroidectomy, in order to decrease the recurrence of both multinodular goiter and associated thyrotoxicosis. Complication rates of thyroidectomy in toxic multinodular goiter are similar to those quoted for thyroidectomy in general. The Mayo Clinic experience with treatment was reviewed for comparison between surgery and radioactive iodine therapy in the period from 1950 to 1974. None of the 446 patients who underwent thyroidectomy versus 24% of those patients treated with radioactive iodine required additional treatment for thyrotoxicosis in the first year after treatment. It should be noted that the incidence of postoperative hypothyroidism was quite high for those patients treated surgically in the later part of the study, perhaps because of more aggressive removal of thyroid tissue.[30] With longer follow-up, the incidence of postoperative hyperthyroidism remains below 20%, and variability is noted in the incidence of postoperative hypothyroidism.[31]

Radioactive iodine may be used to treat toxic multinodular goiter successfully. Elderly patients and those patients with surgical contraindications are excellent candidates. There is considerable active discussion regarding dosages, and variability in success rates. Retreatment for those patients who have not achieved a euthyroid state is acceptable, resulting in some differences in reporting. Success rates from 57% to 100% are described, with 12 month follow-up.[30,32] Rates of posttreatment hypothyroidisms have been reported as approximately 10%. One long term study reported 5 year follow-up figures of 40% recurrence of thyrotoxicosis and 24% incidence of hypothyroidism.[33]

Occasional exacerbation of thyrotoxicosis is noted after administration of radionuclide cause by release of stored thyroid hormone, but this can usually be easily controlled with antithyroid medication. Case reports of exacerbation of obstructive airway symptoms after radioiodine administration have been noted, but serial ultrasound examination of multinodular goiter after radioiodine administration has failed to document any increase in thyroid gland volume.[34]

## Diffuse Non-Toxic Goiter

Diffuse non-toxic goiter is essentially a broad descriptive term, and may include nearly all thyroid pathologies. Worldwide, endemic goiter often presents as a diffuse enlargement of the thyroid gland with euthyroid or hypothyroid function. It is often caused by iodine deficiency, and less often by dietary or other environmental goitrogens. In the United States endemic goiter is uncommon. Instead, sporadic goiter is often caused by autoimmune disease, drugs, iodine excess, or other goitrogens. Common etiologies are listed in Table 24–1, and their management has largely been discussed above, in that they can present in the hyperthyroid patient during the clinical course of the disease.

Several remaining clinical entities include invasive fibrous thyroiditis and various types of thyroid malignancy presenting with diffuse glandular involvement. A very rare disorder, invasive fibrous thyroiditis is also termed by the eponym Reidel's thyroiditis. It is an idiopathic disease characterized by extensive fibrosis of the thyroid gland, capsule, and surrounding fascia, found predominantly in euthyroid women in the third to sixth decade of life. Surgical intervention is relegated to procedures required to obtain a tissue diagnosis in order to rule out malignancy, and provide relief of airway and swallowing symptoms. Surgical planes are often obliterated, and minimal dissection is advocated in order to avoid unwanted morbidity and to avoid inciting additional fibrotic response. Diffuse involvement of the thyroid gland is noted as an uncommon, but well-known presentation of thyroid lymphoma, papillary thyroid carcinoma, and anaplastic thyroid carcinoma.

Thyroid lymphoma may occur de novo or in a background of Hashimoto's thyroiditis. The presence of a rapidly enlarging gland, constitutional symptoms, and an FNA with atypical lymphocytes in a euthyroid or hypothyroid patient with antithyroid antibodies should raise suspicion for thyroid lymphoma. A core needle biopsy or open biopsy may be required for definitive diagnosis, and other sites of origin of lymphoma should be excluded.

Papillary thyroid carcinoma may also present with diffuse glandular involvement. Diagnosis by FNA is usually straightforward. Anaplastic carcinoma may arise de novo or from an existing papillary thyroid carcinoma in a goitrous thyroid gland in an elderly person. Sudden, rapid increase in the size of a pre-existing goiter or sudden, massive, diffuse enlargement of the thyroid gland is characteristic. Patients rapidly progress to airway compromise. Definitive diagnosis must include exclusion of lymphoma as a differential diagnosis. Debate exists as to appropriate management of this tumor, as its extraordinary lethality and tendency to present in an advanced stage have resulted in historical median survivals of 3 months, with a small fraction of patients living greater than one year. In the majority of patients who are elderly, advanced stage patients, conservative and/or palliative management is often advocated. Recently, some authors have advocated aggressive surgical debulking, pre- and postoperative hyperfractionated external beam radiation, and chemotherapy, with 4 out of 33 patients surviving without disease at 2 years.[35]

## Solitary Non-Toxic Thyroid Nodule

Most solitary thyroid nodules remain stable in size, and are usually dominant, benign colloid nodules in a small, clinically unrecognized multinodular goiter.[36,37] Other causes of benign solitary thyroid nodules include follicular and Hürthle cell adenomas, thyroid cysts, and benign nodular disorders, as described in the previous paragraphs. Approximately 5% of solitary thyroid nodules are in fact malignant.

As outlined above, FNA is indicated to obtain adequate diagnosis of a solitary thyroid nodule. A malignant or indeterminate FNA result, or an insufficient sampling on repeated attempts, is an indication for surgery, as is recurrence of cystic nodules despite multiple aspirations.[37] Depending on the biopsy result, the patient should be counseled as to the utility of either hemithyroidectomy or total thyroidectomy. The details and intricacies of this decision making process are substantial, and the reader is referred to the appropriate chapters in this volume for further information. However, the sine qua non for diagnosis of a solitary thyroid nodule is surgical excision, and definitive diagnosis cannot be made on the basis of cystic structure, growth patterns, or response to thyroxine suppression therapy.

As indicated above, ultrasound is useful in delineating the size and location of nodules, and may be used to guide appropriate FNA biopsy. Ultrasound may also be used to follow thyroid nodules that are benign on FNA, with surgery reserved for those nodules that enlarge.

Thyroxine therapy is widely used for non-toxic solitary thyroid nodules, but proof of its efficacy is unclear. Theoretically, benign thyroid nodules are dependent on TSH stimulation for growth, and suppression of TSH secretion by the administration of exogenous thyroid hormone should result in removal of growth stimulus to the offending nodule. Of the four randomized, prospective trials comparing the effect of TSH-suppressive doses of thyroxine on the size of thyroid nodules, two studies showed no benefit.[38,39] The third study showed only a minor difference in the thyroxine-treated group,[40] and the fourth study found a response only in smaller nodules.[41] Based on these data, the utility of thyroxine therapy is questionable.

## Non-Toxic Multinodular Goiter

A non-toxic multinodular goiter in and of itself is not an indication for therapy. The most common indications for therapy include suspicion of malignancy, tracheal or esophageal compression, cosmesis, subjective discomfort, or inaccessibility to surveillance for malignancy

The incidence of malignancy in non-toxic multinodular goiter (NTMNG) has been reported to be as high as 10%,[42] but this number is derived from highly selected series undergoing surgical resection that included papillary microcarcinomas in an elderly patient population. Other series have examined populations presenting to a medical endocrinology clinic, with incidences ranging from 1–4%.[43,44]

Accordingly, minimum yearly follow-up is indicated, with clinical examination and possible ultrasound examination. FNA is indicated when a suspicious nodule is found, ie a rapidly growing nodule; a dominant nodule; a nodule that is firm, hard, or fixed; or a nodule in a patient with prior radiation exposure. Symptomatic goiter should be evaluated for degree of substernal extension. CT scanning is the most widespread modality to delineate substernal extension and also can determine the degree of tracheal compression in the patient with airway symptoms. Iodine containing contrast may induce mild thyrotoxicosis in some patients; if this concern exists MRI is an attractive imaging alternative. The management of substernal goiter is a subject unto itself, the reader is referred to several excellent reviews or elsewhere in this text for further information and management.[45,46]

Treatment of NTMNG includes surgery, radioactive iodine therapy, and levothyroxine suppression. Thyroid hormone suppression therapy has been touted as effective in several nonrandomized studies, but to date only one study has been reported as a randomized, placebo-controlled trial. A decrease in the size of NTMNG was noted in 58% of the patients treated with levothyroxine as compared to 5% of those given placebo. However, size decrease was defined as a decrease in volume of 13% or greater (mean 25%), and the NTMNG in this study were of modest size, with a mean volume of about 50 ml.[47] Furthermore, as in all studies, goiter size returned to prior dimensions after therapy was discontinued. In large goiters, the frequency of autonomously functioning nodules increases, therefore caution should be exercised because of the risk of inducing thyrotoxicosis in patients with autonomously functioning nodules when exogenous thyroid hormone is given. For those patients with borderline low or low normal TSH values, thyroid hormone therapy is relatively contraindicated.

Radioactive iodine therapy is usually used in those patients for whom a contraindication to surgery exists. $I^{131}$ is effective in reducing the size of NTMNG in the majority of patients, with a mean reduction in thyroid volume of approximately 40% after one year and 50 60% after five years.[48 50] The majority of patients reported improvement in compressive symptoms related to goiter. Risk of radiation-induced cancers caused by radioactive iodine therapy has not been explicitly examined in this group, but is likely to be low.

Thyroidectomy, usually subtotal, has been standard therapy for NTMNG. By definition, it is immediately effective in controlling the size of NTMNG. The incidence of recurrence of nodules ranges from near zero to 10%.[51-53] In a large series of 735 patients with multinodular goiter, nodular recurrence was noted in 3.4% of patients.[53] Recurrence was noted to occur steadily over the course of the initial 10 year follow-up, in patients with residual thyroid tissue, with half of all recurrences occurring after 10 years. Postoperative thyroid hormone therapy was noted to delay the onset of recurrence in those patients with residual thyroid gland, but did not prevent eventual recurrence or control growth of recurrent nodules. Surgical risks for uncomplicated NTMNG are comparable to those for subtotal and total thyroidectomy for other thyroid disorders.[54] Extensive substernal extension requires heightened awareness for potential airway compromise and other routine complications, but likely poses little additional risk in experienced hands.[45] Sternotomy is rarely needed to remove substernal goiter, with all series reporting the need for sternotomy in less than 3% of cases. Tracheomalacia may rarely be caused by compressive effects, but can usually be treated by short term stenting with an endotracheal tube for several days. More complex methods of tracheopexy and reinforcement with external graft material have been described, but the critical part of management of tracheomalacia is intraoperative recognition of the problem allowing anticipation of possible complications.

Extent of thyroidectomy has been debated over the past decades, with a trend toward more extensive removal of thyroid tissue caused by reports of significant nodular recurrence over prolonged follow-up intervals. A single prospective, randomized trial has been performed, randomizing 141 patients to either total or subtotal thyroidectomy, with a median follow-up of 14.5 years (range 10–21 years).[55] A 14% recurrence rate was found in the subtotal thyroidectomy group, with no recurrences in the total thyroidectomy group. There were no significant differences in morbidity, although the authors noted a high rate of complication when completion thyroidectomy was performed for recurrent disease, in accordance with other published reports.

## SUMMARY

Thyroid goiter is caused by a plethora of pathophysiologic states resulting in enlargement of the thyroid gland. Appropriate management of goiter requires diagnosis of the underlying etiology of thyroid enlargement, followed by judicious selection of the appropriate therapy for the underlying disease process. Surgical management of goiter is dependent on accurate and appropriate diagnosis of the underlying cause of goiter, followed by application of sound surgical judgment and principles.

## References

1. Delange F, Bastani S, Benmiloud M et al. Definitions of endemic goiter and cretinism, classification of goiter size and severity of endemias, and survey techniques. In: Dunn JT, Pretell EA, Daza CH et al. eds. *Towards the Eradication of Endemic Goiter, Creitnism, and Iodine Deficiency.* Washington DC: Pan American Health Organization Scientific Publication no. 502; 1986: 373.

2. Williams I, Ankrett VO, Lazarus JH, Volpe R. Aetiology of hyperthyroidism in Canada and Wales. *J Epidemiol Community Health.* 1983;37:245–2148.

3. Gaitan E, Nelson NC, Poole GV. Endemic goiter and endemic thyroid disorders. *World J Surg.* 1991;15:205–215.

4. Turnbridge WMG, Evered DC, Hall R et al. The spectrum of thyroid disease in a community: the Whickham survey. *Clin Endocrinol.* 1977;7:481–493.

5. Vander JB, Baston EA, Dawber TR. The significance of non-toxic nodules: final report of a 15 year study of the incidence of thyroid malignancy. *Ann Intern Med.* 1968;69:537–540.

6. Mazzaferri EL. Management of a solitary thyroid nodule. *N Engl J Med.* 1993;328:553–559.

7. Ashcraft MW, Van Herle AJ. Management of thyroid nodule II scanning techniques, thyroid suppressive therapy, and fine needle aspiration. *Head Neck Surg.* 1981;3:297–322.

8. Mazzaferri EL, de los Santos ET, Rofagha-Keyhani S. Solitary thyroid nodule: diagnosis and management. *Med Clin North Am.* 1988;72:1177–1211.

9. Rojeski MT, Gharib H. Nodular thyroid disease: evaluation and management. *N Engl J Med.* 1985;313:428–436.

10. DeGroot LJ, Quintans J. The causes of autoimmune thyroid disease. *Endocr Rev.* 1989;10:537–562.

11. Tamai H et al. The mechanism of spontaneous hypothyroidism in patients with Graves' disease after antithyroid drug treatment. *J Clin Endocrinol Metab.* 1987;64:718–22.

12. Solomon BL, Evaul JE, Burman KD et al. Remission rates with antithyroid drug therapy: continuing influence of iodine intake? *Ann Intern Med.* 1987;107:510–512.

13. Becker DV. Current status of radioactive iodine treatment of hyperthyroidism. *Thyroid Today.* 1979;2:1–5.

14. Okamoto T, Fujimoto Y, Obara T et al. Retrospective analysis of prognostic factors affecting the thyroid functional status after subtotal thyroidectomy for Graves' disease. *World J Surg.* 1992; 16:690–695.

15. Sugino K, Mimura T, Ozaki O et al. Management of recurrent hyperthyroidism in patients with Graves' disease treated by subtotal thyroidectomy. *J Endocrinol Invest.* 1995;18:415–419.

16. Mazzaferri EL. Thyroid cancer and Graves' disease. *J Clin Endocrinol Metab.* 1990;70:826–829.

17. Belfiore A, Garofalo MR, Giuffrida D et al. Increased aggressiveness of thyroid cancer in patients with Graves' disease. *J Clin Endocrinol Metab.* 1990;70:830–835.

18. Aozasa K. Hashimoto's thyroiditis as a risk factor of thyroid lymphoma. *Acta Pathol Jpn.* 1990;40:459–468.

19. Russo D, Arturi F, Wicker R et al. Genetic alterations in thyroid hyperfunctioning adenomas. *J Clin Endocrinol Metab.* 1995;80: 1347–1351.

20. Van Sande J, Parma J, Tonacchera M, Swillens S, Dumont J, Vassart G . Somatic and germline mutations of the TSH receptor gene in thyroid diseases. *J Clin Endocrinol Metab.* 1995;80:2577–2585.

21. Belfiore A, Sava L, Runello F, Tomaselli L, Vigneri R. Solitary autonomously functioning thyroid nodules and iodine deficiency. *J Clin Endocrinol Metab.* 1983;56:283–287.

22. Hamburger JI. Evolution of toxicity in solitary non-toxic autonomously functioning thyroid nodules. *J Coin Endocrinol Metab.* 1980;50:1089–1093.

23. Sandrock D, Olbricht T, Emrich D, Benker G, Reinwein D. Longterm follow-up in patients with autonomous thyroid adenoma. *Acta Endocrinol.* 1993;128:51–55.

24. Smith M, McHenry C, Jarosz H et al. Carcinoma of the thyroid in patients with autonomous nodules. *Am J Surg.* 1988;54:448–449.

25. Ferrari C, Reschini E, Paracchi A. Treatment of the autonomous thyroid nodule: A review. *Eur J Endocrinol.* 1996;135:383–390.

26. Papini E, Panunzi C, Pacella CM et al. Percutaneously ultrasound-guided ethanol injection: a new treatment of toxic autonomously functioning thyroid nodules? *J Clin Endocrinol Metab.* 1993; 76:411–416.

27. Plummer H. The clinical and pathologic relationship of hyperplastic and nonhyperplastic goiters. *JAMA.* 1913;61:650.

28. Brown RS, Jackson IM, Pohl SL, Reichlin S. Do thyroid-stimulating immunoglobulins cause non-toxic and toxic multinodular goiter? *Lancet.* 1978;1:904–906.

29. Paschke R. Constitutively activating TSH receptor mutations as the cause of toxic thyroid adenoma, multinodular toxic goiter and autosomal dominant nonautoimmune hyperthyroidism. *Exp Clin Endocrinol Diabetes.* 1996;104:129–132.

30. Jensen MD, Gharib H, Naessens JM, van Heerden JA, Mayberry WE. Treatment of toxic multinodular goiter (Plummer's disease): surgery or radioiodine? *World J Surg.* 1986;10:637–680.

31. Kinser JA, Roesler H, Furrer T, Grutter D, Zimmermann H. Nonimmunogenic hyperthyroidism: cumulative hypothyroidism incidence after radioiodine and surgical treatment. *J Nucl Med.* 1989;30:1960–1965.

32. Huysmans DAKC, Hermus ARMM, Corstens FHM, Kloppenborg PWC. Long-term results of two schedules of radioiodine treatment for toxic multinodular goitre. *Eur J Nucl Med.* 1993;20: 1056–1062.

33. Danaci M, Feek CM, Notghi A et al. 131-I radioiodine therapy for hyperthyroidism in patients with Graves' disease, uninodular goitre and multinodular goitre. *N Z Med J.* 1988;101:784–786.

34. Mygaard B, Faber J, Hegedu L. Acute changes in thyroid volume and function following 131-I therapy of solitary autonomous thyroid nodules. *Thyroid.* 1994;4:167–171.

35. Tennvall J, Lundell G, Hallquist A, Wahlberg P, Wallin G, Tibblin S. Combined doxorubicin, hyperfractionated radiotherapy, and surgery in anaplastic thyroid carcinoma: report on two protocols. *Cancer.* 1994;74:1348–1354.

36. Vander JB, Gaston EA, Dawber TR. The significance of non-toxic thyroid nodules: final report of a 15-year study of the incidence of thyroid malignancy. *Ann Intern Med.* 1968;69:537–40.

37. Mazzaferri EL. Management of a solitary thyroid nodule. *N Engl J Med.* 1993;328:553–559.

38. Gharib H, James EM, Charboneau JW, Naessens JM, Offord KP, Gorman CA. Suppressive therapy with levothyroxine for solitary thyroid nodules: a double-blind controlled clinical study. *N Engl J Med.* 1987;317:70–75.

39. Reverter JL, Lucas A, Salinas I, Audi L, Foz M, Sanmarti A. Suppressive therapy with levothyroxine for solitary thyroid nodules. *Clin Endocrinol.* 1992;36:25–28.

40. Papini E, Bacci V, Panunzi C et al. A prospective, randomized trial of levothyroxine suppressive therapy for solitary thyroid nodules. *Clin Endocrinol.* 1993;38:507–513.

41. La Rosa GL, Lupo L, Giuffrida D, Gullo D, Vigneri R, Belfiore A. Levothyroxine and potassium iodide are both effective in treating benign solitary solid cold nodules of the thyroid. *Ann Intern Med.* 1995;122:1–8.

42. Rojeski MT, Gharib H. Nodular thyroid disease: evaluation and management *N Engl J Med.* 1985;313:428–436.

43. Belfiore A, La Rosa GL, La Porta GA et al. Cancer risk in patients with cold thyroid nodules: relevance of iodine intake , sex, age, and multinodularity. *Am J Med.* 1992;93:363–369.

44. Franklyn JA, Daykin J, Young J, Oates GD, Sheppard MC. Fine needle aspiration cytology in diffuse or multinodular goiter compared with solitary thyroid nodules. *BMJ.* 1993;307:240.

45. Newman E, Shaha AR. Substernal goiter. *J Surg Onc.* 1995;60:207–212.

46. Singh B, Lucente FE, Shaha AR. Substernal goiter: a clinical review. *Am J Otolaryngol.* 1994;15:409–416.

47. Berghout A, Wiersinga WM, Drexhage HA, Simits NJ, Touber JL. Comparison of placebo with L-thyroxine alone or with carbimazole for treatment of sporadic non-toxic goitre. *Lancet.* 1990;336:193–197.

48. Nygaard B, Hegedus L, Gervil M, Hjalgrim H, Soe-Jensen P, Hansen JM. Radioiodine treatment of multinodular non-toxic goitre. *BMJ.* 1993;307:828–832.

49. Wesche MF, Tiel-v-Buul MM, Smits NJ, Wiersinga WM. Reduction in goiter size by 131-I therapy in patients with non-toxic multinodular goiter. *Eur J Endocrinol.* 1995;132:86–87.

50. Huysmans D, Hermus A, Edelbroek M, Barentsz J, Corstens F, Kloppenborg P. Radioiodine for non-toxic mutinodular goiter. *Thyroid.* 1997;7:235–239.

51. Berghout A, Wiersinga WM, Drexhage HA et al. The long term outcome of thyroidectomy for sporadic non-toxic goitre. *Clin Endocrinol (Oxf).* 1989;31:193–199.

52. Geeerdsen JP, Frolund L. Recurrence of non-toxic goitre with and without postoperative thyroxine medication. *Clin Endocrinol.* 1984;21:529–533.

53. Kraimps JL, Marechaud R, Gineste D et al. Analysis and prevention of recurrent goiter. *Surg Gynecol Obstet.* 1993;176:319–322.

54. De Roy van Zuidewijn DBW, Songun I, Kievit J et al. Complications of thyroid surgery. *Ann Surg Oncol.* 1995;2:56–60.

55. Pappalardo G, Guadalaxara A, Frattaroli FM, Illomei G, Falaschi P. Total compared with subtotal thyroidectomy in benign nodular disease: personal series and review of published reports. *Eur J Surg.* 1998;164:501–506.

# Surgical Treatment of Substernal Thyroid Disease

## Douglas Klotch, M.D.

The management of substernal thyroid disease requires an understanding of anatomy, surgical approach and pathologic process in order to ascertain the management requirements. A tendency would be to address all problems similarly, but this philosophy potentially results in errors in management.

Although the majority of disorders will represent benign substernal thyroid disease, the surgeon must be prepared to extend treatment when malignancy is encountered, especially if these tumors are invasive and involve the trachea, esophagus, great vessels or the vagus, and recurrent laryngeal nerves.

## MEDIASTINAL ANATOMY

The mediastinum is a partition in the thorax which is bordered ventrally (anteriorly) by the sternum, dorsally (posteriorly) by the vertebrae, and laterally by the pleura.[1] It has two major divisions: superior and inferior (Figure 25–1). The superior mediastinum extends from the first rib and the thoracic inlet to a line passing through the sternal angle and the disk between the fourth and fifth thoracic vertebrae. The soft tissue boundary is the superior pericardium. The inferior mediastinum is inferior to the superior mediastinum and superior to the diaphragm. The inferior mediastinum has three subdivisions: anterior, middle, and posterior. The anterior subdivision lies in front (anterior) of the pericardium. The middle subdivision lies between the anterior and posterior pericardium. The posterior is behind (posterior) the pericardium.

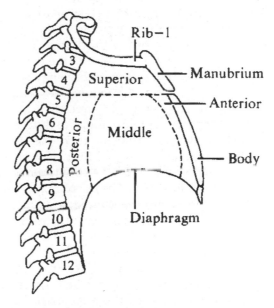

**Figure 25–1.** Although the classic description of the anatomy of the mediastinum is as illustrated, there is not a clear dividing line between the anterior superior mediastinum and the anterior mediastinum. Likewise, the posterior superior mediastinum is contiguous with the posterior mediastinum.

The superior mediastinum is the division most often involved with head and neck pathologic processes. It anatomically includes structures derived from the third and fourth branchial arches. These structures include the origins of the sternohyoid and sternothyroid muscles, the remnants of the thymus gland, the arch of the aorta, the brachiocephalic, left common carotid and left subclavian arteries, the superior vena cava and brachiocephalic veins, and the thoracic duct. The trachea is in the midline with the esophagus located posteriorly. The nerves within the superior mediastinum include the left and right vagus, the left recurrent laryngeal nerves, the phrenic nerves, and the cardiac nerves. The posterior muscle groups are the lower longus colli muscles.

The anterior mediastinum has no major structures except the residual thymus.

The middle mediastinum contains the heart and great vessels. The vessels include the superior vena cava, the termination of the azygos, the ascending aorta, and the pulmonary arteries. The phrenic nerves are in the lateral border of the middle mediastinum.

The posterior mediastinum contains the thoracic aorta, the azygous and hemiazygos veins, the thoracic duct, the esophagus, the trachea and mainstem bronchi, and the vagus and splanchnic nerves.

Although these are anatomic descriptions, there are some important surgical considerations regarding anatomy which offer a more pragmatic approach for surgical anatomic consideration. The superior mediastinum is composed largely of third and fourth branchial derivatives, the third arch structure being the thymus and the inferior parathyroids. The vagus nerve is the neural derivative of the third arch. The fourth arch gives rise to the great vessels and the recurrent laryngeal nerve. A general rule in embryology is that the nerve of the arch is dorsal to the arch vessel and each succeeding arch is dorsal to the preceding arch. The fourth arch structures are more dorsal to third arch derivatives. The recurrent laryngeal nerve passes dorsal (posterior) to the great vessels and third arch structures (ie, thymus). This is of great importance when identifying the inferior parathyroids. The inferior parathyroids, when not associated with the thyroid, are often found in the anterior superior mediastinal structures such as the thymus. The superior parathyroids are often posterior to the trachea and esophagus and will follow the path of the recurrent laryngeal nerves. The left vagus nerve courses anterior to the aortic arch lateral to the ductus arteriosum. It gives off the recurrent laryngeal nerve posteriorly, which wraps around the aortic arch and ascends superiorly in the posterior superior mediastinum. The right vagus passes anterior to the subclavian artery immediately lateral to the take off of the right carotid from the brachiocephalic artery. The recurrent laryngeal nerve exits posteriorly to pass dorsal (posterior) to the brachiocephalic-subclavian junction, ascending in the posterior superior mediastinum to the neck. It is interesting that most anatomic discussions do not consider the right carotid artery and recurrent laryngeal nerve to be a part of the mediastinum, as they clearly are located in the lateral border of the superior mediastinum from a surgical viewpoint.

It is also interesting that anatomy texts consider the superior mediastinum to contain both anterior and posterior structures. The pericardium, which divides the inferior mediastinum, also extends to the aorta and brachiocephalic artery. Similarly, the esophagus and trachea are considered part of the posterior mediastinum. The thymus extends to the anterior mediastinum. For practical purposes, the superior mediastinum can be considered to have anterior and posterior structures. The structures anterior to the trachea, which include the thymus, aberrant inferior parathyroids, and the surrounding fat pad, are distinct from the more posterior tissues. The tracheoesophageal lymphoareolar contents following the recurrent laryngeal nerves contain the aberrant superior parathyroids and the retrotracheal and retroesophageal nodal groups. This area extends beneath the aortic arch and the brachiocephalic artery to the posterior mediastinum with only an arbitrary line dividing these areas. The experienced surgeon may reach nodal groups to the region of the carina, and pulmonary arteries from a transcervical approach in patients with a wide thoracic inlet. Similarly, the division between the anterior superior mediastinum and the anterior inferior mediastinum are quite arbitrary. Generally the inferior border of the great vessels is the limiting dissection plane. This is predicated by the A-P dimension of the mediastinum, the extent of disease and its adherence to surrounding tissues.

## SURGICAL APPROACH TO THE MEDIASTINUM

The superior mediastinum can normally be approached via a transcervical route.[2-7] Occasionally extended access is required and may be provided by resecting the medial third of the clavicle (Lore).[8] Only when tumors are attached to the great vessels or extend inferior to the great vessels is median sternotomy mandated. Obviously the experience of the surgeon influences the decision to use an extended approach. Fastidious dissection with a detailed knowledge of the surgical anatomy is essential to avoid potentially serious complications. Surgery in this region risks injury to a major vessel, pleura, trachea, esophagus, lymphatic, duct, or nerve (vagus, recurrent laryngeal, or more rarely the phrenic).[9-11] Surgical technique requires accurate identification of structures and careful hemostasis using bipolar cautery or suture ligature to control smaller mediastinal vessels.

Access to the mediastinum is best approached by following the carotid sheath structures. If one starts on the right side, the vagus nerve can be identified posterior-lateral to the carotid medial to the internal jugular vein. As the nerve is followed inferiorly it courses more anteriorly as it crosses anteriorly to the right subclavian artery at the take off of the carotid artery from the brachiocephalic artery. The recurrent laryngeal nerve exits the vagus posteriorly and then angles medially to wrap around the brachiocephalic artery and ascend in the posterior tracheoesophageal groove. If not already identified, the recurrent laryngeal nerve needs to be identified before dissecting out the fat pad in this region. It is usually already exposed within the tracheoesophageal grove if the patient has undergone a thyroidectomy. By following the fascia along the anterior superior aspect of the brachiocephalic artery, the aortic arch will be reached. It is preferable to have the left recurrent laryngeal nerve exposed before dissection of the superior mediastinal fat pad. The vagus may be readily dissected to the superior aortic arch but it is more difficult to track the origin of the left recurrent laryngeal nerve since it takes off in the region of the ductus arteriosum which limits complete exposure of the nerve in this region. The left recurrent laryngeal nerve will also traverse a more medial course as it ascends within the tracheoesophageal groove and not infrequently will be attached to the trachea. When these structures have been identified, the fatty tissue with nodes can be dissected freely from the trachea, esophagus, carotid sheath, and the posterior neck muscles. Similarly, the fat pad may be dissected from the anterior attachments. Care must be taken in that the brachiocephalic vein lies slightly anterior-superior to the brachiocephalic artery. Careful dissection cauterizing small veins in this area is essential to prevent tearing of the brachiocephalic vein, which is difficult to repair by this approach. It is possible to displace the trachea and esophagus to one side with a long Kitner dissector to gain access to the posterior mediastinum. This allows the surgeon to assure that the inferior margin of the resection is free of disease.

When patients have a narrow thoracic inlet or disease is bulky with extension to the superior mediastinum, the addition of the resection of the medial third of the clavicle facilitates access.[8] This technique described by Lore not only provides wide access to the involved side but is associated with minimal morbidity. The approach is well adapted to a standard thyroid incision. The skin flap is dissected above the anterior surface of the clavicle to the mid portion of the clavicle. The periosteum is readily dissected from the clavicle with the help of periosteal elevators (Alexander). Careful dissection inferior to the mid clavicle allows one to free the circumference of the clavicle and place a small malleable retractor beneath to protect the vascular structures. One can transect the bone with an oscillating saw. The cut end is grasped with a bone clamp and the soft tissues are freed from the bone to expose the sternoclavicular joint. A scalpel is used to cut the ligamentous attachments and the joint capsule. The bone may then be freed from the posterior joint by using a heavy periosteal elevator. Either the left or right clavicular heads may be removed. The choice depends on the side requiring the greatest exposure. This approach opens the anterior superior mediastinum. It provides excellent exposure of the brachiocephalic (innominate) vein and the anterior aspect of the brachiocephalic artery and the aortic arch. It facilitates the ease of dissection having a wider angle of approach to the posterior aspect of the mediastinum. A wider exposure may be achieved by removing the manubrium. It is usually not required. Removal of the manubrium is best approached by first carefully elevating the posterior periosteum. When reflected this layer helps to prevent possible injury to the mediastinal vessels. If there is surrounding tissue adherence or invasion by the disease process this extended transcervical approach is advantageous for most tumor removal. The transclavicular approach has limitations for disease extending posteriorly to any significant degree below the great vessels.

The median sternotomy is required when tumors extend deep within the inferior mediastinum. This is almost always mandatory when there is extension of malignant thyroid tumors within the posterior mediastinum. Although it is generally possible to remove substernal goiters from a transcervical approach, tumor adherence or invasion within tissues inferior to the great vessels precludes safe removal without wider exposure. This approach is usually performed with a thoracic surgeon to ensure appropriate management of the chest and mediastinal structures.

## SUBSTERNAL GOITER

The substernal goiter represents about 7% of all mediastinal tumors. Published series describe a 3–20% incidence of substernal goiters as the reason for performing thyroid surgery.[2,3,7,12-14] A goiter is defined to be substernal when 50% of the gland is inferior to the thoracic inlet.[4-5] A majority of these tumors are benign, representing either multinodular goiter or thyroiditis.[3] The malignancy rate varies between 5 and 34% among series.[7,11,12,15,16] The majority of these tumors may be removed through a transcervical approach (Figure 25–2). This may be inadequate if there is malignant transformation, which has extended within the mediastinum (Figure 25–3).[1] The mass effect of the goiter within the mediastinum produces a variety of compressive symptoms. The trachea, esophagus, great vessels, and nerves may be displaced or compressed by these tumors (Figure 25–4). Symptoms include airway compromise, difficult or painful swallowing, superior vena cava obstruction, and nerve dysfunction (hoarseness).[2,3,5,7,12,17] Hyperthyroid and hypothyroid states may occur but are not common in most series. Generally, the recurrent laryngeal nerve is displaced posteriorly. One needs to exercise caution when the lobe is bilobed with hypertrophy of the superior section of the gland. Frequently in this circumstance, the recurrent laryngeal nerve may

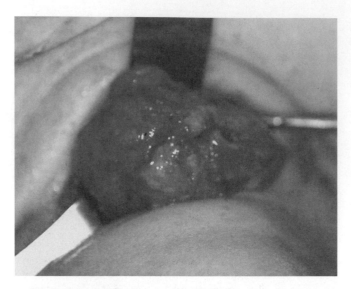

**Figure 25–2.** Substernal goiters can generally be removed via the transcervical route.

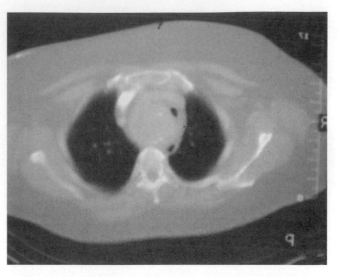

**Figure 25–4.** The substernal goiter represented by this X-ray compresses the trachea, the esophagus, and the major vessels.

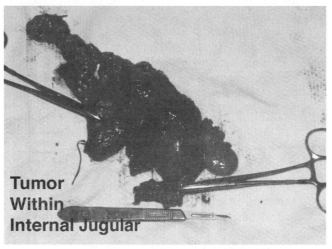

**A**

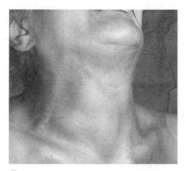

**B**

**Figure 25–3. A.** The specimen was obtained from a patient with a long-standing multinodular goiter. The goiter developed a papillary carcinoma, which metastasized to cervical nodes and also grew within the internal jugular vein. **B.** Patient with long-standing goiter. Cancer developed within the goiter and metastasized to the neck and internal jugular vein.

pass between this upper and lower lobular division. If the surgeon is not careful during dissection on the capsule, the nerve may be either stretched or avulsed. Fortunately this anatomic variation is uncommon. The inferior extent of the disease may be freed by careful finger dissection and delivered from the tracheoesophageal groove and the mediastinum. If there is adherence of the gland to the surrounding soft tissues and increased vasculature, meticulous dissection with careful hemostasis is required. This is often found in patients who have coexisting thyroiditis. Dissection in these situations is slow and tedious and attention to control of bleeding with absolute identification of the recurrent laryngeal nerves is essential. Generally, the nerve will divide into abductor and adductor branches within one centimeter of the posterior edge of the cricothyroid muscle. Occasionally there is extensive branching of the nerve to the trachea and esophagus, as well as subdivisions of the nerve well below the one centimeter zone. Operating with magnification loops or microscopic control can be beneficial for preserving the nerve function in these patients. With careful operating technique the risk to the nerves is minimal. Although uncommon, one must be careful to recognize the anomaly of the non-recurrent laryngeal nerve (<1%). This usually is present on the right side (unless concommitant dextrocardia). It is excluded only when finding the normal anatomy of the recurrent nerve.

As digital dissection proceeds and the mediastinal component of the gland is delivered through the thoracic inlet, bleeding from small and medium sized venous tributaries in the viscero-verterbial angle and inlet may occur as a result of the loss of the compressive effects of the mass within the mediastinum. At times, significant hemorrhage may result, obscuring the surgical field and making dissection of the laryngeal nerves difficult. Every attempt should be made to identify and control these vessels prior to complete removal.

Morselization or decortication of the gland within the mediastinum has been reported, but is generally not recommended and usually not necessary. More recently, decortication for massive substernal benign disease potentially requiring sternotomy has been advocated but remains an unproven and potentially unnecessary modality.[18] If the gland cannot be delivered because of adhesions it is preferable to proceed with a transclavicular or trans-sternal approach to avoid injury to vascular or other mediastinal structures.

## SUBSTERNAL THYROID CANCER MANAGEMENT

The surgeon may be required to resect thyroid cancer within the mediastinum for a variety of reasons. The initial tumor may arise from a substernal goiter. The cancer may have already directly extended into the mediastinum. There may be extensive adenopathy within the substernal region. The surgeon may be resecting recurrent cancer within the mediastinum. A planned therapeutic mediastinal node dissection may be required. Certainly therapeutic node dissection has represented the standard of care for medullary thyroid cancer, and even provides survival benefits for recurrent disease.[18] This treatment approach is more controversial for well-differentiated thyroid cancers occurring in adults unless there is palpable disease.[19-24] Mediastinal dissection is generally mandated for cancers occurring in children since they have a high propensity for mediastinal involvement (Figure 25–5).[11,25]

It is easy for most surgeons to plan for extending the dissection within the mediastinum for obvious gross disease. Fortunately, the primary cancers rarely have a large volume of disease extending extracapsularly within the mediastinum. This is not the case for recurrent disease, which generally has either direct spread or gross nodal involvement of the mediastinum. Although this nodal disease may become extracapsular, the trachea is rarely invaded beneath the fourth tracheal ring. This is not the case for the esophagus, which is more likely to have muscle invasion within the mediastinum. It is uncommon for the mucosa to be involved with tumor. The dissection of the muscularis is facilitated by placing a 50–60 Fr. esophageal dilator. This allows easy identification of the esophagus and ease in dissection of the muscularis from the mucosa. If the mucosa is involved, it generally is only for a small length and can be closed primarily.

To date, only two patients in 237 undergoing resection of well-differentiated thyroid cancers (by the author) over the last twelve years have required median sternotomy to safely remove their cancers. One patient had a Hürthle cell cancer, which extended down the posterior mediastinum and was attached to the superior aspect of the patient's hiatal hernia (Figure 25–6 and

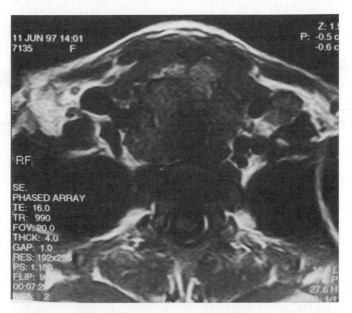

**Figure 25–5.** Extensive papillary thyroid cancer in a 17-year-old girl involving the trachea, esophagus within the mediastinum.

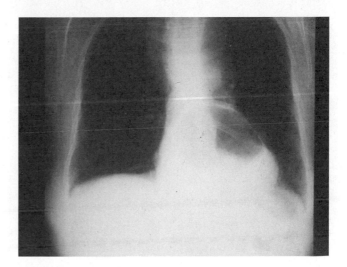

**Figure 25–6.** Patient with a large Hürthle cell carcinoma involving the posterior mediastinum and attaching to the hiatus hernia.

25–7). The other patient had an extensive substernal goiter with de-differentiation to cancer within the inferior-most portion of the gland, which was encasing the brachiocephalic artery and vein. The transclavicular approach previously described may also provide extended access to the mediastinum (Figures 25–8 through 25–10). This approach is somewhat limited if there is substantial tumor beneath the great vessels. These tumors are uncommon but are more safely removed via a median sternotomy approach.

Therapeutic node dissection is somewhat more controversial. There is excellent documentation that nodal metastases influence recurrence rates.[6,20,22,23,25-28]

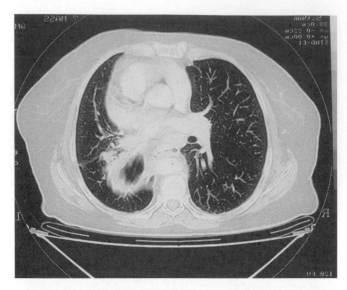

**Figure 25–7.** CT scan of Hürthle cancer attached to the hiatus hernia.

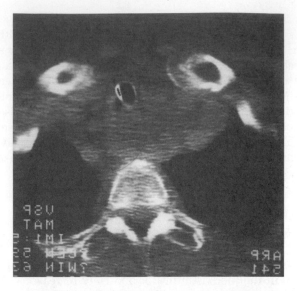

**Figure 25–9.** Disease (HR) involves mediastinum esophagus and trachea.

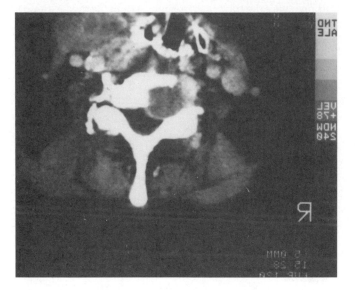

**Figure 25–8.** Patient (HR) with massive invasion of spine with extensive involvement of mediastinum.

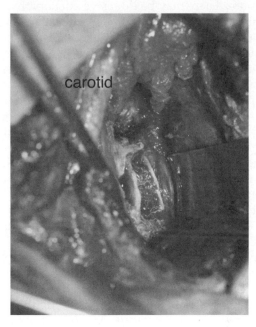

**Figure 25–10.** The tumor (HR) was removed via a transclavicular approach, with the clavicle used to stabilize the defect in the spine.

The effect on survival is less clear; although some authors demonstrate a benefit in lower recurrence and survival for patients undergoing therapeutic nodal dissection,[29-32] I have found 34% involvement of mediastinal nodes in the 237 patients mentioned above. This is similar to that reported in the literature.[24,28,32] It is difficult to predict preoperatively which patients with clinically $N_0$ necks are at risk for nodal disease. Though a variety of tumor markers have been implicated for diagnosing aggressive tumors, they have not been diagnostically exclusive and require more tissue than obtained from needle biopsies to be accurate.[33] These tests have provided no significant clinical application to date. Lymphatic mapping has been described in limited series. The technique appears to identify microscopic disease within nodes with a false negative rate of 17%.[34] The effect on survival and recurrence has not been studied since there is to date limited short term experience with this technique. Indications for mediastinal dissection include the presence of gross positive nodes within the mediastinum or upon finding positive nodes within the tracheoesophageal groove. I routinely sample the tracheoesophageal fat pad on the side of the lesion, since this represents the first echelon nodal basin.[30]

The follow-up of disease within the neck is generally accomplished by means of the routine head and neck exam. Using sonography can enhance the accuracy of the cervical examination. Palpation of the mediastinum is not feasible and sonography of this area is less reliable than in the neck. Magnetic resonance or computerized tomography is useful in detecting recurrence if suspected. Needle biopsies are more difficult to obtain,[12] though possible with CT guidance. Our experience has not shown thyroglobulin or radioactive iodine scans to be reliably sensitive for nodal disease. Patients may have palpable disease in the neck with normal thyroglobulin. Similarly, positive disease justification may exist in the neck despite previous treatment with radioactive iodine. This lends some credence to a primary surgical intervention with mediastinal dissection for patients at risk for substernal disease.

## SUMMARY

Resection of substernal thyroid disease is most often accomplished through a transcervical approach, especially for benign disease. A detailed knowledge of the anatomic relationship of important visceral, neural, and vascular structures within the thoracic inlet and mediastinum, together with meticulous dissection technique aids, is necessary in successful resection and prevention of complications. Malignant mediastinal disease, either primary or nodal, may require sternotomy for an uncomplicated successful removal.

## References

1. *Gray's Anatomy.* Lea & Febinger; 1965; 1194–1196.
2. Moron JC, Singer JA, Sardi A. Retrosternal goiter: a six-year institutional review. *Am Surg.* 1998; 64(9):889-93.
3. Netterville JL, Coleman SC, Smith JC, Smith MM, Day TA, Burkey BB. Management of substernal goiter. *Laryngoscope.* 1998; 108(11 Pt 1):1611–17.
4. Newman E, Shaha AR. Substernal goiter. *J Surg Oncol.* 1995; 60(3):207–12.
5. Shaha A, Jaffe BM. Complications of thyroid surgery performed by residents. *Surgery.* 1988; 104:1109–1114.
6. Chen H, Udelsman R. Papillary thyroid carcinoma: justification for total thyroidectomy and management of lymph node metastases. *Surg Oncol Clin N Amer.* 1998; 7(4):645–63.
7. Torre G, Borgonovo G, Amato A, et al. Surgical management of substernal goiter: analysis of 237 patients. *Am Surg.* 1995; (9): 826–31.
8. Lore JM, Szymula NJ. Superior mediastinal exposure. *Arch Otolaryngol.* 1980; 106(1):6-7.
9. Bergamaschi R, Becouarn G, Ronceray J, Arnaud J. Morbidity of thyroid surgery. *Amer J Surg.* 1998; 176(1): 71–75.
10. Roher HD, Goretzki PE, Hellmann P Witte J. Complications in thyroid surgery. *Chirurg.* 1999; 70(9):999–1010.
11. Hallwirth U, Flores J, Kaserer K, Niederle B. Differentiated thyroid cancer in children and adolescents: the importance of adequate surgery and review. *Eur J Ped Surg.* 1999; 9(6):359–63.
12. Allo MD, Thompson NW. Rationale for the operative management of substernal goiters. *Surgery.* 1983; 94(6):969–977.
13. Nishida T, Nakao K, Hamaji M, Kamiike W, Kurozumi K, Matsuda H. Preservation of recurrent laryngeal nerve invaded by differentiated thyroid cancer. *Ann Surg.* 1997; 226(1):85-91.
14. Wax MK, Briant TD. Management of substernal goiter. *J Otolaryngol.* 1992; 21(3):165-70.
15. Katlie MR, Wang CA, Grillo HC. Substernal goiter. *Ann Thorac Surg.* 1985; 39(4):391–9.
16. Nervi M, Iacconi P, Spinelli C, Janni A, Miccoli P. Thyroid carcinoma in intrathoracic goiter. *Langenbecks Arch Surg.* 1998;383(5):337–9.
17. Mann B, Buhr HJ. Lymph node dissection in patients with differentiated thyroid carcinoma—who benefits? *Langenbecks Arch Surg.* 1998; 383(5):355-8.
18. Machens A, Gimm O, Ukkat J, Sutter T, Dralle H. Repeat mediastinal lymph-node dissection for palliation in advanced medullary thyroid carcinoma. *Langenbecks Arch Surg.* 1999; 384(3):271–6.
19. Ahuja S, Ernst H, Lenz K. Papillary thyroid carcinoma: occurrence and types of lymph node metastases. *J Endocrinol Invest.* 1991; 14(7):543–9.
20. Amar A, Rapoport A, Rosas M. Evaluation of lymph node reactivity in differentiated thyroid carcinoma. *Sao Paulo Medical Journal-Revista Paulista de Medicina.* 1999; 117(3):125–8.
21. DeGroot LJ, Kaplan EL, Straus FH, Shukla MS. Does the method of management of papillary thyroid carcinoma make a difference in outcome? *World J Surg.* 1994; 18(1):123–30.
22. Ducci M, Appetecchia M, Marzetti M. Neck dissection for surgical treatment of lymphnode metastasis in papillary thyroid carcinoma. *J Exp Clin Canc Res.* 1997; 16(3):333–5.
23. Harwood J, Clark OH, Dunphy JE. Significance of lymph node metastasis in differentiated thyroid cancer. *Amer J Surg.* 1978; 136(1):107–12.
24. Noguchi S, Murakami N, Yamashita H, Toda, M, Kawamoto, H. Papillary thyroid carcinoma: modified radical neck dissection improves prognosis. *Arch Surg.* 1998; 133(3): 276–280.
25. Robie DK, Dinauer CW, Tuttle RM, et al. The impact of initial surgical management on outcome in young patients with differentiated thyroid cancer. *J Ped Surg.* 1998; 33(7):1134–8; disc. 1139–40.
26. Kobayashi T, Asakawa H, Komoike Y, Tamaki Y, Monden M. Characteristics and prognostic factors in patients with differentiated thyroid cancer who underwent a total or subtotal thyroidectomy: surgical approach for high-risk patients. *Surgery Today.* 1999; 29(3):200–3.
27. Sellers M, Beenken S, Blankenship A, et al. Prognostic significance of cervical lymph node metastases in differentiated thyroid cancer. *Am Jour Surg.* 1992; 164(6):578–81.
28. Wahl RA, Rimpl I, Luther A, Schabram J. Differentiated thyroid gland carcinoma p-T2/T3—extent of lymphadenectomy. *Langenbecks Archiv fur Chirurgie—Supplement—Kongressband.* 1998;115: 203–11.
29. Busutti L, Blotta AB, Calo-Gabrieli G, dell'Erba L. Transcutaneous radiotherapy after thyroidectomy for differentiated thyroid carcinoma. *Clinica Terapeutica.* 1999; 150(2):103–7.
30. Gimm O, Rath, FW, Dralle H, Pattern of lymph node metastases in papillary thyroid carcinoma. *Brit J Surg.* 1998; 85(2): 252–254.
31. Scheumann GF, Gimm O, Wegener G, Hundeshagen H, Dralle H. Prognostic significance and surgical management of locoregional lymph node metastases in papillary thyroid cancer. *World J Surg.* 1994; 18(4):559–67; disc. 567–8.
32. Tisell LE. Role of lymphadenectomy in the treatment of differentiated thyroid carcinomas. *British J Surg.* 1998; 85(8): 1025–1026.
33. Muro-Cacho CA, Munoz-Antonia T, Livingston S, Klotch D. Transforming growth factor beta receptors and p27kip in thyroid carcinoma. *Arch Otolaryngol—Head Neck Surg.* 1999; 125(1): 76–81.
34. Kelemen, Pond R, Van Herle, AJ, Giuliano AE. Sentinel lymphadenectomy in thyroid malignant neoplasms. *Arch Surg.* 1998; 133(3): 288–292.

# 26

# Treatment Complications in Managing Thyroid Disease

Thomas Kennedy, M.D., F.A.C.S.
Ronald Monsaert, M.D., F.A.C.P., F.A.C.E.

## SURGICAL COMPLICATIONS OF THYROIDECTOMY

The risk of a serious complication from thyroidectomy occurs less frequently with the refinement in surgical technique, a better understanding of the anatomy, and the improved medical treatment for hyperthyroidism. Permanent hypoparathyroidism and recurrent or superior laryngeal nerve paralysis does, however, continue to pose significant morbidity for the patient. This chapter deals strictly with surgical complications and, when necessary, the surgical management of those complications. The discussion of the metabolic treatment of hypothyroidism, hypoparathyroidism, and thyroid crisis or storm is reviewed only briefly as it is a topic of another chapter.

Because of the serious risks related to thyroidectomy even the most skillful surgeon needs regular exposure to the anatomy to remain confident in performing this procedure. Over 100 years ago this fact was recognized in a surgical textbook that read, "If a surgeon should be so foolhardy as to undertake thyroidectomy ... lucky it will be ... if his victim lives long enough to enable him to finish his horrid butchery."[1] Although this is much less the case today, significant surgical complications do occur with a wide range in their incidence at various institutions. Complications of thyroid surgery include laryngeal nerve injuries, hypoparathyroidism, postoperative hemorrhage, seroma, or hematoma, respiratory obstruction, wound infection, sepsis, and hyperthyroid crisis. When cervical metastatic thyroid carcinoma is taken into account, other complications need to be mentioned such as spinal accessory nerve injury and chylous fistula. Because metastatic thyroid disease is usually treated with a modified neck dissection, these risks are uncommon. In this chapter those complications related to thyroidectomy and the treatment of thyroid cancer are discussed in detail, bringing in certain aspects of the anatomy when pertinent. Because of the improved diagnostic techniques in voice analysis and the array of surgical procedures now available to improve vocal quality, it seems logical to add this to our discussion.

## LARYNGEAL NERVE INJURY

### Recurrent Laryngeal Nerve Injury

The two main nerves at risk in thyroid surgery are the recurrent and superior laryngeal nerves (Figure 26–1, A and B). In the majority of patients the recurrent nerve is the one that occupies the surgeon's attention the most during surgery. It is generally found without too much difficulty with proper technique, but can be injured with the slightest of mobilization. This nerve is a mixed nerve with motor and sensory branches to the trachea, esophagus, pharynx, and larynx. As the nerve ascends in the tracheal esophageal groove it gives off pharyngeal branches that supply motor and sensory fibers to

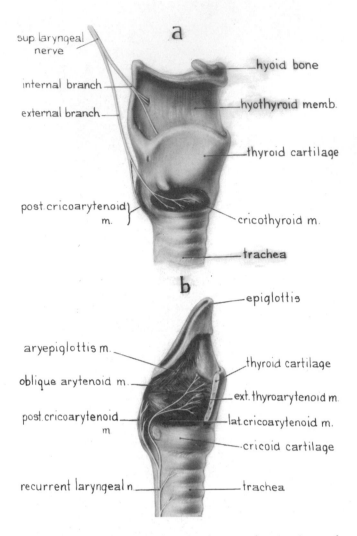

Figure 26-1. **A.** Superior laryngeal nerve showing internal and external branches. **B.** Recurrent laryngeal nerve depicting muscle innervation.

the inferior constrictor muscle and the mucosal surface below the vocal cords, respectively. It continues as the inferior laryngeal nerve supplying all but one of the intrinsic muscles of the larynx. Because of the course of the nerve and the close relationship of the thyroid gland, all these branches are at risk during thyroid surgery.

The reported incidence of injury to the recurrent laryngeal nerve can vary depending on the type of study and the experience of the surgeon to as low as 0.3% and as high as 17%.[2-5] Interestingly, the studies performed at teaching institutions with resident operators reveal low rates of nerve injury.[6,7] It is felt that this is related to the fact that an experienced staff surgeon is usually involved in those cases. Another study compared two surgical specialties to one another and although it found one group to have fewer complications, the reviewer of the article felt that not all variables were considered, and the results were, therefore, suspect.[8] When

reading results from the literature, several other points need to be considered when reporting the incidence of recurrent nerve injury. There is a known higher incidence of five times normal in second thyroid operations, and, therefore, these patients need to be considered separately.[9] Lack of good hemostasis and the need to re-explore the neck for hemorrhage holds an increase in recurrent nerve injury. Other factors that can have a significant effect on the incidence of recurrent nerve injury include the type of surgical approach, the histology or reason for the thyroidectomy, the technique of nerve identification versus the blind technique, and reporting nerves at risk rather than operations performed. The three most significant factors leading to nerve damage, aside from the experience of the operator, comprise the histologic features, second operations, and the failure to identity the nerve.[10] In one study the incidence of nerve injury was noted to be 5.2% versus 1.2% for nerve identification.[4] Although it is far better to identify the nerve during thyroid surgery, the location and the anatomic variation of the nerve in the neck presents a challenge to the surgeon.

The embryology of the vascular structures of the neck and chest results in a different course taken by each of the recurrent nerves as they leave the vagus nerve. On the right the recurrent nerve arises as it loops around the subclavian artery going behind the artery before ascending up the tracheal esophageal groove. This places the nerve more lateral and slightly more superficial than the recurrent nerve on the left. More importantly in regards to risk of injury, however, is the rare event of a nonrecurrent nerve that is reported in 0.3% to 1.0% of cases on the right.[11] This results in the nerve coming directly off the vagus entering at the level of cricothyroid membrane as it enters the larynx. There is also a second variant in which the nerve may act as a partial recurrent nerve when it is seen looping around the inferior thyroid artery. In both of these cases there is an anomalous development of the right subclavian artery from the fourth aortic arch with the subclavian coming off the aorta rather than the brachiocephalic artery. This results in the subclavian artery lying posterior to the esophagus and may cause symptoms in childhood. This vascular anomaly can only occur on the right side and, therefore, a left nonrecurrent laryngeal nerve is not a possibility. The recurrent laryngeal nerve on the left appears as a branch of the vagus nerve and crosses over the aorta just lateral to the ligamentum arteriosum. The nerve then loops around the aorta to ascend closely to the trachea in a more medial and straighter course than on the right.

These variations that the recurrent nerve may take on the two sides of the neck are the reason that the thoracic inlet is one of three potential sites where the nerve is at high risk. The two other areas are at the point of lig-

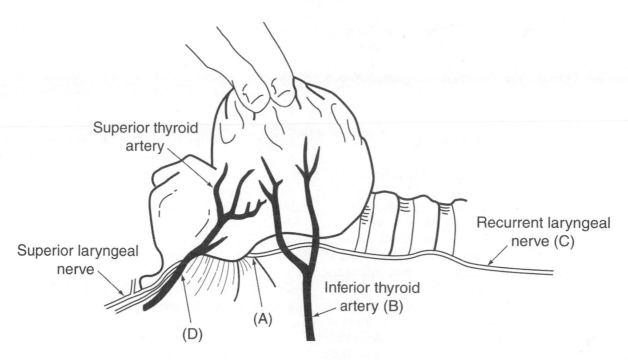

**Figure 26–2.** Risk of recurrent (RLN) and superior (SLN) laryngeal injury at thyroidectomy. **A.** At the ligament of Berry—RLN. **B.** Inferior thyroid artery ligation—RLN. **C.** At the thoracic inlet—RLN. **D.** Superior thyroid pole dissection—SLN.

ation of the branches of the inferior thyroid arteries and at the ligament of Berry (Figure 26–2).[12] After the identification of the inferior thyroid artery most surgeons begin to look for the nerve as it ascends in a triangle formed by the carotid laterally, the trachea medially, and the thyroid lobe superiorly. One thing that the surgeon can rely on is that the nerve has no constant relationship to the inferior thyroid artery and as the nerve nears the artery, it may show one of several variations. The nerve can be found posterior (45%–65%), anterior (18%–26%), or between (18%–36%) the branches of the inferior thyroid artery.[13,14] It, therefore, becomes important not to clamp the inferior thyroid artery until the nerve has been identified and its relationship to the branches of the artery determined. Once past this potential trouble spot, the next region of concern is around Berry's ligament, and the recurrent nerve frequently branches at this time. Care needs to be taken not to cause pressure on the nerve when dissecting under the ligament, and to avoid injury to the terminal branch of the inferior thyroid artery at this location. Any troublesome bleeding should be handled with topical pledgets of adrenaline solution 1/1000. The general rule is to avoid traction on the nerve at all times and to keep the nerve in view throughout the procedure.

With injury to the recurrent nerve, symptoms of hoarseness, mild dysphagia, and airway compromise may occur. The type of injury and whether both recurrent nerves are affected determine the degree of symptoms. When one nerve is involved, the patient usually experiences a breathy, sometimes raspy, voice and some difficulty swallowing liquids (Figure 26–3). However, it is also not uncommon to note a paralyzed vocal cord on clinical exam with little change in one's voice. When both the recurrent nerves have been injured it can be-

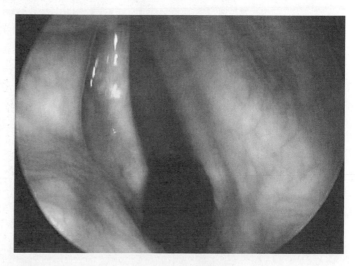

**Figure 26–3.** Laryngeal view showing a left vocal cord paralysis. Note the open glottis and bowing of the left true vocal cord.

come an emergent airway situation requiring the need for surgical intervention. The discussion of bilateral recurrent nerve injury is addressed in more detail under "Treatment Options for Recurrent Laryngeal Nerve Injuries."

## Superior Laryngeal Nerve Injury

The superior laryngeal nerve is probably injured more frequently than reported because of the lack of significant clinical symptoms. With the refinement in voice analysis through such techniques as laryngeal videostroboscopy and EMG, the detection of mild changes in vocal cord movement is now more apparent (Figure 26–4). The superior laryngeal nerve originates high in the neck from the vagus as it descends in close relationship to the carotid sheath. As the nerve lies on the middle constrictor muscle at or past the superior cornu of the hyoid, it divides into an internal and external branch. The internal branch enters the larynx high at the thyrohyoid membrane supplying sensory fibers to the mucous membrane of the supraglottis and the piriform sinus of the hypopharynx. The external branch has a close relationship with the superior thyroid artery as they both descend in the neck towards the superior pole of the thyroid and the cricothyroid muscle. The nerve supplies motor fibers to the inferior constrictor

and cricothyroid muscles.[12] Thyroid surgery is the most common cause of injury to this branch leading to changes in the patient's ability to change pitch. The speaking register lowers, high pitch control is lost, and the patient may experience early voice fatigue. If the injury is bilateral, the effect on the voice may be more significant. The changes on clinical indirect or fiberoptic laryngoscopy may be subtle if the examiner is not familiar with this type of nerve injury. Unless the patient is a professional singer or has a similar profession that places significance on the use of one's voice, injury to this nerve causes little disability. Although there are refined techniques in phonosurgery to help address this complication, they are rarely needed.

## Combined Superior and Recurrent Laryngeal Nerve Injury

A combined loss of both the superior and recurrent nerve is most noticeable when they occur on the same side. Symptoms tend to be more severe than with just a unilateral recurrent injury. The patient experiences a breathier voice, intermittent cough, and occasional aspiration with liquids. The exam reveals the vocal cord to be more lateral, at a slightly lower level, and unable to show any adduction towards the opposite cord during phonation. This is a result of the loss of the cricothy-

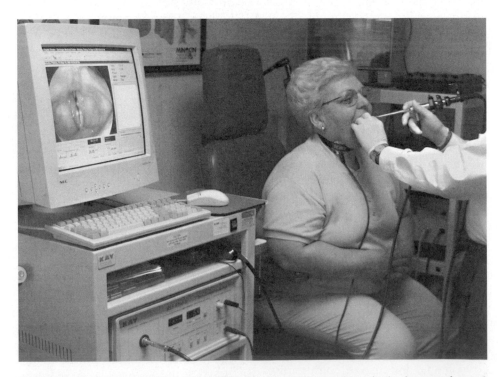

**Figure 26–4.** Patient undergoing a video-laryngostroboscopy with the laryngeal vocal cords viewed on the monitor.

roid muscle. Unilateral recurrent nerve loss with bilateral superior nerve weakness can cause a severe change in the voice requiring several types of phonosurgical procedures. Fortunately, this complication from thyroid surgery is not very common.

## TREATMENT OPTIONS FOR RECURRENT LARYNGEAL NERVE INJURIES

### Unilateral Recurrent Nerve Injury

There are many phonosurgical procedures available to the laryngologist to repair injuries sustained to the laryngeal nerves. It is not the scope of this chapter to describe all these in detail, but we will review the more common approaches. These procedures comprise dynamic or static principles.

The active techniques include primary nerve repair and reinnervation procedures. If during surgery the nerve is sacrificed for tumor control or cut, then a decision needs to be made about primary or interpositional graft microanastomosis of the recurrent nerve. This was a topic of debate in the past because of the possible synkinesis that might occur between the abductor and adductor nerve fibers. However, this does not commonly occur, and repair at the time of surgery has shown excellent restoration of voice quality in some cases. If spastic movement did result, this could be resolved by simply cutting the nerve and carrying out another procedure to deal with the nerve loss. Reinnervation techniques are not as popular as they were when they first came onto the scene. This is partly because the results were not uniform by those performing these procedures and the time for any noticeable improvement was much longer than the static medialization techniques. Probably the first to clinically popularize reinnervation was Harvey Tucker in the 1970s with the ansa hypoglossal nerve muscle pedicle from the omohyoid muscle for laryngeal reinnervation.[15] This nerve muscle pedicle was placed in the posterior cricoarytenoid muscle for bilateral paralysis and in the thyroarytenoid muscle for unilateral recurrent nerve weakness. Crumley described a different technique using a severed ansa hypoglossal branch and connecting it directly into the cut end of the recurrent nerve.[16] In this way one could, if necessary, select out the adductor or abductor branches as the nerve divided before entering the larynx. This procedure requires waiting at least a year to see if normal return of function occurs in a recurrent nerve not originally cut at surgery.

Static or passive phonosurgical procedures are by far the most frequently used surgical correction for a unilateral recurrent nerve injury. The principle behind all these techniques is to move the vocal fold more to the midline and close the glottic gap during phonation. The three commonly used procedures include injection of various materials into the vocal cord or paraglottic space, thyroplasty type 1, and arytenoid adduction. All these techniques have proven successful in the properly selected cases. Gelfoam, Teflon, collagen, and fat are the frequently used injection material. Brunings in 1912 was the first to describe the injection of the vocal cord for medialization.[17] His use of paraffin led to a high rate of failure because of a foreign body granuloma reaction. It was not until 1962 when Arnold used a new substance called Teflon that the procedure became the primary treatment for rehabilitating a unilateral vocal cord paralysis.[18] Although Teflon is still considered a good material for medialization, it has some drawbacks because of its permanence and the difficulty in accurate placement in every case. Gelfoam was popularized in 1978 as a nonpermanent medialization procedure as the Gelfoam usually resorbed in 4 to 5 weeks. Collagen has recently been found to be effective in improving the quality of the voice for patients with Parkinson's disease but is usually not long-lasting enough to help those with a recurrent nerve injury.[19] Fat has been used as an injection material as well as a surgical placed filler to improve the vibrator surface of the true vocal cord.[20] Personally, we have found fat to be an excellent material to inject into the paraglottic space in those patients who need a little more medialization following thyroplasty.

Thyroplasty type 1 has now become the procedure of choice for most surgeons in vocal cord rehabilitation after unilateral vocal cord paralysis. Isshiki popularized the use of Silastic as a laryngeal implant in the late 1970s and started a large wave of others with their own specific variation to his original description. Isshiki described four basic laryngeal framework procedures.[21] These procedures alter the voice by changing the position of the vocal cord with modifications in the laryngeal cartilage. Type 1 refers to a lateral compression technique that is designed to medialize the cord towards the midline. This procedure is usually performed on those symptomatic patients with a permanent vocal cord paralysis, but has also been beneficial in other voice disorders. A review of this subject and various modifications of the technique can be found in a review article by Koufman.[22] This procedure offers the benefit of an implant that can be removed for any reason and, therefore, is reversible. It seems to be more reproducible with better voice results.

### Bilateral Recurrent Nerve Injury

Bilateral vocal cord paralysis after thyroid surgery although rare is one of the more dreaded complications to manage. The condition leads to dyspnea with any exertion, some degree of stridor, and voice weakening. The significance of these symptoms can vary and, therefore, may not be noticed immediately after surgery. Because not all surgeons perform postoperative laryngoscopy, the diagnosis may be delayed in certain cases. Also postoperative hypothyroidism with myxedema of the vocal cords or laryngospasm with hypocalcemia tetany from hypoparathyroidism may lead to further airway obstruction in a patient with bilateral cord paralysis resulting in a delayed airway emergency.[23,24]

Treatment of bilateral vocal cord paralysis is a challenging problem. The first thing to remember in any recurrent nerve injury is that unless the surgeon deliberately cut or sacrificed the nerve in treating the thyroid disease, the nerve may still recover with time. Sometimes, but not always, a tracheotomy may be needed in the acute setting. Placing a suture around the vocal process, secured externally, is another temporizing procedure. If the nerves do not recover or show some return of function in one year then a more permanent procedure can be considered, such as a laser arytenoidectomy or a Woodman procedure.

## METABOLIC COMPLICATIONS

### Hypothyroidism

Hypothyroidism is an expected result in most thyroid procedures and can even occur following a unilateral lobectomy. It can also be a consequence of the disease process that prompted the thyroid surgery in the first place, such as longstanding Graves' disease and Hashimoto's thyroiditis. This as well as other metabolic complications from thyroidectomy are discussed in greater detail later in this chapter.

### Hypocalcemia (Hypoparathyroidism)

The two major complications of thyroid surgery continue to be recurrent laryngeal nerve injury and hypocalcemia. Although damage to the parathyroid tissue is the most common reason for postoperative hypocalcemia, there are several other causes. Thyrocalcitonin may play a role. Patients with hyperthyroidism secondary to Graves' disease may develop hypocalcemia as a result of rapid uptake of calcium into the bones to repair a chemical osteodystrophy. Hypoparathyroidism from thyroid surgery occurs when parathyroid tissue is removed and not reimplanted, the gland infarcts from manipulation, or the blood supply is disrupted. This complication varies in incidence based on many factors and has been reported to occur in from 1.2% to 40% of cases.[25] Transient hypocalcemia tends to be seen more

commonly and is probably caused by the initial vascular shock to the parathyroid tissue. Factors that may play a role in postoperative hypoparathyroidism include the extent of surgery, the experience of the operator, and the number of functioning glands remaining.[26] Most surgeons believe that you should leave at least two functional parathyroids with adequate blood supply to avoid hypoparathyroidism.

Once recognized during the surgeon's learning curve for thyroid surgery, the parathyroid glands become relatively easy to identify. The problem, however, lies in preserving their blood supply. Close to 80% of all parathyroid glands receive their blood from the inferior thyroid artery. As the inferior thyroid artery is identified with the recurrent nerve, care is taken not to ligate the main trunk but rather follow the branches into the gland and preserve the blood supply to the parathyroid tissue. The field should be kept dry and suctioning on the parathyroids avoided. If a gland is felt to have sustained injury by a change in its color, the operator should then remove the gland, mince the tissue into 1 to 2 mm pieces, and autotransplant the material into the sternocleidomastoid muscle. With these techniques, the knowledge of the anatomy, and a meticulous unhurried dissection, the surgeon should be able to achieve a low incidence of permanent hypocalcemia or hypoparathyroidism. This subject is discussed later in this chapter under "Medical Complications of Treatment."

### Thyroid Storm

By the use of antithyroid drugs and propranolol, thyroid storm is usually prevented during thyroid surgery by adequate preoperative preparation in those cases manifesting symptoms of hyperthyroidism. Thyroid crisis occurs in conditions of severe hyperthyroidism such as in thyrotoxicosis of Graves' disease and if untreated holds a high mortality rate. The pathogenesis is thought to occur because of the binding of thyroid stimulating immunoglobulins to thyroid cell receptors. This condition and its treatment is addressed elsewhere in this text.

## OTHER COMPLICATIONS

### Intraoperative

#### Neural Injuries—Lymph Node Dissection

Neural injuries are at a higher risk in the treatment of thyroid carcinoma. In thyroid carcinoma total thyroidectomy is the philosophy of most institutions and as the amount of thyroid tissue removed increases, so does the risk for laryngeal nerve damage. Also nodal metastasis from thyroid carcinoma requires some type of nodal dissection. Most surgeons now favor some type of a modified neck dissection over the "berry picking" technique or the more aggressive radical neck approach. Any form of cervical nodal procedure carries the risk of injury to other neural structures including the ramus branch of the facial nerve, the hypoglossal, the spinal accessory, the vagus and the sympathetic nerves. Probably the nerve most commonly affected by a neck dissection is cranial nerve eleven or spinal accessory. Injury to this nerve is disabling to any patient but much worse for a female because of the cosmetic appearance. The incidence for these complications from neck dissection for thyroid carcinoma is extremely low, especially in the hands of an experienced head and neck surgeon.

## Chyle Leak

A chylous fistula is a rare event from thyroid surgery but does occur in the removal of very large thyroid masses, extensive thyroid carcinoma, and in those cases requiring a cervical neck dissection. At the time of surgery a recognized leak should be repaired with the use of the operating microscope if necessary. Postoperative chylous drainage can be managed with diet control of fatty acids and neck pressure. Rarely does re-exploration of the neck prove helpful.

## Tumor Spillage

Oncologically spilling any tumor cells at the time of surgery is extremely disheartening to the surgeon and may occur more commonly in treating thyroid carcinoma. Although it is hard to predict the effect on tumor control in thyroid cancer patients, the cystic nature of some papillary thyroid carcinoma lesions leads to an increased risk of this complication. Figure 26–5 shows a patient with cystic papillary thyroid carcinoma in the thyroid as well as the neck. At surgery these cystic neck metastases were found to be very thin-walled making the dissection more difficult for fear of tumor spillage. Another rare cystic presentation for thyroid carcinoma was seen in thyroid carcinoma arising in a thyroglossal duct cyst. The CT scan in Figure 26–6 represents such a case with papillary carcinoma. At surgery the structure was multicystic and the walls were very thin, requiring careful meticulous dissection to avoid rupture of any of the cystic contents. Most head and neck surgeons would not hesitate to perform a fine needle aspiration on a solid cervical neck mass. Because cystic lesions in the neck can appear to represent benign congenital lesions, one does not always confirm this with a fine needle biopsy. The authors believe that all cystic neck masses should be needled before removal to limit oncologic mistakes at the time of surgery.

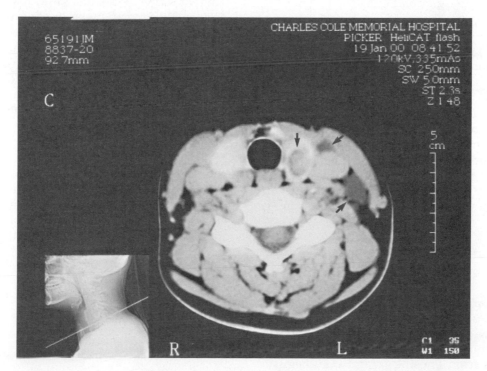

**Figure 26–5.** Patient with a cystic papillary carcinoma in the thyroid and cervical nodes.

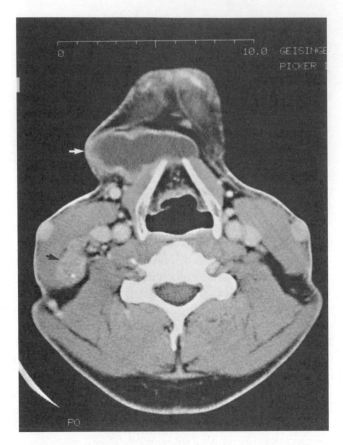

**Figure 26–6.** CT scan showing papillary carcinoma within a thyroglossal duct cyst. Note the cervical metastasis from the thyroglossal duct cyst carcinoma. Total thyroidectomy failed to show any evidence of carcinoma in the gland.

## Tumor Involvement of Adjacent Structures

Sacrifice of surrounding structures because of tumor involvement may not be considered a complication by some surgeons. To the patient, however, it may represent a significant disability when functions of speech and swallowing are affected. Involvement of the recurrent laryngeal nerve, the outer muscle tissue of the esophagus or hypopharynx, the laryngotracheal framework, and the major vessels in the neck can lead to sacrificing these structures and leaving the patient with major morbidity.

## Postoperative

### Hemorrhage

After thyroidectomy, hemorrhage may be immediate or delayed and is usually arterial. Rarely is it a result of an unsuspected hematologic problem. An immediate bleed occurs after or shortly before extubation when the patient lightens from anesthesia and may begin to cough, causing a vessel to open. The neck enlarges rapidly or, if suction drains are used, blood loss through

the drains becomes so significant that it becomes obvious immediately. The treatment is to secure the airway by reintubation if extubation has occurred and re-explore the neck. Delayed hemorrhage may develop slowly and, therefore, may not be recognized at first. Airway compromise from tracheal compression may then occur and require immediate intervention. Spinelli et al found nine immediate and ten delayed hemorrhages in a review of 1800 thyroid procedures with all requiring surgical treatment under general anesthesia.[27] The source of the bleeding was usually the strap muscles and the inferior pole site. Others have found the cause of hemorrhage to be the superior thyroid vessels. As stated earlier, postoperative re-exploration for hemorrhage has shown to result in a higher incidence of recurrent nerve injury.

## Airway Obstruction

Postoperative airway obstruction is a major complication of thyroid surgery which can lead to a high rate of mortality. The reasons for airway compromise include: bilateral recurrent nerve injury, tracheal malacia from longstanding tracheal compression caused by a large thyroid mass, subglottic edema from laryngeal involvement with tumor, tracheal invasion by tumor, and postoperative hemorrhage or hematoma. All of these require quick recognition and treatment to prevent significant mortality or morbidity.

## Wound Complications

Thyroid surgery holds the same postoperative wound problems that can be seen in other cervical head and neck wounds. Infection, hematoma, seroma, and necrosis of skin flaps are a few of the wound complications that can occur but are relatively uncommon. The need for a modified neck dissection or prior radiation therapy may increase the chances for some of these events. Care in planning skin incisions and in wound closure, the use of prophylactic antibiotics, and considering suction drainage in those cases with increased vascularity at the time of surgery, such as in Graves' disease, should lessen the chance of these wound complications. Hypertrophic scarring or keloid formation is seen in younger patients and in the black population. Injecting steroids during the postoperative period will help in these patients and, later, scar revision can be considered if cosmetic improvement is desired.

## MEDICAL COMPLICATIONS OF TREATMENT

### Hypocalcemia

Transient hypocalcemia following thyroid surgery is common. It is often seen following removal of a parathyroid adenoma. Hypocalcemia may be more severe or prolonged, depending on the number of parathyroid glands removed or devitalized. Similarly, patients with parathyroid bone disease may also have prolonged hypocalcemia ("hungry bone syndrome") following removal of a parathyroid adenoma. Unremitting hypoparathyroidism occurs in 5–15% of patients undergoing a total or near-total thyroidectomy.

Symptoms of hypocalcemia include facial and acral paresthesias, nervousness and muscle cramps. If left untreated, patients will have tetany, seizures, cardiac arrhythmia, and may expire. Serum ionized or total calcium levels should be monitored following surgery. Chvostek's sign, twitching of the lip in response to tapping on the ipsilateral facial nerve, is usually positive before other symptoms occur and is helpful in management. Patients should be evaluated for Chvostek's sign preoperatively as some normocalcemic patients may have a positive sign.

Mild symptoms of hypocalcemia can be treated with oral calcium (calcium carbonate 1 gm every 6 hours). More severe symptoms may herald a medical emergency and should be treated promptly with intravenous calcium gluconate, 20 ml of a 10% solution IV over 10–15 minutes. This should be followed by slow intravenous infusion, 60 ml of a 10% solution in 1,000 ml $D_5W$ over 3–4 hours. If hypocalcemia is expected to be transient, the intravenous calcium can be given as needed.

If hypocalcemia is expected to be prolonged or permanent (as following a three-and-a-half gland parathyroid resection or following total parathyroidectomy with autograft) then oral calcium should be started as soon as practical along with vitamin D. Table 26–1 shows the available vitamin D products with their doses, half-life and relative costs. The advantages of using vitamin D metabolites is that they have a rapid onset of action and, if hypercalcemia is experienced, discontinuance or reduction of dose will achieve more rapid lowering of calcium levels. The more polar metabolites of vitamin D, however, are more expensive than native vitamin D.

## Thyroid Storm

Thyroid storm is a rare complication of thyroid surgery. The incidence of this potentially fatal complication has decreased dramatically as patients are usually pretreated for their hyperthyroidism prior to surgery. Storm presumably occurs as a result of "dumping" of preformed thyroid hormone into the circulation during surgical manipulation. Preoperatively, hyperthyroid patients should be treated with thionamides and beta-blockers to avoid this preventable complication.

Thyroid storm should be treated vigorously with high dose thioureas (such as propylthiouracil 200 mg ever 6 hours) with subsequent administration of oral intravenous iodide several hours later. Heart rate should be monitored and oral or intravenous beta-blockers given. Prednisone may also be helpful as it may aid in inhibiting peripheral conversion of thyroxine to triiodothyronine.

## Hypothyroidism

Hypothyroidism is an expected sequelae of total thyroidectomy or radioiodine therapy. It can also be seen during thiourea therapy. Reducing the dose or discontinuing thioureas will relieve the hypothyroidism. In patients in whom hypothyroidism is expected to be permanent, thyroid hormone therapy is appropriate and L-thyroxine (1.6 mcg/kg) should be given once a day.[28] If it is desirable to suppress TSH (as in patients with papillary or follicular carcinoma) a dose of 2.7 mcg/kg of body weight should be given.[29] Thyroid hormone levels (TSH and free $T_4$) should be checked in 5–6 week intervals to ensure that the prescribed dose of hormone is appropriate. If a subtotal thyroidectomy has been performed, waiting 5–6 weeks is also the appropriate interval to see if thyroid hormone will be required.

There are no known side effects of thyroid hormone per se, unless it is given in injudicious doses. A recent study has shown that some patients feel better when combination L-thyroxine and triiodothyronine are ad-

**Table 26–1.** Vitamin D products with their doses, half-life, and relative costs

| Vitamin D Product | Dose/Day | Time for Reversal of Hypercalcemia | AWP/Month |
| --- | --- | --- | --- |
| Ergocalciferol | 25,000 – 100,000 U | 17 – 60 days | $2.40 – 52.20 |
| Dihydrotachysterol | 0.2 – 1.2 MG | 3 – 14 days | $30.00 – 54.00 |
| Calcifediol | 0.05 – 2.0 MCG | 7 – 30 days | $32.33 – 60.50 |
| Calcitriol | 0.5 – 1.0 MCG | 1 – days | $35.91 – 57.40 |

ministered together.[30] At the time of this writing, however, combination $T_4$ and $T_3$ therapy is controversial.

## References

1. Gross SD. *A System of Surgery: Pathological, Diagnostic, Therapeutic and Operative.* (3rd ed.). Philadelphia, PA: Blanchard and Lea; 1866.

2. Martensson H, Terins J. Recurrent laryngeal nerve palsy in thyroid gland surgery related to operations and nerves at risk. *Arch Surg.* 1985;120:475–477.

3. Wagner HE, Seiler CA. Recurrent laryngeal nerve palsy after thyroid gland surgery. *Br J Surg.* 1994;81:226–228.

4. Jatzko GR, Lisborg PH, Müller MG, Wette VM. Recurrent nerve palsy after thyroid operation—principal nerve identification and a literature review. *Surgery.* 1994;115:139–144.

5. Al-Suliman NN, Ryttov NF, Quist N, Blichert-Toft M, Graversen HP. Experience in a specialist thyroid surgery unit: a demographic study, surgical complications, and outcome. *Eur J Surg.* 1997;163:13–20.

6. Lamadé W, Renz K, Willeke F, Klar E, Herfarth CH. Effect of training on the incidence of nerve damage in thyroid surgery. *Br J Surg.* 1999;86:388–391.

7. Mishra A, Agarwal G, Agarwal A, Mishra S. Safety and efficacy of total thyroidectomy in hands of endocrine surgery trainees. *Am J Surg.* 1999;178:377–380.

8. Burge MR, Zeise T, Johnsen MW, Conway MJ, Qualls CR. Risks of complications following thyroidectomy: a retrospective study. *J Gen Intern Med.* 1998;13:24–31.

9. Menegaux F, Turpin G, Dahman M, et al. Secondary thyroidectomy in patients with prior thyroid surgery for benign disease: a study of 203 cases. *Surgery.* 1999;126:479–483.

10. Herranz-Gonzalez J, Gavilan J, Matinez-Videl J, Gavilan C. Complications following thyroid surgery. *Arch Otolaryngol Head Neck Surg.* 1991;117:516–518.

11. Stewart GR, Mountain JC, Colcock BP. Non-recurrent laryngeal nerve. *Br J Surg.* 1972;59:379–381.

12. Kalky MP, Weber RS. Complications of surgery of the thyroid and parathyroid glands. *Surg Clin North Am.* 1993;73:307–320.

13. Reed AF. The relation of the interior laryngeal nerve to the interior laryngeal artery. *Anat Rec.* 1943;85:17–23.

14. Fowler CH, Hanson WA. The surgical anatomy of the thyroid gland with special relation of the recurrent laryngeal nerve. *Surg Gynecol Obstet.* 1929;49:59–65.

15. Tucker HM. Human laryngeal reinnervation. *Laryngoscope.* 1976; 82:769–779.

16. Crumley RL, Izdebsk K. Voice quality following laryngeal reinnervation by ansa hypoglossi transfer. *Laryngoscope.* 1986; 96:611–616.

17. Brunings W. Uber eine neue be handlungs methode der rekurrenslamung. *Verh Verl Dtsch Laryngol.* 1911;18:93–151.

18. Arnold GE. Vocal rehabilitation of paralytic dysphonia, IX. Technique of intracordal injection. *Arch Otolaryngol.* 1962;76:358–368.

19. Ford CN, Bless DM, Campbell D. Studies of injectable soluble collagen for vocal fold augmentation. *Rev Laryngol Otol Rhinol.* 1987; 108:33–36.

20. Wetmore SJ. Injection of fat for soft tissue augmentation. *Laryngoscope.* 1989;99:50–57.

21. Isshiki N, Morita H, Okamura H, et al. Thyroplasty as a new phonosurgical technique. *Acta Otolaryngol.* 1974;78:451–457.

22. Koufman JA. *Laryngoplastic Phonosurgery Instructional Coursers.* St Louis, C.V. Mosby; 1988:339.

23. Holinger PC, Holinger LD, Seibel MS, Holinger PH. Psychiatric manifestations of the post-thyroidectomy bilateral abductor vocal cord paralysis syndrome. *J New Ment Dis.* 1980;168:46–49.

24. Young HA, Ferguson IT. Laryngeal tetany: an unusual presentation of chronic renal failure. *J Laryngol Otol.* 1977;91:373–377.

25. Flynn MB, Lyons KJ, Tarter JW, Ragsdale TL. Local complications after surgical resection for thyroid carcinoma. *Am J Surg.* 1994; 168:404–407.

26. Pattou F, Combemale F, Fabre S, et al. Hypocalcemia following thyroid surgery: incidence and prediction of outcome. *World J Surg.* 1998;22:718–724.

27. Spinelli C, Berti P, Miccoli P. The postoperative hemorrhagic complication in thyroid surgery. *Minerva Chir.* 1994;49:1245–1247.

28. Hennessey JV, Evaul JE, Tseng YC, Burman KD, Wartofsky L. 1986. L-thyroxine dosage: a reevaluation of therapy with contemporary preparations. *Ann Int Med.* 1986;105:11–15.

29. Bartalena L, Martino E, Pacchiarotti A, et. al. Factors affecting suppression of endogenous thyrotropin secretion by thyroxine treatment: retrospective analysis in athyreotic and goiterous patients. *J Clin Endocrinol Metab.* 1987;64:849–855.

30. Banevicius R, Kazanavicius G, Zalinkevicius R, et al. 1999. Effects of thyroxine as compared with thyroxine + triiodothyronine in patients with hypothyroidism. *New Engl J Med.* 1999;340(6):424–429.

# 27

# Congenital Thyroid Cysts and Ectopic Thyroid

Thomas Kennedy, M.D., F.A.C.S.

W. Edward Wood, M.D.

Mark Aferzon, M.D.

## CONGENITAL THYROID CYSTS

Congenital thyroid cysts and ectopic thyroid are, in essence, embryologic malformations and are, therefore, considered together in this chapter. Among the various congenital neck masses confronted by the head and neck surgeon, the thyroglossal duct cyst is, by far, the most frequently found. For this reason and because a small percentage of these cysts may also harbor ectopic thyroid and even a thyroid malignancy, it is essential that the surgeon have a firm understanding of the embryology, anatomy, and treatment of this entity. Ectopic thyroid may imply accessory thyroid that represents a mass of thyroid tissue distant from the normal gland or aberrant thyroid implying that the entire thyroid is located at a location different from the midline of the neck. A thyroglossal duct cyst may do either but is more likely to show ectopic thyroid tissue along with benign cystic contents and a normal thyroid gland at its usual location low in the neck. Any ectopic or accessory thyroid tissue away from the gland should be held with suspicion as possibly indicating a focus of metastatic carcinoma. Thyroid cancer can also be found in a thyroglossal duct cyst in 1% of the cases.[1,2] These and various other developmental abnormalities are discussed along with their treatment.

## Embryology

The anlage of the thyroid develops as a ventral diverticulum from the floor of the pharyngeal gut at the tuberculum impar (foramen caecum) in the 3–4 mm embryo. As the diverticulum descends caudally with the development of the embryo, it stays caudal to the first arch derivative and ventral to the remaining arches. In this manner the future gland descends in the neck anterior to the second and remaining arches that form the hyoid, thyroid, and cricoid cartilages.[3] As the diverticulum or thyroid gland migrates to its final location low in the midline of the neck, it leaves a tract that starts at the foramen cecum and ends at the pyramidal lobe of the thyroid. The foramen cecum is at the junction of the tongue base and the anterior two-thirds of the tongue. In the seventh to eighth week of development the gland has reached its final position in front of the trachea and the duct becomes obliterated.[4] If it remains, it may give rise to cystic masses anywhere along this tract from the tongue base to the pyramidal lobe of the thyroid gland. Aside from benign cysts, sinus tracts or solid thyroid tissue may occur along this duct. These congenital abnormalities most commonly occur below the level of the hyoid, but can be found anywhere from the tongue base to the thyroid gland.[5] David Ellis and Peter van Nostrand found in a large series of adult laryngeal sections, embryonic sections, and surgical specimens that the thyroglossal tract or duct was consistently anterior to the hyoid bone.[6] The tract was shown also to lie inferior and posterior to the hyoid body because of how the tract hooked around the hyoid in development. This finding is also consistent with the origin of the diverticulum of thyroid, which is anterior to the second, third, and fourth arch derivatives.

## Thyroglossal Duct Cyst

Thyroglossal duct remnants are believed to occur in 7% of the population and are the most common congenital anomaly in the neck treated by otolaryngologists and head and neck surgeons. Allard reported prevalence rates from 4 in 10,000 pediatric cases to 26% for a series of 267 children undergoing surgery for neck masses.[4] Some studies show an equal sex distribution while others find males more common at 2:1.[4,7] Over 90% present in the midline of the neck with the lateral location seen more on the left than the right side. Differential diagnosis may include: adenomas or other thyroid masses; dermoid cyst; ectopic or lingual thyroid tissue; cystic hygromas, branchial cysts or laryngoceles when confused with laterally placed thyroglossal duct remnants; and inflammatory cervical nodes. Cervical adenopathy is the most common differential when located above the level of the hyoid in the submental triangle. As discussed earlier, these cysts can occur anywhere along the duct remnant from the tongue base to the thyroid gland.

Clinical presentation is most frequent in children and becomes apparent by the age of 16 years.[7] The finding of a thyroglossal duct cyst in adults, however, is not uncommon and should be in the differential of all patients with midline neck mass. Draining fistulas may occur as a result of infection and the need to incise and drain the mass or from incomplete resection of a tract. The size of the cyst may vary with the average range 2–4 cm in diameter. There also may be movement of the mass with protrusion of the tongue because of its origin from the foramen cecum and the close relationship with the hyoid bone.

Workup of a suspected thyroglossal duct cyst should include studies to confirm the diagnosis and the location of the thyroid gland. An ultrasound of the neck will accomplish both and save the younger patient the effects of ionizing radiation from other scans. However, this will not rule out the possibility of ectopic thyroid tissue or the rare case of a thyroglossal duct cyst carcinoma. Therefore, the author strongly recommends a fine needle aspiration (FNA) of all midline neck masses before the ultrasound study is performed. If the diagnosis of ectopic thyroid within a thyroglossal duct cyst is

suggested by the FNA, a contrast CT scan is ordered rather than an ultrasound. This will enable a complete assessment of the thyroid gland and the cervical neck nodes for the possibility of a thyroid malignancy. The iodine contrast does eliminate the use of a thyroid scan and delays the use of radioactive iodine in malignant thyroid nodules for up to 6 to 8 weeks. This, however, is an acceptable time period.

Treatment for thyroglossal duct remnants is complete surgical excision. The center of hyoid bone should be removed in every case and the tract followed, as much as possible, to the base of the tongue. If necessary the pharynx may be entered at the tongue base and then surgically repaired. It was Sistrunk, in 1920, who pointed out the importance of removing the center portion of the hyoid bone with the tract in order to prevent recurrence.[8] This approach to management leads to a very low rate of recurrent thyroglossal remnants of less than 4%.

The histopathologic findings in thyroglossal duct remnants usually show a squamous lining in both the cyst and the sinus tract. In those cysts that have had repeated infection the mucosal lining may have been lost, resulting in a difficult diagnosis for the pathologist. Ectopic thyroid within the cyst or tract may be found and may explain the rare occurrence of a thyroglossal duct cyst carcinoma.

## Thyroglossal Duct Cyst Carcinoma

Brentano in 1911 and Uchermann in 1915 were the first to describe a neoplasm in a thyroglossal duct cyst.[9,10] Ashurst and White in 1925 reported a case in the American literature of a carcinoma at the tongue base within an aberrant thyroid.[11] Owen and Ingelby are credited with the first English report of a papillary carcinoma in a thyroglossal duct cyst.[12] It is believed that a carcinoma within a thyroglossal duct cyst is found in approximately 1% of all thyroglossal duct remnants. This entity is rarely seen before the age of 14 years and the median age for a thyroglossal duct cyst carcinoma is about 40 years of age.[1,2] Figure 27–1 shows a 43-year-old male who presented with a large multicystic thyroglossal duct cyst carcinoma and a right cervical neck metastasis. Surgery included a total thyroidectomy with the final pathology revealing no evidence of papillary cancer in the thyroid gland.

The histology of reported thyroglossal duct carcinomas are listed in Table 27–1 with papillary adenocarcinoma representing 75 to 85% of the tumors in the literature. Mixed papillary and follicular are the next most common at 7%.[13–16] As a tumor can originate from any one cell from a thyroglossal remnant and the thyroid is an epithelial proliferation from the pharyngeal

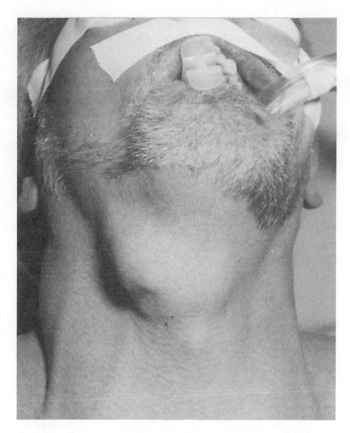

**Figure 27–1.** A 43-year-old male with a large multicystic thyroglossal duct cyst and a right cervical neck metastasis.

**Table 27–1.** Histologic Types of thyroglossal duct carcinoma

Papillary adenocarcinoma

Mixed follicular and papillary adenocarcinoma

Squamous cell carcinoma

Pure follicular

Adenocarcinoma without subclassification

Hürthle cell carcinoma

Hashimoto's disease

Concurrent papillary and squamous cell carcinoma

gut, one would expect a tumor of squamous epithelium to be common and the only true primary thyroglossal duct cyst carcinoma. Squamous cell carcinoma has been found to arise in 5% of thyroglossal duct carcinomas and has the worst prognosis.[13] The two theories that help explain the thyrogenic origin of thyroglossal duct adenocarcinomas include a carcinoma arising within a cyst de novo and tumors representing a metastasis from an occult primary carcinoma of the thyroid gland.[17–19] There are excellent review articles that the reader can refer to on this subject with most authors favoring the de novo theory.

Unfortunately, the diagnosis of a patient with a thyroglossal duct cyst carcinoma is usually not suspected and is discovered at the time of surgery. This can present a management dilemma for the operating surgeon, which may have been avoided if certain steps were taken preoperatively in evaluating a suspected thyroglossal duct cyst as discussed earlier. Controversy still exists, however, regarding what to do with the thyroid gland once the diagnosis of a thyroglossal duct cyst carcinoma is made. Most agree that if disease is also found in the thyroid or cervical nodes during the preoperative workup, a complete thyroidectomy along with a selective neck procedure is performed with the Sistrunk procedure followed by postoperative radioactive iodine. The question arises of what to do in those cases that show no evidence of clinical disease other than within the thyroglossal duct cyst. This author feels that a Sistrunk procedure and a total thyroidectomy should be performed in most cases of thyroglossal duct cyst carcinoma. Surgery, limited to a Sistrunk procedure, is recommended for medically high-risk patients and those cases with only a microscopic focus of thyroid carcinoma in a thyroglossal duct cyst that has not invaded the cyst wall or shown clinical evidence of metastatic spread.[20] Those opposing this view cite the complications of thyroidectomy and the low probability of disease in the thyroid gland that is not picked up clinically. The author refers the reader to those references cited for more discussion on the management of thyroglossal duct cyst carcinoma.[21] Because these patients are relatively young, any management decision should be based on the best potential for long-term surveillance of recurrent disease and the least morbidity for the patient.

## ECTOPIC THYROID

### Lingual Thyroid

Lingual thyroid is characterized by thyroid tissue in the midline base of the tongue anywhere between the circumvallate papilli and the epiglottis. It is a developmental anomaly caused by a failure of the thyroid to descend from its embryologic point of origin just posterior to the tuberculum impar. The pathogenesis of this descent failure is unknown.

The prevalence of symptomatic lingual thyroid is estimated to be 1:100,000[22] and affected individuals have no other functioning thyroid tissue in over 70% of cases.[23] Clinical hypothyroidism is found in up to one-third of cases.[23] A marked female to male preponderance of 4:1 has been reported.[24]

Most patients with lingual thyroid are asymptomatic with lesions being incidentally detected on routine intraoral examination. Symptoms may, however, occur at any point in life from infancy to old age and are in great part related to the size of the gland relative to the airway. Varying degrees of dysphagia, foreign body sensation, dysphonia, and dyspnea may be reported. Stridor with significant airway obstruction may occur in neonates and infants. Juvenile myxedema or cretinism may be found in up to 10% of young patients.[25] Many symptomatic patients present during puberty or pregnancy at a time when elevated TSH levels, which occur secondary to increased metabolic demands, cause lingual gland hypertrophy.[26] The stress of trauma and infection may produce similar physiologic responses.

On physical examination lingual thyroids are typically seen on direct visualization or indirect mirror examination of the tongue base. The usual appearance is that of a raised mass, light pink to bright red or bluish in color. The surface may be smooth or irregular and lobulated. Hemorrhagic changes, ulceration, and bleeding may sometimes be encountered. Fiberoptic examination can be helpful in determining the size of the gland and possible compromise of the airway.

When the diagnosis is suspected, evaluation should include thyroid function tests. Such studies most often reveal normal or marginally diminished gland function as represented by normal or decreased levels of $T_3$ and $T_4$ with normal or elevated levels of TSH and thyroglobulin.[26]

Imaging studies play an invaluable role in the evaluation of lingual and other ectopic thyroid anomalies. Radionuclide technetium-99m scanning with demonstrable activity at the tongue base confirms the diagnosis. Typically there is no associated activity within the neck. Computed tomography and magnetic resonance imaging are helpful in determining gland size and position. In most all cases lingual thyroid tissue interdigitates with tongue musculature. Consequently, sagittal views can be particularly helpful in ascertaining gland depth within the tongue as well as airway patency.

Clinical management of lingual thyroid has been a matter of controversy. Most, however, agree that the decision to treat should be individualized based on the size of the gland, severity of symptoms, and presence of such complications as ulceration and bleeding. Asymptomatic euthyroid patients can be closely observed. Suppressive therapy with exogenous thyroid hormone is the accepted mainstay of medical management. Such therapy suppresses TSH thereby eliminating the stimulus for gland hypertrophy. Therapy should be considered not just for symptomatic patients but for asymptomatic patients with elevated TSH levels as well. This should avoid future hypothyroidism and associated gland enlargement, which will often develop. Interval

thyroid function testing and clinical evaluation of the patient on suppressive therapy would seem prudent.[27]

Surgical intervention is appropriate for select patients. Indications include the development or progression of symptoms concurrent with suppressive therapy. Significant dysphagia, airway obstruction, and recurrent hemorrhage would merit surgery. Surgical approaches include lateral pharyngotomy, suprahyoid or transhyoid excision, and midline split of the tongue.[28] A preoperative tracheotomy or postoperative nasotracheal intubation should be anticipated as significant lingual edema may compromise the airway. Lingual thyroid autotransplantation to various body locations has been reported in an attempt to prevent postsurgical hypothyroidism. Success has, however, been limited.[26]

Radioactive ablation of the thyroid with I-131 may be an alternative to surgical excision for suppressive failures. Outcomes, however, have proven variable and unpredictable. This therapeutic modality is generally reserved for patients who refuse surgery or are considered high surgical risk.[29]

Carcinoma of the lingual thyroid is exceedingly rare. All pathologic types except medullary have been reported with a follicular predominance. There appears to be a propensity for lymphatic metastasis especially to the neck. Treatment is surgical excision with a margin of normal tissue. Neck dissection for surgical metastatic disease would seem appropriate. A therapeutic dose of I-131 after surgery may be needed dependent on completeness of resection and metastatic disease status.[30]

## Midline Cervical Ectopic Thyroid

As discussed previously, the thyroid develops as a midline structure by epithelial proliferation in the floor of the foregut between the tuberculum impar and hypobranchial eminence, the site of the foramen cecum. As the thyroid descends to its normal pretracheal position, it divides into right and left lobes and forms a tubular structure known as the thyroglossal duct. The thyroglossal duct normally atrophies. Ectopic thyroid tissue may, therefore, be found anywhere between the foramen cecum and the normal pretracheal location of the thyroid gland. Thyroid tissue not located anterior to the cervical trachea is considered ectopic. Ninety percent of thyroid ectopia is lingual and represents a descent failure. Less often, ectopic tissue may be found in the sublingual, anterior cervical (thyroglossal area), and possibly the lateral cervical regions. This would seem to represent arrested descent or dispersal of thyroid tissue during the migrational process. Factors regulating thyroid descent are unknown. As ectopic thyroid tissue is usually hypoplastic, this may be the primary factor governing maldescent.

The majority of cervical thyroid ectopia presents as a midline neck mass typically present since birth and often slowly enlarging. The differential diagnosis of a mass in this location includes: thyroglossal duct cyst, dermoid, epidermoid, and lymphadenopathy.

Ectopic thyroid tissue is usually hypoplastic and unable to accommodate increased metabolic demands. Enlargement and goiterous changes may, therefore, become apparent with growth spurts.[31] Hypothyroidism, although common, is not uniform. Further, partial ectopic thyroid, that is, thyroid ectopia in the presence of normally positioned thyroid gland can occur.

There is controversy regarding the appropriate preoperative evaluation of a patient with a midline neck mass. Ectopic midline cervical thyroid may be easily misdiagnosed as a thyroglossal duct cyst. Should the ectopia represent the only functional thyroid tissue, its inappropriate removal would render the patient athyroid. A normally positioned thyroid gland could be established preoperatively with either a thyroid scan or ultrasound of the neck. It would seem prudent to consider either study before the removal of all midline neck masses.[32]

## Lateral Cervical Ectopic Thyroid

The controversial existence and significance of lateral aberrant thyroid ectopia has been debated extensively within the literature. Thyroid tissue lateral to the carotid sheath defines lateral thyroid ectopia.[33] Consensus contemporary thinking is that any thyroid tissue within a lymph node, even with seemingly normal histology, represents not thyroid ectopia, but rather metastatic malignant disease from an occult thyroid tumor. It is somewhat difficult to reconcile lateral thyroid ectopia with the known embryologic midline descent of the thyroid anlage. Embryologically, maldescent or failure of fusion of the ultimobranchial body has been postulated as an explanation for lateral thyroid ectopia. The ultimobranchial contribution to the thyroid is derived from the fourth and fifth branchial pouches providing follicular and C cells.[34] This explanation is not consistent with the uniform absence of radioactive uptake in the lateral neck encountered in patients with undescended thyroid rests such as lingual thyroid. Further, primary extra-thyroidal medullary carcinoma has not been reported in the lateral neck. A more plausible explanation of lateral thyroid ectopia would be an intimate developmental association of the median thyroid anlage with mesodermal neck structures, eg, muscle, fibrofatty tissue, carotid sheath. Conceptually, nodular ectopic thyroid tissue not associated with lymph nodes might also arise as a result of implantation from previous neck trauma or surgery.[33] Such sequestered nodules should not have papillae or psammoma bodies, and should appear normal histologically.

When confronted with lateral cervical thyroid tissue, suspicion of metastatic disease rather than ectopia would seem justified. Most malignancies are of the papillary type. It has been shown that any papillary carcinoma of the thyroid gland, even a microscopic focus less than 1 mm, carries significant metastatic potential.[35] That a clinically normal thyroid gland can harbor occult thyroid carcinoma is supported by the findings of malignancy: 1) coincidentally after surgery for goiter; 2) as part of a surgical procedure for non-thyroid carcinoma of the head and neck, and 3) by necroscopy studies.

Histologic appearance on frozen section of a lateral thyroid nodule is vital to treatment planning. If frozen section reveals conclusive benign thyroid tissue without associated lymph node elements and meticulous detailed visual and digital examination of the thyroid gland is normal, some advocate not performing a thyroidectomy. Batsakis, however, cautions that lymph node tissue may not be identifiable as a result of histologic differentiation of papillary carcinoma in a metastatic site and also by cystic dilation of a metastasis. With the latter, only a rare papillary projection may betray the carcinoma.[36] If thyroid carcinoma is present or equivocal, total thyroidectomy should be performed and consideration given to appropriate neck dissection.

Conversely, a mistaken diagnosis of metastatic thyroid carcinoma might be rendered in cases of lateral aberrant thyroid associated with lymphocytic thyroiditis. In this situation, prominent lymphocytic infiltration including germinal centers could simulate the appearance of a lymph node. However, unlike actual lymph nodes, subcapsular spaces are not evident and the thyroid follicular epithelium demonstrates changes consistent with lymphocytic (Hashimoto's) thyroiditis.

## Laryngotracheal Thyroid

Intra-laryngotracheal thyroid was first described in 1875. Currently well over 120 cases have been reported within the literature. Two theories have been proposed in an attempt to explain this ectopia.

The "malformation" theory was originated by Von Bruns. In his series, there was no apparent connection between the thyroid gland and ectopic, intratracheal thyroid. He speculated the embryonic thyroid gland is encroached upon and divided by the later developing laryngeal and tracheal cartilages with the sequestration of embryonal thyroid within the airway. Paltauf put forth the "ingrowth" theory in 1892. In his series, a bridge of thyroid tissue connected ectopic intraluminal thyroid tissue with normal thyroid gland. This theory proposes a developmental lack of mesenchymal tissue between the thyroid gland and trachea, thus allowing an unusually tight adherence of the two. Originally, Paltauf felt that intratracheal thyroid resulted from the direct ingrowth of mature thyroid through tracheal and laryngeal cartilages.[37]

Laryngotracheal thyroid has been described in newborns and adults. Females are more commonly affected with a gender ratio of 3:1. Most reported adult cases occur in the third to fifth decades of life, with many patients residing in zones of endemic goiter. This would seem to account for the higher number of reported cases within the European literature.[38]

Patients with small airway lesions may be asymptomatic. This is supported by reports of such lesions found incidentally at autopsy. Symptoms of dyspnea and airway obstruction may evolve as the mass enlarges often in association with thyroid goiter. Life-threatening airway obstruction with associated stridor has been reported in newborns.

Laryngotracheal ectopic thyroid tissue most often presents in the lateral subglottis and proximal trachea. Lesions have, however, been reported in various sites ranging from the glottis to the carina. Typically, lesions are smooth, broad-based and submucosal with a reddish brown color. Multiple nodules, ulceration and hemorrhage are unusual and should arouse suspicion of carcinoma.[39] Malignant thyroid tissue within the larynx or trachea most commonly occurs by direct invasion of thyroid carcinoma. Although rare, malignant transformation of laryngotracheal ectopic thyroid has been reported with two described cases.[40,41]

Definitive diagnosis is made by endoscopy and biopsy. CT scan and MRI can be helpful in delineating the extent of the lesion. A thyroid scan may be helpful in the diagnosis; however, uptake in the thyroid gland itself will often obscure laryngotracheal uptake.

The management of intra-laryngotracheal thyroid has not been definitively established. Thyroxin suppression has not been shown to be reliably effective, especially in adults. Consensus opinion is that treatment is primarily surgical. Midline laryngotracheal fissure with submucosal resection is advocated for benign disease. For malignant lesions a more aggressive approach with wide surgical resection including laryngectomy, tracheal resection and reconstruction would seem appropriate. A more conservative surgical approach might include debulking, total thyroidectomy, neck dissection with postoperative radiation and radio-iodine ablation.

## Intraesophageal Thyroid

Only three cases of intraesophageal thyroid ectopia have been reported.[42–44] All involved the cervical esophagus. Ectopic thyroid was incidentally discovered

in two asymptomatic patients and upon evaluating the third patient for odynophagia. Thyroid tissue was apparent intraluminally on esophagoscopy in all cases. Two lesions were removed endoscopically and the other by an open cervical approach.

## Intracardiac Thyroid

Ectopic intracardiac thyroid is a rarity with fewer than 10 cases reported worldwide. The most plausible explanation lies in the close proximity of the thyroid primordium and the heart in early embryologic development. Most all reported intracardiac thyroid tissue has involved the right ventricular outflow tract. It has been postulated that during embryologic development the thyroid primordium uniformly contacts the same side of the primitive heart, the bulbous cordis. The distal part of the bulbous cordis (infundibulum) gives rise to the right ventricular outflow tract. Prolonged contact may allow some thyroid cells to become trapped in the infundibulum.[45–47]

The possibility that intracardiac thyroid tissue represents a solitary metastasis from a well-differentiated carcinoma of the thyroid or as part of a teratoma should be considered. Macroscopic and microscopic examination of the thyroid gland and intracardiac tumor at autopsy in some reported cases confirm the true existence of this lesion. Patients typically present with ventricular tachycardia and signs of right ventricular outflow obstruction. Many patients have been treated successfully with surgery.

## Subdiaphragmatic Thyroid

Thyroid tissue differentiation can occur in the presence of an ovarian teratoma, and represents the most common presentation of thyroid tissue below the diaphragm. Ovarian teratoma, in which 50% of the tissue component is thyroid, is termed struma ovarii. This is not true ectopia and is not embryologically related to the developing thyroid gland. Thyroid neoplasms associated with struma ovarii are rare but do occur; the most common type occurring in this situation is papillary.

Reported presentations of intra-abdominal thyroid tissue include the vaginal wall,[48] duodenum,[49] pancreas,[50] and porta hepatis.[51,52]

The significance of thyroid tissue below the diaphragm is controversial. It is difficult to reconcile subdiaphragmatic thyroid ectopia with thyroid gland embryology. Despite some arguments to the contrary, metastasis from an occult malignancy of the thyroid gland, or struma ovarii, would seem the more plausible explanation.

# References

1. Topf P, Fried MP, Strome M. Vagaries of thyroglossal duct cysts. *Laryngoscope.* 1988;98:740–742.
2. Larovere MJ, Drake AF, Baker SR, Richter HJ, Magielski JE. Evaluation and management of a carcinoma arising in a thyroglossal duct cyst. *Am J Otolaryngol.* 1987;8:351–355.
3. Davies J. *Embryology of the Head and Neck in Relation to the Practice of Otolaryngology.* Rochester, Minn.: American Academy of Ophthalmology and Otolaryngology; 1957.
4. Allard RHB. The thyroglossal cyst. *Head Neck Surg.* 1982;5:134–146.
5. Montgomery WW. *Surgery of the Upper Respiratory System.* Philadelphia: Lea & Febiger; 1973.
6. Ellis TDM, Van Nostrand AWT. The applied anatomy of thyroglossal tract remnants. *Laryngoscope.* 1977;87:765.
7. Batsakis JG. *Tumors of the Head and Neck: Clinical and Pathological Considerations.* Baltimore. Williams & Wilkins Co.; 1974.
8. Sistrunk WE. The surgical treatment of cysts of the thyroglossal tract. *Ann Surg.* 1920;71:121.
9. Weiss SD, Orlich CC. Primary papillary carcinoma of a thyroglossal duct cyst: report of a case and literature review. *Br J Surg.* 1991;78:87–89.
10. Colloby P, Sinha M, Holl-Allen R, Crocker J. Squamous cell carcinoma in a thyroglossal cyst remnant: a case report and review of the literature. *World J Surg.* 1989;13:137–139.
11. Ashurst AP, White C. Carcinoma in an aberrant thyroid at the base of the tongue. *JAMA.* 1925;85:1219.
12. Owen HR, Ingelby H. Carcinoma of the thyroglossal duct. *Ann Surg.* 1927;85:132–136.
13. Boswell WC, Zoller M, Williams JS, Lord SA, Check W. Thyroglossal duct carcinoma. *Ann Surg.* 1994;60:650–655.
14. Fernandez JF, Ordonez NG, Schultz PN, Samaan NA, Hickey RC. Thyroglossal duct carcinoma. *Surgery.* 1991;110:928–935.
15. Trail ML, Zeringue GP, Chicola JP. Carcinoma in thyroglossal duct remnants. *Laryngoscope.* 1997;87:1685–1691.
16. Joseph TI, Komorowski RA. Thyroglossal duct carcinoma. *Hum Pathol.* 1975;6:717–729.
17. LiVolsi VA, Perzin KH, Savetsky L. Carcinoma arising in median ectopic thyroid (including thyroglossal duct tissue). *Cancer.* 1974;34:1303–1315.
18. Crile G Jr. Papillary carcinoma of the thyroid and lateral cervical region: so-called "lateral aberrant thyroid." *Surg Gynecol Obstet.* 1947;85:757–766.
19. Nuttall FQ. Cystic metastasis from papillary adenocarcinoma of the thyroid with comments concerning carcinoma associated with thyroglossal remnants. *Am J Surg.* 1965;109:500–505.
20. Kristensen S, Turel A, Moesner J. Thyroglossal cyst carcinoma. *J Laryngol Otol.* 1984;98:1277–1280.
21. Kennedy TL, Whitaker M, Wadih G. Thyroglossal duct carcinoma: a rational approach to management. *Laryngoscope.* 1998;108:1154–1158.
22. Nienas FW, Colum AG, Devine KD, et. al., Lingual thyroid. *Ann Intern Med.* 1973;79:205–210.
23. Nienas FW, Gorman CA, Devine KD, Woolner LB. Lingual thyroid. Clinical characteristics of 15 cases. *Ann Intern Med.* 1973;79:205–210.
24. Noyek AM, Friedberg J. Thyroglossal duct and ectopic thyroid disorders. *Otolaryngol Clin North Am.* 1981;14:187–201.
25. Kaplan M, Kauli R, Lubin E, Grunebaum M, Laron Z. Ectopic thyroid gland. A clinical study of 30 children and review. *J Pediatr.* 1978;92:205–209.
26. Wertz ML. Management of undescended lingual and subhyoid thyroid glands. *Laryngoscope.* 1974;84:507–521.
27. Williams JD, Slupchinski JO, Sclafani AP, Douge C. Evaluation and management of a lingual thyroid gland. *Ann Otolaryngol Rhinol Laryngol.* 1996;105:312–316.
28. Wislow CP, Weisberger EC. Lingual thyroid and neoplastic change: a review of the literature and description of a case. *Otolaryngol Head Neck Surg.* 1997;117:100–102.
29. Steinwald OP, Muehrcke RC, Economou SG. Surgical correction of complete lingual ectopia of the thyroid glands. *Surg Clin North Am.* 1970;50:1177–1186.
30. Aadiaz-Arias AA, Bickel JT, Loy TS, Croll GH, Puckett EL, Havey AD. Follicular carcinoma with clear cell changes arising in lingual thyroid. *Oral Surg Oral Med Oral Pathol.* 1992;74:206–211.
31. Damiano A, Glickman AB, Reuben JS. Ectopic thyroid tissue presenting as a midline neck mass. *Int J Ped Otorhinolaryngol.* 1996;34:141–148.
32. Pinczowler E, Crockett DM, Atkinson JV, Kun S. Preoperative thyroid scanning and presumed thyroglossal duct cyst. *Arch Otolaryngol Head Neck Surg.* 1992;118:985–988.
33. LiVolsi VA. *Surgical pathology of the thyroid.* Philadelphia, PA: WB Saunders; 1990:8–10.
34. Williams ED, Toyn CE, Harach HR. The otobrachial gland and congenital thyroid abnormalities in man. *J Pathol.* 1989;159:135–141.
35. Chen KTK. Minute (less than 1 mm) occult primary thyroid carcinoma with metastatsis. *Am J Clin Pathol.* 1989;91:746.
36. Batsakis JG, El-Naggar AK, Luna MA. Pathology consultation thyroid gland ectopias. *Ann Otolaryngol Rhinology, Laryngol.* 1996;105;996–1000.
37. Chanin LR, Greenberg LM. Pediatric upper airway obstruction due to ectopic thyroid: classification and case reports. *Laryngoscope.* 1988;98:422–427.
38. Myers EN, Pantangco IP. Intratracheal thyroid. *Laryngoscope.* 1975;85:1833–1839.
39. Donegan JO, Wood MD. Intratracheal thyroid/familial occurrence. *Laryngoscope.* 1985;95:6–8.
40. Fish J, Moore R. Ectopic thyroid tissue and ectopic thyroid carcinoma. Review of the literature and report of a case. *Ann Surg.* 1963;157:212–221.
41. See ACH, Patel SG, Montgomery PQ. Intralaryngotracheal thyroid, ectopic thyroid or invasive carcinoma? *J Laryngol Otol.* 1998;112:673–676.
42. Whale HL. Oesophageal tumour of thyroid tissue. *Br Med J.* 1921;2:987.
43. Porto G. Esophageal nodule of thyroid tissue. *Laryngoscope.* 1960;70:1336
44. Postlethwait RW, Detmer DE. Ectopic thyroid nodule in the esophagus. *Ann Thorac Surg.* 1975;19:98–100.
45. Pollice L, Caruso G. Strumacordis: ectopic thyroid goiter in the right ventricle. *Arch Pathol Lab Med.* 1986;110:452–453.
46. Porqueddu M, Antona C, Polvani G, et al. Ectopic thyroid tissue and the ventricular outflow tract: embryologic implications. *Cardiology.* 1995;86:524–526.
47. Richmond I, Whittaker JS. Intracardiac ectopic thyroid: a case report and review of published cases. *Thorax.* 1990;45:293–294.
48. Kurman RJ, Prabha AC. Thyroid and parathyroid glands in the vaginal wall. *Am J Clin Pathol.* 1973;59:503–507.
49. Takahashi T, Ishikura H, Kato H, Tanabe T, Yoshiki T. Ectopic thyroid follicles in the submucosa of the duodenum. *Virchows Arch Pathol Anat.* 1991;418:547–550.
50. Seelig MH, Schönleben K. Intra-abdominal ectopic thyroid presenting as a pancreatic tumor. *Eur J Surg.* 1997;163:549–551.
51. Schubert W. Uber iene akzessorische Schilddrüse an der Leberpforte. *Zentralbl Allg Pathol.* 1957;96:339–341.
52. Strohschneider T, Timm D, Worbes C. Ektopes Schilddrüsengewewe an der Leberpforte. *Chirug.* 1993;64:751–753.

# 28

# Embryology and Anatomy of the Parathyroid Glands

John T. Hansen, Ph.D.

## EMBRYOLOGY

An understanding of the embryology of the parathyroid gland requires an appreciation for the development of the pharyngeal pouches. Development of the branchial arch and pharyngeal pouch system in the human begins around the fourth week of embryonic development. The branchial arch apparatus consists of: a) branchial arches; b) pharyngeal pouches; c) branchial grooves; and d) branchial membranes.[1]

The parathyroid glands develop directly from the endodermally lined pharyngeal pouch system (Figure 30–1). Paired inferior parathyroid glands develop from the third pair of pharyngeal pouches in concert with the thymus anlage. While thymic development begins near the end of the fourth week, the inferior parathyroids do not form until early in the fifth week. Together, the inferior parathyroid glands and thymus then migrate inferiorly during elongation and differential growth of the neck region. Normally, the inferior parathyroid glands separate from the migrating thymus and pass medially to assume their adult position posteriorly and inferiorly on lateral lobes of the thyroid gland. Superior parathyroid glands actually develop somewhat inferior to the inferior parathyroids as derivatives of the fourth pair of pharyngeal pouches (Figure 28–1). However, the superior parathyroid glands usually migrate only a short distance inferiorly and then become attached to the thyroid diverticulum as it migrates caudally, anterior to the trachea. Superior parathyroid glands come to rest posteriorly and superiorly behind the lateral lobes of the thyroid gland. Because the migratory route of the inferior parathyroid glands is longer and their migration is

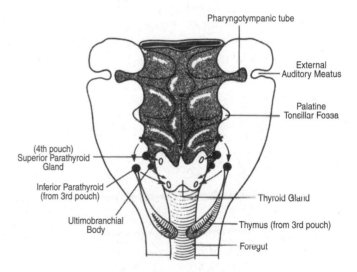

**Figure 28–1.** Schematic illustration of the pharyngeal pouch derivatives, showing the migration of the thyroid, parathyroid and thymus glands. When the thyroid descends from the foramen cecum, the parathyroid glands attach themselves to the passing thyroid. This is a ventral view with the lung bud and future trachea removed. (Reproduced, with permission, from Falk, SA ed., *Thyroid Disease*, Lippincott Williams & Wilkins, 1997.)

associated with that of the thymus gland, the inferior parathyroid glands often are found anywhere along the normal migratory route of the thymus gland, and may even follow the thymus into the superior mediastinum.

Because of their variable location, about 61% of the inferior parathyroid glands are located either inferior, lateral or posterior to the lower pole of the thyroid gland.[2]

Commonly, inferior parathyroids are found in the thyrothymic ligament, a fibrous band of connective tissue that connects the lower thyroid pole and the upper thymic horn.[3] In approximately 26% of cases, parathyroids also are found in the cervical portion of the thymus gland. In anywhere from 2–4% of cases, the inferior parathyroids are located further caudally, associated with the thymus gland where it resides in the superior mediastinum. While a number of studies describe the variable number and anatomic locations of parathyroid tissue, these reports may be suspect because they are garnered from cadaveric material and parathyroids are difficult to discern grossly in fixed material.[4]

In light of the variable positions of the parathyroid glands, especially the inferior pair, their location with respect to the thyroid capsule is important. Generally speaking, the superior parathyroids lie within the prevertebral fascia covering the posterior aspect of the thyroid gland or in the true capsule of the gland itself. The inferior parathyroid glands, on the other hand, either lie below the inferior thyroid artery where this artery lies on the posterior surface of the thyroid gland, or they lie above the inferior thyroid artery (Figure 28–2). Rarely, the inferior parathyroids may be embedded within the thyroid gland itself.[5]

## HISTOLOGY

The parathyroid glands are enveloped in their own thin collagenous connective tissue capsule. This capsule extends septa into the gland which separates the parenchyma into elongated cords or clusters of functional secretory cells. Blood vessels, lymphatics and nerves travel along the septa to reach the interior of the gland.[6]

The major functional parenchymal cells of the parathyroid glands are the slightly eosinophilic-staining chief cells, which measure from 5–8 μm in diameter (Figure 28–3). Chief cells contain numerous small cytoplasmic granules (200–400 nm in diameter) which arise from the Golgi complex and represent the secretory granules.[6] These granules contain parathyroid hormone (PTH), which is synthesized from a precursor of pre-proparathyroid hormone. With increasing age, the secretory cells of the parathyroid glands may be replaced by adipose cells, which can comprise 50–60% of the gland in elderly persons.

The second cell type in the parathyroid gland is the oxyphil cell (Figure 28–3). Although their function is unknown, it is believed that oxyphil cells and a third cell type, sometimes described as intermediate cells, may represent inactive phases of a single cell type.[7]

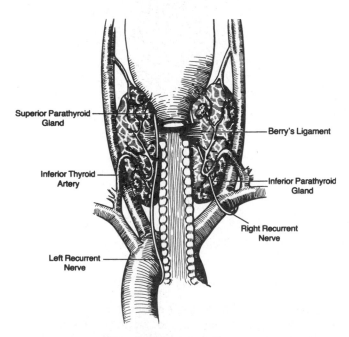

**Figure 28–2.** Posterior aspect of the thyroid gland. Note the blood supply to the gland, the location of the parathyroid glands, and the course of the recurrent laryngeal nerves. (Reproduced, with permission, from Falk, SA ed., *Thyroid Disease*, Lippincott Williams & Wilkins, 1997.)

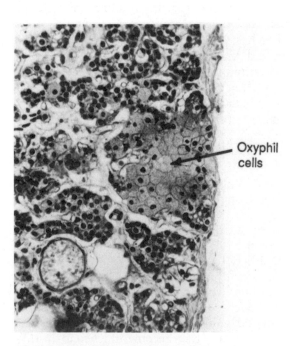

**Figure 28–3.** Histological section of the parathyroid gland. Note the group of large oxyphil cells, and the more numerous and smaller chief cells. (Reproduced, with permission, from Junqueira et al., 1998. *Basic Histology*, Appleton & Lange, and with the permission of The McGraw-Hill Companies.)

However, the chief cells are the actively secreting cell type of the parathyroid gland. Oxyphil cells are less numerous, somewhat larger (6–10 μm in diameter), and stain more deeply with eosin than chief cells.

The PTH produced by the chief cells of the parathyroid glands maintains the proper extracellular fluid concentration of calcium ions. This hormone acts on the cells of bones, kidneys, and indirectly on the intestinal tract, to increase the calcium ion concentration in the body fluids.[6,8] When calcium ion concentration in body fluids falls below normal, the chief cells increase their production and release of PTH quickly. PTH increases both the number and the activity of osteoclasts, and this promotes the resorption of bone matrix and the release of calcium into the blood stream. An increase in plasma calcium levels suppresses PTH secretion. Calcitonin, secreted by the parafollicular cells of the thyroid gland (see Chapter 2), inhibits osteoclast activity and inhibits matrix resorption. The interplay of PTH and calcitonin represents a dual mechanism for regulating calcium levels in the blood. PTH acts to increase calcium levels in the serum while calcitonin has the opposite effect. PTH binds to receptors on the osteoclasts and this signals the cells to increase their secretion of osteoclast stimulating factor. This factor activitates osteoclasts, increasing bone matrix resorption and results in the release of calcium and phosphate into the blood. Additionally, in the kidneys, PTH prevents the loss of calcium in the urine. Finally, PTH controls the rate of calcium uptake in the gastrointestinal tract by indirectly regulating the production of vitamin D in the kidneys, which is necessary for intestinal absorption of calcium.

Phosphate metabolism is closely related to calcium balance and also is critical to many intracellular functions.[8] Phosphate is absorbed with calcium in the gastrointestinal tract and is released from bone during active resorption. The primary route of phosphate excretion is via the kidney and its rate of excretion is dependent upon glomerular filtration and PTH levels.

## ANATOMY

Typically, humans possess two pairs of parathyroid glands, a superior pair and an inferior pair. However, a surgical study of 503 autopsy cases demonstrates that four parathyroid glands are found in only 84% of the cases.[9] More than four glands were found in 13% of the cases and only three parathyroids were identified in 3% of the cases. In the 13% in which more than four glands were found, most were either rudimentary or divided (two split glands lying close to one another). Of the 64 cases that documented more than four glands, 18 cases had five glands, 3 had six, 1 had seven, 1 had eight, and 1 had 11 parathyroid glands.

Anatomically, the superior parathyroid glands are most consistent in location and, this, as described above, is caused by their embryology. About 80% lie within a circumscribed circle of approximately two centimeters in diameter, one centimeter cranial to the intersection of the recurrent laryngeal nerve and the inferior thyroid artery (Figure 28–2).[2] Superior parathyroid glands often lie within the fascial covering of the thyroid gland and are freely movable upon the capsule. Occasionally, a parathyroid lies within the thyroid capsule itself. Alternatively, the inferior parathyroid glands, also because of their embryologic migration with the thymus anlage, are much more variable in their anatomic location. They may be found in the thymus itself, in the superior mediastinum, along the lower pharynx and upper esophagus, or scattered along the trachea just inferior to the thyroid gland.[2,10]

## Blood Supply

The parathyroid glands receive their blood supply from the thyroid arteries, most frequently the inferior thyroid artery. Nevertheless, ligation of the inferior thyroid artery may not always compromise the blood supply to the gland.[4] This may be because of the abundant arterial anastomoses that exist between the parathyroids, and include anastomoses with the thyroid arteries, and with the arteries of the larynx, pharynx, esophagus and trachea. Some surgeons suggest that once the parathyroid gland is identified, the blood supply probably already has been compromised. Therefore, many surgeons prefer dissecting the parathyroids with an attached vascular pedicle to retain a blood supply.[11]

The venous drainage of the glands is via the thyroid veins. Lymphatics from the parathyroids drain with those of the thyroid gland, with lymph ultimately collecting in the deep cervical chain of lymph nodes.

## Relationship to the Recurrent Laryngeal Nerve

The relationship of the parathyroid glands to the recurrent (inferior) laryngeal nerves is of primary importance in the anatomy of this region and is discussed more thoroughly in the chapter on the Embryology and Anatomy of the Thyroid Glands (Chapter 2). Because the relationship of the recurrent laryngeal nerves and the inferior thyroid arteries is variable and it is the inferior thyroid artery that represents the major blood supply to the parathyroid glands, it is important that a surgeon carefully dissect this region and note the relationship of these nerves to the parathyroid glands (Figure 28–2).

# References

1. Carlson BM. *Human Embryology and Developmental Biology*. 2nd ed. St. Louis: Mosby; 1999.

2. Akerstrom G, Malmaeus J, Bergstrom R. Surgical anatomy of human parathyroid glands. *Surgery*. 1984; 95: 14–21.

3. Ashley SW, Wells SA. Parathyroid glands. In: Greenfield LJ, Mulholland MW, Oldham KT, Zelenock GB, eds. *Surgery: Scientific Principles and Practice*. Philadelphia: JB Lippincott; 1993: 1187–1209.

4. Hollinshead WH. *Anatomy for Surgeons, Vol 1. The Head and Neck*. 2nd ed. New York: Harper & Row; 1968.

5. Walton AJ. The surgical treatment of parathyroid tumors. *Br J Surg*. 1931; 19: 285–291.

6. Junqueira LC, Carneiro J, Kelly RO. *Basic Histology*. 9th ed. Stamford, CT: Appleton & Lange; 1998.

7. Gartner LP, Haitt JL. *Histology*. Philadelphia: WB Saunders Co; 1997.

8. Rockwell JC, Baran DT. Parathyroid function and calcium homeostasis. In: Falk SA, ed. *Thyroid Disease: Endocrinology, Surgery, Nuclear Medicine, and Radiotherapy*, 2nd ed. Philadelphia: Lippincott-Raven; 1997.

9. Brennan MF, Doppman JL, Marz SJ, Spiegel AM, Brown EM, Aurbach GD. Reoperative parathyroid surgery for persistent hyperparathyroidism. *Surgery*. 1978; 83: 669-676.

10. Kaplan EL. Thyroid and parathyroid. In: Schwartz SI, ed. *Principles of Surgery*. *Vol 2*. New York: McGraw-Hill; 1989: 1613–1685.

11. Hansen JT. Embryology and surgical anatomy of the lower neck and superior mediastinum. In: Falk SA, ed. *Thyroid Disease: Endocrinology, Surgery, Nuclear Medicine, and Radiotherapy*. 2nd ed. Philadelphia: Lippincott-Raven; 1997.

# 29

# Parathyroid Gland Pathology

## Zubair W. Baloch, M.D., Ph.D. and Virginia A. LiVolsi, M.D.

## INTRODUCTION

Sir Richard Owens first described the parathyroid glands in an Indian Rhinoceros in 1852.[1] Ivar Sandström first published the details about the anatomy and histology of the parathyroid in 1880;[2] however, their significance was not appreciated until Gley showed that their excision led to tetany in rats.[3] Felix Mandl in 1925 demonstrated the first surgical excision of parathyroid from a patient who suffered from a severe bone disease.[4]

Virtually all surgical specimens of parathyroid glands are obtained from patients with hyperparathyroidism; however, a minority of these may be removed in the course of neck exploration for thyroid or laryngeal disease. Almost 12% of patients undergoing thyroid resection have one or more parathyroid glands resected inadvertently. This is usually because of the problems associated with the anatomic location of the glands.

In this chapter a brief review of the embryological development, their anatomy and normal histology is provided. The remainder of the chapter will depict the various pathological conditions affecting parathyroid glands.

## EMBRYOLOGY

The parathyroid glands are endodermal in origin and develop from third and fourth branchial pouches. The superior pair originates from the fourth pouch and descends along with thyroid anlage. These parathyroids are most commonly found close to the posterior and middle of the thyroid. The inferior parathyroids arise from the third branchial pouch along with thymus and come to rest at the inferior poles of thyroid or in the band of fibrous tissue known as thyrothymic ligament.[5,6] Abnormalities in the descent of the parathyroids can cause the glands to reside anywhere along their embryologic pathway from the upper portions of the neck to upper thoracic inlet.[7] Recent embryologic studies have shown that the ablation of the ventral half of the third branchial arch leads to loss of the inferior parathyroid glands.[8] Other investigators have shown that *Hoxa 3* mutant homozygotes exhibit defects in development and migration pathways of thymus, thyroid and parathyroid glands;[9] however, the actual molecular events and importance of this gene in humans still needs to be investigated.

## NUMERICAL AND LOCATION VARIABILITY

Over 80% of normal individuals have at least four parathyroid glands.[10–14] Autopsy studies have shown that from one to twelve glands can be present.[11] The most frequent deviations from normal include three glands (approximately 1 to 7% of cases) and five glands (3 to 6% of studied individuals).[15–16]

The location variability is more commonly encountered in the inferior parathyroids, whereas, the superior parathyroids are situated symmetrically in the neck in about 80% of the individuals.[10–14] The superior parathyroids are often found adjacent to the posterior edge of the thyroid gland close to or in some instances within the thyroid capsule; when ectopically located, the superior parathyroids are found in the posterior neck, retropharyngeal-esophageal space, carotid sheath, and posterior mediastinum.[5,6,10-11,14]

The lower parathyroids are usually located around the lower pole of thyroid; however, they may also be found posterior to the thyroid, in the para-tracheal area, or close to or within the thymus in the thoracic inlet. In some instances the inferior parathyroids may be truly intra-thyroidal.[10-12]

## NORMAL PARATHYROID GLANDS

The parathyroid glands measure between 2 to 7 mm in length, 2 to 4 mm in width, and 0.5 to 2 mm in thickness.[10-11,15-16] They are kidney-shaped, soft and light yellow brown in color. A more yellowish tinge is indicative of higher fat content.[15-16] The color also varies with degree of vascular congestion and amount of oxyphil cells.[16]

The weight of an individual parathyroid gland can range from a few milligrams to more than 70 mg (averages of around 35 to 55 mg) and is highly dependent upon sex, race, and nutritional status of the individual.[17] The combined weight of all the parathyroids in normal adult males ranges around 120 mg and in females around 145 mg.[10-11,15-16]

## Histology

By light microscopy each parathyroid gland is encased by a thin fibrous capsule that extends into parenchyma as thin fibrous septae leading to lobule formation. The glands consist of parenchymal cells, fat cells and fibrovascular stroma (Figure 29–1). The parenchymal cells of the parathyroid are usually of chief cell type, which are identified by their polygonal shape, slightly eosinophilic, or amphophilic cytoplasm and small round nucleus.[10,15-16,17-20] The other population of cells, known as oxyphil cells, exhibit dense eosinophilic cytoplasm and small nuclei. The cells with features intermediate between chief cells and oxyphil cells are termed as transitional oxyphil cells.[15-16,18] In younger individuals, the number of oxyphil and transitional oxyphil cells is small; however, their number increases with age and in certain pathological conditions described later in this chapter. The parenchymal cells are usually arranged in nests and cords, nourished by a rich capillary network.[16]

Early studies reported that the normal acceptable ratio of parathyroid cells to fat cells is 50:50. However, recent autopsy based studies have shown that stromal fat content is significantly lower than 50% in most cases.[17-20] In an adult normal parathyroid, approximately 17% of the cells are adipocytes. The number of fat cells also varies with the age and the body composition: thus, the obese individual often shows higher fat content as compared to lean or cachetic individuals where the glands will show near or total absence of fat cells.[17-20]

By electron microscopy, chief cells show Golgi apparatus, dispersed granular endoplasmic reticulum and few secretory granules. The resting chief cells contain abundant lipid and glycogen, whereas, during active phase the chief cells are smaller in size and contain decreased amount of glycogen and lipid.[21] The oxyphilic cells are characterized by their large size and numerous cytoplasmic mitochondria.[21]

## PATHOLOGY OF PARATHYROID

The pathological evaluation of the parathyroids is a necessary diagnostic step in the evaluation of hypercalcemia. Primary hyperparathyroidism and malignancy account for up to 90% of cases of hypercalcemia. The presence of hypercalcemia for more than a year in an asymptomatic individual usually suggests primary hyperparathyroidism. The patients with malignancy show evidence of tumor with metastases; however, in some, the tumors may be too small to be detected on routine clinical evaluation.[15-16,22]

## Hyperparathyroidism

Hyperparathyroidism is characterized by increased production of parathyroid hormone; serum calcium maybe low, normal or high depending upon other factor such as renal function.[23] Primary hyperparathyroidism is defined as the disease, which is caused by inappropriate secretion of the parathyroid hormone from

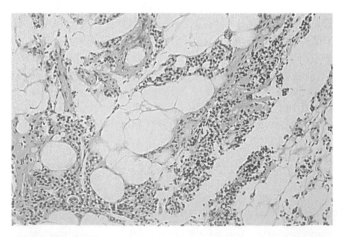

**Figure 29–1.** Normal adult parathyroid showing collection of parenchymal cells intermixed with fat cells.

enlarged parathyroid glands leading to hypercalcemia. Serum calcium ranges from 11 to 18 mg/dl, with most asymptomatic patients found in the lower end of the spectrum.[16,22-23]

Secondary hyperparathyroidism is an increase in parathyroid hormone most commonly in response to hypocalcemia or hyperphosphatemia associated with renal failure. Tertiary hyperparathyroidism refers to autonomous parathyroid hyperfunction in patients with secondary hyperparathyroidism.[15-16]

## Primary Hyperparathyroidism

Primary hyperparathyroidism is a frequently encountered disorder of the parathyroid gland; it is seen in all age groups, although it is rare in children. The prevalence of this disorder in the United States is estimated to be 1–5 cases per 1,000 adults. To date there is no known cause for this disease.[22] In some cases, a history of head and neck irradiation can be elicited.[24-25] Prinz et al documented a history of irradiation in 67% patients with combined thyroid and parathyroid tumors.[25]

In some patients, genetics may play a role. Mutations of MEN-1 gene have been reported in both sporadic and familial parathyroid tumors not related to MEN syndromes.[26-32]

The pathologic lesions responsible for primary hyperparathyroidism include adenoma, hyperplasia, and rarely, carcinoma.

## Parathyroid Adenoma

The parathyroid adenoma is the single most common cause of hyperparathyroidism. However, because of variation in the pathologic interpretation and patient population, the incidence of parathyroid adenoma is reported between 30 to 90%.[15-16,32-36] In larger series of patients, where more generally accepted pathologic criteria were followed, about 80 to 85% of patients with primary hyperparathyroidism were found to have solitary parathyroid adenoma.[16,32-36]

Earlier studies using the isoenzymes of glucose-6-phosphatase dehydrogenase suggested a polyclonal origin for parathyroid adenomas.[37-38] Recent studies have demonstrated that adenomas are clonal proliferations.[32,39-43] Shan et al detected clonality in glands affected by primary hyperparathyroidism by PCR amplification of PGK-1 gene and concluded that clonality was consistent with the diagnosis of parathyroid adenoma.[41-42] Other investigators have reported similar results.[40,43]

Parathyroid adenoma can occur in any of the four parathyroid glands, but it tends to affect lower glands

more commonly than the upper glands. About 10% of the adenomas are found at ectopic sites, including the mediastinum, thyroid, esophagus and within the retroesophageal tissue. They are more common in females with a ratio of about 3 to 1.[16,34-36]

Grossly, the adenomas are oval or bean shaped, red-brown in color and are soft in consistency.[15-16,34,36,44] Sometimes the adenomas are bilobed or multilobated, which may account for instances of incomplete excision.[16] The adenomas usually replace the entire parathyroid gland with a grossly visible yellow-brown rim of residual parathyroid (Figure 29–2A). Some authors have stressed this remaining normal parathyroid rim as one of the criteria for the diagnosis of adenoma. However, this is observed only in 50 to 60% of cases and its absence does not exclude the presence of a parathyroid adenoma.[16] The cut surface of the adenoma may appear smooth, nodular or can show easily discernible areas of cystic degeneration. The weight of parathyroid adenoma is variable and can range from 300 mg to several grams; similarly the size can vary from less than 1 to over 3 cm.[15-16,33-34,36] Some studies have reported a correlation between the weight of the parathyroid adenoma, serum calcium, and severity of bone disease.[15]

By light microscopy, adenomas are usually surrounded by a thin delicate fibrous capsule. The cells are usually arranged in nests and cords invested by a rich capillary network (Figure 29–2B). The other growth patterns seen in adenomas include follicular (Figure 29–2C), pseudopapillary and acinar. Chief cells are the dominant cell types in the majority of parathyroid adenomas. Oxyphil cells and transitional oxyphil cells are usually seen in varying proportions interspersed between the collections of chief cells.[15-16,34,36,44] The chief cells in adenomas can be larger than their normal counterparts and can also exhibit nuclear pleomorphism

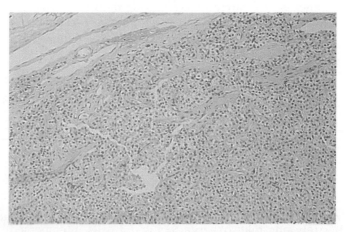

**Figure 29–2A.** Parathyroid adenoma with a thin fibrous capsule and a rim of compressed normal parathyroid containing fat cells.

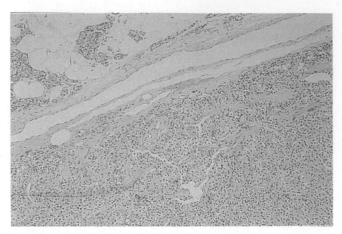

**Figure 29–2B.** Parathyroid adenoma: trabecular and cord like growth pattern.

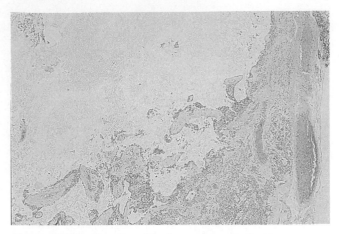

**Figure 29–2D.** Parathyroid adenoma: cystic change.

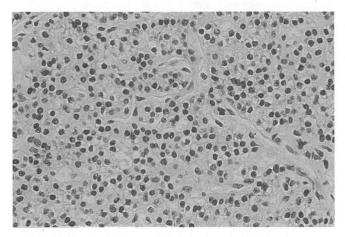

**Figure 29–2C.** Parathyroid adenoma: follicular growth pattern.

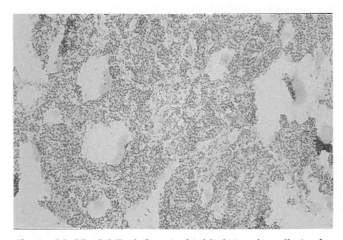

**Figure 29–2E.** Oil Red O stain highlighting fat cells in the compressed rim of normal parathyroid.

and giant cell formation.[45-46] However, nuclear atypia is of limited value in distinguishing between parathyroid adenoma and carcinoma.[16] Mitotic figures are uncommon in adenomas; however, they can be seen in a small percentage of cases.[47] Some authors have suggested that presence of mitoses is indicative of malignancy in parathyroid adenoma,[48] however, this idea is still debatable and needs further examination.

Cystic changes are common in parathyroid adenoma and can appear as large areas of cyst formation filled with PAS positive material (Figure 29–2D). Larger tumors may undergo degenerative changes which may be prominent, including: fibrosis, hemorrhage, cholesterol clefts, hemosiderin and calcification.[15-16,34] Some tumors may rarely show collections of lymphocytes.[49]

Fat cells are virtually absent within adenomas. Rarely one may observe foci of fat cells interspersed within an adenoma, which may cause some parts of the tumor to appear as normal parathyroid.[15-16,34,36] The

normal rim of the compressed parathyroid usually shows normal to increased fat content.[16]

Some adenomas are composed exclusively of oxyphil cells, "oxyphil adenomas." These tumors tend to be larger than the chief cell adenomas and the serum calcium tends to be minimally elevated.[50-55]

Parathyroid adenoma is a single gland disease; however, double adenomas have been reported.[56-58] This concept is still a subject of controversy.[58-61] Most patients who have been diagnosed with double adenoma will, over a period of time, return with recurrent hyperparathyroidism and four-gland hyperplasia.[58-61] The proposed criteria for this diagnosis include presence of two enlarged hypercellular glands each weighing more than 70 mg and the identification and preservation of two other normal sized parathyroids.[61] Using these criteria, Verdon and Edis reported double adenomas in 1.9% of their cases with primary hyperparathyroidism.[61] In our view, if double adenomas do exist they are extremely rare and this diagnosis should be entertained with caution.

## Parathyroid Hyperplasia

Primary parathyroid hyperplasia is defined as proliferation of the parenchymal cells leading to increase in gland weight in multiple parathyroid glands in the absence of a known stimulus for parathyroid hormone secretion.[15-16,36]

Two types of parathyroid hyperplasia are seen: the more common chief cell hyperplasia and the rare water cell or clear cell hyperplasia.[15-16]

### Chief Cell Hyperplasia

In 1958 Cope et al first demonstrated chief cell hyperplasia as a cause of primary hyperparathyroidism.[62] It accounts for 15% of hyperparathyroidism in most series; however, some reports have indicated that about half of primary hyperparathyroidism is produced by hyperplasia. These variable results point to discrepancies in pathologic interpretation. The stimulus for this disorder is unknown; however, some studies have indicated a role of a possible circulating factor that can induce proliferation of parathyroid cells in culture. About 30% of patients with chief cell hyperplasia have familial hyperparathyroidism or one of the syndromes of multiple endocrine neoplasia (MEN).[15-16,31,63-69] Molecular studies have demonstrated that hyperplasias are monoclonal proliferations. Hyperplasias associated with MEN I involve allelic deletions on chromosome 11, and such lesions are larger than those without deletions. Similar deletions have also been encountered in sporadic parathyroid adenomas.[28-32] These results suggest that the monoclonal proliferations may develop after a phase of polyclonal hyperplasia.

Grossly, there is enlargement of all four glands. The glands may be of the same or different size. The combined weight of all four glands can range from 150 mg to over 20 g, but usually is in the range of 1 to 3 g. The cut surface may appear homogeneous, nodular and can show cystic changes.[15-16]

By light microscopy, the dominant cell types are chief cells; however, one may also observe intermixed oxyphil cells and transitional oxyphil cells. The cells are usually arranged in a solid, trabecular or nodular pattern (Figure 29–3). The cellular proliferations may also give rise to nodule formation, and this can cause asymmetrical gland enlargement.[15,16]

The amount of cytoplasmic fat in the chief cells is either reduced or absent.[15-16] The chief cell in the nodular areas may be totally devoid of fat, whereas, the ones between the nodules may contain fat. Bizarre nuclei are rarely found in primary hyperplasia. Mitoses are rare.[16]

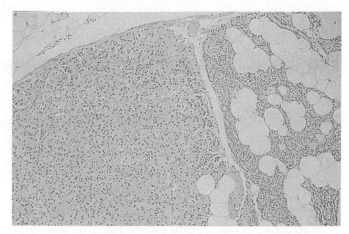

**Figure 29–3.** Nodular hyperplasia of the parathyroid. The periphery of the gland is compressed and gives rise to pseudo-rim formation. The other glands removed in this case displayed the similar histologic picture.

### Water-Clear Cell Hyperplasia

This rare condition is characterized by proliferation of vacuolated water-clear cells in multiple parathyroid glands. It shows a female predilection and leads to pronounced hypercalcemia and severe clinical disease. This is the only parathyroid disorder in which the superior glands are larger than the lower pair of glands. The affected glands tend to be larger and irregular in shape and the proliferating cells may extend into the surrounding tissue of the neck. By light microscopy, the glands are composed of diffuse proliferations of clear cells characterized by clear cytoplasm on scanning or low power magnification with small dense nuclei. However, on higher power magnification the cytoplasm is filled with small vacuoles. Some studies have shown that the amount of parathyroid hormone in clear cell hyperplasia is much lower than the normal glands or chief cell adenomas.[70-73]

## PARATHYROID CARCINOMA

Parathyroid carcinoma accounts for 0.5 to 2% of cases of primary hyperparathyroidism.[74-90] As compared to adenomas which are most commonly seen in females, parathyroid carcinoma does not show any sex predilection. Patients with parathyroid carcinoma tend to be younger than those with adenoma, and virtually always symptomatic, often with pronounced hypercalcemia, and/or with systemic manifestation related to elevated calcium, eg nephrolithiasis, renal failure and bone disease. Rarely parathyroid carcinoma can develop in the setting of familial endocrine disorders[91-95] or in cases of secondary parathyroid hyperplasia.[96-100] Many patients present with a palpable neck mass on initial examination, which may be mistaken for a primary thyroid neoplasm.[15-16,75-78]

Grossly, parathyroid carcinoma presents as an ill-defined large tumor (average weight 12 g) which is adherent to the surrounding soft tissues of neck, thyroid and peri-esophageal soft tissues.[15-16,75-78] This invasion into the surrounding soft tissues serves as an important surgical finding and may lead to an en bloc resection of the tumor mass with surrounding adherent structures.[15-16,78] However, some tumors can be encapsulated and grossly resemble parathyroid adenoma.[15-16] Parathyroid carcinoma is a single gland disease, and rarely has been reported to arise in ectopic locations.[15-16,75-77]

The microscopic diagnosis of parathyroid carcinoma is a difficult task. The entire gland is traversed by broad fibrous bands, which seem to originate from the capsule and extend into the substance of tumor leading to a lobulated appearance[15-16,75-77,101] (Figure 29–4A). The cells can be clear or rarely oxyphilic[102] and are arranged in nests and trabeculae. The cell may be uniformly bland or may demonstrate frank anaplasia (Figure 29–4B); the cases with minimal atypia may be difficult to distinguish from an adenoma.[15-16,75-76,101]

Mitoses can be seen in most cases; this feature has been suggested as of great importance in diagnosing parathyroid carcinoma.[47] However, mitotic figures can also be seen in parathyroid adenoma and hyperplasia and their absence does not rule out a diagnosis of carcinoma.[15-16,48,103] We believe, although not definite indicators of malignancy, mitoses in parathyroid lesion should be of concern since the follow-up in reported benign cases of parathyroid tumor with mitoses is limited. Increased mitotic activity in unequivocal carcinomas is an indicator of poor prognosis.[80]

Recent studies have shown that the only reliable indicator of malignancy in parathyroid carcinoma is invasion of the surrounding structures and metastases.[80] While other features such as desmoplastic reaction, mitotic activity, nuclear atypia and necrosis were more common in carcinoma than in benign lesions, none of these is diagnostic of malignancy.[80] Some authors have suggested that if some features of malignancy, including mitoses, are present without an infiltrative growth pattern or metastases, those cases should be designated as "atypical adenoma."[107] However, long-term follow-up studies are not available to assess the clinical relevance of this diagnostic term.

Rarely, non-functioning parathyroid carcinomas have been described. These lesions tend to be large and consist of clear or oxyphil cells.[55,104,105] Such tumors may be confused diagnostically with primary thyroid

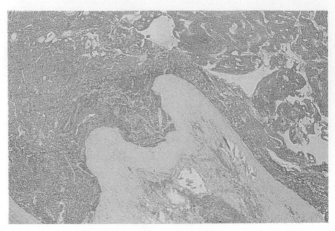

**Figure 29–4A.** Parathyroid carcinoma: the tumor shows dense area of fibrosis.

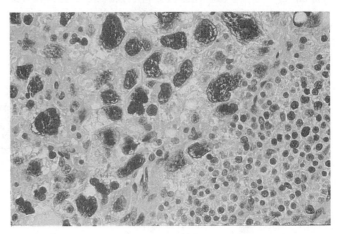

**Figure 29–4B.** Parathyroid carcinoma: marked cellular pleomorphism.

cancers, such as Hürthle cell lesions or medullary carcinoma. Proof of the parathyroid origin of such lesions includes positive immunohistochemical staining for parathyroid hormone, and negative reaction for thyroglobulin and calcitonin.[55,104,105]

Parathyroid carcinoma usually grows slowly and is an indolent tumor. Metastases can be seen in up to one-third of patients and are found in regional lymph nodes, bone, lung and liver. Multiple recurrences are common and can occur over a 15 to 20 year period.[15-16,75-78] Patients with parathyroid carcinoma often succumb to the effects of excessive parathyroid hormone secretion and uncontrolled hypercalcemia rather than to the tumor mass effect. Therefore, surgical excision of recurrences or metastases can provide excellent palliation by lessening the tumor burden and concomitant hormone production.[78,106]

## Familial Hyperparathyroidism

Primary hyperparathyroidism can present as a part of MEN I and II or as a familial disease without proliferative lesions of other endocrine organs.

## Multiple Endocrine Neoplasia Syndromes (MEN)

Parathyroids can display pathologic changes in most patients with MEN I (Wermer's syndrome) and in about 10 to 20% of individuals with MEN II (Sipple syndrome).[16]

Wermer in 1954 described MEN I characterized by lesions of pituitary, parathyroid, endocrine pancreas, foregut carcinoid tumors and adrenocortical tumors.[108] The pathologic changes in parathyroid are similar to those in pseudo-adenomatous or nodular chief cell hyperplasia.[15-16] The parathyroid involvement is perceived as the earliest and prevalent manifestation and is usually detectable at ages of 20 to 30 years in 90% of affected patients.[28,30,31,109-110] However, other studies[111] have shown that pancreatic involvement is the most common and earlier manifestation of this syndrome. Clonality studies have shown that MEN I lesions represent monoclonal proliferations possibly originating in the background of polyclonal hyperplasia.[28,30-32] Wermer described a "ribbon-like" pattern to the parathyroid nodules in MEN I.[108]

MEN II is an autosomal dominant inherited disease first described by Sipple in 1961, consisting of medullary thyroid carcinoma (often bilateral), C-cell hyperplasia, unilateral or bilateral pheochromocytoma and primary hyperparathyroidism in 10–20% of patients characterized by this syndrome.[112] In MEN II, the parathyroid exhibit diffuse hyperplasia but in some cases one gland is affected, suggesting an "adenoma." MEN II patients usually show less severe hypercalcemia than MEN I patients and may show normal serum calcium and parathyroid hormone levels despite gland enlargement.[16] Genetic studies have demonstrated the MEN II locus to be on chromosome 10q11.2, the region of ret proto-oncogene.[113] Point mutations within the cysteine-rich extracellular region of the ret proto-oncogene have been detected in MEN II and familial MTC, and specific mutations have been revealed in families with parathyroid involvement.[114-115]

## Familial Isolated Primary Hyperparathyroidism

This condition usually shows an autosomal dominant mode of inheritance, but a few families show autosomal recessive inheritance.[91-94,116-118] The affected glands often display chief cell hyperplasia and some families may show adenomas, an increased risk for parathyroid carcinoma and other nonendocrine tumors. The autosomal dominant form has been found to be related to MEN I locus; however, other studies have disputed these findings.[117-118]

## Unusal Lesions of the Parathyroid

### Parathyroid Cysts

Parathyroid cysts are uncommon lesions and can be seen in the cervical region or mediastinum.[119-131] They are more commonly observed in the neck and can be mistaken for a thyroid lesion.[119] Parathyroid cysts are more common in females and usually are large, ranging from 1 to 6 cm with a propensity to occur in lower glands.[119-120] Mediastinal parathyroid cysts can be mistaken for superior/anterior mediastinum tumors. These cysts may also contain fragments of thymic tissue and are sometimes referred as third pharyngeal pouch cysts.[121,130]

Grossly, these cysts are always unilocular and smooth walled and contain watery clear fluid, which is high in parathyroid hormone content. The cyst wall is lined by a single layer of glycogenated epithelium and also contains nests of normal parathyroid. Some authors have suggested that these cysts arise by fusion of the smaller microcysts often seen in normal parathyroids. Alternatively, these cysts may also represent embryologic remnants of pharyngeal pouches, which undergo cystic degeneration with entrapped parathyroid tissue.[119-123] However, many experts believe that the cysts are degenerating adenomas and in fact some of these cases present with or are associated with hyperparathyroidism.[124-127]

Parathyroid cysts can be encountered at fine-needle aspiration, and may be mistaken for a cystic thyroid nodule. The aspiration sample almost always consists of watery clear fluid which can be assayed for parathyroid hormone to confirm the cytologic impression.[127,131]

### Lipoadenoma—So Called " Hamartoma of the Parathyroid"

These are rare parathyroid tumors, which are composed of mature adipose tissue or myxoid stroma and nests of parathyroid parenchyma.[132-135] Most of these are functional tumors and are associated with hyperparathyroidism.[132,135] They are circumscribed, rarely encapsulated, yellow-tan in color and show a lobulated cut surface. In some cases one may notice other mesenchymal elements including metaplastic bone. The parenchymal component of the lipoadenomas includes chief cells and some oncocytic cells, which are usually arranged in thin cords, tubules and abortive acini[132-135]

(Figure 29–5). These tumors have also been found in ectopic locations.[132]

## Parathyromatosis

Rarely, small deposits of parathyroid cells, mainly chief cells, can be seen outside the parathyroid gland capsule embedded within the surrounding soft tissue of the neck and mediastinum. This is usually seen in association with primary and secondary chief cell hyperplasia. Normally these lesion are not detectable; however, in cases of diffuse hyperplasia of parathyroids, all functional tissue may become hyperplastic and appear as separate fragments on histologic examination.[136-139]

Parathyromatosis can occur because of two main reasons: seeding of hypercellular parathyroid glands during surgical excision, and overgrowth of parathyroid rests left behind during ontogenesis. Both forms of parathyromatosis can be the cause of recurrent hyperparathyroidism following excision of abnormal parathyroid glands.[136,139] A word of caution, these fragments should not be confused with local invasion by parathyroid carcinoma. An examination of parathyroids along with clinical history should be helpful in arriving at the correct diagnosis.

## Spontaneous Infarction of Parathyroid Adenomas

To date, 12 cases of spontaneous infarction of parathyroid adenomas have been documented in the literature.[140] This is usually observed in association with remission of hypercalcemia. Although the exact etiology is unclear, some cases have been seen in patients taking drugs which may predispose to vascular damage, thrombosis or hemorrhage.[81]

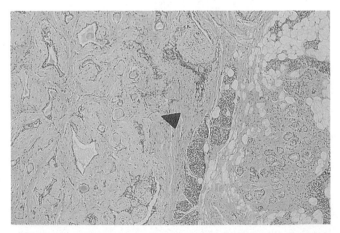

**Figure 29–5.** Lipoadenoma (Hamartoma): cells forming cords and tubules embedded in a myxoid stroma (arrow head).

## Intraoperative Assessment of Parathyroid—Old and New

Parathyroidectomy via cervical exploration is an effective treatment for hyperparathyroidism, with cure rates of greater than 95%. Frozen section is widely used to identify parathyroids during parathyroidectomy.[141-147] In short, the frozen section procedure usually involves correct labeling, gross examination measurement and weighing the specimen. The representative sample is frozen and stained with hemotoxylin and eosin stains.[15-16,147] Usually the parathyroid tissue is not difficult to identify; however, in some cases it may be difficult to distinguish from other neck tissues, including lymph node, thyroid and ectopic thymus.[142] Some authors have also advocated the use of intraoperative touch imprints in conjunction with frozen section for identification of parathyroid tissue.[148]

Despite its effectiveness, frozen section error and failure to localize the abnormal parathyroid gland can be a cause of failed parathyroidectomy.[141-147] A rapid parathyroid hormone assay in conjunction with frozen section can be helpful in indicating the successful excision of abnormal parathyroid gland(s). The samples for parathyroid hormone assay are taken preoperatively from the thyroid veins. The samples are procured again after the removal of suspected abnormal parathyroid gland(s); a successful removal of the abnormal gland is accompanied by a rapid fall in parathyroid hormone.[149-150]

In normal parathyroid glands, 80% of cells are in the nonsecretory phase and contain intracytoplasmic fat, whereas, hyperfunctioning chief cells contain much less or no intracytoplasmic fat.[15-16] Therefore, demonstration of fat by stains (Sudan IV or oil Red O) has become a method of choice in distinguishing between adenoma and hyperplasia.[151-157] However, many authors have shown that fat stain is only helpful in 80% of cases and should be interpreted in conjunction with gross findings, gland weight, and size.[147,151-157] We have recently found that a rapid (30 seconds) toluidine blue stain performed on frozen sections of parathyroid can easily highlight the intracellular fat. In addition, this method is faster to perform and interpret than oil Red O.[158]

The ratio of parenchymal to fat cells can also be assessed by density gradient measurements. This technique is rapid and provides an objective evaluation of the parenchymal mass. This technique involves taking samples from the abnormal (preferably center) and normal rim of the gland and determining their densities in a 25% mannitol solution. Abnormal parathyroid tissue will sink because of decreased fat content and high parenchymal mass. The surgeon can perform this test in the operating room to distinguish between normal and abnormal parathyroid glands.[159]

In light of the above mentioned techniques of intraoperative assessment of parathyroid pathology, it is prudent that there be close communication between the surgeon and the pathologist during surgery.[146-147] In summary, the recommended procedure of intraoperative and histologic assessment of parathyroid gland is as follows: the largest gland resected first should be weighed, measured and examined histologically. In case of diffuse proliferation of chief cells, presence of normal rim, lack of intracellular lipid and presence of second normal gland, a diagnosis of adenoma can be rendered.[15-16,147] We cannot stress too much the need for sampling another parathyroid gland to distinguish between single and multi-gland disease. Some of the hyperplastic glands may closely resemble adenomas and only up to 70% of adenomas will show a normal rim of tissue.[15-16]

## Other Types of Hyperparathyroidism

### Secondary Hyperparathyroidism

Progressive renal disease is the most common cause of secondary hyperparathyroidism. Other causes include gastrointestinal absorption defects, dietary vitamin D deficiency, liver disease and long-term lithium administration.[15-16,160-162] The role of the pathologist is usually that of identifying the parathyroid at intraoperative frozen section. This allows the surgeon to procure a portion of parathyroid tissue for auto-transplantation. The histologic picture is similar to that seen in primary hyperplasia.[160-162]

The pathologist can also encounter transplanted parathyroid tissue in cases of recurrent hyperparathyroidism caused by hyperplasia of the transplanted tissue. Tissue samples from these usually show nests of parathyroid tissue growing in muscle and adipose tissue.[163-166]

### Tertiary Hyperparathyroidism

This term has been used to define autonomous function of parathyroid in patients previously diagnosed with secondary hyperparathyroidism. The pathology resembles that of secondary hyperparathyroidism, although one of the four glands is usually much larger than the other glands.[167]

### Familial Hypocalciuric Hypercalcemia

This condition is inherited in an autosomal dominant fashion, and is characterized by moderate to minimally elevated serum calcium, and reduced urinary calcium excretion.[168-169] Several studies have shown that inactivating mutations in the calcium-sensing receptor cause familial hypocalciuric hypercalcemia and lead to neonatal hypoparathyroidism.[170-171] The parathyroid glands appear normal to mildly hypercellular. Subtotal parathyroidectomy does not cure this familial condition.[168-169]

## Special Studies and the Parathyroid

### Cytology

A majority of parathyroid lesions are not palpable therefore it is unlikely that a fine-needle aspiration (FNA) will be performed on a parathyroid tumor.[172] However, as mentioned, some parathyroid adenomas, especially the ones located in the capsule of thyroid, can be mistaken for thyroid nodules and, hence, will undergo FNA.[173] These samples usually show a monotonous population of small round cells, with even chromatin arranged in organoid or trabecular arrangement (Figure 29–6). Some cases may also show presence of vascular cores. Immunostain for parathyroid hormone may help in distinguishing these lesions from primary thyroid tumors.[172]

### Proliferative Markers

Several reports have shown that cell proliferation markers (MIBI/Ki67) can be helpful in distinguishing between parathyroid adenomas and hyperplasia[174-178] However, other studies have shown similar proliferative indices for adenomas and hyperplasias. Some authors have explored the role of proliferating cell nuclear antigen (PCNA) in differentiating between adenoma and hyperplasias.[179] Loda et al noted higher numbers of labeled nuclei in adenomas than hyperplasias.[176]

Cyclin-dependent kinase inhibitor p27 helps regulate the transition from the G1 to the S phase of the cell

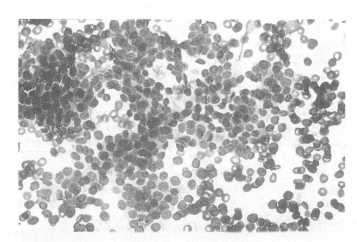

**Figure 29–6.** Parathyroid cytology: FNA of parathyroid lesion showing a monotonous population of small and round cells (Diff-Quik® stain).

cycle. Normal tissue shows higher levels of this protein than its neoplastic counterpart.[181-182] Erickson et al, by doing *in situ* hybridization for p27 mRNA, have shown that normal parathyroids express higher levels of p27 than hyperplasia, adenomas and carcinomas.[182]

## Flow Cytometry

Both image and flow cytometry techniques have been used to assess the nuclear DNA content of normal and abnormal parathyroid glands.[183-191] A majority of normal parathyroid gland shows diploid patterns; however, some normal glands associated with adenomas also reveal tetraploid peak, indicating multi-glandular abnormality. Both diploid and tetraploid DNA patterns are observed in adenomas as well as hyperplastic glands. Aneuploidy is reported in up to 25% of adenomas and considerably higher in parathyroid carcinoma.[187-188] It has been shown that aneuploidy in parathyroid carcinoma is associated with poor prognosis; however, hyperplastic glands can also show aneuploid DNA content.[188-189,191] Therefore, similar to other endocrine organs, the finding of aneuploidy does not imply a diagnosis of malignancy.

## Clonality

The role of clonal studies has been discussed earlier in this chapter in the description of various pathologic entities.

## Genetics

It has been shown that the over-expression of PRAD1 (for *parathyroid adenoma*)/cyclin *D1* induced by a DNA rearrangement of the parathyroid hormone (PTH) gene can be seen in parathyroid adenomas. This rearrangement is created by a break in the vicinity of the parathyroid gene on the short arm of chromosome 11 (band 11p 15), second break in the long arm (band 11q 13), rotation of the central fragment around the axis of the centromere, and rejoining.[192-193] Tominga et al also showed that besides adenomas this gene was also over-expressed in nodular hyperplasia, as compared to diffuse hyperplasia of parathyroid.[194]

The retinoblastoma gene (Rb) is a tumor suppression gene that has growth inhibitory properties. Allelic deletion of the Rb gene on chromosome 13 has been reported in parathyroid tumors.[195-201] It has been shown that a majority of parathyroid carcinomas show abnormal expression of Rb protein, a complete or predominant absence of nuclear staining for protein; whereas, parathyroid adenoma show positive nuclear staining for Rb protein (Figure 29–7).[196,198,200] Thus, this differential staining for Rb protein can assist in the distinction

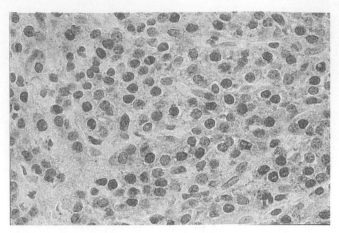

**Figure 29–7.** RB immunostain showing positive nuclear stain in a case of parathyroid adenoma.

between parathyroid adenomas and carcinomas. However, caution must be exerted in interpretation of these results since some parathyroid adenomas do not show loss of Rb protein and a few adenomas do.[198]

## Humoral Hypercalcemia of Malignancy (HHM) or Pseudo-Hyperparathyroidism

Hypercalcemia can be recognized in patients with cancers of various sites. In most of these cases, the elevated serum calcium is produced by skeletal metastases. However, in some patients with non-metastatic, localized tumors, hypercalcemia is found, which disappears following tumor resection and reoccurs when the tumor recurs.[16,202-206] Initial studies suggested that these non-parathyroid tumors were ectopically producing PTH. Various assay studies indicated this was not true; indeed, serum PTH levels were suppressed. It has now been proved by serum and tumor assay, as well as immunohistochemical studies, that these cancers produce parathyroid hormone-related protein (PTHRP).[16,203-204] The gene encoding PTHRP has been localized to the short arm of chromosome 12, which is thought to belong to the same gene family as the PTH gene on chromosome 11.[207-208] PTHRP exerts its action by binding to the parathyroid hormone receptors on bone and kidney and mimics the action of parathyroid hormone itself.[204] The types of tumors commonly associated with HHM include squamous cell carcinoma (lung, head and neck, and vulva), clear cell tumors (renal or ovarian origin) and small cell tumors of the ovary.[205-206] The few studies of the histologic appearance of the parathyroid glands have shown that they are normal or atrophic.[16]

## Hypoparathyroidism

The surgical pathologist does not see glands from hypoparathyroid patients. The most common cause of hypoparathyroidism is inadvertent removal or damage to the vascular supply of normal glands during head and neck surgery.[14] Other causes include infiltration by iron, amyloid, or, rarely, metastatic tumors.[209-214] Autoimmune parathyroiditis, either as an isolated lesion or as part of systemic polyglandular endocrinopathy, is another significant cause of parathyroid failure.[213-214]

## References

1. Owen R. On the anatomy of the Indian rhinoceros (*Rh. Unicornis, L*). *Trans Zool Soc Lond.* 1862;iv:31–58.
2. Sandström IV. On a new gland in man and several mammals—glandulae parathyroideae. *Proc Ups Soc Phys.* 1879–1880;15:441–471.
3. Gley E. Sur les fonctions du corps thyroide. *C R Seances Soc Biol.* 1891;43:841–43.
4. Mandl F. Therapeutischer Versuch bei Ostitis fibrosa generalisata mittels Extirpation eines Epithelköperchentumors. *Wein Klin Wochenschr.* 1925;50:1323–44.
5. Gilmour JR. The embryology of the parathyroid glands, the thymus and certain associated remnants. *J. Pathol Bacteriol.* 1937;45:507–522.
6. Boyd JD. Development of thyroid and parathyroid glands and the thymus. *Ann R Coll Surg Engl.* 1950;7:455–71.
7. Edis AJ, Purnell DC, van Heerden JA. The undescended "parathymus": an ocassional cause of failed neck exploration for hyperparathyroidism. *Ann Surg.* 1979;190:64–68.
8. Merida-Velasco JA, Sanchez-Montesinos I, Espin-Ferra J, et al. Ectodermal ablation of the third branchial arch in chick embryos and the morphogenesis of the parathyroid III gland. *J. Craniofac Genetics and Develop Biol.* 1999,19.33–40.
9. Manley NR, Capecchi MR. Hox group 3 paralogs regulate the development and migration of the thymus, thyroid and parathyroid glands. *Develop Biol.* 1998;195:1–15.
10. Grimelius L, Akerstrom G, Johansson H, Bergstrom R. Anatomy and histopathology of human parathyroid glands. *Pathol Annu.* 1981;16 (part 1):1–24.
11. Akerstrom G, Malmaeus J, Bergstrom S. Surgical anatomy of human parathyroid glands. *Surgery.* 1984;95:14–21.
12. Wang CA. The anatomic basis of parathyroid surgery. *Ann Surg.* 1976;183:271–175.
13. Alveryd A. Parathyroid glands in thyroid surgery. *Acta Chir Scand (Suppl)* 1968;389:9–36.
14. Lee NJ, Blakey JD, Bhuta S, Calcaterra TC. Unintentional parathyroidectomy during thyroidectomy. *Laryngoscope.* 1999;109:1238–1240.
15. Castleman B, Roth SI. *Tumors of the Parathyroid Glands.* Fascicle 14, Series 2, Washington, DC: Armed Forces Institute of Pathology; 1978.
16. DeLellis, RA. *Tumors of the Parathyroid Glands.* Fascicle 6, series 3, Washington, DC; Armed Forces Institute of Pathology; 1993.
17. Dufour DR, Wilkerson SY. Factors related to parathyroid weight in normal persons. *Arch Pathol Lab Med.* 1983;107:167–172.
18. Dufour DR, Wilkerson SY. The normal parathyroid revisited: percent of stromal fat. *Hum Pathol.* 1982;13:717–721.
19. Dekker A, Dunsford HA, Geyer SJ. The normal parathyroid gland at autopsy: the significance of stromal fat in adult patients. *J Pathol.* 1979;128:127–132.
20. Akerstrom G, Grimelius L, Johansson H, et al. Estimation of parathyroid parenchymal cell mass by density gradients. *Am J Pathol.* 1980;99:685–694.
21. Johannessen JV. Parathyroid glands. In: Johannessen JV, ed. *Electron Microscopy in Human Medicine.* New York: McGraw Hill; 1981;vol.10:111.
22. Heath H, Hodgson SF, Kennedy MA. Primary hyperparathyroidism: incidence morbidity and potential economic impact in a community. *N Engl J Med.* 1980;302:189–193.
23. Marcus R. Laboratory diagnosis of primary hyperparathyroidism. *Endocrinol Metab Clin North Am.* 1989;18:647–58.
24. Russ JE, Scanlon EF, Sener SF. Parathyroid adenoma following irradiation. *Cancer.* 1979;43:1078–1083.
25. Prinz RA, Barbato AL, Braithwaite SS, et al. Prior irradiation and the development of coexistent differentiated thyroid cancer and hyperparathyroidism. *Cancer.* 1982;49:874–877.
26. Dotzenrath C, Goretzki PE, Farnebo F, et al. Molecular genetics of primary and secondary hyperparathyroidism. *Exp Clin Endocrinol Diab.* 1996;104:Supp. 4:105–107.
27. Farnebo F, Teh BT, Dotzenrath C, et al. Differential loss of heterozygosity in familial sporadic and uremic hyperparathyroidism. *Hum Genet.* 1997;99:342–349.
28. Heppner C, Kester MB, Agaroval SK, et al. Somatic mutation of the MEN-1 gene in parathyroid tumors. *Nature Genetics.* 1997;16:375–378.
29. Farnebo F, Teh BT, Kytola S, et al. Alterations of the MEN-1 gene in sporadic parathyroid tumors. *J Clin Endocrinol Metab.* 1998;83:2627–2630.
30. Carling T, Correa P, Hessman O, et al. Parathyroid Men-1 gene mutations in relation to clinical characteristics of nonfamilial primary hyperparathyroidism. *J Clin Endocrinol Metab.* 1998;83:2960–2963.
31. Ohye H, Sato M, Matsubara A, et al. Germline mutations of the MEN-1 gene in a family with primary hyperparathyroidism. *Endocrine J.* 1998;45:719–723.
32. Arnold A, Staunton CE, Kim HG, et al. Monoclonality and abnormal parathyroid hormone genes in parathyroid adenomas. *N Engl J Med.* 1988;318:658–662.
33. Dolgin C, LoGerfo P, LiVolsi V, Feind C. Twenty-five year experience with primary hyperparathyroidism at Columbia Presbyterian Medical Center. *Head Neck Surg.* 1979;2:92–98.
34. Ghandur-Mnaymneh L, Kimura N. The parathyroid adenoma: a histopathologic definition with a study of 172 cases of primary hyperparathryoidism. *Am J Pathol.* 1984;115:70–83.
35. Grimilius L, Johansson H. Pathology of parathyroid tumors. *Semin. Surg Oncol.* 1997;13:142–154.
36. Fialkow PJ, Jackson CE, Block MA, Greenwald KA. Multicellular origin of parathyroid "adenomas." *N Engl J Med.* 1977;297:695–698.
37. Jackson CE, Cerny JC, Block MA, Fialkow PJ. Probable clonal origin of aldosteronomas versus multicellular origin of parathyroid "adenomas." *Surgery.* 1982;92:875–879.
38. Arnold A, Kim HG. Clonal loss of one chromosome II in a parathyroid adenoma. *J Clin Endocrinol Metab.* 1989; 69:496–499.
39. Arnold A, Kim HG, Gaz RD, et al. Molecular cloning and chromosomal mapping of DNA rearranged with the parathyroid hormone gene in a parathyroid adenoma. *J Clin Invest.* 1989;83:2034–2040.
40. Shan L, Nakamura Y, Nakamura M, et al. Genetic alterations in primary and secondary hyperparathyroidism. *Pathol International.* 1998;48:569–574.

41. Shan L, Nakamura M, Nakamura Y, et al. Comparative analysis of clonality and pathology in primary and secondary hyperparathyroidism. *Virch Arch.* 1997;430: 241–251.

42. Koshiishi N, Chong JM, Fukasawa T, et al. Microsatellite instability and loss of heterozygosity in primary and secondary proliferative lesions of the parathyroid gland. *Lab Invest.* 1999;79:1051–1058.

44. Williams ED. Pathology of the parathyroid glands. *J Clin Endocrinol Metab.* 1974;3:285–303.

45. Lloyd HM, Jacobi JM, Cooke RA. Nuclear diameter in parathyroid adenomas. *J Clin pathol.* 1979;32:1278–1281.

46. Rudberg C, Grimelius L, Johansson H, et al. Alterations in density, morphology, and parathyroid hormone release of dispersed parathyroid cells from patients with hyperparathyroidism. *Acta Pathol Microbiol Immunol Scand (A).* 1986;94:253–61.

47. San-Juan J, Monteagudo C, Fraker D, Norton J, Merino MJ. Significance of mitotic activity and other morphologic parameters in parathyroid adenomas and their correlation with clinical behavior [Abstract]. *Am J Clin Pathol.* 1989;92:523.

48. Snover DC, Foucar K. Mitotic activity in benign parathyroid disease. Am *J Clin Pathol.* 1981;75:345–347.

49. Lawton TJ, Feldman M, LiVolsi VA. Lymphocytic infiltrates in solitary parathyroid adenomas. *Intl J Surg Pathol.* 1998;6:5–10.

50. McGregor DH, Lotuaio LG, Chu LH. Functioning oxyphil adenoma of parathyroid gland. an ultrastructural and biochemical study. *Am J Pathol.* 1978;92:691–703.

51. Ordonez NG, Ibanez ML, MacKay B, et al. Functional oxyphil cell adenomas of parathyroid gland: evidence of hormonal activity in oxyphil cells. *Am J Clin Pathol.* 1982;78:681–689.

52. Rodriquez FH, Sarma DP, Lunseth JH, Guileyardo JM. Primary hyperparathyroidism due to an oxyphil adenoma. *Am J Clin Pathol.* 1983;80:878–880.

53. Bedetti CD, Dekker A, Watson CG. Functioning oxyphil cell adenoma of the parathyroid gland: a clinicopathologic study of ten patients with hyperparathyroidism. *Hum Pathol.* 1984;15:1121–1126.

54. Jones SH, Dietler P. Oxyphil cell adenoma as a cause of hyperparathyroidism. *Am J Surg.* 1981;141:744–745.

55. Baloch ZW, LiVolsi VA. Oncocytic lesions of the neuroendocrine system. *Sem Diagn Pathol.* 1999;16:190–199.

56. Low, RA Katz AD. Parathyroidectomy via bilateral cervical explotation: a retrospective review of 866 cases. *Head & Neck.* 1998; 20:583–587.

57. Kakimoto, K, Shiba M, Matsuoka, Y, Hara, T, Oda M, Yoshioka T, Koide T. Nonsynchronous double adenoma of the parathyroid gland. *Int J Urol.* 1998;5:490–492.

58. Harness JK, Ramsbury SR, Nishiyama RH, Thompson NW. Multiple adenomas of the parathyroids; do they exist? *Arch Surg.* 1979;114:468–474.

59. Seyfar AE, Sigdestad JB, Hirata RM. Surgical considerations in hyperparathyroidism: reappraisal of the need for multigland biopsy. *Am J Surg.* 1976;132:38–340.

60. Schwindt WD. Multiple parathyroid adenomas. *JAMA.* 1967;199: 945–946.

61. Verdon CA, Edis AJ. Parathyroid "double adenomas." Fact or fiction? *Surgery.* 1981;90:523–526.

62. Cope O, Keynes WM, Roth SI, Castleman B. Primary chief-cell hyperplasia of the parathyroid glands: a new entity in the surgery of hyperparathyroidism. *Ann Surg.* 1958;28:163–215.

63. Wang CA, Castleman B, Cope O. Surgical management of hyperparathyroidism due to primary hyperplasia. a clinical and pathologic study of 104 cases. *Ann Surg.* 1982;195:384–392.

64. Adams PH, Chalmers TM, Peters N, et al. Primary chief cell hyperplasia of the parathyroid glands. *Ann Intern Med.* 1965;63:454–467.

65. Edis AJ, vanHeerden JA, Scholz DA. Results of subtotal parathyroidectomy for chief cell hyperplasia. *Surgery.* 1979;86:492–469.

66. Scholz DA, Purnell DC, Edis AJ, et al. Primary hyperparathyroidism with multiple parathyroid gland involvement. Review of 53 cases. *Mayo Clin Proc.* 1978;53:792–797.

67. Castleman B, Schantz A, Roth SI. Parathyroid hyperplasia in primary hyperparathyroidism. *Cancer.* 1976;38:1668–1675.

68. Herfart KK, Wells SA. Parathyroid glands and the multiple endocrine neoplasia syndromes and familial hypocalciuric hypercalcemia. *Semin Surg Oncol.* 1997;13:114–124.

69. Prinz RA, Gamuros OI, Sellu D, Lynn JA. Subtotal parathyroidectomy for primary chief cell hyperplasia of the multiple endocrine neoplasia type 1 syndrome. *Ann Surg.* 1981;193:26–29.

70. Dorado AE, Hensley G, Castleman B. Water clear hyperplasia of parathyroid. *Cancer.* 1976;38:1676–1683.

71. Dawkins RL, Tashjian AH, Castleman B, Moore EW. Hyperparathyroidism due to clear cell hyperplasia. *Am J Med.* 1973;54:119–126.

72. Persson S, Hansson G, Hedman I, et al. Primary parathyroid hyperplasia of water clear cell type. Transformation of water clear cells into chief cells. *Acta Pathol Micrbiol Scand Sect A.* 1986; 94:391–395.

73. Hedback G, Oden A. Parathyroid water clear cell hyperplasia, an O-allele associated condition. *Hum Genet.* 1994;94:195–197.

74. Sandelin K, Auer G, Bondeson L, et al. Prognostic factors in parathyroid cancer: a review of 95 cases. *World J Surg.* 1992; 16:724–731.

75. Wynne AG, van Heerden J, Carney JA, Fitzpatrick LA. Parathyroid carcinoma: clinical and pathologic features in 43 patients. *Medicine.* 1992;71:197–205.

76. Schantz A, Castleman B. Parathyroid carcinoma: a study of 70 cases. *Cancer.* 1973;31:600–605.

77. Shane E, Bilezikian JP. Parathyroid caricnoma: a review of 62 patients. *Endocr Rev.* 1982;3:218–226.

78. Van Heerden JA, Weiland LH, ReMine NH, et al. Cancer of the parathyroid glands. *Arch Surg.* 1979;114:475–480.

79. Aldinger KA, Hickey RC, Ibanez ML, Samaan NA. Parathyroid carcinoma. A clinical study of seven cases of functioning and two cases on nonfunctioning parathyroid cancer. *Cancer.* 1982;49:388–397.

80. Bondeson L, Sandelin K, Grimelius L. Histopathological variable and DNA cytometry in parathyroid carcinoma. *Am J Surg Pathol.* 1993;17:820–829.

81. DePapp AE, Kinder B, LiVolsi VA, et al. Parathyroid carcinoma arising from parathyroid hyperplasia: autoinfarction following intravenous treatment with pamidronate. *Am J Med.* 1994;97: 399–400.

82. Holmes EC, Morton DL, Ketcham AS. Parathyroid carcinoma: a collective review. *Ann Surg.* 1969;169:631–640.

83. Ellis HA, Floyd M, Herbert FK. Recurrent hyperparathyroidism due to parathyroid carcinoma. *J Clin Pathol.* 1974;24:596–604.

84. Anderson BJ, Samaan NA, Vassilopoulou-Sellin R, et al. Parathyroid carcinoma: features and difficulties in diagnosis and management. *Surgery.* 1983;94:906–915.

85. Wand C, Gaz RD. Natural history of parathyroid carcinoma. *Am J Surg.* 1985;149:522–527.

86. Inoue H, Ishihara T, Fukai S, et al. Parathyroid carcinoma with tracheal invasion and airway obstruction. *Surgery.* 1980;87: 113–117.

87. Cohn K, Silverman M, Corrado J, Sedgewick C. Parathyroid carcinoma: the Lahey Clinic experience. *Surgery.* 1985;98:1095–1100.

88. Favia G, Lumachi F, Polistin F, D'Amico DF. Parathyroid carcinoma: sixteen new cases and suggestions for correct management. *World J Surg.* 1998;22:1225–1230.

89. Obara T, Okamoto T, Kanbe M, Ishara M. Functioning parathyroid carcinoma: clinicopathologic features and rational treatment. *Sem Surg Oncol.* 1997;13:134–141.

90. Hundahl SA, Fleming ID, Fremgen AM, Menck HR. Two-hundred eighty-six cases of parathyroid carcinoma trated in the U.S. between 1985–1995; a National Cancer Data Base Report. *Cancer.* 1999;86:538–544.

91. Mallette LE, Bilezikian JP, Ketcham AS, Aurbach GD. Parathyroid carcinoma in familial hyperparathyroidism. *Am J Med.* 1974;57:642–648.

92. Dinnen JS, Greenwood RH, Jones JH, et al. Parathyroid carcinoma in familial hyperparathyroidism. *J Clin Pathol.* 1977;30:966–975.

93. Streetin EA, Weinstein LS, Norton JS, et al. Studies in a kindred with parathyroid carcinoma. *J Clin Endocrinol Metab.* 1992;75:362–366.

94. Yoshimoto K, Endo H, Tsuyuguchi M, et al. Familial isolated primary hyperparathyroidism with parathyroid carcinomas: clinical and molecular features. *Clin Endocrinol.* 1998;48:67–72.

95. Jenkins PJ, Satta MA, Simmgen M, et al. Metastatic parathyroid carcinoma in the MEN2A syndrome. *Clin Endocrinol.* 1997;47:747–751.

96. Berland Y, Olmer M, Lebreuil G, Grisoli J. Parathyroid carcinoma, adenoma and hyperplasia in a case of chronic renal insufficiency on dialysis. *Clin Nephrol.* 1982;18:154–158.

97. Ireland J, Fleming S, Levison D, et al. Parathyroid carcinoma associated with chronic renal failure and previous radiotherapy to the neck. *J Clin Pathol.* 1985;38:1117–1118.

98. Kodama M, Ikegami M, Kmanishi M, et al. Parathyroid carcinoma in a case of chronic renal failure on dialysis. *Urol Int.* 1989;44:110–112.

99. Krishna GG, Mendez M, Levy B, et al. Parathyroid carcinoma in a chronic hemodialysis patient. *Nephron.* 1989;52:194–195.

100. Boyle NH, Ogg CS, Hartley RB, Owen WJ. Parathyroid carcinoma secondary to prolonged hyperplasia in chronic renal failure and in cardiac disease. *Europ J Surg Oncol.* 1999;25:100–103.

101. Evans HL. Criteria for diagnosis of parathyroid carcinoma. *Lab Invest.* 1992;66:35A (Abstract).

102. Obara T, Fujimoto Y, Yamaguchi K, et al. Parathyroid carcinoma of the oxyphil cell type. *Cancer.* 1985;55:1482–1498.

103. Chaitin BA, Goldman RL. Mitotic activity in benign parathyroid disease (letter). *Am J Clin Pathol.* 1981,76.363–364.

104. Merlano M, Conte P, Scarsi P, et al. Nonfunctioning parathyroid carcinoma. A case report. *Tumori.* 1985;71:193–196.

105. Yamashita H, Noguchi S, Nakayama I, et al. Light and electron microscopic study of nonfunctioning parathyroid carcinoma. *Acta Pathol Jpn.* 1984;34:123–132.

106. Zisman E, Buckle RM, Deftos LJ et al. Production of parathyroid hormone by metastatic parathyroid carcinoma. *Am J Med.* 1968;45:619–623.

107. Levin KE, Galante M, Clark OH. Parathyroid carcinoma versus parathyroid adenoma in patients with profound hypercalcemia. *Surgery.* 1987;101:649–660.

108. Wermer P. Genetic aspects of adenomatosis of endocrine glands. *Am J Med.* 1954;16:363–371.

109. Larsson C, Skogseid B, Öberg K, et al. Multiple endocrine neoplasia type I gene maps to chromosome 11 and is lost for insulinoma. *Nature.* 1988;332:85–87.

110. Chandrasekharappa SC, Guru SC, Manickam P, et al. Positional cloning of the gene for multiple endocrine neoplasia-type 1. *Science.* 1997;276:404–407.

111. Skogseid B, Eriksson B, Lundqvist G, et al. Multiple endocrine neoplasia type I—a ten year prospective screening study in four kindreds. *J Clin Endocrinol Metab.* 1991;73:281–287.

112. Sipple JH. The association of pheochromocytoma with carcinoma of the thyroid gland. *Am J Med.* 1961;31:163–166.

113. Gardner E, Papi L, Easton DF, et al. Genetic linkage studies map the multiple endocrine neoplasia type 2 loci to a small interval on chromosome 10q11.2. *Hum Mol Genet.* 1993;2:241–246.

114. Mulligan LM, Eng C, Healey CS et al. Specific mutations of the RET proto-oncogene are related to disease phenotype in MEN 2A and FMTC. *Nat Genet.* 1994;6:70–4.

115. Eng C, Clayton D, Schuffenecker I, Lenoir G, Cote G, Gagel RF. The relationship between specific RET proto-oncogene mutations and disease phenotype in multiple endocrine neoplasia type 2: international RET mutation consortium analysis. *JAMA.* 1996; 20:1575–79.

116. Goldsmith RE, Sizemore GW, Chen IW, et al. Familial hyperparathyroidism, Description of a large kindred with physiologic observations and a review of the literature. *Ann Intern Med.* 1976;84:36–43.

117. Marx SJ, Speigel AM, Brown EM, Aurbach GD. Family studies in patients with primary parathyroid hyperplasia. *Am J Med.* 1977;62:698–706.

118. Wassif WS, Moniz CF, Friedman E, et al. Familial isolated hyperparathyroidism: a distinct genetic entity with an increased risk of parathyroid cancer. *J Clin Endocrinol Metab.* 1993;77:1485–89.

119. Wang CA, Vickery AL, Maloof F. Large parathyroid cysts mimicking thyroid nodules. *Ann Surg.* 1972;175:448–453.

120. Ginsberg J, Young JEM, Walfish PG. Parathyroid cysts. *JAMA.* 1978;240:1506–1507.

121. Thacker WC, Wells VH, Hall ER. Parathyroid cysts of the mediastinum. *Ann Surg.* 1971;174:969–975.

122. Hoehn JG, Beahrs OH, Woolner LB. Unusual surgical lesions of the parathyroid gland. *Am J Surg.* 1969; 118:770–778.

123. Troster M, Chiu HF, McLarty TD. Parathyroid cysts: report of a case with ultrastructural; observations. *Surgery.* 1978;83:238–242.

124. Earll JM, Cohen A, Lundberg GD. Functional cystic parathyroid adenoma. *Am J Surg.* 1969;118:100–103.

125. Albertson DA, Marshall RB, Jarman WT. Hypercalcemic crisis secondary to a functioning parathyroid cyst. *Am J Surg.* 1981; 141:175–177.

126. Clark OH. Hyperparathyroidism due to primary cystic parathyroid hyperplasia. *Arch Surg.* 1978;113:748–750.

127. Silverman JF, Khazanie PG, Norris T, Fore WW. Parathyroid hormone (PTH) assay of parathyroid cysts examined by fine needle aspiration biopsy. *Am J Clin Pathol.* 1986;86:708–776.

128. Marco V, Carrasco MA, Marco C, Bauza A. Cytomorphology of a mediastinal parathyroid cyst. *Acta Cytol.* 1983;27:688–692.

129. Gough IR. Parathyroid cysts. *Aust NZ J Surg.* 1999;69:404–406.

130. Shields TW, Immerman SC. Mediastinal parathyroid cysts revisited. *Ann Thorac Surg.* 1999;67:581–590.

131. Shi B, Guo H, Tang N. Treatment of parathyroid cysts with fine needle aspiration. *Lancet.* 1999;11:797–798.

132. Wolff M, Goodman EN. Functioning lipoadenoma of supernumerary parathyroid gland in the mediastinum. *Head Neck Surg.* 1980;2:302–307.

133. Grimelius L, Johansson H, Lindquist B. A case of unusual stromal development in a parathyroid adenoma. *Acta Chir Scand.* 1972;138:628–629.

134. Ober WB, Kaiser GA. Hamartoma of the parathyroid. *Cancer.* 1958;11:601–606.

135. Perosio P, Brooks JJ, LiVolsi VA. Orbital brown tumor as initial manifestation of parathyroid lipoadenoma. *Surg Pathol.* 1988; 1:77–82.

136. Stehman-Breen C, Murihead N, Thorning D, Sherrard D. Secondary hyperparathyroidism complicated by parathyromatosis. *Am J Kidney Dis.* 1996; 28:502–507.

137. Reddick RL, Costa JC, Marx SJ. Parathyroid hyperplasia and parathyromatosis. *Lancet.* 1977;1:549.

138. Fitko R, Roth SI, Hines JR, et al. Parathyromatosis in hyperparathyroidism. *Hum Pathol.* 1990;21:234–237.

139. Kollmorgen CF, Aust MR, Ferreiro JA, et al. Parathyromatosis: a rare yet important cause of persistent or recurrent hyperparathyroidism. *Surgery.* 1994;116:111–115.

140. Kovacs KA, Gay JDL. Remission of primary hyperparathyroidism due to spontaneous infarction of a parathyroid adenoma: case report and review of the literature. *Medicine.* 1998;77:398–402.

141. Low RA, Katz AD. Parathyroidectomy via bilateral cervical exploration: a retrospective review of 866 cases. *Head Neck.* 1998;20:583–7.

142. Westra WH, Pritchett DD, Udelsman R. Intraoperative confirmation of parathyroid tissue during parathyroid exploration: a retrospective evaluation of the frozen section. *Am J Surg Pathol.* 1998;22:538–44.

143. Summers GW. Parathyroid update: a review of 220 cases. *Ear Nose Throat.* 1996;75:434–9.

144. Wang CA. Parathyroid reexploration. *Ann Surg.* 1977;186:140–145.

145. Paloyan E, Lawrence AM, Strauss FH. *Hyperparathyroidism.* New York: Grune & Stratton; 1973.

146. Roth SI, Wang CA, Potts JT. The team approach to primary hyperparathyroidism. *Hum Pathol.* 1975;6:645–658.

147. LiVolsi VA, Hamilton R. Intraoperative assessment of parathyroid gland pathology. A common view from the surgeons and the pathologist. *Am J Clin Pathol.* 1994;102:365–373.

148. Bloustein PA, Silverberg SG. Rapid cytologic examination of surgical specimens. *Pathol Annu.* 1977;12 (Pt 2):251–78.

149. Irvin GL 3rd, Molinari AS, Figueroa C, Carneiro DM. Improved success rate in reoperative parathyroidectomy with intraoperative PTH assay. *Ann Surg.* 1999;229:874–8.

150. Saharay M, Farooqui A, Farrow S, Fahie-Wilson M, Brown A. Intra-operative parathyroid hormone assay for simplified localization of parathyroid adenomas. *J Royal Soc Med.* 1996;89:261–4.

151. Dufour DR, Durkowski C. Sudan IV staining: its limitations in evaluating parathyroid functional status. *Arch Pathol Lab Med.* 1982;106:224–227.

152. King DT, Hirose FM. Chief cell intracytoplasmic fat used to evaluate parathyroid disease by frozen section. *Arch Pathol Lab Med.* 1979;103:609–312.

153. Kasden EJ, Cohen RB, Rosen S, Silen W. Surgical pathology of hyperparathyroidism: usefulness of fat stains and problems in interpretation. *Am J Surg Pathol.* 1981;5:381–384.

154. Ljungberg O, Tibblin S. Perioperative fat staining of frozen sections in primary hyperparathyroidism. *Am J Pathol.* 1979;95:633–642.

155. Dekker A, Watson CG, Barnes EL. The pathologic assessment of primary hyperparathyroidism and its impact on therapy: a prospective evaluation of 50 cases with Oil-Red-O stain. *Ann Surg.* 1979;190:671–675.

156. Monchik JM, Farrugia R, Teplitz C, Brown S. Parathyroid surgery: the role of chief cell intracellular fat staining with osmium carmine in the intraoperative management of patients with hyperparathyroidism. *Surgery.* 1983;94:877–886.

157. Bondeson AG, Bondeson L, Ljundberg O, Tibblin S. Fat staining in parathyroid disease—diagnostic value and impact on surgical strategy. *Hum Pathol.* 1985;16:1255–1263.

158. Lyle S, LiVolsi VA, Tomaszewski J. Intraoperative frozen-section evaluation of intracytoplasmic fat in parathyroid glands using toluidine blue [Abstract]. *Mod Pathol.* 2000;13:224A.

159. Wang CA, Ryder SV. A density test for the intraoperative differentiation of parathyroid hyperplasia from neoplasia. *Ann Surg.* 1978;187:63–67.

160. Roth SI, Marshall RB. Pathology and ultrastructure of human parathyroid glands in chronic renal failure. *Arch Intern Med.* 1969;124:397–407.

161. Malmaeus J, Grimelius L, Johansson H, et al. Parathyroid pathology in hyperparathyroidism secondary to chronic renal failure. *Scan J Urol Nephrol.* 1984;18:75–84.

162. Akerstrom G, Malmaeus J, et al. Histological changes in parathyroid glands in subclinical and clinical renal disease. *Scand J Urol Nephrol.* 1984:18:75–84.

163. Rattner DW, Marrone GC, Kasdon E, Silen W. Recurrent hyperparathyroidism due to implantation of parathyroid tissue. *Am J Surg.* 1985;149:745–748.

164. Akerstrom G, Rudberg C, Grimelius L, Rastad J. Recurrent hyperparathyroidism due to preoperative seeding of neoplastic or hyperplastic parathyroid tissue. *Acta Chir Scand.* 1988:154–219.

165. Jansson S, Tisell LE. Autotransplantation of diseased parathyroid glands into subcutaneous abdominal adipose tissue. *Surgery.* 1987;101:549–556.

166. Max MH, Flint LM, Richardson JD, et al. Total parathyroidectomy and parathyroid autotransplantation in patients with chronic renal failure. *Surg Obstet Gynecol.* 1981;153:177–180.

167. Krause MW, Hedinger CE. Pathologic study of parathyroid glands in tertiary hyperparathyroidism. *Human Pathol.* 1985;16:772–784.

168. Law WM, Carney JA, Heath H. Parathyroid glands in familial benign hypercalcemia (familial hypocalciuric hypercalcemia). *Am J Med.*1989;76:1021–1026.

169. Thorgeirsson U, Costa J, Marx SJ. The parathyroid glands in familial hypocalciuric hypercalcemia. *Hum Pathol.* 1981;12:229–237.

170. Chikatsu N, Fukumoto S, Suzawa M et al. An adult patient with svere hypercalcemia and hypocalciuria due to novel homozygous inactivating mutation of calcium sensing receptor. *Clin Endocrinol.* 1999;50:537–543.

171. Okazaki R, Chikatsu N, Nakatsu M, Takeuchi Y, Ajima M, Miki J. A novel activating mutation in calcium-sensing receptor gene associated with a family of autosomal dominant hypocalcemia. *J Clin Endocrinol Metab.* 1999;84:363–366.

172. Abati A, Skarulis MC, Shawker T, Solomion D. Ultrasound-guided fine needle aspiration of parathyroid lesions: a morphological and immunocytochemical approach. *Hum Pathol.* 1995;26:338–343.

173. Spiegel AM, Marx SJ, Doppmann JL, et al. Intrathyroidal parathyroid adenoma or hyperplasia. *JAMA.* 1975;234:1029–1033.

174. Abbona GC, Papotti M, Gasparri G, Bussoloti G. Proliferative activity in parathyroid tumors as detected by Ki67 immunostaining. *Hum Pathol.* 1995;26:135–138.

175. Karak AK, Sarkar C, Chumber S, Tandon N. MIB-1 proliferative index in parathyroid adenoma and hyperplasia. *Indian J Med Res.* 1997;105:235–238.

176. Loda M, Lysman J, Cukor B, et al. Nodular foci in parathyroid adenomas and hyperplasias: an immunohistochemical analysis of proliferative activity. *Hum Pathol.* 1994;25:1050–1056.

177. Karak AK, Sarkar C, Chumber S, Tandon N. MIB-1 proliferative index in parathyroid adenoma and hyperplasia. *Indian J Med Res.* 1997;105:235–238.

178. Wang Q, Palnitkar S, Parfitt AM. The basal rate of cell proliferation in normal human parathyroid tissue: implications for the pathogenesis of hyperparathyroidism. *Clin Endocrinol.* 1997;46:343–349.

179. Yamaguchi S, Yachicku S, Morikawa M. Analysis of proliferative activity of the parathyroid glands using proliferating cell nuclear antigen in patients with hyperparathyroidism. *J Clin Endocrinol Metab.* 1999;82:2681–2688.

180. Parfitt AM, Wang Q, Palnitkar S. Rates of cell proliferation in adenomatous, suppressed and normal parathyroid tissue: implications for pathogenesis. *J Clin Endocrinol Metab.* 1998;83:863–899.

181. Lloyd RV, Jin L, Qian X, Kulig E. Aberrant p27 (Kipi) expression in endocrine and other tumors. *Am J Pathol*. 1997;150:401–407.

182. Erickson LA, Jin L, Wollan P, et al. Parathyroid hyperplasia, adenomas and carcinomas: differential expression of p27 Kip1 protein. *Am J Surg Pathol*. 1995;23:288–295.

183. Bengtsson A, Grimelius L, Johansson H, Ponten J. Nuclear DNA content of parathyroid cells in adenomas, neoplastic and normal glands. *Acta Pathol Microbiol Scand*. 1977;85:455–460.

184. Bowlby LS, DeBault LE, Abraham SR. Flow cytometric DNA analysis of parathyroid glands. *Am J Pathol*. 1987;128:338–344.

185. Harlow S, Roth SI, Bauer K, Marhsal RB. Flow cytometric DNA analysis of normal and pathologic parathyroid glands. *Mod Pathol*. 1991;4:310–315.

186. Mallette LE. DNA quantiation in the study of parathyroid lesions: a review. *Am J Clin Pathol*. 1992;98:305–311.

187. Joensuu H, Klemi PJ. DNA aneuploidy in adenomas of endocrine organds. *Am J Pathol*. 1988;132:145–151.

188. Obara T, Fujimoto Y, Hirayama A, et al. Flow cytometric DNA analysis of parathyroid tumors with special reference to its diagnostic and prognostic value in parathyroid carcinoma. *Cancer*. 1990;65:1789–1793.

189. Levin KE, Chew KL, Ljung BM, et al. Deoxyribonucleic acid cytometry helps identify parathyroid carcinomas. *J Clin Endocrinol Metab*. 1988;67:779–784.

190. Xioa-Lin P, Koide N, Kobayashi S, et al. Assessment of proliferative activity of glandular cells in hyperfunctioning parathyroid gland using flow cytometric and immunohistochemical methods. *World J Surg*. 1996;20:361–366.

191. Bocsi J, Perner F, Szucs J, et al. DNA content of parathyroid tumors. *Anticancer Res*. 1998;18:2901–2904.

192. Hsi EP, Zukerberg LR, Yang WI, Arnold A. Cyclin D1/PRAD 1 expression in parathyroid adenomas. An immunohistochemical study. *J Clin Endocrinol Metab*. 1996;81:1736–1739.

193. Vasif MA, Bynnes RK, Sturm M, et al. Expression of cyclin D1 in parathyroid adenomas and hyperplasia: a paraffin immunhistochemical study. *Mod Pathol*. 1999;12:412–416.

194. Tominaga Y, Tsuzuki T, Uchida K et al. Expression of PRAD1/cyclin D1, retinoblastoma gene products, and Ki67 in parathyroid hyperplasia caused by chronic renal failure versus primary adenoma. *Kidney Intern*. 1999;55:1375–83.

195. Cryns VL, Thor A, Xu HJ, et al. Loss of retinoblastoma tumor-suppressor gene in parathyroid carcinoma. *N Engl J Med*. 1994; 330:757–761.

196. Subramiam P, Wilkinson S, Shepherd JJ. Inactivation of retinoblastoma gene in malignant parathyroid growths: a candidate genetic trigger? *Aust NZ Surg*. 1995;65:714–716.

197. Lloyd RV, Carney JA, Ferreiro JA, et al. Immunohistochemical analysis of the cell-cycle associated antigens Ki67 and retinoblastoma protein in parathyroid carcinoma and adenoma. *Endocr Pathol*. 1995;6:279–287.

198. Dotzenrath C, Teh BT, Farnebo F, et al. Allelic loss of the retinoblastoma tumor suppressor gene: a marker for aggressive parathyroid tumors? *J Clin Endocrinol Metab*. 1996;81:3194–3196.

199. Farnebo F, Auer G, Farnebo LO, et al. Evaluation of retinoblastoma and Ki67 immunostaining as diagnostic of benign and malignant parathyroid disease. *World J Surg*. 1999;12:68–74.

200. Vargas MP, Vargas HI, Kleiner DE, Merino MJ. The role of prognostic markers (MiB-1, RB, and bcl-2) in the diagnosis of parathyroid tumors. *Mod Pathol*. 1997;10:12–7.

201. Pearce SH, Trump D, Wooding C, Sheppard MN, Clayton RN, Thakker RV. Loss of heterozygosity studies at the retinoblastoma and breast cancer susceptibility (BRCA2) loci in pituitary, parathyroid, pancreatic and carcinoid tumors. *Clin Endocrinol*. 1996;45:195–200.

202. Strewler GJ, Stern PH, Jacobs JW, et al. Parathyroid hormone like protein from human renal cell carcinoma cells. *J Clin Invest*. 1987;80:1803–1807.

203. Stewart AF, Horst R, Deftos LJ, et al. Biochemical evaluation of patients with cancer associated hypercalcemia. *N Engl J Med*. 1980;303:1377–1383.

204. Burton PBJ, Moniz C, Knight DE. Parathyroid hormone related peptide can function as an autocrine growth factor in human renal cell carcinoma. *Biochem Biophys Res Commun*. 1990;167: 1134–1138.

205. Mallette LE, Beck P, Vandepol C. Malignancy hypercalcemia. *Am J Med Sci*. 1991;302:205–210.

206. Tachimori Y, Watanabe H, Kato H, et al. Hypercalcemia in patients with esophageal carcinoma. *Cancer*. 1991;61:2625–2629.

207. Capen CC, Rosol TJ. Pathobiology of parathyroid hormone and parathyroid hormone related protein. In: LiVolsi VA, DeLellis RA, eds. *Pathobiology of the Parathyroid and Thyroid Glands*. Baltimore: Williams and Wilkins; 1993:1–33.

208. Lanske B, Kronenberg HM. Parathyroid hormone-related peptide (PTHrP) and parathyroid hormone (PTH)/PTHrP receptor. *Critical Rev Eukaryotic Gene Expres*. 1998;8:297–320.

209. Sherman LA, Pfeffernbaum A, Brown EB. Hypoparathyroidism in a patient with longstanding iron storage disease. *Ann Intern Med*. 1970;73:259–261.

210. Eipe J, Johnson SA, Kiamko RT, Bronsky D. Hypoparathyroidism following 131 I therapy for hyperparathyroidism. *Arch Intern Med*. 1968;121:270–272.

211. Kleerekoper M, Basten A, Penny R, Posen S. Idiopathic hypoparathyroidism with primary ovarian failure. *Arch Intern Med*. 1974;143:944–947.

212. Marieb NJ, Melby JC, Lyall SS. Isolated hypoaldosteronism associated with idiopathic hypoparathyroidism. *Arch Int Med*. 1974;134:424–429.

213. Van de Casseye M, Gepts W. Primary (autoimmune?) parathyroiditis. *Virchows Arch Pathol Anat*. 1973;361:257–261.

214. Neufeld M, Maclaren NK, Blizzard RM. Two types of autoimmune Addison's disease associated with polyglandular autoimmune (PGA) syndromes. *Medicine*. 1981;60:335–357.

# 30

# Perspectives on the Etiology, Demographics, and History of Hyperparathyroidism

## Phillip K. Pellitteri, D.O., F.A.C.S.

## HISTORY

The recorded history of hyperparathyroidism in modern medicine is relatively recent. Sir Richard Owen, a renowned British anatomist and curator, is generally acknowledged as being the first to describe the existence of the parathyroid glands in 1852.[1] This discovery occurred subsequent to the death of the Zoological Society of London's Indian rhinoceros, the postmortem of which was conducted by Owen and subsequently reported to the Zoological Society. In 1877, the Swedish histologist Ivar Sandstrom, reported the existence of distinct glandular tissue adjacent to the thyroid in a dog.[2] Over the subsequent two years, similar findings in other small mammals led to the search for, and ultimate discovery of, a similar organ in humans (glandulae parathyroideae), which Sandstrom reported on in 1880.

The earliest reports of clinical hyperparathyroidism involved bone disease, or osteitis fibrosa cystica, as termed by von Recklinghausen.[3] These reports, however, did not associate the characteristic changes in bone from hyperparathyroidism with parathyroid gland abnormalities. Askanazy, in 1903, reported on an autopsy performed on a patient with osteomalacia and non-fusing long bone fractures upon whom a large (>4cm) tumor was seen adjacent to the thyroid gland, noting that it might represent a parathyroid tumor.[4] It was not until Jacob Erdheim, a Viennese pathologist, discovered parathyroid gland morphologic and histo-

logic abnormalities in patients with bone disease that an association between osteomalacia and parathyroid gland function was suspected. Erdheim studied the parathyroid glands at autopsy on all patients who died with bone disease, and noted that many patients with osteomalacia and osteofibrosis cystica demonstrated enlarged parathyroid glands. He postulated that these glandular enlargements were secondary to compensatory hyperplasia and that the bone disease was the primary initiating factor.[5] Following up on initial experiments performed in rats by Eugene Gley, a French physiologist, Erdheim demonstrated that cautery destruction of the parathyroid glands in rats produced not only tetany, as shown by Gley, but also the typical dental changes consistent with calcium not being laid down.

Numerous reports of large parathyroid glands and bone disease followed until Schlagenhaufer suggested at a meeting in Vienna in 1915 that if only a single parathyroid gland was thought to be enlarged it should be excised.[6] The event which followed this suggestion years later would usher in the future treatment of parathyroid disease. Anton von Eiselberg, a pupil of Theodor Billroth, is noted as having performed the first parathyroid transplant. After performing total thyroidectomy in cats, von Eiselberg autografted half of the thyroid gland and a parathyroid gland into the animal's abdominal wall. Postoperatively, the animals showed no sign of tetany and, when subjected to histologic examination, these grafts demonstrated evidence of neovascularization.[7] William Halsted's experience with chronic hypocalcemia and thyroidectomy prompted him to study parathyroid transplantation experimentally in dogs. He demonstrated that even very small portions of parathyroid tissue surviving autograft could be lifesaving in these animals and would result in tetany and death following removal. In addition, he used intravenous calcium gluconate solution to treat animals following experimental thyroidectomy. These experiments and others sparked his ever present mandate to perform thyroidectomy carefully and meticulously avoiding injury to the parathyroid glands and their blood supply (see Chapter 1).[8]

Halsted worked with Herbert Evans, a medical student at Johns Hopkins, to define the blood supply to the parathyroid glands using vascular casting technique and emphasized that tetany following thyroidectomy was caused more by interruption of the vascular supply to the parathyroid glands than by their inadvertent removal.

From a clinical standpoint, the treatment of parathyroid disease was to change significantly with the work of Felix Mandle. Albert Gahne, the tram conductor, lived in Vienna following a bout with tuberculosis, which he acquired while serving in the army during the years 1914–1918. He subsequently developed bone pain and muscle fatigue in 1921 from which he became disabled. In 1924, following a fall which resulted in a fractured femur, he came under the treatment of Mandle, who recognized these events as being consistent with parathyroid abnormality. Believing that this might represent compensatory parathyroid hyperplasia, as postulated by Erdheim, Mandle administered fresh parathryoid extract to Albert without improvement. Subsequently, Mandle transplanted fresh parathyroid glands obtained from the victim of a street accident into Albert, which, again, did not result in any resolution of symptoms. Recalling Schlagenhaufer's suggestion of nearly 10 years earlier, Mandle explored the neck of the now severely crippled tram conductor and removed a parathyroid tumor.[9] Albert experienced a remarkable and immediate improvement in bone pain and nearly 4 years later, was walking with a cane free of pain. The disease recurred and the patient was subsequently re-explored but did not survive following the procedure.[10] This experience illustrated several important issues which would come to influence future work with surgical parathyroid disease, including clinical use of parathyroid transplantation in humans and the treatment of recurrent disease by re-exploration.

That same year (1924), Hanson developed a potent extract of the parathyroid glands, which when injected into animals, led to increased serum calcium, decreased phosphate and elevated output of calcium in the urine. When used chronically, this extract would produce os-

teoporosis in the animals.[11] The association of elevated blood calcium levels and parathyroid dysfunction was well acknowledged when Charles Martell, a sea captain, was evaluated at the Massachusetts General Hospital in 1927, found to have hypercalcemia and generalized demineralization of the skeleton felt to be caused by hyperparathyroidism. The first two of a total of six operations performed on Captain Martell was by Dr. E. Richardson, chief of surgery at MGH. These first two neck explorations yielded only a single normal parathyroid gland on each side without identification of abnormal tissue.[12] A third neck exploration was performed in New York in 1929 by Dr. Russell Patterson without success. As renal function began to deteriorate with increasing symptoms of parathyroidism, he returned to MGH under the care of Fuller Albright and Oliver Cope. Cope had experience in several parathyroid explorations under the supervision of Churchill and began cadaver dissections in preparation for re-exploration of Martell, which he did on 3 occasions in 1932 without success. At the urging of Captain Martell, who had read extensively about his own disease and the potential locations of ectopic parathyroid tissue, a mediastinal exploration, the seventh surgical procedure on Martell, was planned by Churchill. With Cope assisting, Churchill identified and removed the majority of a 3 cm tumor from the mediastinum, leaving an attached remnant portion with its vascular pedicle intact in order to avoid profound hypocalcemia. In spite of these measures, tetany developed postoperatively, which required treatment with calcium supplementation. Several weeks following surgery, Captain Martell experienced renal colic from an impacted ureteral stone, which required surgery. Unfortunately, this remarkable patient died from laryngospasm following an operation to relieve obstruction from the impacted stone. Interestingly, although the series of procedures performed on Captain Martell predated it and received more notoriety, the first successful parathyroidectomy performed in the United States took place in 1928 at Barnes Hospital of Washington University by Dr. Isaac Olch. In this instance, a large adenoma was removed precipitating a profound fall in serum calcium, which required massive doses of parathyroid extract[12,13] and intravenous calcium to save the patient.

The Nobel work of Berson and Yalow in 1963 paved the way for accurate identification of parathyroid hormone levels in serum, and heralded a new era in the presentation of patients with parathyroidism. Coupled with this, multichannel autoanalyzing systems rapidly assess blood chemical components, including calcium, in a routine fashion, thus changing the manner in which patients with hyperparathyroidism present for treatment. Instead of renal stones and bone abnormalities, patients now present in an asymptomatic fashion without significant subjective complaints and very few (if any) clinical signs. In most instances, the only abnormality facing the surgeon is an elevated serum calcium and parathyroid hormone level. It is upon these findings and the assessment of risk of developing end organ damage, that the modern day surgeon treating parathyroid disease must base his/her management decisions.

## INCIDENCE OF HYPERPARATHYROIDISM

The diagnostic evidence of primary hyperparathyroidism is based upon repetitive assessments of serum calcium elevation in concert with increased serum levels of parathyroid hormone. The incidence of hyperparathyroidism has changed dramatically over the past three decades. In the early 1970s, before the widespread use of multichannel autoanalysis of blood chemistry, Heath reported an annual incidence of 7.8 cases per 100,000 persons in Rochester, Minnesota.[15] Following the introduction of routine serum calcium assessment later in the 1970s, the incidence rate rose dramatically to 51 cases per 100,000 persons per year. After the most prevalent or clinically significant cases were managed, the incidence declined to 27 cases annually per 100,000, and recent reports indicate that within the population associated with this area of Minnesota, a steady decline in the incidence of hyperparathyroidism since the late 1970s has been noted. This can not be easily explained by the more limited routine use of multichannel autoanalyzing of blood, which has become part of cost-saving measures in the late 1990s; nor has this declining incidence been similarly experienced in other populations nationally or internationally. A higher rate of incidence was noted in the "Stockholm Study" which examined over 15,000 subjects over a 2-year period (1971–1973) with a follow-up at 10 years. The early rate was assessed at 6 cases per 1,000 persons which, at the 10-year follow-up, was verified to be 4.4 cases per 1,000 persons. This rate has not changed appreciably over a 20 year period, in contrast to the Rochester experience.[16] One may postulate that the Rochester experience is unique in that after securing a very high incidence rate promulgated by routine calcium screening, higher prevalence cases were eliminated to reveal a lower base incidence rate in a population that receives its treatment at a single major center, thus explaining the steady decline in this fixed population base.

There appears to be a distinct predilection for this disease to have a higher incidence in females, especially those patients beyond the menopause. The highest prevalence rate among females in the Stockholm experience confirmed at the 10 year follow-up was approximately 13 per thousand, which represented a female to male ratio of about 4:1. This experience is similar to that of other published reports.[15,17,18,19,20] The limitation in widespread routine multichannel screening of blood, which is currently being experienced by health providers in the United States as mandated by managed care organizations and insurers, is certain to affect the rate at which hyperparathyroidism is detected. The anticipated decline in the incidence of this disease as a result of this occurrence may herald an era in which physicians are initially exposed to the disorder at a point when patients actually present with symptoms of the disease, instead of abnormal serum chemistry. In this scenario, the manner by which hyperparathyroidism is diagnosed and managed may be expected to come full circle with respect to its historical beginnings.

## ETIOLOGY AND PATHOGENESIS

Parathyroid adenomas appear to be monoclonal or oligoclonal neoplasms, whereby the mechanism of propagation is felt to be clonal expansion of cells which have an altered sensitivity to calcium.[21] Arnold's work indicates that the molecular events which appear to trigger clonal propagation are heterogeneous. The genetic mutational events which occur in hyperparathyroidism have been characterized in a minority of tumors. Among those events identified are genetic rearrangements of the PRAD 1, or parathyroid adenomatosis 1 oncogene, which is also known as cyclin D1. This proto-oncogene is located in the vicinity of the regulatory region of the gene for PTH production[22,23] (Figure 30–1). The subsequent realignment of DNA in this event now combines a growth promoter (PRAD 1) with a regulatory region that would ordinarily control only PTH synthesis. This genetic realignment has not been uniformly demonstrated in a majority of parathyroid adenomas, with only a minimal number having been shown to manifest the rearrangement.

A more common molecular event, postulated to occur in parathyroid neoplasia, is alteration in tumor suppressor gene expression (Figure 30–2). In order for this gene to be inactivated and thus product deficient, both alleles on the gene must be affected by the mutational event. Thus, tumorigenesis occurs as a sequential event by inactivation of both copies of the suppressor gene.[24] The most well known of these is the MEN 1 tumor suppressor gene which demonstrates somatic mutations in both gene copies in 20% of patients with primary hyperparathyroidism.[25] Not surprisingly, this gene was initially recognized in patients with the MEN 1 syndrome.[26] Evidence of loss of suppressor gene function on chromosome 1p has been postulated as being an even more common event in the development of sporadic parathyroid adenomas. It has been suggested that

## Pericentromeric Inversion of Chromosome 11 in Parathyroid Adenomas

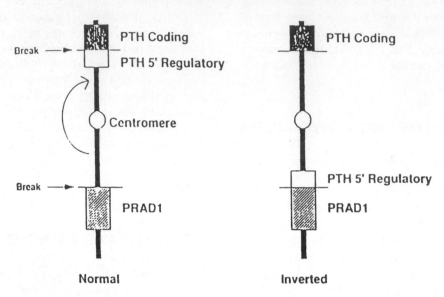

**Figure 30–1.** Genetic rearrangement of the parathyroid hormone gene in primary hyperparathyroidism. Pericentromeric inversion of chromosome 11 illustrating PRAD 1 and PTH gene rearrangement. (From Arnold A. Molecular genetics of parathyroid gland neoplasia. *J Clin Endocrinol Metab.* 1993;77:1108–1112. ©The Endocrine Society; reprinted with permission.)

## Postulated Roles of Tumor Suppressor Genes in Parathyroid Neoplasia

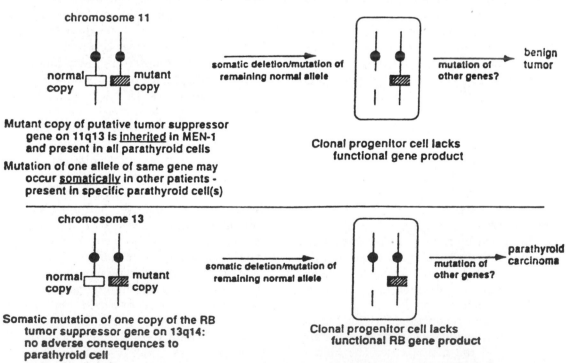

**Figure 30–2.** Hypothesized roles of inactivated tumor suppressor genes in the development of parathyroid neoplasia. (From Arnold A. Molecular genetics of parathyroid gland neoplasia. *J Clin Endocrinol Metab.* 1993;77:1108–1112. ©The Endocrine Society; reprinted with permission.)

patients with this chromosomal abnormality may be subject to developing the same constellation of endocrine changes found in MEN 1 syndrome and perhaps at an earlier age.[24] Suspected loss of tumor suppressor gene function has been identified in other chromosomal loci in patients with parathyroid adenomas, including the sites 15q, 9p, 6q and 1q.[24]

Point mutations in the calcium sensing receptor gene which reduce the activity of this gene have been elucidated as the basis for familial hypocalciuric hypercalcemia (FHH) and neonatal severe hyperparathyroidism.[27] Thus, it would seem that this gene would represent a likely candidate for molecular rearrangement and altered calcium sensing function in patients with hyperparathyroidism. To date, however, a calcium-sensing receptor gene mutation or allelic inactivation has not been demonstrated in these patients. It has been postulated that alterations in the calcium-sensing function in primary hyperparathyroidism may represent post-genomic events related to reduced RNA transcript or the actual protein receptor in the parathryoid cell clone.[28] Whether this may represent the primary cause for, or secondary effect of, hypercalcemia remains to be determined. Abnormalities in the parathyroid cell's vitamin D receptor similarly may represent changes occurring secondary to hypercalcemia and not a primary genetic event. An inactivating mutation in the gene coding for this receptor has been postulated in primary hyperparathyroidism, but results from these investigations are conflicting.[29]

Firm evidence supports the theory that ionizing radiation can represent the etiologic factor in several solid and humoral human cancers. Tisell observed that there appears to be an association between exposure to ionizing radiation to the head and neck at an early age and the late development of hyperparathyroidism.[30] This finding is supported by other independent observations where hyperparathyroidism has developed, presumably as a late complication of radiation therapy to the head and neck, similar to the finding noted with differentiated thyroid cancer.

## SUMMARY

The management of parathyroid disease has enjoyed a brief but nevertheless "storied" evolution involving the combined effort of pioneers in anatomy, pathology, physiology, medicine and surgery. Technological advances in screening large populations of patients ushered in a new era of surgical care for patients with hyperparathyroidism which, for the most part, was not associated with the symptom complex which inspired the work of von Recklinghausen, Mandle, Hanson, Cope, and others. Modern day forces, which have

shaped medical practice around cost containment, may indeed bring back the period in which patients present, again, with "bones, groans and stones." Regardless, the history of hyperparathyroidism is a fascinating documentary of medical science at its best, reflecting all that inspires physicians and surgeons to discovery in the care of their patients.

## References

1. Taylor S. Hyperparathyroidism: retrospect and prospect. *Ann R Coll Surg.* 1976; 58:255–265.
2. Seiple C. *On a New Gland in Man and Several Mammals* (Glandulae Parathyroideae). Sandström I, (transl.) Baltimore: Johns Hopkins Press, 1938.
3. Von Recklinghausen F. Die fibrose oder deformierende ostitis, die osteomalacie und die osteoplastiche Karzinosk in ihren gegenseitigen Beziehumgen. Excerpted from Taylor S, history of hyperparathyroidism. In: *Progr Surg.* 1986;18:1–11.
4. Askanazy M. Uber ostitis deformans ohne osteideo Genebe. *Arb Pathol Inst Tübingen.* 1904;4:398–422.
5. Erdheim J. Tetania parathyreopriva. *Mih Grenzes Mes Chir.* 1906; 16:632–744.
6. Schlagenitaufer F. Zwei Fälle von Parathyreoideatumoren. *Wien. Klin. Wschr.* 1915;28:1362.
7. Von Eiselsberg A. Über Erfolgreiche Einbeilung der Katzenshilddrüse in die Bauchdecke und Autreten von Tetanie nach deren extirpation. *Wien Klin Wochenschr.* 1892;5:81–85.
8. Halsted W, Evans H. The parathyroid glandules: their blood supply and their preservation in operation upon the thyroid gland. *Ann Surg.* 1907; 46:489–506.
9. Mandle F. Attempt to treat generalized fibrous osteitis by extirpation of parathyroid tumor. *Zentiabl F. Chir.* 1926;53:260–264. Orgara C, transl., 1984.
10. Bauer W, Albright F, Aub J. A case of osteitis fibrosa cystica (osteomalacia) with evidence of hyperactivity of the parathyroid bodies: metabolic study. *J Clin Invest.* 1930;8:229–248.
11. Collip J. Extraction of a parathyroid hormone which will prevent or control parathyroid tetany and which regulates the levels of blood calcium. *J Biol Chem.* 1925;63:395–438.
12. Richardson E, Aub J, Bauer W. Parathyroidectomy in osteomalacia. *Ann Surg.* 1929; 90:730–741.
13. Hanson A. An elementary chemical study of the parathyroid glands of cattle. *Milit Surgeon.* 1923;52:280–284.
14. Barr D, Bulger H, Dixon H. Hyperparathyroidism. *J Am Med Assoc.* 1929;92:951–952.
15. Heath H, Hodgson S, Kennedy M. Primary hyperparathyroidism. Incidence, morbidity, and potential economic impact in a community. *New Engl J Med.* 1980; 302:189.
16. Christensson T, Hellström K, Wengue B, Alveryd A. Prevalence of hypercalcemia in a health screening in Stockholm. *ALDA Med Scand.* 1976;200:131–137.
17. Boonstra C, Jackson C. Serum calcium survey for hyperparathyroidism: results in 50,000 clinic patients. *Am J Clin Path.* 1971;55: 523.
18. Haff R, Black W, Ballinger W. Primary hyperparathyroidism: changing clinical, surgical and pathologic aspects. *Ann Surg.* 1970; 171:85.
19. Johasson H, Thoren L, Werner I. Hyperparathyroidism. Clinical experiences from 208 cases. *Upsal J Med Sci.* 1972;77:41.
20. Williamson E, Van Peevan H. Patient benefits in discovering occult hyperparathyroidism. *Arcot Intern Med.* 1974;133:430.
21. Arnold A, Staunton C, Kim H, et al. Monoclonality and abnormal parathyroid hormone genes in parathyroid adenomas. *N Engl J Med.* 1988;318:658–662.

22. Arnold A, Kim H, Gaz R, et al. Molecular cloning and chromosomal mapping of DNA rearranged with the parathyroidal hormone given in parathyroidal adenoma. *J Clin Invest.* 1989;83: 2034–2040.

23. Friedman E, Bale A, Marx S, et al. Genetic abnormalities in sporadic parathyroid adenoma. *J Clin endocrinol Metab.* 1990;71: 293–297.

24. Arnold A. Genetic basis of endocrine disease 5: molecular genetics of parathyroid gland neoplasia. *J Clin Endocrinol Metab.* 1993; 77:1108–1112.

25. Heppner C, Kester M, Agarwal S, et al. Somatic mutation of the men 1 gene in parathyroid tumors. *Nat Genet.* 1997; 16:375–378.

26. Tahara H, Smith A, Gaz B, et al. Genetic localization of novel candidate tumor suppressor gene loci in human parathyroid adenomas. *Cancer Res.* 1996;56:599–605.

27. Pollak M, Brown E, Chou Y-Hw, et al. Mutations in the human $Ca^{2+}$-sensing receptor gene cause familial hypocalciuric hypocalcemia and neonatal severe hyperparathyroidism. *Cell.* 1993;75: 1297–1303.

28. Kifor O, Moore F, Wang P, et al. Reduced immunosustaining for the extra cellular calcium sensing receptor in primary and uremic secondary hyperparathyroidism. *J Clin Endocrinol Metab.* 1996;81: 1598–1606.

29. Carling T, Ridefelt P, Hellman P, et al. Vitamin D receptor polymorphisms correlate to parathyroid cell function in primary hyperparathyroidism. *J Clin Endocrinol Metab.* 1997;82:1772–1775.

30. Tisell L, Carlson S, Lindberg S, Ragnhult I. Kan Strålterapi iducera hyperparathyroidism. *Svensk Kirurgi.* 1975;32:83–85.

# 31

# Evaluation of Hypercalcemia and the Diagnosis of Hyperparathyroidism

## Bart L. Clarke, M.D., F.A.C.P., F.A.C.E.

## EVALUATION OF HYPERCALCEMIA

Hypercalcemia has been reported as occurring in 1–3.9% of the general adult population, and 0.2–2.9% of hospitalized populations.[1] Patients with hypercalcemia present with widely variable clinical symptoms, depending on the severity of the hypercalcemia. Most commonly, mild hypercalcemia is asymptomatic, but severe hypercalcemia may become life threatening, especially when the serum calcium is greater than 14.0 mg/dL. Serum ionized calcium is essential for numerous physiological processes, and is therefore tightly regulated by homeostatic mechanisms (see chapter 30).

The definition of hypercalcemia is dependent on the range of normal serum calcium. In most assays, this is reported as 8.5–10.5 mg/dL. Variation in the normal range reported by different laboratories depends largely on differences in assay method. Circulating serum calcium binds to proteins (47%), primarily albumin, and complexes to circulating anions such as bicarbonate, phosphate, citrate or sulfate (10%). The remainder of serum calcium is found as the free ionized form (43%). Only free ionized calcium exerts physiological effects. Free ionized calcium is the major regulator of parathyroid hormone (PTH) secretion.

Several factors may influence measured serum total or ionized calcium. Commonly, alterations in serum albumin level increase or decrease serum total calcium without affecting the ionized calcium level. Albumin binds about 70% of the circulating calcium bound to protein, and has roughly twelve calcium-binding regions per molecule. Under normal circumstances only 20% of these calcium-binding sites are occupied by serum calcium. Decreases in serum albumin below 4.0 g/dL decrease total calcium by 0.8 mg/dL for each 1.0 g/dL decrease in serum albumin. Correspondingly, increases in serum albumin above 4.0 g/dL increase serum total calcium by 0.8 mg/dL for each 1.0 g/dL increase in serum albumin. Occasionally, monoclonal proteins may bind serum calcium sufficiently to increase the total serum calcium but leave ionized calcium in the normal range. Dehydration may increase total serum calcium because of the resulting hemoconcentration. Acidemia increases serum ionized calcium by decreasing binding of calcium to albumin, and alkalemia decreases ionized calcium by increasing binding of calcium to albumin, without affecting serum total calcium. Under most circumstances, measurement of serum total calcium is appropriate and adequate, but serum ionized calcium should be measured in complex situations associated with changes in albumin concentration or blood pH.[2]

Serum calcium reflects the balance between calcium influx into and calcium efflux from extracellular fluid. Calcium influx into extracellular fluid is derived from intestinal absorption, skeletal resorption, and renal reabsorption, and calcium efflux from extracellular fluid is determined by intestinal secretion, skeletal uptake, and renal excretion. Hypercalcemia, therefore, usually results when the rate of calcium influx into the extracellular fluid exceeds the rate of calcium efflux from extracellular fluid.

Under pathological conditions, hypercalcemia usually results from increased skeletal resorption or intestinal absorption with normal or decreased renal excretion. Hypercalcemia may also result from normal calcium influx into the extracellular fluid, with decreased renal excretion or defective skeletal mineralization. Increased skeletal resorption typically is caused by accelerated osteoclast recruitment and activation, most often under the influence of parathyroid hormone (PTH), parathyroid hormone-related protein (PTHrp), or 1,25-dihydroxyvitamin D.[3] Other cytokines that may stimulate osteoclast recruitment or activation include interleukin (IL)-1α, IL-1β, IL-6, tumor necrosis factor (TNF)-α, lymphotoxin, or transforming growth factor (TGF)-β. Increased intestinal absorption of calcium is a less common cause of hypercalcemia, although this may occur with increased 1,25-dihydroxyvitamin D production by extra-renal 1α-hydroxylase activity or absorptive hypercalciuria. Under most circumstances associated with increased calcium influx into extracellular fluid, the kidneys normally compensate appropriately by increasing urinary calcium excretion. Serum calcium levels do not typically increase unless the kidneys fail to clear the filtered calcium load.

Other factors may indirectly affect serum calcium. Increased levels of PTH or PTHrp directly stimulate renal tubular reabsorption of filtered calcium, thereby decreasing renal calcium excretion to some degree. Hypercalcemia inhibits the normal action of antidiuretic hormone (ADH) to increase free water reabsorption in the distal renal tubule, resulting in nephrogenic diabetes insipidus. Nausea and vomiting directly resulting from hypercalcemia may lead to further hemoconcentration. Significant volume depletion of any cause may eventually limit renal calcium excretion. Immobilization, especially when patients have Paget's disease of bone, but also with spinal cord injuries, space flight, or any other cause of prolonged bed rest, may directly increase bone resorption caused by decreased gravitational biomechanical effects on the skeleton.

The recently reported G-protein-coupled extracellular calcium-sensing receptor (CaSR) plays a major role in regulation of extracellular calcium.[4] The CaSR is found on parathyroid, renal tubular, osteoblast, and intestinal mucosal cells, as well as many other cells. This receptor interacts with ionized calcium and other cations in extracellular fluid in a classic hormone-receptor G-protein-linked signal transduction mechanism. Interactions between ionized calcium and the CaSR specifically regulate PTH secretion by parathyroid cells and renal tubular calcium resorption, and probably regulate bone turnover and intestinal calcium absorption as well. The CaSR is a 7-transmembrane segment receptor with a large extracellular portion that binds ionized calcium and other cations, and a shorter intracellular portion that interacts with a variety of G-proteins and signal-transduction pathways. It is thought to be part of a larger family of not yet described calcium- or cation-binding receptors.

Hypercalcemia may cause a variety of clinical symptoms. Neurologic dysfunction is often reported, and may range from subtle cognitive impairment or drowsiness to depression, confusion, delirium, or obtundation.[5] Muscle weakness may be prominent if the hypercalcemia is severe. Constipation is commonly reported, and anorexia, nausea, or vomiting may be present, caused by more severe hypercalcemia. Pancreatitis or peptic ulcer disease have been associated with hypercalcemia, especially that caused by primary hyperparathyroidism, but the pathophysiological mechanism of this association remains uncertain. Frequent urination and thirst are not uncommon with moderate hypercalcemia, and result from the increased renal water clearance necessary to excrete the filtered calcium load. Kidney stones or nephrocalcinosis may occur eventually, especially if the hypercalcemia is persistent. A variety of cardiac manifestations of hypercalcemia have been described, including decreased repolarization time associated with shortened QT interval. Bradycardia, first-degree atrioventricular block, and other cardiac dysrhythmias may also occur. Chronic hypercalcemia may eventually be associated with osteopenia or osteoporosis and subsequent increased fracture risk. Most patients with hypercalcemia remain asymptomatic unless the serum calcium increases above a threshold of about 12 mg/dL, or the serum calcium is rapidly increasing. Virtually all patients become symptomatic when the serum calcium exceeds 14 mg/dL, although occasional patients with excessively high serum calcium levels may remain impressively asymptomatic or only mildly symptomatic.

The differential diagnosis of hypercalcemia is broad. It is still true that the most common cause of outpatient hypercalcemia is primary hyperparathyroidism, and that the most common cause of hypercalcemia in hospitalized patients is malignancy. Fortunately, the differential diagnosis of hypercalcemia can be broadly divided into PTH-mediated and non-PTH-mediated hypercalcemia (Tables 31–1, 31–2, and 31–3).

PTH-mediated hypercalcemia is most frequently caused by primary hyperparathyroidism (Table 31-1). However, it may be caused by physiologic secondary hyperparathyroidism, defined as hyperparathyroidism caused by a recognized physiologic cause without associated renal insufficiency, or pathologic secondary hyperparathyroidism, with associated renal insufficiency. Tertiary hyperparathyroidism may occur in patients with long-standing renal insufficiency or failure.

Physiologic secondary hyperparathyroidism most commonly occurs in patients with insufficient calcium intake, decreased intestinal calcium absorption, insufficient vitamin D intake or malabsorption, or renal

**Table 31–1.** Causes of PTH-Mediated Hypercalcemia

---

Primary Hyperparathyroidism

    Parathyroid adenoma

    Parathyroid lipoadenoma

    Parathyroid hyperplasia

    Parathyroid carcinoma

    Neck or mediastinal parathyroid cyst

Secondary Hyperparathyroidism

Tertiary Hyperparathyroidism

---

hypercalciuria, and represents the homeostatic attempt to maintain normal serum calcium at all costs. It is important to distinguish physiologic secondary hyperparathyroidism from primary hyperparathyroidism prior to embarking on surgical correction of presumed primary hyperparathyroidism. The biochemical distinction between primary and physiologic secondary hyperparathyroidism will be further discussed later in this chapter in the section on diagnosis of primary hyperparathyroidism.

Pathologic secondary hyperparathyroidism and tertiary hyperparathyroidism occur because of renal insufficiency or failure. It is thought that the hyperparathyroidism associated with these conditions results from subtle ionized hypocalcemia persisting over months to years, resulting in chronic stimulation of the parathyroid glands. Eventually, after long-standing renal insufficiency or failure, parathyroid glands may become autonomous and no longer respond to regulation by serum ionized calcium, and develop tertiary hyperparathyroidism. Secondary and tertiary hyperparathyroidism are further addressed in Chapters 39–40.

Familial hypocalciuric hypercalcemia (FHH)[6,7] may mimic the serum biochemical appearance of primary hyperparathyroidism, and should not be confused with primary hyperparathyroidism, as this may result in unnecessary parathyroid surgery. This autosomal dominant disorder, linked to chromosomes 3q, 19p, and 19q, is largely caused by inactivating mutations in the parathyroid cell CaSR linked to chromosome 3q,[8] and results in mild hypercalcemia associated with high normal or mildly increased intact PTH levels. Cases linked to chromosomes 19p and 19q are thought to be caused by mutations in as yet unknown genes. Patients with FHH have low 24-hour urinary calcium excretion relative to their hypercalcemia. The best current test to distinguish FHH from primary hyperparathyroidism is the 24-hour urinary calcium to creatinine clearance ratio.[6] Calculation of this ratio requires knowledge of the 24-hour urinary calcium and creatinine, with simultaneously measured serum calcium and creatinine. The ratio is derived as $U_{Ca} \times S_{Cr} / S_{Ca} \times U_{Cr}$. Patients with FHH typically have ratios of less than 0.01, whereas patients with primary hyperparathyroidism have ratios greater than 0.01.

The second most common cause of hypercalcemia is malignancy (Table 31–2). The most common cause of malignancy-associated hypercalcemia is humoral hypercalcemia of malignancy (HHM) caused by excessive PTHrp secretion by tumors of various types.[9] A wide range of solid tumors has been reported to secrete excessive PTHrp, including cancers of the lung, esophagus, head and neck, kidney, ovary, bladder, breast, and pancreas. In addition, thymic carcinoma, islet cell carcinoma, malignant carcinoid tumors, and sclerosing hepatic carcinomas have been reported to secrete excessive PTHrp. Various patients with adult T-cell leukemia or lymphoma or B-cell lymphoma have also been shown to produce excess PTHrp.[10,11]

Ectopic PTH secretion has been well documented in single cases of small cell lung cancer, small cell ovarian carcinoma,[12] squamous cell lung carcinoma, ovarian adenocarcinoma, thymoma, papillary thyroid carcinoma,[13] hepatocellular carcinoma, and undifferentiated neuroendocrine tumor. Ectopic 1,25-dihydroxyvitamin D may be produced in excess by B-cell lymphomas,[14–16] Hodgkin's disease,[17] or lymphomatoid granulomatosis.[18] A variety of tumor cells produce other cytokines in excess that may cause hypercalcemia. T-cell lymphomas and leukemias, non-Hodgkin's lymphomas, and other hematologic malignancies are most likely to produce these bone-resorbing cytokines.

Hypercalcemia caused by malignancy may be caused on occasion by extensive lytic bone metastases caused by multiple myeloma, lymphomas, breast can-

**Table 31–2.** Causes of hypercalcemia of malignancy

---

PTHrp secretion by lung, esophagus, head and neck, renal cell, ovary, bladder, and pancreatic cancers, thymic carcinoma, islet cell carcinoma, carcinoid, sclerosing hepatic carcinoma

Ectopic PTH secretion by small cell lung cancer, small cell ovarian carcinoma, squamous cell lung carcinoma, ovarian adenocarcinoma, thymoma, papillary thyroid carcinoma, hepatocellular carcinoma, undifferentiated neuroendocrine tumor

Ectopic 1,25-dihydroxyvitamin D production by B-cell lymphoma, Hodgkin's disease, lymphomatoid granulomatosis

Lytic bone metastases caused by multiple myeloma, lymphomas, breast cancer, invasive sarcoma

Tumor production of other cytokines by T-cell lymphomas/leukemias, non-Hodgkin's lymphoma, and other hematologic malignancies

---

cer, or invasive sarcomas.[19] In most cases where extensive bone destruction is the mechanism, patients are late in the course of their malignancy and the underlying diagnosis is not often in doubt.

There are many non-malignant causes of non-PTH-mediated hypercalcemia (Table 31–3). Benign

**Table 31–3.** Causes of non-PTH-mediated, non-malignant hypercalcemia

---

Benign Tumors: PTHrp-secreting ovarian dermoid cyst or uterine fibroid

Endocrine Disease
   Thyrotoxicosis
   Pheochromocytoma
   Addison's disease
   Islet cell pancreatic tumors
   VIPoma

Granulomatous Disorders
   Sarcoidosis
   Wegener's granulomatosis
   Berylliosis
   Silicone- and paraffin-induced granulomatosis
   Eosinophilic granuloma
   Tuberculosis (focal, disseminated, MAC in AIDS)
   Histoplasmosis
   Coccidioidomycosis
   Candidiasis
   Leprosy
   Cat-scratch disease

Drugs
   Vitamin D excess (oral or topical)
   Vitamin A excess
   Thiazide diuretics
   Lithium
   Estrogens and antiestrogens
   Androgens
   Aminophylline, theophylline
   Gancyclovir
   Recombinant growth hormone treatment of AIDS patients
   Foscarnet
   8-chloro-cyclic AMP

Miscellaneous
   Familial Hypocalciuric Hypercalcemia
   Immobilization with or without Paget's disease of bone
   End-stage liver failure
   Total parenteral nutrition
   Milk-alkali syndrome
   Hypophosphatasia
   Systemic lupus erythematosus
   Juvenile rheumatoid arthritis
   Recent hepatitis B vaccination
   Gaucher's disease with acute pneumonia
   Aluminum intoxication (chronic hemodialysis)
   Manganese intoxication
   Primary oxalosis

---

tumors, including ovarian dermoid cysts or uterine fibroids, may occasionally secrete PTHrp or other bone-resorbing cytokines.[20] Non-PTH-mediated hypercalcemia may be caused by a variety of endocrine disorders including thyrotoxicosis (resulting from increased bone resorption),[21] pheochromocytoma (caused by coexisting primary hyperparathyroidism in multiple endocrine neoplasia II-A, or increased secretion of PTHrp or catecholamines),[22,23] adrenal insufficiency or crisis (caused by volume depletion or hemoconcentration),[24] and VIPomas (resulting from excess secretion of vasoactive intestinal peptide causing dehydration and metabolic acidosis).[25]

Granulomatous diseases not infrequently cause hypercalcemia when malignancy or endocrine disorders are not present, especially in younger and middle-aged adults, and may occasionally present with hypercalcemia. Granuloma macrophages may produce extra-renal 1α-hydroxylase activity, which causes increased total body 1,25-dihydroxyvitamin D synthesis.[26] Case reports of hypercalcemia caused by overproduction of 1,25-dihydroxyvitamin D have come from patients with sarcoidosis,[27] Wegener's granulomatosis,[28] berylliosis,[29] silicone-[30] or paraffin-induced[31] granulomatosis, eosinophilic granuloma,[32] focal or disseminated tuberculosis[33] and *Mycobacterium avium-intracellulare* complex in AIDS, histoplasmosis,[34] coccidioidomycosis,[35] Candidiasis,[36] leprosy,[37] and cat-scratch disease.[38]

Certain medications may cause hypercalcemia by a variety of mechanisms. Excess vitamin D intake may stimulate intestinal calcium absorption,[39] and thiazide diuretics may directly inhibit renal calcium excretion.[40] Lithium therapy may interfere with the ability of calcium to interact with parathyroid and renal CaSRs, thereby increasing PTH secretion by the parathyroid glands.[41] Vitamin A excess may stimulate bone resorption by uncertain mechanisms.[42] A variety of other agents, including estrogens,[43] antiestrogens or androgens,[44] aminophylline or theophylline,[45] gancyclovir, recombinant growth hormone in AIDS patients,[46] foscarnet,[47] and 8-chloro-cyclic AMP[48] may affect other physiologic mechanisms resulting in hypercalcemia. A variety of other miscellaneous disorders may also be associated with hypercalcemia, as listed in Table 31–3.

Hypercalcemia should be treated initially with rapid normal saline rehydration as tolerated, followed by saline diuresis induced by furosemide or other loop diuretics. Thiazide diuretics should be specifically avoided in patients with hypercalcemia, but may be used if hypercalcemia has resolved and is not recurrent. If rehydration and diuresis are not sufficient to normalize serum calcium or maintain normalization, intravenous pamidronate 30–90 mg over 3–4 hours or intravenous etidronate 5 mg/kg are usually effective. Other options include intravenous plicamycin (mithramycin) at 15–25 μg/kg over 4–6 hours, intramuscular or subcutaneous salmon calcitonin 4–8 units/kg every 6–8 hours, or intravenous gallium nitrate at 200 mg/m²/day over 5 days. Glucocorticoid therapy, given as hydrocortisone 200–300 mg/day or equivalent for 3–5 days, may also be used to decrease hypercalcemia, especially if it is caused by lymphoma, multiple myeloma, granulomatous disease, or vitamin D excess. Intravenous phosphate should never be used to lower serum calcium because of the potential for resulting severe organ dysfunction and death. Oral phosphate is not normally useful as an intestinal calcium binder in chronic hypercalcemic states because of the risk of ectopic calcium phosphate deposition caused by alterations in the tissue calcium phosphate product. Hemodialysis with low or zero calcium dialysate may be appropriate in extreme circumstances.

## DIAGNOSIS OF PRIMARY HYPERPARATHYROIDISM

Primary hyperparathyroidism is the most common cause of outpatient hypercalcemia.[49,50] The incidence of this disorder is estimated to be 1:1,000 in men and 2–3:1,000 in women. Primary hyperparathyroidism occurs at all ages, but most commonly in postmenopausal women in the 6th decade. The incidence of primary hyperparathyroidism has been declining in Olmsted County, Minnesota, but it is not yet clear whether this reflects a national trend.[51] Restriction of routine measurement of serum calcium in the modern health care environment will likely further reduce recognized cases of primary hyperparathyroidism.

Primary hyperparathyroidism is caused by inappropriate secretion or oversecretion of PTH. Solitary parathyroid adenomas are responsible for primary hyperparathyroidism in 80–85% of cases, whereas four-gland hyperplasia is responsible in 15–20% of cases, and parathyroid cancer in less than 0.5% of cases. Histologic diagnosis of parathyroid carcinoma is difficult, and is usually based on evidence of local tissue or vascular invasion or metastatic disease.[52] The majority of single adenomas represent sporadic disease, whereas four-gland hyperplasia implies a familial disorder, most commonly multiple endocrine neoplasia (MEN) types I or IIA. It appears that parathyroid adenomas secrete excess PTH because of loss of feedback control of PTH secretion by extracellular calcium at the cellular level, caused by an increased set point for suppression of PTH secretion. Hyperplastic parathyroid glands are thought to secrete excess PTH because of the increased number of parathyroid cells, with each parathyroid cell maintaining a normal calcium set point for suppression of PTH secretion.

The etiology of sporadic primary hyperparathyroidism is not well understood. Previous neck irradiation contributes in a minority of cases, typically causing primary hyperparathyroidism 20–30 years after exposure. More commonly, parathyroid adenomas represent clonal expansion of a single or several abnormal cells, caused by a genetic abnormality resulting either in stimulation of cell proliferation or loss of inhibition of cell proliferation.[53] A small number of adenomas have been found with a PRAD1 (cyclin D1) proto-oncogene rearrangement, in which the PRAD1 gene was inserted adjacent to PTH gene enhancer elements, resulting in stimulation of parathyroid cell division whenever PTH secretion was stimulated by hypocalcemia. PRAD1 protein expression has been reported to be increased in about 20% of parathyroid adenomas. Up to 17% of parathyroid adenomas have been found to have mutations in the MEN-I (menin) gene. The MEN-I gene normally functions as a tumor suppressor gene, and it is thought that mutations in this gene result in loss of control of parathyroid cell division. Evaluation of parathyroid adenomas by techniques assessing for loss of allelic heterozygosity has shown a number of other potential sites for parathyroid oncogenes on chromosomes 16p and 19, and loss of tumor suppressor genes on chromosomes 1p, 1q, 6q, 13q, and other sites. It is evident that sporadic parathyroid tumors do not have common genetic mutations responsible for the majority of tumors. Interestingly, no study to date has shown parathyroid adenomas to have detectable CaSR abnormalities.

Most patients currently diagnosed with primary hyperparathyroidism present with asymptomatic mild hypercalcemia, typically with serum calcium levels in the 10.0–11.0 mg/dL range. Many patients have osteopenia at diagnosis, which may be caused predominantly by age or menopausal status. More severely affected cases may have classical bone features, including osteitis fibrosa cystica, with distal phalangeal subperiosteal bone resorption, distal clavicular resorption, "salt and pepper" skull, bone cysts, and long bone brown tumors, or osteoporosis, predominantly at cortical sites such as the mid- or distal one third radius. Patients with osteoporosis commonly also have osteoporosis at skeletal trabecular sites. One recent study demonstrated increased fracture risk in patients with primary hyperparathyroidism.[54] Classical osteitis fibrosa cystica is currently recognized in fewer than 5% of patients. Kidney disease, including renal insufficiency caused by chronic or relatively acute hypercalciuria, nephrocalcinosis, or calcium-containing nephrolithiasis, may be seen in up to 20% of patients. Hypercalciuria has been reported in up to as many as 30% of patients. Neuropsychiatric imbalances are often reported, typically as mild fatigue or weakness with subtle cognitive impairment.[55] Previously reported associations with peptic ulcer disease or pancreatitis are probably not causally related to hypercalcemia, unless associated with MEN syndromes. Some patients, usually more symptomatic, may have mild hypertension, coronary artery or cardiac valvular calcifications, or septal and left ventricular hypertrophy. Other classically described abnormalities of primary hyperparathyroidism, such as gout or pseudogout, anemia of chronic disease, ocular band keratopathy, or tooth loss caused by lamina densa resorption, are only infrequently or rarely seen today. Occasional patients may present with severe hypercalcemia caused by acute primary hyperparathyroidism or parathyroid crisis, but this usually represents previously unrecognized primary hyperparathyroidism with supervening dehydration associated with exacerbation of another medical condition.

Diagnosis of primary hyperparathyroidism is usually straightforward based on minimal criteria involving the serum total calcium and intact PTH levels. Patients classically present with increased serum total calcium with frankly increased or inappropriately high-normal PTH levels. Some patients with surgically proven primary hyperparathyroidism present with high-normal serum total calcium, with inappropriately high-normal or increased PTH levels. It is important to recognize that patients with primary hyperparathyroidism almost always have documented increased serum total or ionized calcium sometime during their course, with the acknowledgment that serum calcium exhibits some variation over time.

It is difficult to be certain that patients with serum calcium documented over time to be mostly in the mid- to lower-normal range have primary hyperparathyroidism, even if they are found to have increased intact PTH levels, because of the possibility of physiologic secondary hyperparathyroidism discussed earlier in this chapter. Patients with mid- to lower-normal serum calcium levels associated with increased intact PTH levels should be further evaluated to ensure that they do not have low calcium or vitamin D intake, calcium or vitamin D malabsorption, inability to convert 25-hydroxyvitamin D to biologically active 1,25-dihydroxyvitamin D, or significant hypercalciuria. Each of these situations, independently or in combination, could explain the findings of mid- to low-normal serum calcium and increased intact PTH. Patients with low calcium intake of less than 600 mg/day or intestinal calcium malabsorption will usually maintain serum total calcium in the normal range at the expense of skeletal calcium, and have normal serum 25-hydroxyvitmin D levels, but have 24-hour urinary calcium below 100 mg/day, often below 50 mg/day. Patients with low vitamin D intake or intestinal vitamin D malabsorption will usually have serum 25-hydroxyvitamin D levels

below 20 ng/mL (normal range, 14–80 ng/mL) and often have low 24-hour urinary calcium values. Patients unable to convert serum 25-hydroxyvitamin D to biologically active 1,25-dihydroxyvitamin D because of renal insufficiency or specific inhibitors of renal 1α-hydroxylase activity (as in oncogenic osteomalacia) typically have normal serum 25-hydroxyvitamin D but low or undetectable serum 1,25-dihydroxyvitamin D levels (normal range, 15–60 pg/mL). Patients with idiopathic hypercalciuria typically have 24-hour urine calcium values in excess of 400 mg/day. Since patients with primary hyperparathyroidism are expected to have at least relative hypercalciuria, it may be difficult to distinguish patients with true primary hyperparathyroidism from those with idiopathic hypercalciuria and high-normal serum total calcium.

Patients with primary hyperparathyroidism usually have serum phosphate in the low-normal to mildly decreased range. Patients with simultaneously high-normal or increased serum calcium and high-normal or increased serum phosphate should be investigated further for intestinal hyperabsorptive states or vitamin D excess.

Serum total or bone alkaline phosphatase may be normal or mildly increased in patients with primary hyperparathyroidism. Chronic intact PTH stimulation of osteoblasts is the likely cause of increased alkaline phosphatase in most patients. Unless renal insufficiency is present, serum creatinine should be within normal limits in asymptomatic primary hyperparathyroidism. Secondary hyperparathyroidism may begin to develop as soon as the creatinine clearance decreases below 50 cc/min, so increased intact PTH levels may be found in some patients with only mildly increased serum creatinine.

Intact PTH, measured by current two-site immuno-radiometric (IRMA) or immuno-chemiluminometric (ICMA) assays, is mildly increased or inappropriately high-normal for the level of simultaneously measured serum calcium in patients with primary hyperparathyroidism. There is no cross-reactivity between PTH and PTHrp in current assays, making the distinction between primary hyperparathyroidism and PTHrp-mediated hypercalcemia of malignancy certain. Patients with primary hyperparathyroidism almost always have suppressed PTHrp levels when checked, and patients with PTHrp-mediated hypercalcemia of malignancy almost always have suppressed intact PTH levels. Patients treated with thiazides or lithium may have mild hypercalcemia and increased intact PTH levels without coexisting primary hyperparathyroidism, so it is essential to discontinue these medications for at least one month before reassessing the levels of serum total calcium and intact PTH to make the correct diagnosis. Hypercalcemic patients treated with thiazides or lithium that have coexisting primary hyperparathyroidism will have persistent hypercalcemia and increased intact PTH after discontinuing thiazides or lithium.

Some patients with primary hyperparathyroidism may have mildly increased serum chloride or decreased serum bicarbonate caused by renal tubular effects of intact PTH. Serum 1,25-dihydroxyvitamin D levels are typically upper normal or mildly increased becasue of the stimulation of renal 1$\alpha$-hydroxylase by intact PTH, whereas serum 25-hydroxyvitamin D levels may be normal to low-normal. 24-hour urinary calcium is frankly increased in 25–30% of patients, but the 24-hour urine calcium to creatinine clearance ratio ($U_{Ca}$ x $S_{Cr}/S_{Ca}$ x $U_{Cr}$) will typically be greater than 0.01 when measured. Markers of bone turnover may be high normal or increased in primary hyperparathyroidism without obvious bone disease, possibly driven by increased IL-6 or TNF$\alpha$.

Once the diagnosis of primary hyperparathyroidism is confirmed, surgical intervention is usually necessary in patients with symptomatic primary hyperparathyroidism, provided patients are surgical candidates. Surgical decisions about patients with asymptomatic primary hyperparathyroidism are more difficult. The 1991 NIH Consensus Development Conference recommended surgery for patients with asymptomatic primary hyperparathyroidism when the serum calcium was routinely more than 1.0 mg/dL above the upper limit of the normal range, or in patients with acute primary hyperparathyroidism with life-threatening hypercalcemia. Patients with asymptomatic primary hyperparathyroidism with recognized complications, such as nephrolithiasis or overt bone disease, hypercalciuria defined as 24-hour urine calcium greater than 400 mg/day, bone loss defined as one third distal radial bone mineral density Z-score of less than –2.0, or age younger than 50 years were also advised to seek surgical intervention.[56] Roughly half of patients with newly diagnosed primary hyperparathyroidism meet at least one of these surgical criteria, and of these patients, the majority are asymptomatic but have either increased serum or urine calcium or low bone mass. Patients not meeting criteria for surgical intervention are generally thought to have stable mild hypercalcemia without progression over time, although a recent study showed approximately 25% of a cohort of patients with asymptomatic primary hyperparathyroidism followed conservatively for 10 years developed hypercalciuria or bone loss over this interval sufficient to meet criteria for surgery.[57] This study may imply that patients with asymptomatic primary hyperparathyroidism are best served with elective parathyroidectomy at the time of diagnosis, because of the risk of developing complications requiring surgery over subsequent years of follow-up,

provided the patient is anticipated to live for more than 10 years.

Patients with symptomatic hypercalcemia unable to tolerate surgery have limited options for medical treatment.[58] These patients usually do best by maintaining adequate hydration and remaining physically active. Thiazide diuretics and lithium should generally be avoided. Dietary calcium intake of 800–1,000 mg/day is usually advised to minimize bone loss and avoid aggravation of the persistent hypercalcemia or hypercalciuria. Patients should specifically be advised to avoid decreasing their dietary calcium intake below 600 mg/day because of the likelihood of precipitating physiological secondary hyperparathyroidism described earlier in the chapter. Oral or intravenous phosphate is not indicated and should be generally avoided because of the risk of precipitation of ectopic calcification.

Postmenopausal estrogen replacement therapy has been reported to improve hypercalcemia and prevent bone loss in candidates suitable for this therapy, although intact PTH and phosphate levels do not change. Oral bisphosphonates, such as alendronate or risedronate, or intravenous pamidronate, may potentially be beneficial in women not able to take postmenopausal estrogen or men, but etidronate and clodronate have not shown long-term benefit. Alendronate, risedronate, pamidronate, raloxifene, and salmon calcitonin by nasal spray or injection have not been investigated or approved for this indication. CaSR agonists (calcimimetics) show promise and are under active investigation, and may be the best hope for adequate medical management of these patients in future years.[59] Patients with parathyroid tumors localized on ultrasound who do not desire, or are not candidates for, surgery may benefit from alcohol ablation of their tumor under ultrasound guidance.

Accurate diagnosis of primary hyperparathyroidism is essential prior to surgical exploration and attempted parathyroidectomy. Careful attention to the biochemical parameters described, especially the serum total calcium, phosphate, and intact PTH levels, is essential in making the correct diagnosis. Thoughtful attention to these details, while sometimes time-consuming, will significantly increase chances for surgical success with the initial neck exploration.

# References

1. Frolich A. Prevalence of hypercalcemia in normal and hospitalized populations. *Danish Med Bull.* 1998;45:436–439.
2. Shane E. Hypercalcemia. In: Favus MJ, ed. *Primer on the Metabolic Bone Diseases and Disorders of Mineral Metabolism.* 4th ed. Philadelphia, PA: Lippincott Williams and Wilkins; 1999.183–187.
3. Mundy GR, Guise TA. Hormonal control of calcium homeostasis. *Clin Chem.* 1999.45;1347–1352.

4. Brown EM, Vassilev PM, Quinn S, Hebert SC. G-protein-coupled, extracellular Ca$^{2+}$-sensing receptor: a versatile regulator of diverse cellular functions. *Vitamin Horm*. 1999;55:1–71.

5. Bushinsky DA, Monk RD. Calcium. *Lancet*. 1998;352:306–311.

6. Marx SJ, Attie MF, Levine MA, et al. The hypocalciuric or benign variant of familial hypercalcemia: clinical and biochemical features in fifteen kindreds. *Medicine*. 1981;60:397–412.

7. Law WM Jr, Heath H III. Familial benign hypercalcemia (hypocalciuric hypercalcemia): clinical and pathogenetic studies in 21 families. *Ann Intern Med*. 1985;102:511–519.

8. Brown EM, Pollak M, Seidman CE, et al. Calcium-ion-sensing cell-surface receptors. *New Engl J Med*. 1995;333.234–240.

9. Grill V, Ho P, Body JJ, et al. Parathyroid hormone-related protein: elevated levels in both humoral hypercalcemia of malignancy and hypercalcemia complicating metastatic breast cancer. *J Clin Endocrinol Metab*. 1991;73:1309–1315.

10. Ikeda K, Ohno H, Hane M, et al. Development of a sensitive two-site immunoradiometric assay for parathyroid hormone-related peptide: evidence for elevated levels in plasma from patients with adult T-cell leukemia/lymphoma and B-cell lymphoma. *J Clin Endocrinol Metab*. 1994;79:1322–1327.

11. Nagai Y, Yamato H, Akaogi K, et al. Role of interleukin 6 in uncoupling of bone *in vivo* in a human squamous carcinoma co-producing PTHrp and interleukin 6. *J Bone Miner Res*. 1998;13:664–672.

12. Nussbaum SR, Gaz RD, Arnold A. Hypercalcemia and ectopic secretion of parathyroid hormone by an ovarian carcinoma with rearrangement of the gene for PTH. *New Engl J Med*. 1990;323.1324–1328.

13. Iguchi H, Miyagi C, Tomita K, et al. Hypercalcemia caused by ectopic production of parathyroid hormone in a patient with papillary adenocarcinoma of the thyroid gland. *J Clin Endocrinol Metab*. 1998;83:2653–2657.

14. Breslau NA, McGuire JL, Zerwekh JE, et al. Hypercalcemia associated with increased serum calcitriol levels in three patients with lymphoma. *Ann Intern Med*. 1984;100:1–7.

15. Rosenthal NR, Insogna KL, Godsall JW, et al. Elevations in circulating 1,25(OH)$_2$D in three patients with lymphoma-associated hypercalcemia. *J Clin Endocrinol Metab*. 1985;60:29–33.

16. Adams JS, Fernandez M, Gacad MA, et al. Vitamin D metabolite mediated hypercalcemia and hypercalciuria in patients with AIDS and non-AIDS-associated lymphoma. *Blood*. 1989;73:235–239.

17. Seymour JF, Gagel RF. Calcitriol: the major humoral mediator of hypercalcemia in Hodgkin's disease and non-Hodgkin's lymphomas. *Blood*. 1993;82:1383–1394.

18. Schienman SJ, Kelberman MW, Tatum AH, Zamkoff KW. Hypercalcemia with excess serum 1,25-dihydroxyvitamin D in lymphomatoid granulomatosis/angiocentric lymphoma. *Am J Med Sci*. 1991;301:178–181.

19. Mundy GR, Yoneda T, Guise TA. Hypercalcemia in hematologic malignancies and in solid tumors associated with extensive localized bone destruction. In: Favus MJ, ed. *Primer on the Metabolic Bone Diseases and Disorders of Mineral Metabolism*. 4th ed. Philadelphia, PA: Lippincott Williams and Wilkins; 1999.183–187.

20. Knecht TP, Behling CA, Burton DW, et al. The humoral hypercalcemia of benignancy. A newly appreciated syndrome. *Am J Clin Pathol*. 1996;105:487–492.

21. Burman KD, Monchick JM, Earll JM, Wartofski L. Ionized and total serum calcium and parathyroid hormone in hyperthyroidism. *Ann Intern Med*. 1976;84:668–671.

22. Stewart AF, Hoecker J, Segre GV, et al. Hypercalcemia in pheochromocytoma: evidence for a novel mechanism. *Ann Intern Med*. 1985;102:776–779.

23. Mune T, Katakami H, Kato Y, et al. Production and secretion of parathyroid hormone-related protein in pheochromocytoma: participation of an α-adrenergic mechanism. *J Clin Endocrinol Metab*. 1993;76:757–762.

24. Vasikaran SD, Tallis GA, Braund WJ. Secondary hypoadrenalism presenting with hypercalcemia. *Clin Endocrinol*. 1994;41:261–265.

25. Verner JV, Morrison AB. Endocrine pancreatic islet disease with diarrhea. *Arch Intern Med*. 1974;133:492–500.

26. Rizzato G. Clinical impact of bone and calcium metabolism changes in sarcoidosis. *Thorax*. 1998;53:425–429.

27. Adams JS, Singer FR, Gacad MA, et al. Isolation and structural identification of 1,25-dihydroxyvitamin D3 produced by cultured alveolar macrophages in sarcoidosis. *J Clin Endocrinol Metab*. 1985;60:960–966.

28. Edelson GW, Talpos GB, Bone HG III. Hypercalcemia associated with Wegener's granulomatosis and hyperparathyroidism: etiology and management. *Am J Nephrol*. 1993;13:275–277.

29. Stoeckle JD, Hardy HL, Weber AL. Chronic beryllium disease: long-term follow-up of sixty cases and selective review of the literature. *Am J Med*. 1969;46:545–561.

30. Kozeny GA, Barbato AL, Bansal VK, et al. Hypercalcemia associated with silicone-induced granulomas. *New Engl J Med*. 1984;311:1103–1105.

31. Albitar S, Genin R, Fen-Chong M, et al. Multisystem granulomatous injuries 28 years after paraffin injections. *Nephrol Dial Transplant*. 1997;12:1974–1976.

32. Jurney TH. Hypercalcemia in a patient with eosinophilic granuloma. *Am J Med*. 1984;76:527–528.

33. Gkonos PJ, London R, Hendler ED. Hypercalcemia and elevated 1,25-dihydroxyvitamin D levels in a patient with end stage renal disease and active tuberculosis. *New Engl J Med*. 1984;311:1683–1685.

34. Walker JV, Baran D, Yakub YN, Freeman RB. Histoplasmosis with hypercalcemia, renal failure, and papillary necrosis: confusion with sarcoidosis. *JAMA*. 1977;237:1350–1352.

35. Parker MS, Dokoh S, Woolfenden JM, Buchsbaum HW. Hypercalcemia in coccidioidomycosis. *Am J Med*. 1984;76:341–343.

36. Khantarijian HM, Saad MF, Estey EH, et al. Hypercalcemia in disseminated Candidiasis. *Am J Med*. 1983;74:721–724.

37. Hoffman VH, Korzeniowski OM. Leprosy, hypercalcemia, and elevated serum calcitriol levels. *Ann Intern Med*. 1986;105:890–891.

38. Bosch X. Hypercalcemia due to endogenous overproduction of active vitamin D in identical twins with cat-scratch disease. *JAMA*. 1998;279:532–534.

39. Pettifor JM, Bikle DD, Cacalerso M, et al. Serum levels of free 1,25-dihydroxyvitamin D in vitamin D toxicity. *Ann Intern Med*. 1995;122:511–513.

40. Porter RH, Cox BG, Heaney D, et al. Treatment of hypoparathyroid patients with chlorthalidone. *New Engl J Med*. 1978;298:577–581.

41. Haden ST, Stoll AL, McCormick S, et al. Alterations in parathyroid dynamics in lithium-treated subjects. *J Clin Endocrinol Metab*. 1979;82:2844–2848.

42. Bourke JF, Berth-Jones J, Hutchinson PE. Hypercalcemia with topical calcipotriol. *Br Med J*. 1993;306:1334–1335.

43. Valentin-Opran A, Eilon G, Saez S, Mundy GR. Estrogens and antiestrogens stimulate release of bone-resorbing activity in cultured human breast cancer cells. *J Clin Invest*. 1985;75:726–731.

44. Legha SS, Powell K, Buzdar AU, Blumen-Schein GR. Tamoxifen-induced hypercalcemia in breast cancer. *Cancer*. 1981;47:2803–2806.

45. McPherson ML, Prince SR, Atamer E, et al. Theophylline-induced hypercalcemia. *Ann Intern Med*. 1986;105:52–54.

46. Sakoulas G, Tritos NA, Lally M, et al. Hypercalcemia in an AIDS patient treated with growth hormone. *AIDS*. 1997;11:1353–1356.

47. Gayet S, Ville E, Durand JM, et al. Foscarnet-induced hypercalcemia in AIDS (letter). *AIDS*. 1997;11:1068–1070.

48. Saunders M, Salisbury AJ, O'Byrne KJ, et al. A novel cyclic adenosine monophosphate analog induces hypercalcemia via production

tion of 1,25-dihydroxyvitamin D in patients with solid tumors. *J Clin Endocrinol Metab*. 1997;83:4044–4048.

49. al Zahrani A, Levine MA. Primary hyperparathyroidism. *Lancet*. 1997;349:1233–1238.

50. Bilezikian JP. Primary hyperparathyroidism. In: Favus MJ, ed. *Primer on the Metabolic Bone Diseases and Disorders of Mineral Metabolism*. 4th ed. Philadelphia, PA: Lippincott Williams and Wilkins; 1999.187–192.

51. Wermers RA, Khosla S, Atkinson EJ, et al. The rise and fall of primary hyperparathyroidism: a population-based study in Rochester, Minnesota 1965–1992. *Ann Int Med*. 1997;126:433–440.

52. Wynne AG, Van Heerden J, Carney JA, Fitzpatrick LA. Parathyroid carcinoma: clinical and pathological features in 43 patients. *Medicine*. 1992;71:197–205.

53. Tominaga Y, Takagi H. Molecular genetics of hyperparathyroid disease. *Curr Opin Nephrol Hyperten*. 1996;5:336–341.

54. Khosla S, Melton LJ III, Wermers RA, et al. Primary hyperparathyroidism and the risk of fracture: a population-based study. *J Bone Miner Res*. 1999;14:1700–1707.

55. Okomoto T, Gerstein HC, Obara T. Psychiatric symptoms, bone density and non-specific symptoms in patients with mild hypercalcemia due to primary hyperparathyroidism: a systematic overview of the literature. *Endocrine J*. 1997;44:367–374.

56. Consensus Development Conference Panel. Diagnosis and management of asymptomatic primary hyperparathyroidism: Consensus Development Conference Statement. *Ann Intern Med*. 1991;114:593–597.

57. Silverberg SJ, Shane E, Jacobs TP, et al. A 10-year prospective study of primary hyperparathyroidism with or without parathyroid surgery. *New Engl J Med*. 1999;341:1249–1255.

58. Silverberg SJ, Bilezikian JP, Bone HG III, et al. Therapeutic controversies in primary hyperparathyroidism. *J Clin Endocrinol Metab*. 1999;84:2275–2285.

59. Silverberg SJ, Bone HG III, Marriott TB, et al. Short-term inhibition of parathyroid hormone secretion by a calcium-receptor agonist in patients with primary hyperparathyroidism. *New Engl Journal Med*. 1997;337:1506–1510.

# 32

# Complications of Untreated Hyperparathyroidism

Sofia Garcia-Buder, M.D. and Michael Friedman, M.D.

Since the introduction of multichannel biochemical screening in the 1970s led to increased and early detection of primary hyperparathyroidism (PHPT), the clinical spectrum of the disease presentation has widened from the asymptomatic majority (50–80%) to that of the rarer, classical debilitating disease presentations.

Manifestations of primary hyperparathyroidism are related to the effects of hypercalcemia per se, the resultant hypercalciuria, or to the biochemical effects of parathyroid hormone (PTH). The symptomatology has been traditionally described as "stones, bones, (abdominal) groans, and (psychic) moans."

## CENTRAL NERVOUS SYSTEM

Patients with PHPT may present with a variety of neuropsychiatric symptoms. These may include weakness, fatigue, lethargy, irritability, emotional lability, difficulty concentrating, memory loss, or depression. Adolescents and young adults most commonly present with nonspecific CNS complaints. Patients with more severe disease may present with dementia, psychosis, mental obtundation, or coma.[1-4] Elderly patients are more susceptible to CNS manifestations even in the absence of severe hypercalcemia. Because the milder CNS complaints are not infrequent in the general population, especially the elderly, it is often difficult to ascertain its significance in the patient presenting with mild degrees of hypercalcemia. Neuropsychiatric disturbances are often improved after parathyroidectomy. Depression and anxiety are relieved in about 50% of patients, with dementia and organic brain syndrome improved in about 50% of cases.[5]

## PERIPHERAL NERVOUS SYSTEM

Neuromuscular manifestations have been reported in up to 70–80% of certain study populations. There may be sensory abnormalities involving decreased vibration in the feet, glove and stocking diminished pain sensation, or hyperpathic sensitivity to stimuli. Cranial nerve abnormalities could result in abnormal tongue movements (tremors), glossal atrophy, hoarseness, diplopia, decreased hearing, dysphagia, or anosmia. Respiratory muscle weakness has been described, with one reported death from respiratory failure attributed to PHPT. Easy fatigability and proximal muscle weakness, lower extremity involvement preceding and more severe than upper extremity, is common and is often associated with aches, pains, and sensation of heaviness. These may progress to muscle atrophy confirmed on muscle biopsy, with abnormal electromyographic findings but normal motor nerve conduction velocities. There may be abnormalities of gait, hyperactive reflexes, or positive Babinski sign, sometimes bilaterally.[1,2,6,7] Surgery reduces vague musculoskeletal pains in about 50% of patients, with complete resolution of malaise, fatigue, and muscular weakness in 80% of patients.[5]

## CARDIAC

PHPT is associated with increased risk of premature death from cardiovascular disease, especially in those with more severe hypercalcemia ($\geq$ 11.2 mg/dl) and in those with renal impairment. Hypertension is found in 20–70% of patients, compared with 23% in the general population. Proposed mechanisms include increased peripheral vascular resistance from hypercalcemia, enhanced myocardial contractility, calcium mediated increase in adrenaline release and in plasma renin activity, role of PTH acting synergistically with calcium to elevate blood pressure, and in some cases, the contributing role of renal damage from hypercalcemia. Hypertension, and possibly the hypertrophic effect on cardiomyocytes of elevated calcium and PTH that have been described, may lead to left ventricular hypertrophy, a strong and independent predictor of cardiovascular morbidity and mortality. There is a high incidence of calcified deposits in the myocardium, calcification of the coronary arteries and valves, hypercontractility of the heart muscle, and cardiac arrythmias including ventricular fibrillation. There may be bradycardia, shortened Q-T interval, and potentiation of digitalis intoxication.[8-13] Metabolic effects of insulin resistance that may be associated with PHPT, and a disorder of triglyceride metabolism described in men, may further contribute to the increased risk for cardiovascular morbidity.[14]

There is controversy whether or not parathyroidectomy results in resolution of HTN, with some studies showing irreversibility and others showing reversibility or at least amelioration in HTN. Left ventricular hypertrophy is reversible in normotensive patients but not in hypertensive patients. Sclerosis of aortic and mitral valves are stabilized with successful parathyroidectomy.[4,5,8,9,10,15,16] The increased risk of death continues for the first 5–10 years after surgery, with observed to expected death ratio of 1.67. However, comparison of untreated with treated patients indicates diminished long-term extra mortality, approaching the normal death rate 5–15 years after the operation.[5]

## RENAL

Hypercalcemia may lead to hypercalciuria (<50% of patients), which predisposes to calcium nephrolithiasis (10–25% of patients) and, more rarely, nephrocalcinosis. Functional abnormalities range from impaired concentrating or acidifying ability, reduction in creatinine clearance, to end-stage renal failure. Associated symptoms include polyuria, polydipsia, hematuria, and recurrent flank pain. Loss of renal function can be stabilized and sometimes reversed by successful parathyroidectomy, which also prevents further stone disease in 90% of patients.[1,2,5,17,18,19]

## GASTROINTESTINAL

Anorexia, nausea and vomiting can occur with severe hypercalcemia and aggravate dehydration. Constipation is common. There may be dyspepsia. Acute or chronic pancreatitis, possibly caused by calcium deposits in the pancreatic ducts or in the pancreatic vessels, among various hypotheses, is a rare complication. Peptic ulcer disease may be present, which may also be related to the association of PHPT with the Zollinger-Ellison syndrome in MEN-1 (Multiple Endocrine Neoplasia) patients.[1,2,20] Surgery improves or resolves constipation in 60–70% of patients,[5] while peptic ulcer disease is unlikely to remit.[17]

## SKELETAL

The skeletal manifestations of advanced or classic PHPT are now rare. These include osteitis fibrosa cystica, bone cysts (usually multiple) containing brownish serous or mucoid fluid, osteoclastomas or brown tumors composed of numerous multinucleated osteoclasts (giant cells) admixed with stromal cells and matrix, and pathologic fractures. Joint pain caused by chondrocalcinosis, gout, or pseudogout is seen in some patients. There is generalized demineralization of the bone, primarily cortical bone, with trabecular or cancellous bone as in the vertebral bodies least if at all affected. This leads to increased risk of fractures of the wrist, radius, hip, and other appendicular bones but not of vertebral fractures. Characteristic subperiosteal resorption is most evident in the distal phalanges of the hands, distal third of the clavicles, distal ulna, inferior margin of the femoral neck and pubis, and the medial aspect of the proximal tibia. These changes may result in bone pain and tenderness, "bowing" of the shoulders, kyphosis and loss of height, "pigeon breast" caused by collapse of the lateral ribs, or collapse of the pelvis with triradiate deformities. Skull films may reveal finely mottled, ground glass, "salt and pepper" appearance with loss of definition of the inner and outer cortices. There may be erosion or disappearance of the lamina dura with extension into the adjacent mandibular bone seen on dental radiographs.[1,2,3,5,17,18,19,21]

Since osteopenia may not be evident on plain skeletal films until there is advanced disease with at least 30–50% bone loss, its presence is best assessed by bone densitometry testing, especially by DEXA (Dual Photon Absorptiometry). This test should be part of the evaluation of all patients with PHPT to determine the severity of skeletal involvement, and to identify the "asymptomatic" patients who do have osteoporosis and therefore may need parathyroidectomy. Subsequent 1–2 year follow-up DEXA is useful to determine the extent of disease reversal and the possible need for the introduction of anti-resorptive therapy, especially in post-menopausal women. Successful parathyroidectomy leads to improvement in bone mineral density (BMD) of up to 6–8% ($\pm$1–2%) in certain skeletal sites after 1 year and 12–14% ($\pm$3–4%) after 10 years.[1,5,17,22]

## METABOLIC

Parathyroid hormone (PTH) decreases renal resorption of phosphate and bicarbonate, which may cause hypophosphatemia and mild metabolic acidosis with hyperchloremia. Increased renal calcium resorption contributes to hypercalcemia which, above a certain threshold, may result in compensatory hypercalciuria (<50% of patients). PTH increases the conversion of 25-(OH) vitamin D to the more metabolically active form 1,25-$(OH)_2$ vitamin D, which enhances calcium absorption in the gut. This contributes to the hypercalcemia from PTH-induced bone resorption and from increased renal calcium resorption. PHPT may lead to reversible elevations in uric acid level, and in men in triglyceride level.[14]

Impaired glucose tolerance (IGT), independent of other risk factors, has been demonstrated in patients with PHPT, with frank diabetes mellitus observed in 7.8% to 8.2% in certain studies, three times greater incidence compared to an age-matched population. Although the mechanism is unclear, increased circulatory concentration of amylin has been found, as in patients with NIDDM. There are suggestions that either the chronic hypercalcemia or the increased levels of PTH may result in insulin resistance, which can lead to overt hyperglycemia in patients with underlying deficiency in pancreatic insulin secretory reserve. IGT is often reversible with successful parathyroid surgery. Although pre-existing diabetes mellitus is generally not reversed, there has been a reported case of remission of DM following resection of a parathyroid adenoma.[23-26]

## MISCELLANEOUS

Metastatic calcifications may result in conjunctival calcifications, calcific keratitis, band keratopathy, or pruritus. Anemia has been attributed to PHPT, possibly caused by a presumed toxic effect of high levels of PTH.[1,2]

## CLINICAL COURSE OF UNTREATED PRIMARY HYPERPARATHYROIDISM

There have been several 8–10 year prospective studies which have demonstrated a relatively benign course of untreated mild hyperparathyroidism in the majority of patients, with no significant progression of symptoms, hypercalcemia, bone mineral density (BMD) loss, or renal function impairment. No fractures or kidney stones developed during these observation periods.[27,28] However, there was evidence of disease progression in up to 27% of patients, including marked hypercalcemia, hypercalciuria, or BMD loss of up to 10%.[22]

Thus, patients who do not undergo surgery need to be monitored closely with bi-annual serum calcium levels, blood pressure, and serum creatinine and creatinine clearance. Further recommendations from the NIH Consensus Statement include annual abdominal radiographs, 24–hour urinary calcium determination, and repeat bone mass measurement after 1 to 2 years. Once the lack of progression of the disease has been established over 1 to 3 years with stability of the various parameters, the intervals between the follow-up testing can be safely extended.[29]

## References

1. Deftos LJ. Primary hyperparathyroidism. In: Deftos LJ, ed. *Clinical Essentials of Calcium and Skeletal Disorders*. Caddo, OK: Professional Communications, Inc.; 1998:97–116.
2. Bringhurst FR, Demay MB, Kronenberg HM. Hormones and disorders of mineral metabolism. In: Wilson JD, Foster DW, Kronenberg IIM, Larsen PR, eds. *Williams Textbook of Endocrinology*. Philadelphia, PA:W.B. Saunders Co.; 1998: 1172–1174.
3. Lundgren E, Ljunghall S, Akerstrom G, et al. Case-control study on symptoms and signs of "asymptomatic" primary hyperparathyroidism. *Surgery*. 1998;124(6):980–986.
4. Loh KC, Duh QY, Shoback D, et al. Clinical profile of primary hyperparathyroidism in adolescents and young adults. *Clin Endocrinol*. 1998;48:435–443.
5. Sivula A, Pelkoken R. Long-term health risk of primary hyperparathyroidism: the effect of surgery. *Ann Med*. 1996;28: 95–100.
6. Patten BM, Bilezikian JP, Mallette LE, et al. Neuromuscular disease in primary hyperparathyroidism. *Ann Int Med*. 1974;80: 182–193.
7. Gentric A, Pennec YL. Fatal primary hyperparathyroidism with myopathy involving respiratory muscles in an old woman. *J Am Geriatr Soc*. 1994;42:1306.
8. Dalberg K, Brodin LA, Juhlin-Dannfelt A, Farnebo LO. Cardiac function in primary hyperparathyroidism before and after operation. *Eur J Surg*. 1996;162:171–176.
9. Raue F. Increased incidence of cardiovascular disease in primary hyperparathyroidism—a cause for more aggressive treatment? *Eur J Clin Invest*. 1998;28:277–278.
10. Stefenelli T, Abela C, Frank H, et al. Cardiac abnormalities in patients with primary hyperparathyroidism: implications for follow-up. *J Clin Endocrinol Metab*. 1997;82(1):106–112.

11. Hedback G, Oden A. Death risk factor analysis in primary hyperparathyroidism. *Eur J Clin Invest.* 1998;28:1011–1018.

12. Hedback G, Oden A. Increased risk of death from primary hyperparathyroidism—an update. *Eur J Clin Invest.* 1998; 28:271–276.

13. Wermers RA, Khosla S, Atkinson EJ, et al. Survival after the diagnosis of hyperparathyroidism: a population-based study. *Am J Med.* 1998;104:115–122.

14. Valdemarsson S, Lindblom P, Bergenfelz A. Metabolic abnormalities related to cardiovascular risk in primary hyperparathyroidism: effects of surgical treatment. *J Intern Med.* 1998;244:241–249.

15. Nainby-Luxmoore JC, Langford HG, Nelson NC, et al. A case-comparison study of hypertension and hyperparathyroidism. *J Clin Endocrinol Metab.* 1982;55(2):303–306.

16. Diamond TW, Botha JR, Wing J, et al. Parathryoid hypertension. A reversible disorder. *Arch Intern Med.* 1986;146:1709–1712.

17. Silverberg SJ. Diagnosis, natural history, and treatment of primary hyperparathyroidism. In Arnold A, ed. *Endocrine Neoplasms.* Boston, MA: Kluwer Academic Publishers; 1997:163–181.

18. Mitlak BH, Daly M, Potts JT, et al. Asymptomatic primary hyperparathyroidism. *J Bone Miner Res.* 1991;6(suppl 2): S103–S124.

19. Silverberg SJ, Shane E, Jacobs TP, et al. Nephrolithiasis and bone involvement in primary hyperparathyroidism. *Am J Med.* 1990; 89:327–334.

20. Shimizu H, Kodama A. Severe acute pancreatitis as a first symptom of primary hyperparathyroid adenoma: a case report. *J Laryngol Otol.* 1996;110:602–603.

21. Silverberg SJ, Shane E, De La Cruz L, et al. Skeletal disease in primary hyperparathryoidism. *J Bone Miner Res.* 1989;4(3):283–291.

22. Silverberg SJ, Shane E, Jacobs TP, et al. A 10-year prospective study of primary hyperparathryoidism with or without parathyroid surgery. *N Engl J Med.* 1999;341:1249–1255.

23. Kumar S, Olukoga AO, Gordon C, et al. Impaired glucose tolerance and insulin insensitivity in primary hyperparathyroidism. *Clin Endocrinol.* 1994;40:47–53.

24. Ljunghall S, Palmer M, Akerstrom G, Wide L. Diabetes mellitus, glucose tolerance and insulin response to glucose in patients with primary hyperparathryoidism before and after parathyroidectomy. *Eur J Clin Invest.* 1983;13:373–377.

25. Taylor WH. The prevalence of diabetes mellitus in patients with primary hyperparathryoidism and among their relatives. *Diab Med.*1991;8:683–687.

26. Quin JD, Gumpert JRW. Remission of non-insulin dependent diabetes mellitus following resection of a parathyroid adenoma. *Diab Med.* 1997;14:80–81.

27. Parfitt AM, Rao DS, Kleerekoper M. Asymptomatic primary hyperparathyroidism discovered by multichannel biochemical screening: clinical course and considerations bearing on the need for surgical intervention. *J Bone Miner Res.* 1991;6(Suppl 2):S97–S101.

28. Rubinoff H, McCarthy N, Hiatt RA. Hypercalcemia: long-term follow-up with matched controls. *J Chron Dis.* 1983;36(12):859–868.

29. Diagnosis and Management of Asymptomatic Primary Hyperparathyroidism. (Reprinted from NIH Development Conference Consensus Statement, 1990; Oct 29–31; 8(7).)

# 33

# Parathyroid Gland Imaging and the Application of Localization Studies

## Robert A. Sofferman, M.D. and Anil Ahuja, M.D.

## INTRODUCTION

The traditional method of resolving primary hyperparathyroidism is bilateral four site surgical exploration. A knowledge of anatomy, differentiation of parathyroid tissue from fat and lymph nodes, and a thorough understanding of embryology and its relationship to ectopic parathyroid locations requires considerable experience. However, the ability to perform a complete cervical exploration for parathyroid adenoma or hyperplasia does not guarantee identification of pathologic glands in ectopic locations, such as the mediastinum or carotid sheath above the bifurcation. Some very skilled surgeons have advocated a unilateral approach with biopsy of both identified glands, one presumably hyperplastic and the other normal. With this pathologic sequence suggesting a parathyroid adenoma, the major potential management error is that of missing a second adenoma on the opposite side. Although parathyroid imaging has been available for many years in the form of ultrasound and technetium-thallium scanning, their marginal interpretative abilities did not allow the potential for minimal access surgery. Since the development of better imaging methods which allow site prediction at or above the 90% level, most of the aforementioned problems with focused or unilateral exploration can be eliminated. Although a comprehensive bilateral exploration of all appropriate parathyroid sites in the surgical management of hyperparathyroidism is still the gold standard and must be fundamental to the armamentarium of all parathyroid surgeons, newer imaging technologies permit the same surgical results utilizing focused, more limited proce-

dures. All these procedures are dependent on pre-operative imaging, and some, such as the use of gamma probe technology, require the adjunctive use of the same radioactive infusion for surgical intervention as that required for parathyroid imaging. A review of these imaging techniques will be summarized and representative scans illustrated. Finally, the interaction of these imaging tools with actual surgical decisions will be presented with a bias toward focused, minimal access surgery.

## METHODS OF PRE-OPERATIVE LOCALIZATION

### Pertechnetate (Tc 99m)/Thallous Chloride (Tl201) Scan

The patient is positioned under the scintillation counter after intravenous injection of 2–3mCi of 201 thallium. The agent concentrates in both thyroid tissue and parathyroid adenoma. A cervico-thoracic anterior image is then obtained 15–20 minutes later and counts taken for 10 minutes. The gamma counter is then re-calibrated, 5mci of Tc-Pertechnetate injected, and a second image acquired. Using the stored computerized data, the Pertechnetate (thyroid) image is subtracted leaving the parathyroid image for view. Thallium 201 may not be the optimum element for imaging with a gamma counter, because of low radiation energy and thus lower target-to-background ratio. Additionally, a requirement for prolonged patient immobilization between the two imaged sequences may further compromise image quality. Identification results of hyperplastic parathyroid glands have been inconsistent. For these reasons, pre-operative Tc/Th scanning has not received acceptance as an adequate pre-operative imaging tool and has justifiably served as an argument in favor of routine four site surgical exploration without pre-operative imaging.

## Technetium 99m-Sestamibi-Cervico-Thoracic Planar Images

In 1992[1] Taillefer, proposed a dual phase scan utilizing Technetium 99m Sestamibi and cervico-thoracic planar parathyroid scintigraphy. The patient is intravenously injected with 20–25 millicuries of Tc-99m-Sestamibi, a cationic lipophilic substance which concentrates in both thyroid and hyperplastic parathyroid tissue. After two to three hours, a second scintigraph is obtained when the radioactive tracer has left the thyroid gland but persists in the enlarged parathyroid(s). Jofre[2] has demonstrated that 70% of delayed images are best seen at 2 hours, and only 15% at 4 hours. In certain circumstances, oblique or lateral images can be obtained to attempt to add a third dimension to the study. This dual phase Technetium-99m-Sestamibi scan is simple and does not require patient immobilization. With this scanning technique, single or double parathyroid adenomas can be identified in 80–90% of cases before surgical intervention (Figures 33–1, 33–2). This is the current most

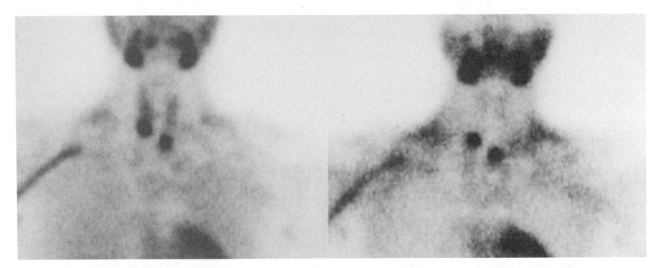

**Figure 33–1.** This patient demonstrates uptake after washout with Tc99m-Sestamibi on each side, proven at surgery with demonstration of two other normal glands. This is a typical appearance of bilateral double parathyroid adenomas. (Courtesy of *Arch Otolaryngol Head and Neck*, 1996, 122:371. Copyrighted 1996; American Medical Association.)

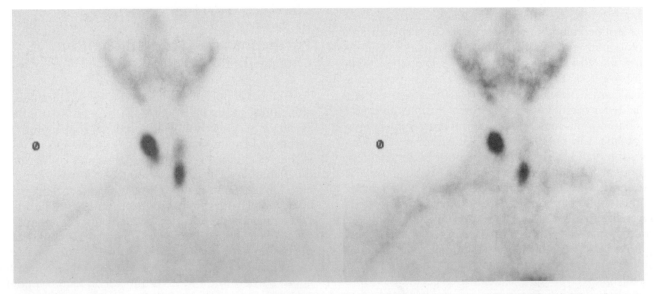

**Figure 33–2.** This second case of confirmed double adenomas shows little change between the initial and delayed acquisitions with Sestamibi scan.

widely utilized pre-operative imaging tool in initial and re-operative parathyroid surgery.

Tc99m-Sestamibi has been combined with I[123] and recorded simultaneously in non-overlapping windows and subtraction. In a series by Hindie et al ,[3] 25 of 27 solitary adenomas were identified with a sensitivity of 94%. In the same population examining with the Tc99m-Sestamibi as a single tracer, only 22 of these 27 patients were correctly imaged for a sensitivity rate of 79%. Neumann[4] has employed Tc99m-Sestamibi/I[123] subtraction and SPECT in patients with secondary hyperparathyroidism for a sensitivity of 77%. More importantly, in recurrent secondary hyperparathyroidism, all hyperplastic parathyroids were predicted and correctly identified in the 13 patient series.

## Technetium 99m-Sestamibi with SPECT

Some experienced endocrine centers recommend the addition of SPECT (single photon emission computerized tomography) as an elective pre-operative study with both primary and re-operative surgical hyperparathyroidism (Figure 33–3). This technology utilizes a camera collimator which rotates 360 degrees around the patient in the axial plane and in essence portrays a three dimensional image as the sequence progresses from mandible through the thorax (Figure 33–4). Some authors[5] have demonstrated a superior sensitivity/localization in the early phase compared with planar images, whereas the delayed images are approximately equivalent. The images do appear to have higher resolution and have two definite recognized advantages over planar Sestamibi scans[6]: 1) anatomical localization in ectopic adenomas within the carotid sheath and 2) localization of mediastinal lesions to the anterior or posterior segment, allowing planning of surgery via thoracotomy versus median sternotomy. The most evident disadvantage is its increased cost above that of routine Technetium Sestamibi scanning.

## CT and MRI Scan

These conventional tools are rarely used as initial pre-operative imaging studies. Neither of these techniques selectively illuminates endocrine tissue and can only lend anatomical information (Figures 33–5, 33–6). For example, small masses identified in the anterior mediastinum, which are suspected ectopic or thymic related parathyroid adenomas, are often proven to be enlarged lymph nodes at surgery and subsequent pathologic assessment. Although pre-operative imaging has now become an important concern in this era of limited access surgery, and these two methods do offer some localization advantages, once again the *relative costs, inconsistent*

*results, and limited availability (outside developed countries)* preclude universal use before the first surgery. However, they are indispensable tools in patients who have recurrent hyperparathyroidism and require re-operative exploration. Because the risks of a second failed exploration are substantial without comprehensive imaging, these studies are usually considered in the re-operative workup.

## Ultrasound

Of all imaging methods, ultrasound is the best for characterization of thyroid anatomy, pathology, and relationship to adjacent thyroidal masses (Figure 33–7). Grey scale ultrasound with high resolution linear array transducers in the range of 7 to 12MHz is the ideal modality for parathyroid study. Enlarged parathyroid glands in the vicinity of the thyroid are clearly visualized. However, ectopic parathyroids and those that are low in the neck may not be demonstrated. Both transverse and longitudinal scans are required. Transverse scans are useful in identifying the adenoma whereas longitudinal scans better demonstrate its relationship to the thyroid and its internal architecture and vascularity. A parathyroid adenoma typically appears as a hypoechoic mass posterior or inferior to the thyroid gland in its usual extracapsular location. Retrothyroid lesions tend to be oval or flat whereas infrathyroid lesions are usually spherical. Some adenomas may demonstrate cystic portions within but calcification is rare. The most common false positive image with Technetium-Sestamibi scan is that of a thyroid adenoma (Figure 33–8). This particular problem may be better clarified and resolved with adjunctive ultrasound. A discrete blood supply to the mass identified by color Doppler may suggest a diagnosis of intrathyroidal adenoma rather than a lesion of thyroid origin (Figure 33–9).

## DISCUSSION

In 1989, Coakley et al[7] demonstrated that Tc-99m-Sestamibi could be used as an imaging agent for parathyroid adenoma in addition to its efficacy in examining myocardial perfusion. Prior to that time, thallous chloride Tl201-Tc-99m pertechnetate subtraction parathyroid imaging was the standard. However, results with this imaging technology had been marginal with localization rates as low as 50%.[8,9] In comparison a meta analysis of the literature has now estimated an 87% sensitivity of Tc-99m-Sestamibi in localizing solitary adenomas.[10] The reason for concentration of the agent in both myocardium and parathyroid adenoma is the respective high volume of tissue mitochondria.[11,12] Takehayashi et al[13] have suggested that gland weight and vascularity

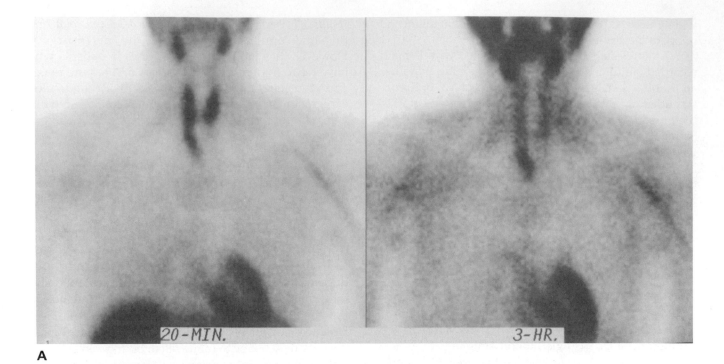

**A**

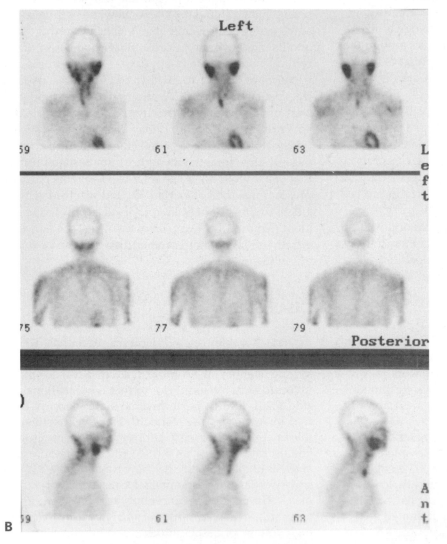

**B**

**Figure 33–3A, B.** A Tc99m-Sestamibi scan (A) shows a right inferior parathyroid adenoma. This patient also underwent a SPECT Sestamibi scan (B), which demonstrates its ability to localize the tumor in the anterior position. However, for cervical imaging, the simple planar images are usually adequate as demonstrated in this comparison between planar and SPECT Sestamibi imaging.

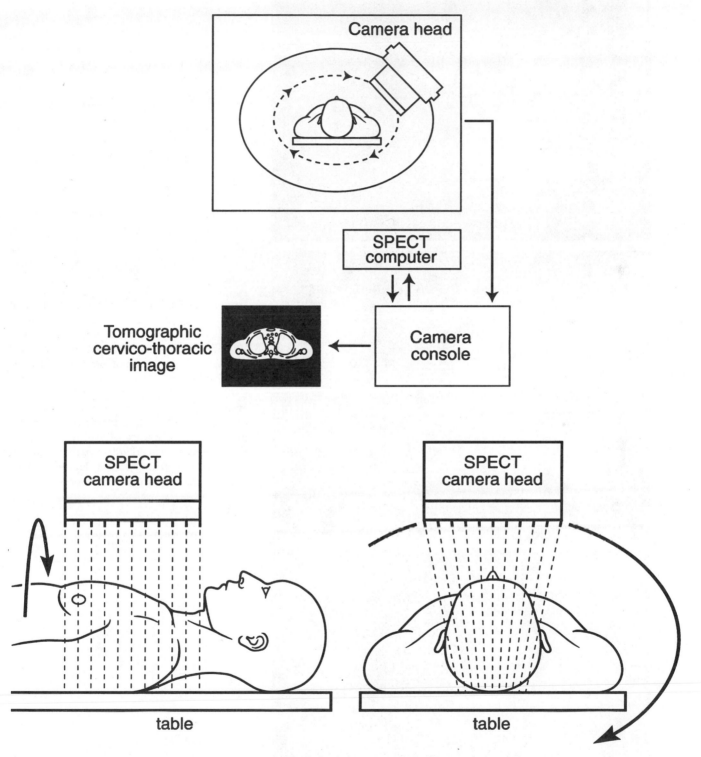

**Figure 33–4.** The basic technique of SPECT Sestamibi scan is outlined in these schematic representations.

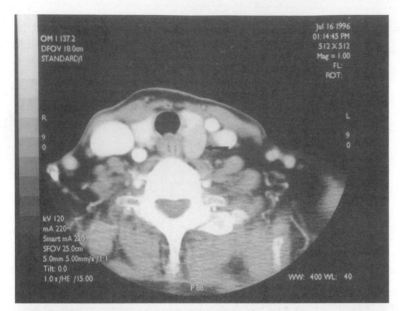

**A**

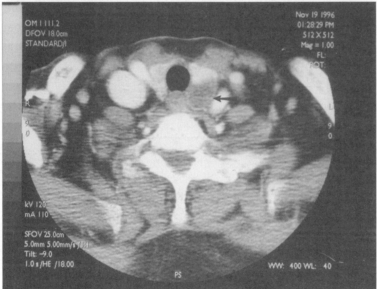

**B**

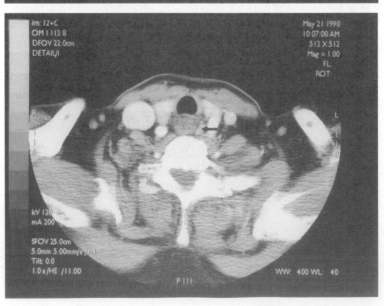

**C**

**Figure 33–5A, B, C.** This elderly patient shows a large parathyroid adenoma on the left side behind the normal thyroid gland (July, 1996, Figure 33–12A). The patient developed spontaneous resolution of her primary hyperparathyroidism and CT scan at that time (November, 1996, Figure 33–3B) demonstrated cystic degeneration of the mass, perhaps representing spontaneous infarction of the adenoma. A mild recurrence of the hyperparathyroid state is correlated with a partial regrowth of the adenoma (May, 1998, Figure 33–12C) but it is smaller than the initial mass.

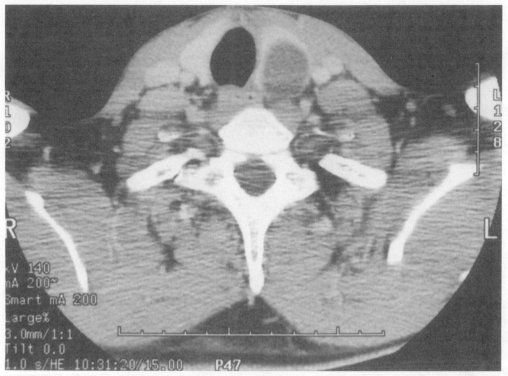

**A**

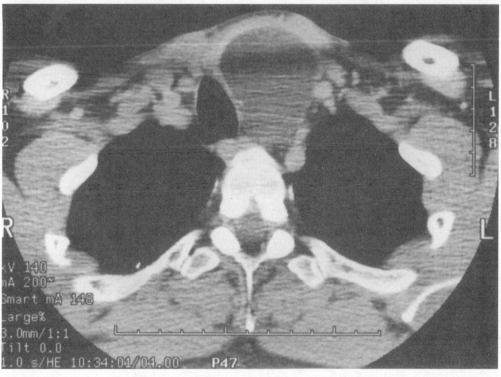

**B**

**Figure 33–6A, B.** A cystic mass within the left lobe of thyroid is aspirated and contains clear fluid (A). The fluid has a markedly elevated parathyroid hormone level consistent with a parathyroid cyst. Interestingly, the patient is eucalcemic which excludes the diagnosis of cystic degeneration of a parathyroid adenoma. Occasionally, these cysts can become quite large and extend well into the anterior mediastinum as illustrated in this Figure (B). (Courtesy of the *Laryngoscope*, 2001, 1111:1576. Lippincott Williams and Wilkins.)

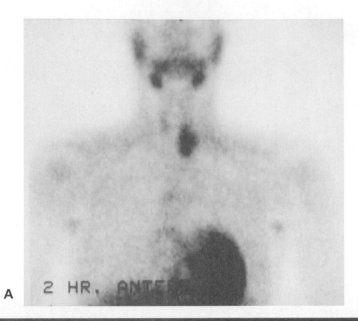

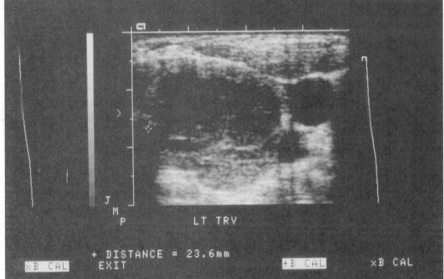

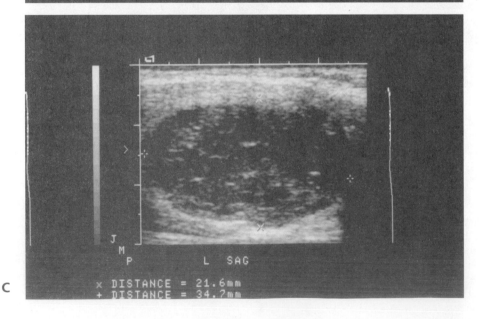

**Figure 33–7A, B, C.** This 14 year-old female with primary hyperparathyroidism demonstrates a mass effect of the left thyroid gland on physical examination consistent with a large thyroid adenoma. A Tc99m-Sestamibi washout scan (A) suggested a large inferior thyroid uptake, and ultrasound demonstrated a mass intrinsic to and virtually replacing the entire left lobe. (B = transverse ultrasound and C = sagittal ultrasound). The mass proved at surgery and pathology to be a large intra-thyroidal parathyroid adenoma.

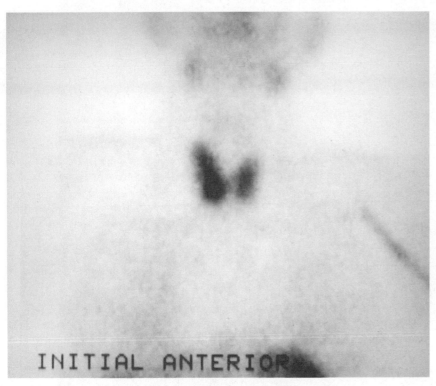

INITIAL ANTERIOR

**A**

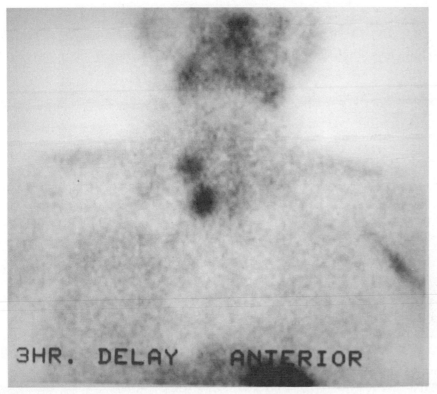

3HR. DELAY ANTERIOR

**B**

**Figure 33–8A, B.** This patient demonstrates apparent two gland persistent ipsilateral uptake after Tc-Sestamibi washout, but the images are of differing densities. The lower image (A) is the parathyroid adenoma, and the upper image (B) a thyroid adenoma. Thyroid adenoma is the most common false positive element in Technetium-Sestamibi scanning.

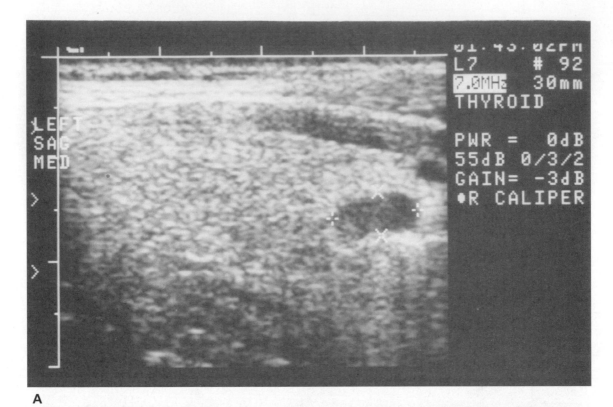

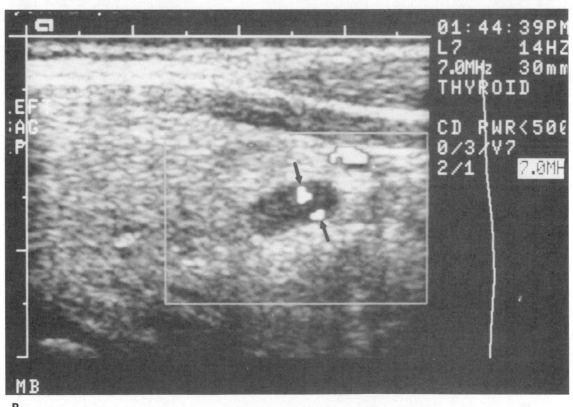

**Figure 33–9A, B.** A small but hyperfunctioning parathyroid adenoma is demonstrated on sagittal ultrasound (A) to be completely within the thyroid gland. Color Doppler (B) shows a discrete blood supply (black arrows) which differs from the more diffuse *perinodular* vascular support for a thyroid adenoma from its surrounding parent gland. This parathyroid adenoma was removed by a thyroidotomy and removal of only the adenoma, assisted by pre-operative localization of the mass. (Courtesy of *Arch Otolaryngol Head and Neck Surg*, 1998, 124:651. Copyrighted 1998, American Medical Association.)

are also important predictors of Sestamibi uptake. Conversely, normal parathyroid tissue and multi-glandular hyperplasia do not consistently demonstrate uptake. Tc-99m-Sestamibi parathyroid gland scintigraphy can be combined with SPECT acquisition and re-projection providing three-dimensional localization relative to the thyroid gland. In ectopic adenoma below the clavicle, SPECT-MIBI is extremely valuable in determining its mediastinal position. In a series comparing convention planar Tc-99m-Sestamibi with the addition of SPECT in the same patient, the latter technology increased the sensitivity by 10%.[14] The added cost of SPECT and adequate information gleaned from conventional planar Sestamibi keeps SPECT in a reserve position for most parathyroid imaging. However, Irvin[14] now uses SPECT-Sestamibi as his preferred pre-operative localization method in all cases. High resolution ultrasound has been favored as a low cost non-invasive localization method. Pearl[15] reported identification of 23 of 25 parathyroid adenomas with ultrasound. However, others report an accuracy far below that of Tc-99m-Sestamibi; Hasslegren[16] has demonstrated a 58% correct side identification in 40 single adenomas studied with ultrasound.

The cost of Sestamibi has been cited as a reason for many surgeons to continue with classic bilateral exploration without the need for this technology. At the University of Vermont, a cost analysis of the first 59 consecutive patients studied with pre-operative Tc-99m-Sestamibi localization has been performed.[17] Three mediastinal adenomas could not have been identified at the initial surgery (Figures 33–10, 33–11) and an additional two intrathyroidal tumors would have posed special problems adding to intra-operative cost. In that series, the cost of missing ectopic adenomas was roughly equivalent to routine Tc-99m-Sestamibi scanning in all 59 patients.

In spite of the inadequate reported pre-operative localization result of ultrasound in identifying enlarged parathyroid glands and adenomas, we have employed it routinely between the Tc-99m-Sestamibi early and late acquisition times. It is particularly helpful in anticipating intra-thyroidal adenomas (Figure 33–12). If the Sestamibi shows adenoma at the thyroid and ultrasound does not demonstrate an extra-thyroidal region mass, an intra-thyroidal location may be suspected. Additionally, the ultrasound often demonstrates the intra-thyroidal position of the parathyroid adenoma on its own. Another important justification for ultrasound is identification of potential coexistent thyroid pathology. Since the surgeon will be in the precise vicinity of the thyroid gland, surgical intervention of the thyroid can be anticipated, discrete masses aspirated, and the patient appropriately counseled. With this algorithm, several occult malignancies of the thyroid gland have been detected

and appropriately managed with better planning. One large series[18] demonstrates a 7% false positive rate with Tc-99m-Sestamibi, but in 14 of 17 of these cases concurrent thyroid pathology was identified. Perhaps this very issue is another compelling argument in favor of combining Tc-99m-Sestamibi and ultrasound. The latter study, if demonstrating a thyroid mass, adds a special dimension to the accurate interpretation of the concomitant Tc-99m-Sestamibi scan. In a 1995 study of 49 patients, DeFeo et al[19] have indicated that ultrasound and Sestamibi represent the best pre-operative imaging combination, including consideration of MRI and CT scanning.

From 1994 through 1999, 106 consecutive author cases of new primary hyperparathyroidism at the University of Vermont have been studied with Tc-99m-Sestamibi pre-operative localization. In this series, an 83% sensitivity (true positive/true positive plus false negative) and 96% specificity have been demonstrated, consistent with other contemporary results. Additionally, the test reveals a 97% positive predictive value. Of these 106 cases, only 47% had ultrasound mainly as a result of Tc-99m-Sestamibi scans having already been ordered by referring primary care and endocrinology physicians. A sensitivity of 72% in this ultrasound series indicates a lower degree of accuracy as a *stand-alone* pre-operative localization study.

High resolution ultrasound has been employed as a relatively inexpensive, non-invasive imaging tool. The results have been variable with reported sensitivities of 28 to 85%.[20] Ultrasound has some potential limitations. Although it may demonstrate tumors in the vicinity of the thyroid gland, tumors that are in the upper mediastinum behind the sternum and those behind air containing structures, such as trachea or esophagus, may not be identifiable. In addition, ultrasound is very often operator dependent. Results may be improved with the use of high frequency linear transducers. We have demonstrated a significant potential to predict the size of parathyroid adenomata with high resolution ultrasound in a limited series of ten patients, comparing the anticipated volumes on ultrasound with those measured at pathologic assessment.[20] This same study demonstrated that the volume of the adenoma can be correlated with the ability of the Tc-99m-Sestamibi scan to recognize it. The average volume of positively imaged tumors was 1.75 cc, whereas three false negative tumors were small at 0.82 cc. This small pilot study suggests that small parathyroid adenomas or hyperplasia lesions are less likely to illuminate on Tc-99m-Sestamibi scan.

Shaha[21] has reported a 96% success rate in resolving hyperparathyroidism with bilateral surgical intervention and pre-operative localization study. Unilateral exploration, which encompasses biopsy of both ipsilateral glands, should detect all cases of diffuse hyperplasia and single non-ectopic adenoma. Although a con-

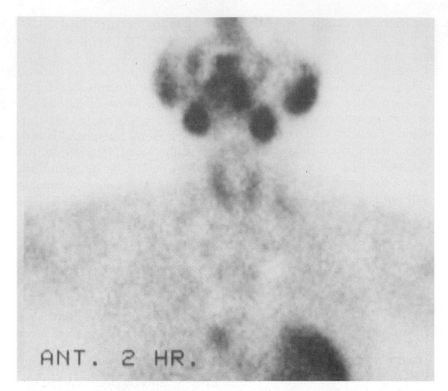

**A**

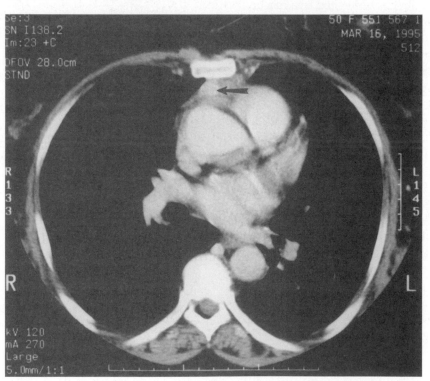

**B**

**Figure 33–10A, B.** Technetium-99m-Sestamibi scan demonstrates a superior mediastinal uptake, which faintly persists after washout (A). Another form of imaging is required to confirm the suspect ectopic mediastinal parathyroid adenoma. The arrow points to the same mass in the retrosternal anterior mediastinum demonstrated on axial CT scan (B). (Courtesy of *Arch Otolaryngol Head and Neck Surg*, 1996, 122:373. Copyrighted 1996, American Medical Association.)

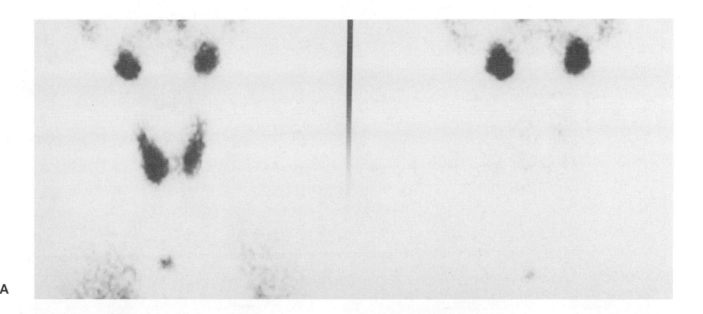

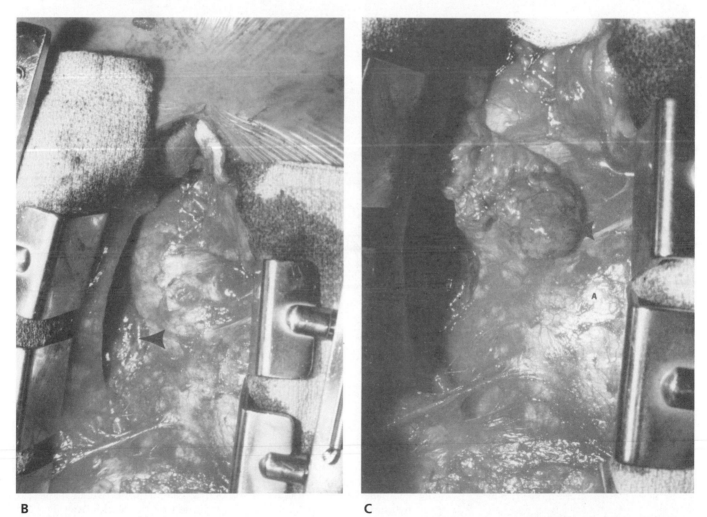

**Figure 33–11A, B, C.** A deep anterior mediastinal parathyroid adenoma is identified on delayed washout of Tc99m-Sestamibi (A). At surgery the mass rested between the root of the aorta and right mediastinal pleura (B). Figure 33–11C demonstrates the adenoma after it has been partially retrieved and rotated onto the aorta (C). (Courtesy of *Arch Otolaryngol Head and Neck Surg*, 1996, 122:372. Copyrighted 1996, American Medical Association.)

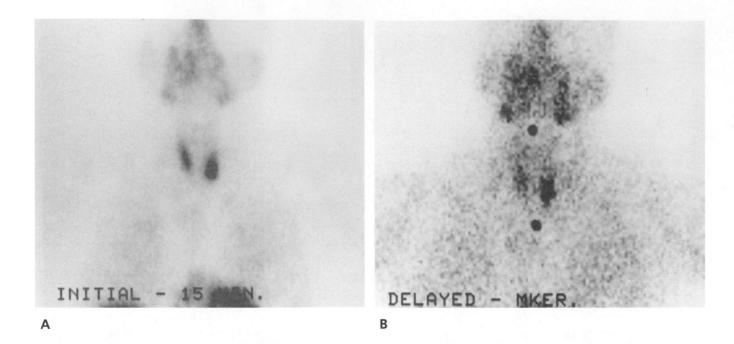

A

B

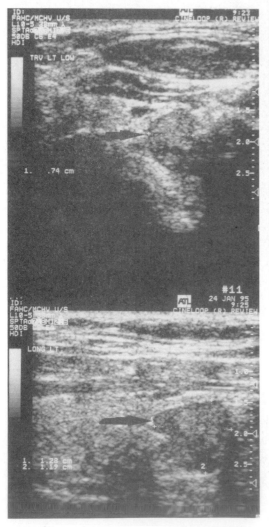

C

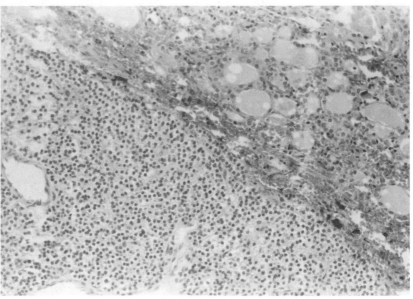

D

**Figure 33–12A, B, C, D.** This patient's Technetium-Sestamibi scan demonstrates the usual persistence in focal imaging after washout (A and B) confined to the left inferior thyroid region. Ultrasound (C) demonstrates the completely intra-thyroidal location of this mass, which is oval in shape and measures 1.28 x 1.19 x 0.74 cm, as indicated by the black arrow. The top image is in the transverse plane and the lower image in the longitudinal plane. The photomicrograph at low power (D) is from the same patient after thyroid lobectomy and demonstrates the normal thyroid gland with its follicular appearance surrounding the uniform parathyroid adenoma void of fat and discretely encapsulated.

tralateral double adenoma would be missed with unilateral exploration, this incidence is low and consistent with a potential limited failure rate. At the University of Vermont, we theoretically would have failed to cure 2.5% of cases with unilateral exploration, since this is our incidence of bilateral double adenomata. Attie[21] has reported an incidence of 3.8% double adenoma. Criteria for the diagnosis of double adenoma are:

1. More than one and fewer than four enlarged parathyroid glands at surgery
2. At least one normal parathyroid gland
3. No evidence of MEN or familial hyperparathyroidism
4. Permanent normocalcemia after resection of the enlarged parathyroid glands.

From December 1995 to the present, all patients with surgical intervention for primary hyperparathyroidism have had pre-operative Tc-99m-Sestamibi scan and intra-operative PTH assay. This technologic marriage has been an orderly progression from the use of pre-operative imaging alone and offers an opportunity for focused surgical intervention. From traditional four site exploration it is now possible, and usually preferable, to approach the usual single enlarged parathyroid gland under local anesthesia, to terminate the procedure without the requirement for frozen section, and to send the patient to the recovery room with a high degree of confidence that the surgical goals have been reached. Prior to the use of intra-operative PTH and reliance on the imaging algorithm previously described, only one failure occurred in 59 cases, which was actually more an error in management than scan interpretation. This case,

early in our experience, was misinterpreted as bilateral adenoma, when in fact the patient had multi-gland hyperplasia and should have undergone comprehensive bilateral multiple site exploration (Figure 33–13). Today with the advent of intra-operative PTH assay, the patient would have been managed differently. In the initial 59 patient series, three cases of mediastinal adenoma beyond the reach of cervical exploration (Figures 33–10, 33–11) and two deep intra-thyroidal parathyroid adenomata were all identified on the pre-operative Sestamibi scans. With the use of intra-operative PTH and focused surgery, localization studies take on an additional level of importance. In 96 of these 106 patients (91%) the correct side of adenoma was approached initially by the surgical team, which added efficiency and reduced morbidity to the procedure. The reason for this improved intra-operative localization anticipation beyond the 83% sensitivity of Tc-99m-Sestamibi scan reported by the radiologist, is surgeon interpretation of the scans in the operating room. Frequently, a suspected image for parathyroid adenoma will be present at the 15 minute scan, but will wash out on the delayed two or three hour images. In nearly every circumstance, these suspicions have been confirmed at surgical exploration, allowing accurate entry to the correct side of the neck. We have now encountered four intra-thyroidal adenomata and all have been anticipated on combined Tc-99m-Sestamibi scan and ultrasound. In one case, color Doppler identified a discrete blood supply which is not usually seen in thyroid adenoma. In three of these cases, a thyroidotomy was performed and the adenoma discretely removed without the need for thyroid lobectomy.

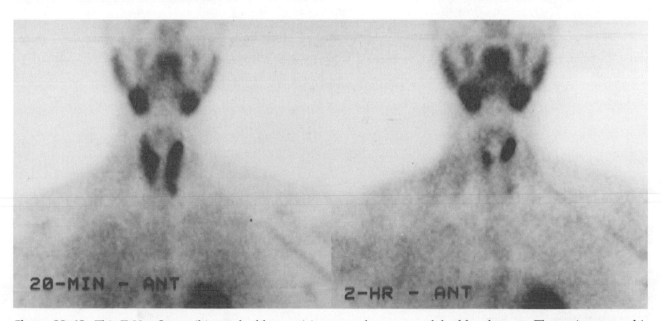

**Figure 33–13.** This Tc99m-Sestamibi scan had been misinterpreted as a case of double adenoma. The patient was ultimately proven to have diffuse hyperplasia of at least five parathyroid glands. Therefore, in bilateral imaging uptake, *all* parathyroid glands must be inspected.

In our experience SPECT imaging is reserved for special circumstances, ie revision procedures, mediastinal adenoma, and on occasions when the patient or surgeon wants the most possible pre-operative information. One patient in this series presented with a suspect mediastinal adenoma and it was preferable to confirm the presence with another imaging study prior to planned sternotomy (Figure 33–14). A chest CT scan and MRI were both negative, whereas the subsequent SPECT Sestamibi study clearly localized to the anterior mediastinum. Another patient with a faintly positive image on initial Sestamibi underwent SPECT, which clarified the same location of the adenoma and allowed focused intervention under local anesthesia.

In summary, single and double adenomata are likely to be positively imaged with Tc-99m-Sestamibi, unless one of the tumors is unusually small. In the unilateral circumstance, removal of the adenoma and biopsy of the ipsilateral adjacent normal gland will usually cure

the condition. Similarly, the bilateral adenoma requires examination and biopsy of at least one additional normal gland to avoid confusing this circumstance with diffuse hyperplasia. In the unusual situation where only one adenoma is visualized on Sestamibi scan and a contralateral smaller adenoma is missed, the patient will, in all likelihood, require re-exploration at some future date. The contralateral side will not have been previously violated, placing the recurrent nerve and blood supply to normal parathyroid at no more than conventional surgical risk. All patients undergoing unilateral exploration should be counseled at the initial surgery about this possibility. Patients demonstrating either no uptake or bilateral uptake must have bilateral exploration. Biopsy of normal appearing glands or intra-operative PTH are important adjuncts to the bilateral condition (Figure 33–15). Intra-operative PTH is especially helpful if supernumerary ectopic hyperplastic glands are present. Although not as important as Tc-99m-Sestamibi, high

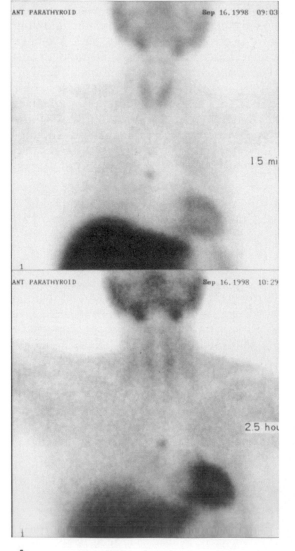

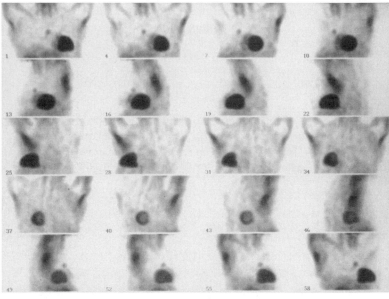

**Figure 33–14A, B.** A cervico-thoracic planar Tc99m-Sestamibi scan (A) demonstrates a suspected mediastinal parathyroid adenoma. Prior to surgery, chest CT and MRI scans were obtained but failed to demonstrate a discrete mass. A SPECT Sestamibi scan (B) similarly confirmed a mediastinal mass, and on lateral views indicated a specific anterior mediastinal location.

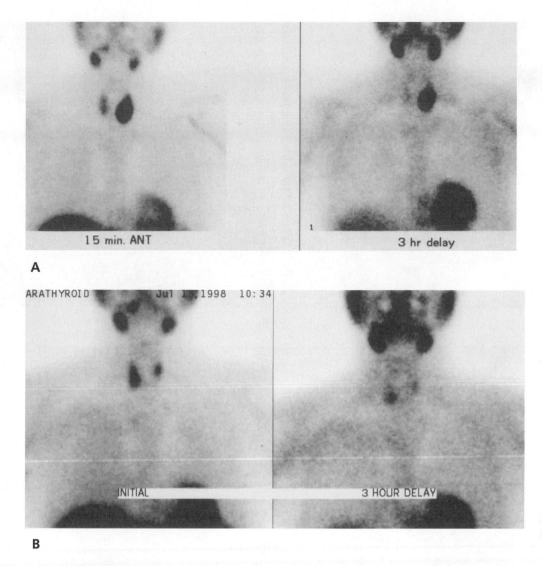

**Figure 33–15A, B.** The Sestamibi scan (A) suggests a left parathyroid adenoma which was confirmed within the left thyroid lobe requiring a lobectomy. Intra-operative PTH reduced from 315 pg/ml to 44 pg/ml and, by the standards of a 14% decrease from baseline, should have resolved the hyperparathyroid state. Mild hypercalcemia persisted after surgery but the patient wanted to defer revision surgery. Six months later, repeat Sestamibi scan (B) then showed concentrated uptake on the opposite side which was not apparent even retrospectively on the first scan. This was confirmed at surgery to be a second contralateral adenoma with resolution in the patient's hypercalcemia after revision surgery. This case graphically illustrates on Sestamibi scan that second adenomas can be unmasked after initial surgery. Additionally, a cap of normal parathyroid on the second adenoma is very convincing for a diagnosis of double adenoma rather than diffuse hyperplasia. Attie,[21] in a series of 865 patients, identified five patients who maintained normocalcemia for three to 18 years, only to develop a second metachronous parathyroid adenoma.

resolution ultrasound adds a dimension to pre-operative localization. Concomitant thyroid pathology can be anticipated and its management discussed with the patient prior to surgical intervention. Additionally, intra-thyroidal parathyroid adenoma can be easily identified with a combination of ultrasound and Tc-99m-Sestamibi. Interestingly, of the six failures in the first 1,000 cases explored at Massachusetts General Hospital, all were cases of intra-thyroidal parathyroid adenoma.[22] Finally, imaging studies are always required in cases of failed exploration or recurrence of hyperparathyroidism. In these circumstances, careful examination of the neck and thorax is required. CT and MRI scans of the neck and mediastinum with contrast are potential adjunctive imaging studies in addition to SPECT Sestamibi (Figure 33–16). Rodriquez et al[23] have reported a series of 152 re-operative parathyroidectomies and reviewed the studies most helpful in correlating the surgical findings. In their experience, the most useful combination is MRI of the neck and chest, ultrasound, and Tc-99m-Sestamibi. Although with only one single study true positive correlation was less than ideal (ultrasound 53%, Sestamibi 70%, MRI 69%), the three studies together gave the best pre-operative information and correlation with surgical findings.

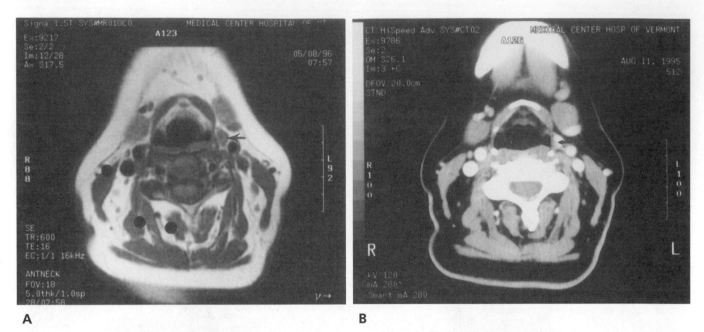

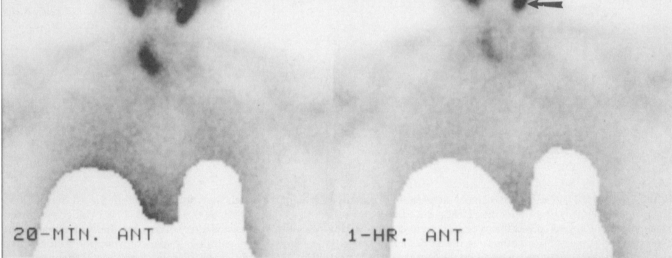

**Figure 33–16A, B, C.** This 65 year-old female was referred for re-operative management of a failed cervical exploration in primary hyperparathyroidism. A planar Sestamibi scan was interpreted as a negative study, but MRI (A) and CT scans (B) demonstrated a mass consistent with an adenoma of an undescended left upper parathyroid gland. At surgery, the parathyroid adenoma was found just inferior to the submandibular gland. A retrospective review of the Sestamibi scan (C) suggests the ectopic site (arrow) can be identified on the original Sestamibi scan.

CT scans were less informative with a true positive rate of only 42%. Ultrasound identified 12 of 14 intra-thyroidal tumors and Technetium-Sestamibi located three of four ectopic glands (one intra-thyroidal, one mediastinal, and one deep cervical).

It is apparent that much controversy remains regarding traditional four site exploration versus pre-operative localization and directed exploration. The improved accuracy of these studies in combination with intra-operative PTH assay has made unilateral focused surgery an exciting capability with a high rate of success and very low morbidity.

## References

1. Taillefer R, Boucher Y, Potvin C, Lambor R. Detection and localization of parathyroid adenomas in patients with hyperparathy-

roidism using a single radionuclide imaging procedure with technetium 99m sestamibi (double phase) *J Nucl Med.* 1992;33:1801–1809.

2. Jofre J, Gonzalez P, Massardo T, Zavola A. Optimal imaging for delayed images in the diagnosis of abnormal parathyroid tissue with Tc-99m-Sestamibi. *Clin Nucl Med.* 1999;24:594–596.

3. Hindie E, Melliere D, Jeannguillaume C, Perlemater L, Chehade F, Galle F. Parathyroid imaging using simultaneous double window recording of technetium-99m-sestamibi and iodine–123. *J Nucl Med.* 1998;39:1100–1105.

4. Neumann D, Esselstyn C, Madera A. Sestamibi/iodine subtraction single photon emission computed tomography in re-operative secondary hyperparathyroidism. *Surgery.* 2000;128:22–34.

5. Carty S, Worsey J, Virji M, Brown M, Watson C. Concise parathyroidectomy and the impact of preopreative SPECT 99mTc-sestamibi scanning and intra-operative quick parathormone assay. *Surgery.* 1997;122:1107–1116.

6. O'Doherty M. Radionuclide parathyroid imaging. *J Nucl Med.* 1997;38:840–841.

7. Coakley AJ, Kettle AG, Wells CP et al. 99m-Tc-sestamibi: a new agent for parathyroid imaging. *Nucl Med Commun.* 1989;10:791–794.

8. Sananta A, Wilson B, Igbal J et al. A clinical audit of Thallium-technetium subtraction parathyroid scans. *Postgrad Med. J.* 1990;66:441–445.

9. Roe SM, Burns RP, Graham LD, Brock, WB, Russell WL. Cost effectiveness of pre-operative localization studies in primary hyperparathyroid disease. *Am Surg.* 1994;219:582–586.

10. Palton F, Huglo D. Proye C. Radionuclide scanning in parathyroid disease. *Br J Surg.* 1998;85:1605–1616.

11. Chiu ML, Kronage JP, Piwnica-Worms D. Effect of mitochondrial and plasma-membrane potentials on accumulations of lexakis (2-methoxyisolutylisonitrile) technetium in cultured mouse fibroblasts. *J Nucl Med.* 1990;31:1646–1653.

12. Sandrock D, Merino M, Norton J, Naumann D. Ultrastructural histology correlates with results of thallium-99m parathyroid subtraction scintigraphy. *J Nucl Med.* 1993;34:24–29.

13. Takebayashi S, Hidai H, Chiba T, Takagi Y, Nagatami Y, Matsubara S. Hyperfunctional parathyroid glands with 99mTc-MIBI scan: semiquantitative analysis correlated with histologic findings. *J Nucl Med.* 1999;40: 1792–1797.

14. Sfakianakis GN, Irvin GL, Mallin W et al. Efficient parathyroidectomy guided by SPECT-MIBI and hormonal measurements. *J Nucl Med.* 1996;37:798–804.

15. Pearl A, Chapnik J, Freeman J et al. A pre-operative localization of 25 consecutive adenomas: a prospective imaging/surgical correlative study. *J Otolaryngology.* 1993;22:301–306.

16. Hasselgren P, Fidler JP. Further evidence against the routine use of parathyroid ultrasonography prior to initial neck exploration for hyperparathyroidism. *Amer J Surg.* 1992;164:337–340.

17. Sofferman RA, Nathan MH. The ectopic parathyroid adenoma: a cost justification for routine pre-operative localization with Technetium 99m sestamibi scan. *Arch Orolaryngol-Head Neck Surg.* 1998;124:649–654.

18. Patton F, Torres G, Mondragon-Sanchez A et al. Correlation of parathyroid scanning and anatomy in 261 unselected patients with sporadic primary hyperparathyroidism. *Surgery.* 1999;126:1123–1131.

19. DeFeo M et al. Parathyroid glands: combination of 99mTcMIBI scintigraphy and US for demonstration of parathyroid glands and nodules. *Radiology.* 2000;214:393–402.

20. Sofferman R et al. Pre-operative technetium Tc-99m-Sestamibi imaging: paving the way to minimal-access parathyroid surgery. *Arch Otol Neck Surg.* 1996;122:369–374.

21. Attie J, Bock G, Auguste LJ. Multiple parathyroid adenomas: report of thirty-three cases. *Surgery.* 1990;108:1014–1020.

22. Wang CA. Surgical management of parathyroid disorders. In: Cummings CW, ed. *Otolaryngology—Head and Neck Surgery*, 2nd ed. St. Louis, MO: Mosby-Yearbook Inc.; 1993.

23. Rodriquez JM, Tezelman S, Siperstein AE et al. Localization procedures in patients with persistent or recurrent hyperparathyroidism. *Arch Surg.* 1994;129:870–875.

# 34

# Parathyroidectomy

James I. Cohen, M.D., Ph.D.
Peter E. Andersen, M.D.

## INTRODUCTION

Parathyroidectomy differs fundamentally from most other operations performed in the head and neck region. The primary concerns of the surgeon as he or she approaches the operation have more to do with whether or not the disease process can be found, rather than the technical aspects of ensuring that it can be removed. This difference is also reflected in the preoperative work-up which is, again, focused on locating the parathyroid tissue of concern rather than studying its margins with respect to normal tissue. This fundamental difference produces an anxiety in most head and neck surgeons as they begin to learn the operation, for while they may be experienced in head and neck anatomic relationships and techniques of tumor removal they are naïve to the art of systematic exploration of an anatomic region. This anxiety is best countered by a dogmatic adherence to a step-by-step pedantic approach; short-cuts tend to create problems. Parathyroid exploration has a steep learning curve, which predominantly has to do with issues surrounding the relative location of the parathyroid glands, their patterns of migration if in an abnormal position, and the ability to distinguish between parathyroid tissue, surrounding fat and lymph nodes without the need for extensive frozen section.

The purpose of this chapter is not to discuss the relative merits of the various preoperative localization studies, or the pros and cons of minimal access surgery, unilateral exploration or bilateral exploration. Rather, it will present a system of unilateral exploration that can be tailored or extended to the situation at hand, de-pending upon the availability of preoperative localization studies, intra-operative PTH assays, surgeon preference and other factors.

## GENERAL CONSIDERATIONS

The key elements to this operation are enhanced if the field is kept dry, as even a small amount of blood staining can make distinguishing normal parathyroid tissue from surrounding fat very difficult. Our preference is to use cautery dissection, both monopolar and bipolar, to facilitate this. Loupe magnification is also helpful in the early identification of the subtle color differences and small vascular pedicles that supply the parathyroid glands and distinguish them from the surrounding tissue.

From a parathyroid exploration standpoint, the neck should be regarded as having two distinct sides. The goal is to systematically explore a side completely before moving to the contralateral side so that it is never necessary to operate in a previously explored area. Exploration continues until either both glands on that side of the neck have been located or all possible locations, approachable transcervically, are excluded. Re-operation, whether later returning to the original side in the same operation where blood staining will have obscured the normal color differences, or at a second operation where scarring obscures not only color changes but also the tissue planes and vascular pedicles normally relied upon for parathyroid identification, is exponentially more difficult. By contrast, the minimal access operations, discussed in detail elsewhere in this book, are not explorations but rather targeted excisions that rely on preoperative localization studies to create a map for a very anatomically focused operation. Dissection of the normal surrounding tissue is kept to a minimum so that should the operation prove unsuccessful, formal re-exploration can be done through a predominantly virgin field.

## PREOPERATIVE CONSIDERATIONS

Proper planning can help reduce much of the anxiety that is normally experienced in the early phases of learning this operation. All possible steps should be taken to decrease the likelihood of being distracted from the surgical plan. The length of time required for the operation is difficult to predict unless localization studies are secure. Time pressures create extra anxiety, and encourage shortcuts from a systematic plan, resulting in increased blood loss which, although minimal, is sufficient to result in problematic tissue staining. Therefore, early in the surgeon's experience, these cases should be scheduled as a last case with no time deadlines to follow. As surgical expertise becomes more secure and the institutional accuracy of localization studies better defined, this may be modified.

Informed consent also deserves special consideration. In addition to the expected small risks of anesthesia, bleeding, infection, and recurrent laryngeal nerve injury, the patient must be introduced to the concept that the offending gland might not be found and that this may not reflect a lack of surgical expertise but rather an aberrant position of the gland. Although in theory a mediastinal adenoma is always a possibility, we do not prepare our patients for a simultaneous cervical and chest exploration, including sternotomy, unless preoperative localization studies have identified an adenoma there. Rather, we tell them that the neck will be explored as completely as necessary to identify an adenoma if it is present in the neck. If it is not found transcervically, the operation will be terminated and after further confirmatory work-up, the chest explored at a later time. We have found that patients, if properly prepared, are more accepting of the small uncertainty of the operation in terms of its potential duration and the possibility of a failed transcervical exploration than they are of the possibility of the added morbidity of a median sternotomy.

Finally the surgeon must be sure the diagnosis is secure. The apprehension encountered during a difficult exploration should not be compounded by sudden doubts about whether or not the disease process is actually present. If the hypercalcemia is relatively mild and/or the localization studies ambiguous, or any other issues raise doubt, this should be sorted out preoper-

atively by appropriate testing or consultation. Operation for hyperparathyroidism is designed to cure not diagnose the disease.

## INTRAOPERATIVE ISSUES

### Guiding Principles

As mentioned above, a dogmatic adherence to a systematic approach works best for this operation, and while experience may temper this, more errors are made because of omission rather than commission in this endeavor. A guiding principle is that a parathyroid gland is not considered identified at surgery, regardless of how sure the surgeon is, unless there is a biopsy confirming the presence of parathyroid tissue. Unfortunately, on frozen section, the pathologist can only reliably determine whether or not parathyroid tissue is present in the tissue sample. He or she cannot distinguish histologically at the time of operation between normal parathyroid tissue, hyperplastic parathyroid tissue, and an adenoma in the vast majority of circumstances. Hyperparathyroidism is at its core a biochemical condition rather than a histologic one; until the recent advent of intra-operative PTH assays, the only criteria the surgeon has been able to rely upon in terms of intra-operative decision making, has been the macroscopic appearance of the identified parathyroid gland(s). Thus, intellectual honesty about what is being seen is required. Size variation among normal glands is very common, and only at its extreme can it be relied upon to accurately label adenoma or hyperplasia. For these reasons, excluding the minimal access approach or the use of intra-operative parathyroid hormone assays, the operation must proceed until an abnormal and a normal gland are identified on the first side and pathologically confirmed as parathyroid tissue; or both sides have been similarly completely explored.

### Technique

The technique of a unilateral operation will be discussed as the basic operation, with the assumption that the principles are easily adapted to the bilateral or minimal access approach.

### Exposure

Peri-operative antibiotics are not necessary for this operation. At the time of induction, the potential need for bilateral exploration must be taken into account in every operation even if the preoperative localization studies seem secure. Thus, the endotracheal tube should be secured in a position, such that both sides of the neck are available for exploration. We prefer to bring the tube up over the top of the patient, taping it to the forehead, and turn the table 90 degrees so that we can position ourselves around the table while operating (see Figure 34–1). This also facilitates superior retraction.

A standard thyroid incision is outlined, which is placed in a horizontal neck crease just below the cricoid cartilage at approximately the level of the thyroid isthmus. This relatively low incision facilitates upper mediastinal exploration, which is critical in following the migration of abnormally positioned inferior glands, whereas superior exposure is seldom an issue in exploring for aberrant superior glands as they tend to migrate into the posterior mediastinum. It is also important to remember that a short incision shifted from side to side by appropriate retraction, if necessary for sequential bilateral exposure, will give adequate exposure. Monopolar cautery is then used in the subplatysmal elevation of the skin flaps up to the hyoid bone and down to the sternal notch. The wound is kept "shallow" after the skin flaps are elevated by ensuring that retraction is pulling parallel to the skin and not upwards, as this latter maneuver can artificially deepen the wound and make things unnecessarily difficult in terms of exposure.

From this point the operation can proceed in one of two ways: the medial approach, where the strap muscles are split in the midline and retracted laterally, thereby working all the way around the anterior aspect of the thyroid lobe to rotate it medially and expose the parathyroids on its posterior lateral surface; or the lateral approach, where the fascia along the anterior border

of the sternocleidomastoid muscle and between the lateral border of the strap muscles and carotid sheath is incised thereby exposing the lateral edge of the thyroid lobe that is then rolled medially with the attached strap muscles.

While this latter approach is certainly faster and involves less dissection (and therefore well suited to the minimal access operation with a significantly enlarged normally positioned adenoma), it offers a slightly distorted and more limited view of the anatomy, particularly with respect to the lower thyroid pole and upper mediastinum. Therefore, we believe that unilateral parathyroid exploration is best learned by the medial approach, as a modification of thyroid lobectomy. The only difference between the operation and a hemithyroidectomy is that in one operation the ipsilateral lobe is removed and the parathyroids identified and left in situ, while in the other the thyroid lobe is dissected and left in situ with the normal parathyroid gland identified and the parathyroid adenoma removed. As one's comfort with the anatomy of the area and familiarity with parathyroid tissue increases, significant time can be saved by selectively adopting the lateral approach, particularly if preoperative localization seems secure.

The medial approach (Figure 34–2) will therefore be described first. As with thyroid lobectomy, the key to this operation is working along the capsule of the gland, freeing it up completely so that it can be easily rotated medially and retracted superiorly, and the soft tissues that surround its posterior and inferior aspects brought up into the field. Division of the sternothyroid muscle, so that it can be completely dissected off the underlying thyroid and superior mediastinal fat, and ligation of the superior thyroid pedicle with complete mobilization of the superior pole of the thyroid gland, greatly facilitates this medial rotation of the thyroid lobe. Prior to rotating the gland forward, the middle thyroid vein and inferior thyroid veins are ligated as closely as possible to the capsule of the gland. Special attention should be paid to the fat on the posterior surface of these inferior veins at their junction with the capsule as the inferior gland may be located there. If the veins are divided too low, a parathyroid gland may be rotated forward with the lobe and missed; if they are divided on the capsule and released without inspection, the inferior gland may retract inferiorly and be more difficult to locate. Bipolar cautery and/or ligation is used in this part of the dissection.

The gland is then grasped on its lateral edge with two Babcock clamps placed carefully, so as not to include a parathyroid in their teeth, and rotated medially and superiorly with appropriate traction.

In the lateral approach (Figure 34–3), the skin incision and flap elevation are identical to that of the medial approach. After elevation of the skin flaps, the fascia

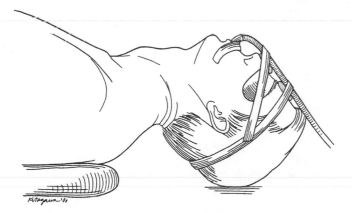

**Figure 34–1.** Patient/Endotracheal Tube Positioning—The neck is extended with a shoulder roll placed vertically between the scapulae. The eyes are protected with eye shields and the endotracheal tube and breathing circuit brought over the top of the patient's head, securing it to the forehead over foam rubber padding. This allows equal access to both sides of the patient's neck.

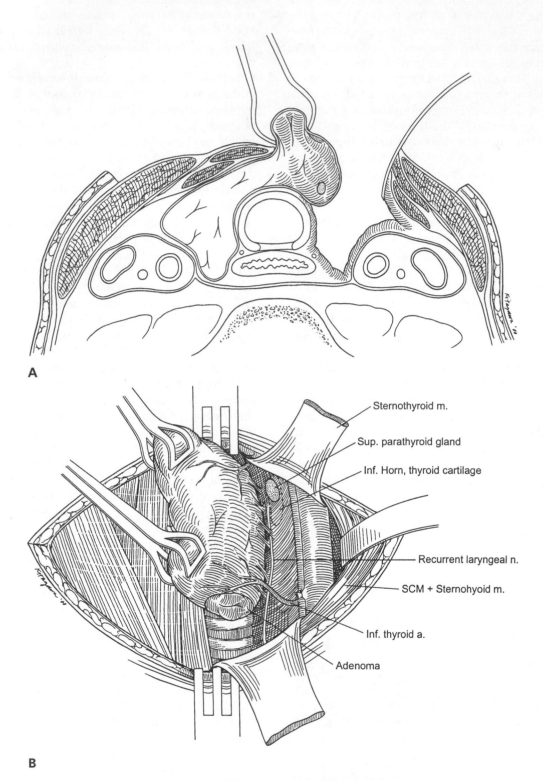

**A**

**B**

**Figure 34–2A and 34–2B.** Parathyroid Exploration—Medial Approach—The sternohyoid muscle is retracted laterally and the sternothyroid muscle is either similarly retracted or divided. The superior and inferior thyroid pedicle are then divided and the gland rolled forward exposing its posterior lateral surface and the parathyroid glands.

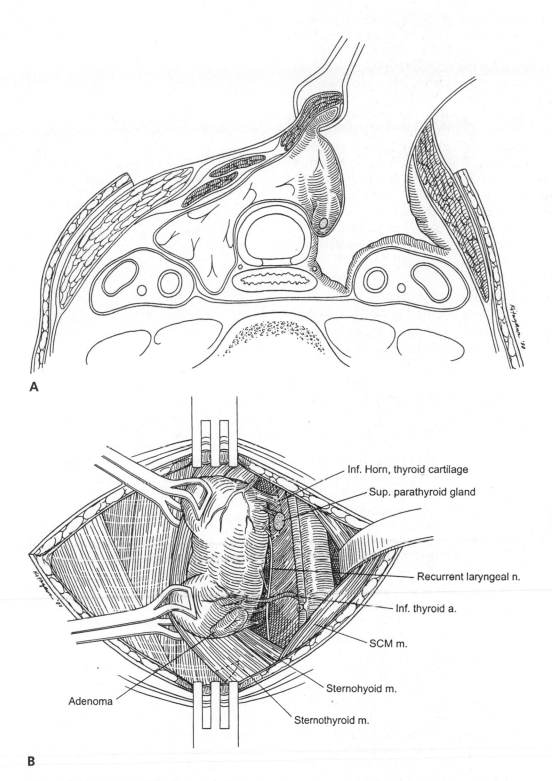

**A**

**B**

Inf. Horn, thyroid cartilage

Sup. parathyroid gland

Recurrent laryngeal n.

Inf. thyroid a.

SCM m.

Sternohyoid m.

Sternothyroid m.

Adenoma

**Figure 34–3A and 34–3B.** Parathyroid Exploration—Lateral Approach—The fascia between the sternocleidomastoid muscle and sternohyoid/sternothyroid muscles is divided allowing the sternohyoid, sternothyroid and thyroid gland to be grasped as a single unit and rolled forward, exposing the posterior lateral surface of the thyroid gland and the parathyroid glands. A relaxing incision in the lateral half of the inferior aspect of the sternothyroid muscle is sometimes necessary for complete exposure.

along the medial border of the sternocleidomastoid muscle, and between the carotid sheath and lateral border of the strap muscles, is incised. The middle thyroid vein is once again ligated on the thyroid capsule and two Babcocks grasp the upper pole and the lower pole of the thyroid in conjunction with the overlying strap muscles and rotate the two together medially as a unit. The presence of the strap muscle limits the ability to rotate and pull the thyroid superiorly to some degree so that inferior exposure is more difficult. With this in mind, one can incise at least half of the lateral aspect of the sternothyroid muscle inferiorly, to facilitate retraction. However in considering this approach for an inferiorly situated adenoma as part of a unilateral exploration or minimal access surgery, this limitation of inferior exposure must be recognized.

## Searching for the Parathyroids

Dissection continues medially on the posterior capsule in a vertically oriented straight line gradually releasing the surrounding soft tissues and looking for the parathyroids. Staying on the capsule is important as it ensures identification of a parathyroid gland trapped and compressed within the capsule and therefore harder to distinguish on color grounds from the thyroid. In addition, it allows early identification and preservation of the inferior thyroid artery and its small branches which, if followed, can lead to the parathyroid glands. It also prevents accidental forward displacement of the recurrent laryngeal nerve on the capsule and allows it to be easily identified in its most stable position adjacent to the inferior thyroid cornu where it enters the larynx. Identification of this nerve is mandatory as part of an exploration to prevent accidental injury, and helpful as it represents a line that can help distinguish between the superior and inferior parathyroid gland. A gland located above and lateral to the nerve is most likely to be the superior gland; below and medial to it the gland in association with the inferior thyroid pole veins is most likely to be an inferior gland (Figure 34–4).

Although an adenoma may be immediately obvious, one must avoid the temptation to immediately excise it, as this may distort normal anatomic relationships; rather, one should proceed carefully with the rest of the exploration. In general, it is the normal gland that is the most difficult to find, as it is often smaller than normal as a result of chronic suppression by the patient's hypercalcemia.

There are a number of clues that can be used to identify parathyroid tissue without extensive biopsies and frozen section. Parathyroid tissue is darker and browner than the surrounding yellow fat or the whiter tissue of the thymus. It is not as red as para-tracheal lymph nodes which also tend to be firmer and rounder. Parathyroids have a distinct vascular pedicle, best seen

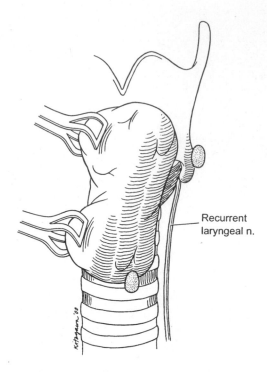

Recurrent laryngeal n.

**Figure 34–4.** Recurrent Laryngeal Nerve/Parathyroid Gland Anatomy—The recurrent laryngeal nerve is most reliably identified where it enters the larynx on the lateral cricothyroid membrane just anterior to the inferior thyroid cartilage cornu. The superior parathyroid gland is normally situated superior and lateral to this position. The inferior parathyroid gland is normally situated anterior and inferior to this location.

with loupe magnification, which may be very useful in distinguishing glands from surrounding tissue. Parathyroid tissue sinks when placed in saline; fat tends to float.

With time, these tissues are not difficult to distinguish from each other, but this is not a substitute for frozen section confirmation. Therefore, when both parathyroid glands on one side have been identified, they are biopsied. Biopsies are done from the end of the gland farthest from the vascular pedicle in an attempt to save as much normal tissue and blood supply as possible. The cut bleeding surface is allowed to stop bleeding spontaneously, rather than risk injuring the remaining tissue with cautery. Realistically however, parathyroid biopsy often results in temporary gland dysfunction, and this must be acknowledged as one determines the risk for postoperative hypoparathyroidism.

To avoid accidental wasting of parathyroid tissue, a gland is only completely removed if it is clearly abnormal in size relative to the normal gland. Otherwise a small confirmatory biopsy is performed and, prior to excision, the contralateral side explored in order to help determine which gland(s) are clearly abnormal. Glands that are accidentally removed or become compromised at the time of surgery, particularly as a result of venous congestion, should be cut into small pieces and immediately reimplanted into the sternocleidomastoid muscle. When there is an uncertainty about whether or not excised parathyroid tissue is abnormal, it should be kept on ice in saline while frozen section is done. If uncertainty persists, tissue should be cryopreserved, after a sufficient amount has been sent to pathology, for later reimplantation should it prove necessary.

## The Missing Gland

A common clinical situation occurs when, after complete exploration of one side of the neck, only one seemingly normal parathyroid gland can be found. At this point a systematic search is begun based upon which gland is missing and the typical pattern of aberrant migration is considered. Superior glands tend to migrate towards the posterior mediastinum and, if enlarged, may have the recurrent laryngeal nerve draped over them. Inferior glands, by contrast, migrate toward the anterior mediastinum and may be found in a superior thymic extension anterolateral to the trachea (Figure 34–5). All vascular pedicles, particularly those leading

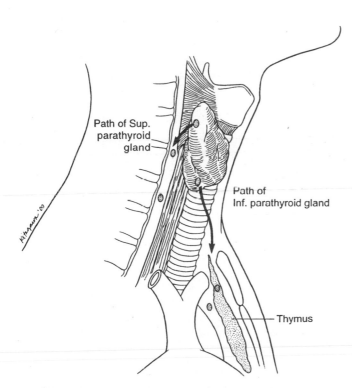

**Figure 34–5.** Aberrant Parathyroid Gland Position—In general the superior gland, if abnormally descended, travels into the posterior mediastinum. The recurrent laryngeal nerve may be draped over its superior and lateral surface. The inferior parathyroid gland if abnormally descended, migrates into the anterior mediastinum and is situated anterior to the recurrent laryngeal nerve.

toward the thymus, are followed and explored. The superior thymus should, at a minimum, be removed and examined on the back table to look for the presence of parathyroid tissue. If the inferior gland is judged to be missing, the majority of the tissue in the superior mediastinum down to the level of the innominate artery can be excised by careful traction on the thymic tissue as it is pulled superiorly. The exploration of the upper mediastinum is greatly facilitated by being sure that the patient's neck is fully extended and placing the initial incision low enough that one is not working under a long inferior flap. The recurrent laryngeal nerve, which will be posterior to this dissection, must be traced inferiorly to ensure that it is not accidentally injured. The retroesophageal region is explored if the superior gland is missing, particularly posterior to where the recurrent laryngeal nerve enters the larynx. While the carotid sheath can be palpated and visualized, it is generally not incised unless there are abnormalities detected. Avoiding disuption of the neck lateral to the carotid sheath will make subsequent imaging studies for localization more useful.

Everything short of removal of the ipsilateral thyroid lobe is done prior to exploring the opposite side. The concept of identifying an abnormal gland, not finding the normal gland, and therefore going to the opposite side to do so is to be condemned, because if the patient remains hyperparathyroid, then both sides have been partially explored unsuccessfully and both must be re-explored.

Methylene blue may be helpful in the setting of the unidentified gland. Five mg/kg IV is given in a 200 cc bolus of saline. Its effect is to darken the parathyroid glands relative to the surrounding tissue, peaking at about 10–20 minutes after infusion and lasting for 60 minutes. Therefore, it is not given preoperatively, but if required, may be given intra-operatively, without significant delay in the procedure.

Following a complete bilateral exploration, and then only if a single gland is missing, should the ipsilateral thyroid lobe be excised to exclude the possibility of an intra-thyroidal gland.

## The Operative Note

Whether the operation is successful or unsuccessful, the operative note is critically important should future management be necessary. This will provide the best clues as to the likely position of a missing gland if it is properly dictated. The operative note must include a complete listing of all regions explored, the size and location of all glands found, and the position and status of the recurrent laryngeal nerves. Most importantly, the intra-operative pathology record must be examined and the source and result of every frozen or permanent section reviewed.

## Postoperative Management

This wound is generally not drained unless there has been extensive dissection or an extremely enlarged thyroid lobe, which results in a larger wound bed. Unilateral explorations do not need to be kept in hospital overnight postoperatively, as even in the case of extreme bone hunger resulting from long term hyperparathyroidism, the remaining two undisturbed parathyroid glands prevent the patient from becoming dangerously hypocalcemic. Mild symptoms may develop when the serum calcium level falls to the 7–8 mg/dl range, however this does not represent any significant risk to the patient. Serum total or ionized calcium levels are monitored on a q6–8hr basis initially (6–18 hrs) to ensure an appropriate drop, indicating a successful operation and later (12–24 hr) in the case of bilateral exploration to rule out postoperative hypoparathyroidism.

## CONCLUSION

Exploration for hyperparathyroidism requires rigorous, systematic exploration of the neck and extreme honesty with oneself regarding the operative findings; there are no shortcuts possible if one hopes to achieve a high cure rate with initial surgical management. However, by careful attention to detail and this strict adherence to a systematic approach, a successful parathyroid exploration can be accomplished in the majority of cases. As the surgeon's experience grows he or she will become facile with the identification of abnormal hyperfunctional parathyroid glands in all their myriad forms and locations, and the initial anxiety associated with the operation will be replaced by the comfort of knowing that if abnormal parathyroid tissue is present it will be found.

# 35

# Surgical Management of Primary Hyperparathyroidism

Phillip K. Pellitteri, D.O., F.A.C.S.
Pranay Patel, M.D., F.A.C.S.

## INTRODUCTION

Surgical exploration with removal of the hyperfunctioning parathyroid gland(s) represents the only available definitive treatment for primary hyperparathyroidism.[1] The approach to surgical exploration is predicated upon the disease entity involved and the skill, experience, and management philosophy of the surgeon. In general, the optimal surgical approach is individualized to offer the best chance for cure while minimizing the potential for morbidity and cost.

This discussion offers perspectives on the surgical management of sporadic primary hyperparathyroidism relative to the indications for exploration and the issues that influence surgical technique and decision-making. A detailed discussion of primary hyperparathyroidism associated with inherited disorders (MEN, severe neonatal hyperparathyroidism) can be found in Chapter 36 and will not be addressed here.

## PRIMARY HYPERPARATHYROIDISM

Primary hyperparathyroidism results from hyperfunctioning of parathyroid glands without the influence of a proven physiologic stimulus. Parathyroid hormone secretion is elevated and, consequently, patients are rendered hypercalcemic. The incidence in patients over age 50 has been determined to be approximately 4 to 6 per thousand, with female to male ratios varying from 2:1 to 4:1. This incidence appears highest in postmenopausal women over 65 years old.

The prevalence of the diagnosis of primary hyperparathyroidism has increased, largely as a result of widespread use of routine blood chemistry screening in ambulatory and hospitalized patients over the last three decades. The usual offending lesion in primary hyperparathyroidism is the parathyroid adenoma, occurring in a solitary manner in approximately 85% of patients with primary hyperparathyroidism in large studies. Hyperplasia has been judged to occur in approximately 12% to 15% of patients, the chief cell variety being more common than the clear cell.

The incidence of multiple adenomas is low, occurring in approximately 1% to 2% of patients with hyperparathyroidsm.[2] Some of these may actually represent nodular hyperplasia. Carcinomatous parathyroid glands producing hyperparathyroidism is rare, occurring in less than 1% to 2% of patients with the disorder.

## CLINICAL CHARACTERIZATION

### Presentation

The majority of patients treated for hyperparathyroidism in recent years have not manifested symptoms as a result of their disease. The usual presenting abnormality in these patients is an abnormally elevated serum calcium detected on routine blood chemistry screening. Despite the lack of obvious abnormalities noted at the time of diagnosis, caution should be exercised before declaring that a patient is asymptomatic. A number of seemingly asymptomatic patients may manifest subtle or even "silent sequelae" of hyperparathyroidism at presentation. These patients may, in fact, be more appropriately described as minimally symptomatic in that nonspecific symptoms and unidentified complications of hyperparathyroidism would be eliminated by parathyroidectomy.[3] Some of these nonspecific entities include: emotional complaints, muscular fatigue, constipation, bone and joint pain, and silent objective findings such as renal calculi and decreased bone density. In the majority of patients with asymptomatic or minimally symptomatic hyperparathyroidism, these symptoms are subtle and may be so common in the general population that they preclude establishment of a causal relationship to primary hyperparathyroidism.

Among patients in whom symptoms are present or evolving at the time of diagnosis, two populations may be identified. In the first group, the disease progresses insidiously over several years and eventually presents as renal colic. The second group manifests symptoms over a considerably shorter period of time with marked elevations in serum calcium leading to weight loss, acute GI symptoms, anorexia, bone pain, and occasionally pathologic fracture. Traditionally, clinical manifestations are described according to the organ system affected.

## Kidney/Urinary Tract

Historically, greater than 50% of patients with hyperparathyroidism developed renal symptoms manifested by nephrolithiasis and nephrocalcinosis. This percentage decreased significantly to approximately 4% following the widespread use of screening tests for serum calcium levels.[4] Most stones are composed of calcium oxalate; however, calcium phosphate stones may also occur. The symptoms associated with urolithiasis include renal colic, hematuria, and pyuria. Metabolic acidosis may also be a part of the clinical syndrome.

## Skeletal System

Abnormalities of the skeletal system in the form of osteitis fibrosa cystica, once a common malady in patients with primary hyperparathyroidism, are now rarely encountered (less than 10%). These changes include subperiosteal erosion of the distal phalanges, bone wasting and softening, and chondrocalcinosis as a result of bone demineralization. Bone disease may present as bone pain, pathologic fracture, cystic bone changes, or focal areas of bone swelling (epulis of the jaw or "brown" tumors) representing accumulations of osteoclasts, os-

teoblasts, and fibrous matrix. Symptoms attributable to joint pathology include gout and pseudogout.

Bone loss in hyperparathyroidism occurs at cortical bone sites, generally sparing trabecular bone.[5] Because of this finding, the role of hyperparathyroidism in osteoporosis is not clear, especially for patients in whom symptoms are minimal or absent and in whom the disease is mild.

Postmenopausal women with primary hyperparathyroidism exhibiting early signs of osteoporosis appear to be at significant risk for developing more severe bone disease and resultant sequelae, ie, vertebral and hip fractures. It is in this population of patients that the benefit of parathyroidectomy is most apparent.[6]

## Neuromuscular

Muscle weakness, particularly in the proximal extremity muscle groups, together with progressive fatigue and malaise, may occur in symptomatic primary hyperparathyroidism. Electromyographic changes may be seen in these patients together with atrophy of skeletal muscle on biopsy. Although the severe symptoms are rarely encountered, subtle signs of muscle fatigue and weakness may be present in as many as 40% of patients with mild primary hyperparathyroidism. Usually these subtle symptoms are manifested as muscle aches and fatigue on rising from a chair or climbing stairs. Progression of the disease may ultimately result in weakness that limits activity and ambulation over a short period of time (weeks to months). The weakness is noted to improve following parathyroidectomy.

## Neurologic

Neurologic manifestations of primary hyperparathyroidism are represented by a spectrum of symptoms ranging from anxiety and mild emotional disturbance to frank psychosis. Depression, nervousness, and cognitive dysfunction may commonly occur to varying degrees in primary hyperparathyroidism. Cerebral dysfunction characterized by organic brain syndrome is more common in elderly patients with an underlying mild cognitive abnormality exposed to hypercalcemia. Other neurologic changes occasionally seen in patients with hyperparathyroidism include deafness, dysphagia, dysosmia, and dysesthesia.

## Gastrointestinal

Gastrointestinal disorders that may occur in hyperparathyroidism include acid peptic disease, pancreatitis, and cholelithiasis. Peptic ulceration occurs with increased frequency in these patients secondary to increased serum gastrin and gastric acid secretion stimulated by hypercalcemia. Hyperparathyroidism may be the heralding manifestation of endocrine disease in patients with MEN-1. Those patients exhibiting the Zollinger-Ellison syndrome demonstrate the highest incidence of peptic ulceration. The lower gut may be affected by hyperparathyroidism. Frequently, patients with "asymptomatic disease" complain of sluggish bowels or constipation, which improves following surgery and achievement of normocalcemia.

## Cardiovascular

Hypertension may occur in as many as 50% of patients with hyperparathyroidism. Convincing evidence of a pathogenic mechanism does not exist, however, and parathyroidectomy results in a reduction in blood pressure in only a few of these patients. Swedish investigators reported an association with myocardial ischemia and left ventricular dysfunction in patients with hyperparathyroidism of varying symptomatology, which exhibited reversibility following parathyroidectomy.[7]

## Hypercalcemic Abnormalities

Hypercalcemic syndrome occurring as a result of hyperparathyroidism includes polydipsia and polyuria, anorexia, vomiting, constipation, muscle weakness and fatigue, mental status changes, and skin abnormalities.

Those patients developing markedly elevated serum calcium levels approaching 15 mg/dl may present with severe mental status changes or coma, a so-called hypercalcemic crisis. If untreated, this condition may progress to acute renal failure and the onset of dysrhythmias, which may precipitate sudden death. Other abnormalities include metastatic calcifications at the corneal/scleral junction, so-called "band" keratopathy, shortened Q–T interval on electrocardiogram, ectopic calcium deposits in various organs, and pruritis. Additionally, some patients may present with a nonspecific debility manifested by anorexia, fatigue, anemia, weight loss, and advancing osteitis, all of which are reversible following parathyroidectomy.

## HISTOPATHOLOGIC CHARACTERISTICS

### Single Glandular Enlargement or Parathyroid Adenoma

Single glandular enlargement, or adenoma, is the etiology of primary hyperparathyroidism approximately 85% of the time. Adenomas may be composed of chief cells, transitional forms of oxyphilic cells resembling chief cells and, rarely, pure oxyphilic cells. The typical adenoma displays a monomorphic proliferation of

chief cells within the morphologically enlarged parathyroid gland. In up to 70% of adenomas, a rim of normal parathyroid tissue may be found around the hypercellular portion of the gland (Figure 35–1). However, considerable pleomorphism may be found in both adenomas and multiple enlarged hyperplastic glands. As a result, morphologic criteria alone may not be used to differentiate between the two entities. Cellular mitotic activity is rarely found in adenomas but may frequently be seen in carcinoma. Pure oxyphilic adenomas have been described but are usually nonfunctional and thus are usually noted at autopsy. Occasionally, they are found to produce parathormone and may rarely result in clinical hyperparathyroidism.

The concentration of stromal fat is useful in distinguishing between hyperfunctional and normal parathyroid tissue in that hypercellular tissue in adenoma or hyperplasia is noted to contain little or no stromal fat as compared to normal tissue. This is helpful provided

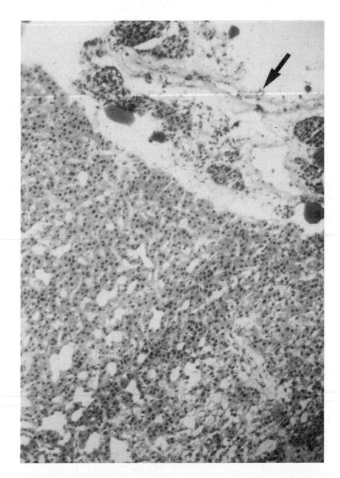

**Figure 35-1.** Parathyroid adenoma, frozen section with oil red O stain. Large dark arrow indicates rim of suppressed parathyroid tissue with abundant inter- and intra-cytoplasmic fat, which is compressed by the adenoma.

the sample of normal gland provided is of sufficient size/volume to determine fat content. In most instances, the histologic evaluation of a single gland cannot differentiate between an adenoma and the presence of a single hyperlastic gland. Typical parathyroid adenomas weigh between 0.1 and 5 gm but may be as large as 20 gm. Grossly, they are indistinguishable from enlarged hyperplastic glands. Larger adenomas may display cystic changes or focal areas of hemorrhage. Rarely, multiple adenomas may occur with the remaining glands being histologically normal (not hypercellular). This has been reported as occurring in 1% to 2% of patients with hyperparathyroidism and is associated with supernumerary glands which are ectopically located. In reality, these may represent instances of nodular hyperplasia occurring in both enlarged and normal-sized glands (see next section, Multiple Enlarged Glands or Parathyroid Gland Hyperplasia).

## Multiple Enlarged Glands or Parathyroid Gland Hyperplasia

Hyperplasia of the parathyroid glands accounts for approximately 12% to 15% of patients with primary hyperparathyroidism. The typical presentation is characterized by enlargement of all four glands. The most common histologic finding is that of chief cell hyperplasia with the predominant cell type being the chief cell. Chief cell hyperplasia may occur in parathyroid glands exhibiting nodules of hyperplastic cells or nodular hyperplasia. Nodular hyperplasia may account for the reports of multiple adenomas.[2] Although hyperplasia affects all four glands, uniform enlargement of the glands may not be seen. In pseudoadenomatous hyperplasia, a single grossly enlarged gland may exist with minimal enlargement of the remaining glands.[8] The smaller, normal appearing glands possess an abnormal histologic appearance characterized by nodularity and an increased cell-to-fat ratio.

Chief cell hyperplasia represents the pathologic entity found in patients with multiple endocrinopathy syndromes (MEN-1 and 2A) and in familial hyperparathyroidism, but generally not in MEN-2B.[9] It is also the predominant lesion found in patients with secondary hyperparathyroidism produced by renal disease.

Water-clear cell hyperplasia is the second variant of primary hyperparathyroid hyperplasia. It is characterized by large vacuous cells arranged in a monotonous pattern and is rarely encountered in primary lesions and not at all in familial and secondary hyperparathyroidism.

## Parathyroid Carcinoma

The true incidence of parathyroid carcinoma is difficult to accurately assess, primarily because of the difficulty in establishing a histologic diagnosis. Most series place the incidence at approximately 1% to 2% of all patients with primary hyperparathyroidism.[10-12] The gross morphologic appearance at surgery is perhaps more distinctive than the histologic evidence in suggesting the diagnosis. The lesions are noted to be hard and fibrous with a grayish-white color, demonstrating adherence to and invasion of, surrounding structures. Carcinomatous glands demonstrate an inflammatory-like reaction that is characteristic and distinct from benign glandular enlargement.

Histologic features considered characteristic include invasion of the fibrous capsule and vascular elements, with trabeculated regions of cells separated by thick fibrous septa. Mitotic figures, rarely seen in benign disease, are usually present. Clinically, a firm palpable mass may be appreciated in the neck. Total serum calcium levels are usually elevated, in excess of 14 to 15 mg/dl, with markedly elevated levels of serum parathyroid hormone being characteristic.

Malignant disease is more common in males than females (in whom benign disease predominates). Death from malignant disease is usually a result of persistent hypercalcemia and associated sequelae. Overall survival is noted to be poor regardless of treatment, with 5- and 10-year survival rates of approximately 50% and 10%, respectively.

## Miscellaneous Parathyroid Lesions

Lipoadenoma is a unique neoplasm composed of parenchymal cells separated by adipose tissue and a myxoid stroma. The tumors are large and solitary and may be functional or nonfunctional. When functional, they are a rare cause of clinical hyperparathyroidism.[13]

Parathyroid cysts are usually noted to be solitary, unilocular, thin-walled structures located low in the neck. The cystic lining is composed of cuboidal or low columnar cells with parathyroid cells present in the wall lining. A few of these cysts have been found to be functional and, in these instances, cystic degeneration of an adenoma or hyperplastic gland must be considered.

## CLINICAL AND DIAGNOSTIC EVALUATION

### History and Physical Examination

Initial efforts at establishing the diagnosis of primary hyperparathyroidism should be aimed at determining the duration of hypercalcemia, if possible, and what symptomatic manifestations have occurred. In the absence of overt symptomatology, subtle historical aspects concerning the patient's level of activity, sense of well-being, and constitutional status should be sought.

A thorough family history of medical and surgical illness should be obtained in order to determine the possible existence of any familial endocrinopathies suggestive of familial hypercalcemia syndromes. A history of previous malignancies should be absolutely ruled out. Inquiries should be made in order to eliminate from the differential diagnosis other etiologies of hypercalcemia, such as sarcoidosis, milk alkali syndrome, hypervitaminosis D, hyperthyroidism, and thiazide diuretic ingestion.

The physical manifestations of hyperparathyroidism are few and when present are usually subtle. The examiner may observe the presence of band keratopathy, calcium deposits located in the medial and lateral limbic region of the cornea. The patient may manifest subtle neuromuscular findings with proximal muscle weakness, predominantly noted in the lower extremities. Rarely, fasciculations of the tongue may be noted. Palpation and pressure on the prominence of the iliac crest and shin may produce pain indicative of bone involvement. A palpable cervical mass representing an enlarged parathyroid gland is almost never appreciated except on the rare occasion that the disease is caused by parathyroid carcinoma or cystic degeneration of an adenoma or hyperplastic gland. A palpable mass usually suggests the presence of a thyroid nodule in most instances.

Preoperative assessment and documentation of vocal cord mobility is advisable, given the risk of recurrent nerve injury during the surgery. Also, baseline presence or absence of Chvostek's sign (contraction of the facial musculature in response to tapping the facial nerve anterior to the tragus) should be noted. Postoperative hypocalcemia is associated with increased neuromuscular excitability and a positive Chvostek's sign, but as many as 15% of normal subjects may have a positive sign without hypocalcemia.

## Laboratory Evaluation

Whereas the physical examination provides clues to the severity of hyperparathyroidism upon which a therapeutic decision may be based, the laboratory investigation and biochemical findings establish the diagnosis.

The definitive diagnosis of primary hyperparathyroidism depends on the concurrent demonstration of persistently elevated serum calcium together with evidence of hyperfunctioning parathyroid tissue represented by elevation of circulating parathyroid hormone or PTH.

Because total serum calcium levels may vary according to the general health of the individual patient, measurements of serum calcium alone are not sufficient to make the diagnosis of hyperparathyroidism. Approximately 40% of total serum calcium is protein bound with a portion of the remaining 60% complexed to anions. The biologically active ionized component represents approximately 50% of the measurable serum calcium. Thus, alterations and total protein levels will strongly influence measured serum calcium and may, under certain conditions, yield an underestimation of the hypercalcemia. In general, about 1 mg/dl of calcium may be added for each gram of total protein by obtaining a serum albumin, especially where nutritional status is in question or in patients with an underlying metabolic disorder. The most accurate indication of hypercalcemia is measurement of the ionized calcium level; however, it is also the most difficult to accurately assess. Provided the protein status of the individual is normal, a series of three determinations of total calcium demonstrating persistent elevation (greater than 10.5 mg/dl) is sufficient to establish the presence of hypercalcemia.

Normocalcemic or subtle hyperparathyroidism is a definite rare entity that must be considered in patients with symptoms or complications of hyperparathyroidism.[14] Minimal elevation, no elevation or intermittent elevation of total serum calcium can still be associated with elevated parathyroid hormone levels and complications, especially nephrolithiasis.[15] Ionized calcium determination in conjunction with intact PTH levels and oral calcium loading has an important role in targeting patients with normocalcemic hyperparathyroidism.[16]

Determination of serum parathyroid hormone represents the most efficient method of assessing parathyroid function. Parathyroid hormone is metabolized rapidly in the circulation into a biologically active N-terminal fragment and an inactive C-terminal fragment. Older assays developed to assess biologically active hormone have been replaced by site-specific immunoassay of "intact" parathyroid hormone. This assay utilizes two region-specific antibodies directed to the N-terminus and mid-molecular region and is now the method of choice for measurement of parathyroid hormone. Because of the variance in both circulating serum calcium and parathyroid hormone levels, both entities should be assessed concurrently.

In the absence of renal disease, it is important to assess the status of urinary calcium in order to eliminate the possibility of familial hypocalciuric hypercalcemia (FHH).[17] FHH is an autosomal dominant disorder that represents a rare cause of hypercalcemia (less than 1%). The disorder results from mutation in the calcium-sensing receptor gene yielding increased renal tubular absorption of calcium.[18] Urinary calcium is noted to be less than 100 to 150 mg over a 24-hour period in the majority of patients affected with FHH. Serum parathyroid hormone may be normal or minimally elevated. Urinary calcium levels in primary hyperparathyroidism are found to be normal or elevated, despite the direct action of PTH on the kidney to influence reabsorption. This is primarily caused by the increased calcium burden in the circulation presented to the kidney. Additional studies should be performed and may prove helpful in establishing the diagnosis and eliminating other causes of hypercalcemia. In addition to the albumin, creatinine and phosphorus levels should be assessed concurrently with serum calcium. Thyroid function studies should be obtained because of the effect of dysthyroid conditions on serum calcium.

## Imaging Studies

The value of imaging studies in establishing the diagnosis of hyperparathyroidism is questionable. However, these studies are often useful in providing evidence in support of the diagnosis and also in eliminating the possibility of other etiologies of hypercalcemia.

Skeletal surveys may provide evidence of direct bone involvement. Radiographs of the skull in affected individuals demonstrate a moth-eaten or salt-and-pepper appearance. Brown tumors may be seen in the skull, mandible, and facial skeleton, or along the long bones of the extremities. Subperiosteal resorption may be seen involving the distal phalangeal tufts on the hands. Generalized demineralization of the axial skeleton may be noted, especially in postmenopausal women exhibiting osteopenia of the spine. The skeletal effects of hyperparathyroidism in presumed asymptomatic patients may be further addressed by bone densitometry studies. This method assesses the density of cortical and trabecular bone at several sites including the lumbar spine, femoral neck, and radius. Comparison is made to normal age and gender matched density values at the same sites, and differences are noted in terms of standard deviation from the mean for age. Patients judged to be at risk for pathologic fracture demonstrate density scores which are two standard deviations or more below the mean for age at these sites.

A chest X-ray is important in order to eliminate the possibility of primary or metastatic malignant disease or granulomatous disease as an etiology for hypercalcemia. A flat plate of the abdomen or urogram is helpful in determining the presence of renal calculi.

## Differential Diagnosis

In distinguishing the hypercalcemia of primary hyperparathyroidism from hypercalcemia caused by other etiologies, the foremost cause to be eliminated is malignancy. Primary hyperparathyroidism, together with malignancy, account for 90% of patients with hypercal-

cemia. In hospitalized patients, malignancy represents the most common etiology for hypercalcemia, while the most prevalent cause in the outpatient setting is hyperparathyroidism. The hypercalcemia of malignancy is produced by parathyroid hormone related peptide (PTHrP) producing nonparathyroid malignant tumors.[19,20] Generally, the hypercalcemia of malignancy is acute in onset and rapidly progressive, attaining serum calcium levels in excess of 13 mg/dl over a short period of time. There may be associated hypoproteinemia, anemia, and elevated erythrocyte sedimentation rates. The serum PTH level is usually normal in these patients, indicating a discordant measurement between serum calcium and PTH. In some malignancies, however, the serum PTH levels may be slightly elevated, creating a scenario favoring hyperparathyroidism. Thus, eliminating malignancy as the underlying cause for hypercalcemia may be a formidable diagnostic challenge requiring an exhaustive investigation.

Other important etiologies that need to be excluded from consideration include sarcoidosis and thiazide diuretic ingestion as well as the aforementioned FHH. In sarcoidosis, hypercalcemia may be accompanied by hypercalciuria but serum PTH is depressed because of increased calcium absorption by the gut. Thiazide ingestion carries with it a history of medication usage but also demonstrates a normal ionized calcium and a normal or depressed serum PTH. FHH may be distinguished by a depressed urinary calcium level below 100 to 150 mg over 24 hours.

In spite of the problems encountered in reconciling the differential diagnosis, the demonstration of a persistently elevated serum calcium level with a concurrent elevation in parathyroid hormone level remains the most reliable indicator for the presence of hyperparathyroidism.

## Indications for Surgery

The decision to perform surgical exploration in the medically stable patient with primary hyperparathyroidism is predicated upon the potential for development of complications from prolonged exposure to hypercalcemia and the long-term benefit of surgery. In general, patients should be assessed for the risk of developing complications on the basis of disease severity at the time of diagnosis, and those previously diagnosed in whom complications have arisen over a short interval since diagnosis and are at significant risk of developing further problems.

Patient age should not be an absolute derminant of candidacy for surgery; rather, general medical condition and the potential for pursuing an active lifestyle should play a more prominent role in determining candidacy. In general, younger patients who potentially will have longer exposure to hypercalcemia are at a substantially greater risk for developing complications.

The severity of hypercalcemia represents a consideration in the decision to perform surgery. Although no absolute level of serum calcium provides stringent criteria for surgery, most endocrine surgeons consider a serum calcium level of 11.5 mg/dl or greater as an absolute indication for surgery. Surgery in post-menopausal women should be given special consideration independent of the severity of hypercalcemia and/or absence of symptoms. Women in this population are at greater risk for development of long-term skeletal complications from generalized demineralization and osteopenia, ie, hip and vertebral fractures.[21]

A major factor to be considered in determining the need for surgery is the potential for long-term benefit and prospects for cure. In 85% to 90% of patients, hyperparathyroidism occurs as a result of a single adenoma. Exploration and removal of the adenoma is curative in greater than 95% of patients, and the long-term benefit and potential for cure is high. Primary hyperplasia occurs in approximately 10% to 12% of patients with hyperparathyroidism. Surgery in these patients involves subtotal parathyroidectomy, with the amount of tissue left ultimately determining the long-term benefit of surgery. Because of the variable amount of parathyroid tissue left in the neck and thus potential for variable activity, the prospect for cure is less reliable than for patients with adenoma. These patients have cure rates significantly reduced from those in whom an adenoma is removed.[22]

Given the considerations mentioned above, the decision to perform surgery on patients who appear asymptomatic and who have no obvious metabolic complications is somewhat problematic. Although early surgical intervention seems to be favored, stringent criteria as to whether or not these patients should undergo surgery have not been defined. About 50% of asymptomatic patients will go on to develop metabolic complications from hyperparathyroidism within 5 to 7 years of the onset of hypercalcemia.[23] As a result of some of the uncertainties about the indications for surgery in asymptomatic patients, a Consensus Conference held by the National Institutes of Health in 1990 addressed the question of management in this clinical situation. The recommendations from that conference have been summarized and published.[1] The following is a review of the indications for surgery as suggested by the conference:

1. Serum calcium is greater than 11.5 to 12 mg/dl.
2. Creatinine clearance is reduced more than 30% for age in the absence of another cause.
3. Twenty-four hour urinary calcium is greater than 400 mg/dl.
4. Bone mass is reduced more than two standard deviations compared with age, gender, and race-matched controls.
5. Patients request surgery, or patients are unsuitable for long-term surveillance.
6. Patients are younger than 50 years of age.

These recommended indications are conservative; they provide a framework for surgical decision-making but are not absolute or universal. The decision to perform surgery on a patient with primary hyperparathyroidism and metabolic complications is straightforward. The decision is less clear in asymptomatic patients and must be guided by the potential benefits of surgery, the patient's risk of developing complications from disease, the wishes of the patient and, importantly, the experience of the surgeon. The success rate of surgery and the incidence of complications following parathyroidectomy have been documented to vary greatly, depending upon the surgeon's experience. In one study, experienced Swedish surgeons achieved normocalcemia in greater than 90% of patients with recurrent laryngeal nerve complications realized in less than 1%. However, surgeons who perform fewer than 10 parathyroidectomies per year had a success rate of 70%, with 15% of patients remaining hypercalcemic and 14% becoming permanently hypocalcemic.[24] Therefore, in weighing potential benefits of surgery against risk for patients with asymptomatic hyperparathyroidism, the experience of the surgeon should be of primary consideration.

Although patients with mild to moderate hypercalcemia seldom experience rapid elevation in serum calcium level, hypercalcemia, and thus the risk of developing subclinical symptoms and risk for potential end organ damage, increases with time. As a result, patients with untreated primary hyperparathyroidism are at increased risk for major morbidity and mortality from cardiovascular diseases.[7,25]

A number of studies have documented the benefits of parathyroidectomy in stabilizing or reversing the clinical sequelae of primary hyperparathyroidism. Parathyroidectomy in these patients has been shown to improve psychiatric and emotional disturbances as well as neuromuscular function within a short period of time following surgery.[26-28] Disturbances in left ventricular function secondary to hypertrophy and dysrhythmia have also been shown to improve following successful parathyroidectomy,[7,29] although the same may not be declared for patients with arterial hypertension, the etiology of which appears to be multifactorial.[30] Mineral disturbances related to kidney and bone have also been noted to improve in patients with primary hyperparathyroidism following parathyroidectomy. Renal lithiasis decreases from a rate of 70% to less than 5% within the first year following surgery,[29] while bone mineral density scores exhibit sustained improvement for a minimum of 4 years after parathyroidectomy.[31,32] Finally, parathyroidectomy appears to offer a distinct and measurable advantage in patients with mild asymptomatic primary hyperparathyroidism as indicated by the results of a randomized trial in which patients were subjectively surveyed using a standardized health survey instrument.[33] In this study, patients with mild asymptomatic hyperparathyroidism were randomized to surgery or observation and then assessed every six months following randomization for two years using the SF-36 Health Survey, an instrument which measures wellness.[34] Significantly improved function was noted in patients following parathyroidectomy when compared with patients who were observed.

## SURGICAL STRATEGY

### General Considerations

The optimal surgical approach in managing primary hyperparathyroidism is one in which normocalcemia is achieved while minimizing potential surgical morbidity, including: recurrent laryngeal nerve injury, post-exploration hypocalcemia, and persistent/recurrent hyperparathyroidism requiring re-operation. Additionally, the approach selected should be individualized to the patient and disease entity (suspected single vs. multiple gland disease) and should be time and cost-efficient.

Exploration of the neck for hyperparathyroidism, regardless of the pathology suspected, requires meticulous dissection, maintenance of a bloodless field, attention to anatomic detail, and, most importantly, a thorough understanding of regional anatomy and embryology.

It is worthwhile to review the embryologic derivation of the parathyroid glands (Figure 35–2). Parathyroid tissue originates from primordial pharyngeal endoderm formed in the third and fourth pharyngeal pouches. During embryonic development, the parathyroid tissue destined to become the superior glands originates in the fourth pharyngeal pouch and descends with elements of the thyroid gland to assume a characteristic position in the neck. The future inferior glands derive from the third pharyngeal pouch and descend with thymic elements over a long course to eventually rest low in the neck. This embryologic pattern has significant implications for the identification of ectopic or normal glandular variance during the course of parathyroidectomy. Ectopic superior glands will often follow a path of descent posteriorly behind the esophagus or carotid sheath into the posterior superior mediastinum (Figure 35–3). Because of a shared common primordium in the fourth pharyngeal pouch with the thyroid, a missing superior gland may be located within the thyroid parenchyma. These intrathyroidal

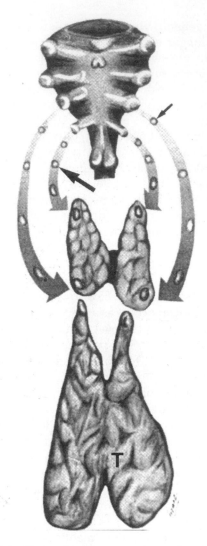

**Figure 35–2.** Illustration demonstrating embryologic derivation and subsequent descent of the parathyroid glands with associated structures. Large arrow—superior parathyroid gland; small arrow—inferior parathyroid gland; T—thymus. (From Clark. *Endocrine Surgery.* W. B. Saunders: 1997, p. 278.)

parathyroid lesions may appear as "cold" thyroid nodules on radio-iodine scanning. Failure to locate a missing superior gland suspected to be an adenoma mandates thyroid lobotomy or lobectomy to exclude intrathyroidal parathyroid tissue. Inferior glands tend to follow the course of the thymus into the anterior superior mediastinum, although their ectopic locations are less predictable as a result of a longer pathway during embryonic development.

### Surgical Approach

The surgical approach to patients with primary hyperparathyroidism has in recent years evolved from the routine performance of bilateral cervical exploration to a more directed unilateral approach. In theory, as the

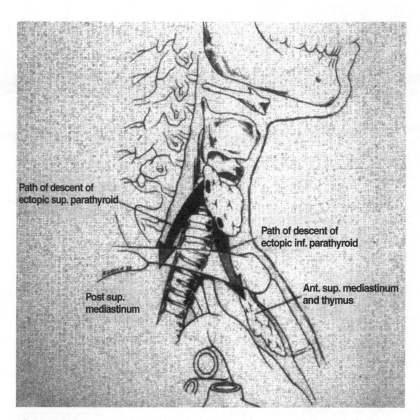

**Figure 35–3.** Schematic demonstrating paths of ectopic parathyroid gland migration.

vast majority of patients with primary hyperparathyroidism have a single hyperfunctioning adenoma as the offending lesion, it follows that the ideal surgical approach would involve directed removal of the solitary abnormal gland in the least invasive and potentially traumatic manner. Incorporating this theoretic ideal into a practical and reliable surgical approach has been limited until recently by two constraints. The first of these was accurate preoperative localization of the abnormal gland and the second was an inability to intraoperatively confirm removal of all hyperfunctioning parathyroid tissue without performing a bilateral cervical exploration and examining all four parathyroid glands.

Traditionally, the argument for a bilateral cervical exploration in patients with suspected adenoma has been the high success rate in achieving normocalcemia with a conventional bilateral approach in experienced hands (>95% cure), the inability to accurately predict which side to selectively explore and the potential risk of missing unsuspected multiple gland disease such as double adenoma or unsuspected hyperplasia.[35-40] Recent technologic advances have helped address these areas of concern and there is now growing consensus for a less extensive and directed exploration in the approach to primary hyperparathyroidism. The first impetus to this shift in surgical philosophy was provided by improvements in preoperative imaging for the accurate localization of hyperfunctioning solitary adenomas. Previous localization techniques which primarily relied on either ultrasound or thallium-201/technetium-99m subtraction scanning, were not noted to be sufficiently accurate in predicting the location of the abnormal parathyroid gland.[41-43] With Coakley's (1989) description of parathyroid tissue demonstrating avid uptake of technetium–99m sestamibi, the stage was set for an improved, accurate preoperative localization study.[44] Subsequent investigators have demonstrated that technetium–99m sestamibi imaging is more than 90% accurate in localizing a hyperfunctioning solitary adenoma.[45-48] In 1998, Denham and Norman further reinforced these studies when they reported their results on a meta-analysis of 784 patients having undergone preoperative technetium–99m sestamibi imaging prior to exploration for primary HPT.[49] They found the sensitivity of technetium–99m sestamibi imaging to be 91% with a specificity of 99%. They also concluded that technetium–99m sestamibi imaging was cost-effective when it allowed greater than 51% of patients with suspected adenoma to undergo a unilateral cervical exploration.[49]

The improvement in preoperative localization offered by using this technique has led to increasing support for a directed unilateral exploration for suspected parathyroid adenoma. Several investigators have reported their results with unilateral cervical exploration following preoperative localization using this technique.[50-52] These investigators have reported excellent success rates (>94%) while also noting significant reductions in operative time, cost and potential surgical morbidity. More recently, promising experience with radio-guided parathyroid surgery for adenoma involving intravenous injection of technetium–99m sestamibi 1 to 2.5 hours prior to surgery and the intraoperative use of a hand-held gamma probe to direct surgical exploration to a specific quadrant of the neck have further strengthened the arguments for directed unilateral cervical exploration in cases of suspected parathyroid adenoma.[53,54]

Some surgeons, however, remain concerned about the possibility of missing unsuspected multi-glandular disease with a unilateral cervical approach.[55] It is in this context that intraoperative assays for parathyroid hormone (IOPTH) have proven to be most valuable. The intraoperative use of rapid PTH assays to confirm removal of all hyperfunctioning parathyroid tissue has greatly reduced the possibility of missing multiple gland disease caused by double adenomas or unsuspected hyperplasia, thereby enhancing the performance of directed cervical exploration for primary hyperparathyroidism. A number of studies have documented the effectiveness of intraoperative assays in accurately reflecting removal of all hyperfunctioning parathyroid tissue.[56-59] With the ability to biochemically confirm removal of all hyperfunctioning parathyroid tissue intraoperatively, the theoretic advantages of a directed unilateral cervical approach have increasingly become reality.[56,60,61]

We advocate a directed unilateral cervical exploration utilizing both preoperative localization with technetium–99m sestamibi and IOPTH for the surgical management of primary hyperparathyroidism secondary to anticipated parathyroid adenoma. In our experience this surgical approach has yielded not only excellent success rates but also decreases in operative time, cost, and potential surgical morbidity.[56] In the initial screening process, all patients with disease entities exhibiting multiple gland hyperplasia, such as those with familial hyperparathyroidism and MEN types 1 or 2A, are determined to be candidates for a standard bilateral cervical exploration and do not have localizing studies performed prior to initial operation. A preoperative technetium–99m sestamibi scan is obtained on all other patients with primary hyperparathyroidism, which represents the overwhelming majority (>85%). If the scan is inconclusive or equivocal, as judged by both the surgeon and nuclear medicine specialist, a standard bilateral cervical exploration is planned and performed, whether or not an enlarged gland is found on the side explored first. Failure to localize with an optimally performed technetium–99m sestamibi scan, in the absence of significant thyroid disease, is strongly suggestive of sporadic diffuse hyperplasia.[56,60] If the nuclear scan identifies a discrete area of delayed uptake, suggestive of adenoma, a directed exploration to the side localized is performed, and biochemical confirmation of removal of all hyperfunctioning parathyroid tissue is obtained

through the use of IOPTH. It has been previously demonstrated that the most precipitous decease in PTH levels occurs five minutes following removal of all hyperfunctioning parathyroid tissue.[62] The short half-life of PTH (roughly 2–5 minutes) allows peripheral blood samples to be obtained intraoperatively for rapid PTH testing 7–10 minutes following excision of all suspected hyperfunctioning parathyroid tissue.[56] Accordingly, a peripheral blood sample for rapid PTH assay is drawn at the time of abnormal gland identification and subsequently at 10 minutes following removal of all suspected hyperfunctioning parathyroid tissue. A decrease in excess of 50% noted in the post-excision PTH level as compared to the pre-excision level indicates biochemical confirmation of removal of all hyperfunctioning parathyroid tissue, and the procedure is concluded without identification or biopsy of any other glands. If the post-excision PTH level is greater than 50% of the pre-excision level suggesting the presence of residual hyperfunctioning parathyroid tissue, a standard bilateral cervical exploration is performed.

IOPTH may be performed by a number of methodologies. For our explorations we employ a rapid PTH radioimmunoassay developed within our institution. This radioimmunoassay was developed through a simple, previously described modification of an intact PTH overnight assay method.[63] Results of this rapid PTH assay are generally available within 20 minutes. Our experience is consistent with that of other investigators in that a decrease of 50% or greater between the post-excision and pre-excision PTH values is indicative of removal of all hyperfunctioning parathyroid tissue.[56,59,61] There is 100% correlation between the IOPTH post-excision level and the standard intact PTH postoperative level in patients who experience the minimum 50% decline (Figure 35–4). All these patients have achieved sustained normocalcemia.

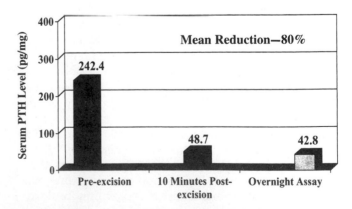

## Parathyroid Hormone Level N=240

**Figure 35–4.** Intact parathyroid hormone levels as assessed intraoperatively by rapid PTH (IOPTH) and standard overnight radio immunoassay in 240 patients.

In situations where localization studies are inconclusive or equivocal (lacking mutual agreement by both surgeon and radiologist), or where clinical circumstances suggest multiple gland disease (MEN, familial hyperparathyroidism), a traditional bilateral cervical exploration is advocated. Specifically, both sides of the neck are explored in an attempt to identify at least four parathyroid glands, independent of whether or not the first side explored yields an enlarged gland. We do not routinely biopsy all normal appearing parathyroid glands but rather selectively perform incisional biopsy of glands sparingly. IOPTH remains an important adjunct in the bilateral approach to patients with primary hyperparathyroidism in that this modality serves to biochemically confirm removal of all hyperfunctioning parathyroid tissue and thus reduce the chance of missing ectopic multi-glandular disease, whether as a result of "double adenoma" or ectopic supernumerary glands. It is our belief, as well as others, that the use of this technique in all explorations for primary hyperparathyroidism, independent of etiology, will result in achieving improved rates of normocalcemia at initial operation, fewer re-operations, and, as a corollary, reduced morbidity and cost.[52,54,56,64]

Our experience with the directed cervical approach has yielded a positive predictability rate of 97% for accurate localization, together with a predictability of achieving postoperative normocalcemia in 100% of patients where IOPTH has been noted to decrease greater than 50%. This strategy, summarized in Figure 35–5, has led to an overall *initial* operative success rate of 98% in our hands.

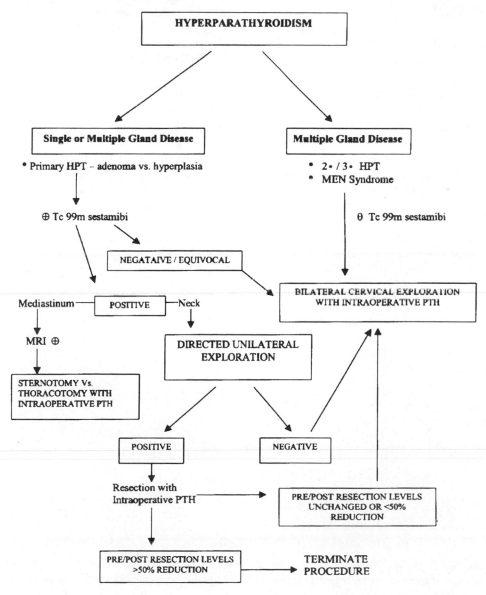

**Figure 35–5.** Algorithm describing surgical strategy for directed parathyroid exploration.

Problems encountered with inaccurate or failed localization using the technetium-99m sestamibi usually occur as a result of the presence of multi-nodular thyroid disease or unanticipated diffuse four gland hyperplasia. In these circumstances, the results of nuclear scanning have served as a guide in determining the surgical approach, directed vs. bilateral. These methodologies are not intended to supplant sound surgical judgment, experience and meticulous technique in order to expedite the performance of an operation for which the surgeon is ill prepared to undertake. Rather, they should serve to increase the capability of the surgeon to safely and efficiently manage a potentially formidable surgical problem.

## SPECIAL CIRCUMSTANCES

### Failure To Localize

In most situations, failure to localize to a discrete area of the neck following sestamibi imaging occurs as a result of unrecognized multi-nodular thyroid disease (Figure 35–6). In the absence of a nodular thyroid gland, one must suspect diffuse hyperplasia or less likely, an ectopically located gland, either cervical or mediastinal. One must be careful that an appropriately dosed (25 millicuries) and correctly performed nuclear scan has been carried out in all studies. Single positron emission computed tomography (SPECT) technetium–99m ses-

tamibi imaging may be helpful in reconciling equivocal planar images.[56,60] A failure to localize on delayed nuclear imaging mandates the performance of a standard bilateral exploration.

### False Positive Scan

Although rare in our experience, discrete areas of delayed nuclear uptake representing false positive locations at operation do occur. Without exception, this occurs as a result of unsuspected nodular thyroid disease. We have encountered both subcapsular and intra-thyroidal abnormal parathyroid glands which have imaged correctly so all nodularity within or associated with the thyroid gland should be subjected to biopsy in this circumstance. More likely, these findings are consistent with an adenomatous thyroid nodule and a bilateral exploration is necessary.

### Mediastinal Localization

Mediastinal localization on initial technetium–99m sestamibi imaging is rare but may occur (Figure 35–7). A suspected mediastinal location should be confirmed with a correlative anatomic/physiologic study series whereby either CT or MRI are used to complement the physiologic nuclear scan. Sternotomy/thoracotomy should not be performed without this correlation, and

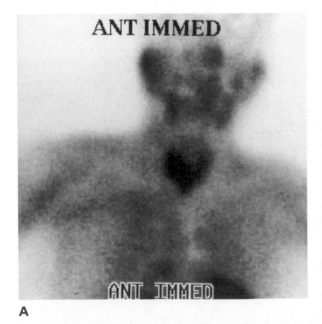

**A**

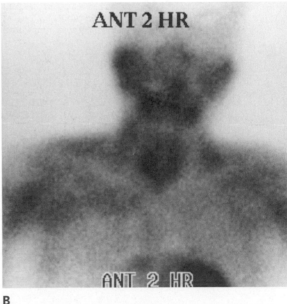

**B**

**Figure 35–6.** Initial (A) and delayed (B) Technetium–99m sestamibi nuclear imaging in a patient with hyperparathyroidism and multi-nodular thyroid disease. Nuclear uptake in right lower cervical region on delayed image represents uptake by thyroid nodule.

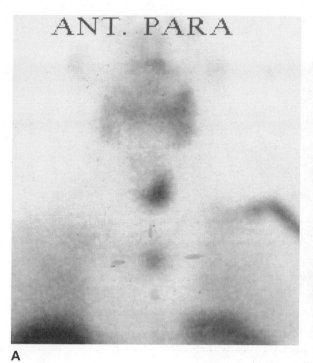

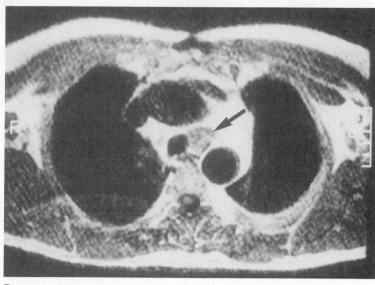

**Figure 35–7. A.** Technetium–99m sestamibi imaging and **B.** magnetic resonance scan in a patient with a mediastinal parathyroid adenoma. The area of nuclear uptake noted on the sestamibi scan correlates anatomically with the nodule demonstrated in the aorto-pulmonary window on MRI (see arrow). Adenoma was removed via left lateral thoracotomy.

the surgeon should be prepared to perform a standard bilateral cervical exploration concurrently in the event that IOPTH does not biochemically confirm removal of all hyperfunctional tissue.

## True Double Adenoma

The incidence of double adenomas appears to increase with age. Synchronous double adenomas have been variably reported at rates ranging from 1% to 2% to as high as 10% in patients older than 60 years of age.[65,66] In our experience, synchronous homolateral double adenomas have not been encountered, although one re-exploration has yielded a second adenoma on the neck side where a previous adenoma had been removed. All synchronous double adenomas in our series have been noted bilaterally.

Approximately 50% of true double adenomas will image accurately to each of the two locations (Figure 35–8). Bilateral exploration is required despite high suspicion on localization because of the possibility of asymmetric hyperplasia. IOPTH is confirmatory in that a sequential drop in PTH levels will be noted after successive excision of the first and then second enlarged gland (Figure 35–9). We identify at least one other normal gland but do not biopsy any further glands provided the final post-excision PTH level ultimately decreases beyond 50% of the pre-excision level intraoperatively.

## Hyperplasia

Multiglandular disease secondary to diffuse hyperplasia of the parathyroid glands may occur in as many as 10% to 15% of patients with sporadic primary hyperparathyroidism and those with the multiple endocrine neoplasia syndromes, types 1 and 2A. In our series, primary hyperparathyroidism occurred as a result of diffuse multi-glandular hyperplasia (minimum 4 glands) in 8% of patients explored.

The approach to these patients includes performance of a nuclear imaging study using technetium–99m sestamibi preoperatively unless the patient is known to have one of the MEN disorders. (A complete discussion of these disorders is found in Chapter 36.)

A scan which does not indicate an unequivocal area of nuclear uptake on delayed images raises the surgeon's suspicion of diffuse hyperplasia. Forty percent of equivocal scans were associated with the ultimate finding of multi-glandular hyperplasia at exploration in our series (Figure 35–10). The presence of an equivocal scan demonstrating the absence of a distinct focus of delayed uptake of nuclear material mandates the performance of a bilateral exploration with histologic identification of at least one abnormal and one normal gland and the assurance that no additional grossly enlarged glands exist on either side. Following removal of all enlarged glands (either single or multiple) and the

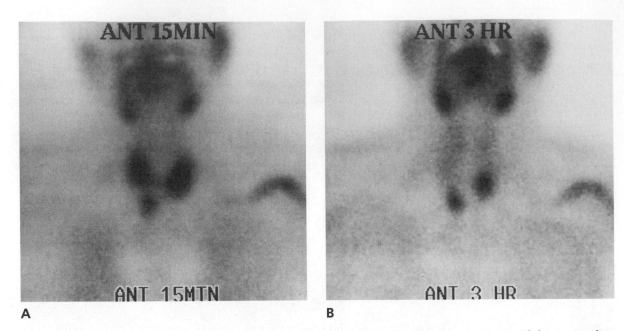

**Figure 35–8.** Initial (A) and delayed (B) technetium–99m sestamibi nuclear scans in a patient with hyperparathyroidism secondary to double parathyroid adenomata. Nuclear uptake is clearly demonstrated bilaterally on the delayed image indicating the location of both adenomas confirmed at surgery.

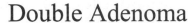

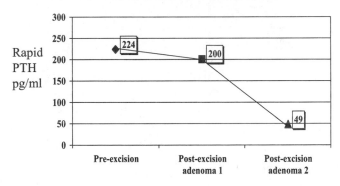

**Figure 35–9.** Sequential serum parathyroid hormone levels assessed by intraoperative rapid PTH immunoassay (IOPTH) following removal of the first and then second parathyroid adenoma in a patient with hyperparathyroidism and double adenomata (see Figure 35–7).

demonstration of a histologically normal gland (in the event of less than four gland disease), rapid PTH assessment (Figure 35–11) is performed in order to confirm the removal of all hyperfunctional parathyroid tissue, per the same protocol used in the directed exploration strategy (see Figure 35–4). Failure to achieve this decrement threshold mandates further exploration, either for an ectopically located gland or, uncommonly, a supernumerary gland.

Once all hyperplastic glands have been located in situ, the three largest glands are removed and histologically confirmed. Subtotal excision of the remaining gland follows, leaving at least one-third to one-half of the gland as a viable vascularized remnant. Titration of PTH level is helpful using rapid PTH assessment. Should the post-excision level fall below 10 pg/ml, consideration should be given to cryopreservation of parathyroid tissue excised from the fourth gland. Although we have not found this to be necessary, we would favor this approach over routine forearm autotransplantation of parathyroid tissue in that additional surgery is avoided and because a measurable PTH level detected intraoperatively has been predictive of normocalcemia.

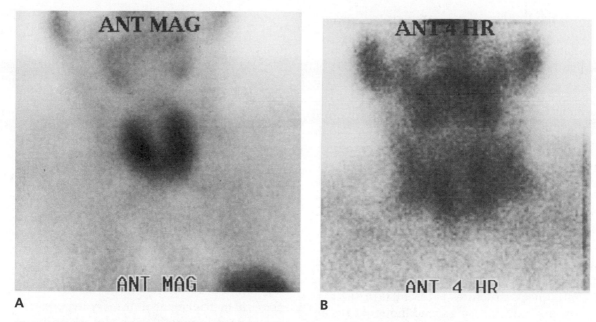

**Figure 35–10.** Initial (A) and delayed (B) technetium–99m sestamibi nuclear scans performed on a patient with hyperparathyroidism secondary to diffuse 4-gland hyperplasia. Note the absence of any focus of nuclear uptake on the delayed image.

## Diffuse Hyperplasia

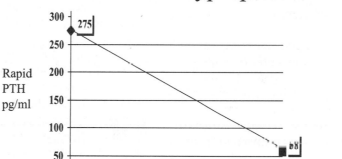

**Figure 35–11.** Sequential serum parathyroid hormone levels as assessed by intraoperative rapid PTH immunoassay comparing hormone level obtained before and 10 minutes following a 3½ gland subtotal parathyroidectomy in a patient with diffuse 4-gland hyperplasia (see Figure 35–9).

## The Missing Adenoma: Ectopic Locations

The failure to locate and identify a fourth parathyroid gland thought to represent an adenoma, after identifying three normal glands, is perhaps the most frustrating and humbling experience encountered by the surgeon performing parathyroid surgery. A systematic strategy is required to investigate all possible locations accessible via a trancervical approach, through which the vast majority (90%) of missed adenomas may be removed.

The embryologic basis of parathyroid origin and subsequent descent into the lower neck weighs heavily in determining the likely location of a missing adenoma. By way of its origin as a third branchial pouch derivative, a suspected missing inferior gland is most likely to be found in the region extending from the inferior thyroid pole into the anterior superior mediastinum. In this manner it may be located in the path of descent associated with the thymus. Ectopically located inferior parathyroid glands may be found in the subcapsular plane associated with the inferior thyroid pole, the thyrothymic ligament and the thymic soft tissue and fat of the anterior superior mediastinum. Less likely locations for the inferior gland are more superior in location, ie, the hyoid or carotid sheath regions. The superior parathyroid gland, because of its origin as a fourth branchial pouch derivative and less extensive descent, is generally less likely to be ectopic in location. However, a missing superior gland may be more difficult to find as its path of ectopic progression may allow it to migrate in a retroesophageal manner into the posterior superior mediastinum. Superior glands may also be found within the thyroid gland itself.

A thorough knowledge of the embryologic–anatomic relationship of the parathyroid glands and associated central neck structures is essential in successfully locating an ectopic missing gland thought to be an adenoma. When confronted with this situation, the first order of business is to determine which gland, superior or inferior, is missing. Using the predictive potential ectopic pathways described above, an orderly methodologic search is carried out addressing each region.

We usually begin by thoroughly dissecting the region extending from the inferior thyroid pole to the anterior mediastinum. This includes opening the thyroid capsule, dissecting the thyrothymic ligament (more prominent in younger patients) and anterior superior mediastinal fat and remnant thymic tissue. Transcervical thymectomy may be performed at this time. One must be careful to identify and trace the recurrent laryngeal nerve well into the mediastinum in order to protect this structure. If not already accomplished, the superior thyroid pole is mobilized next together with blunt dissection of the retroesophageal plane anterior to the spine. Palpation in this area will often disclose an ectopic enlarged superior parathyroid gland. Digital dissection is carried well into the upper mediastinum quite safely in this plane. Next, the carotid sheath is opened and its structures identified and traced as high as the hyoid bone. Finally, palpation of the thyroid gland itself is accomplished to determine the presence of any dominant nodularity. If identified, thyroidotomy may be performed and the nodule either excised totally or biopsied. If no nodules are apparent, it has been our practice to perform thyroid lobectomy on the side where both parathyroid glands have not been identified. This practice has yielded three intrathyroidal glands which were not palpable, all of which represented the superior gland.

Should all maneuvers prove unsuccessful in identifying a fourth gland, the operation is terminated and further studies are planned in an attempt to localize the missing gland. No attempt should be made to perform a mediastinal exploration at the time of initial surgery and before localization studies have identified the ectopic location, in part because considerable time has elapsed during cervical exploration making tissue edema and staining more problematic in identifying parathyroidal tissue. Mediastinal exploration is generally not required in more than 2% of patients with primary hyperparathyroidism and should be done only after appropriate correlative localization studies have identified the mediastinum as the suspicious site. It has been our practice to perform approach to the mediastinum in conjunction with a thoracic surgeon, although this is not necessary for general surgeons who regularly perform chest procedures.

## SUMMARY

Surgical management of primary hyperparathyroidism mandates a thorough, methodologic approach to diagnosis, patient evaluation, and the development of a surgical strategy. Advances in nuclear imaging and the ability to rapidly assess the serum level of parathyroid hormone has allowed the fundamental surgical approach to become accurately directed, more refined, and less extensive, leading to improvements in outcome and reductions in treatment time, morbidity, and cost.

Although these changes have revolutionized the manner in which surgeons approach this disorder, they may not be universally applicable and thus should not serve as a substitute for a well-founded and traditional knowledge base in surgical embryology, anatomy, and technique. The majority of patients with primary hyperparathyroidism who undergo parathyroid surgery benefit symptomatically as well as metabolically.

## References

1. National Institutes of Health Conference. Diagnosis and management of asymptomatic primary hyperparathyroidism: consensus development conference statement. *Ann Intern Med.* 1991;114: 593–597.
2. Bartsch D, Mies C, Hasse C, et al. Clinical and surgical aspects of double adenoma in patients with primary hyperparathyroidism. *Br J Surg.* 1995;82:926–929.
3. Thalpos G, Bowe H III, Kleerekoper M, et al. Randomized trial of parathyroidectomy in mild asymptomatic primary hyperparathyroidism: patient description and effects on the SF-36 health survey. *Surgery.* 2000;128:1013–1021.
4. Heath H III, Hodgson S, Kennedy N. Primary hyperparathyroidism incidence, mortality and potential economic impact in a community. *N Engl J Med.* 1980;302:189–193.
5. Strewer G. Indications for surgery in patients with minimally symptomatic primary hyperparathyroidism. *Surg Clin North Am.* 1995;75:439–447.
6. Silverberg S, Shane E, de la Cruz L. Skeletal disease in primary hyperparathyroidism. *J Bone Miner Res.* 1989;4:283–295.

7. Nilsson I, Aberg J, Rastad J, Lind L. Left ventricular systolic and diastolic function and exercise testing in primary hyperparathyroidism—effects of parathyroidectomy. *Surgery*. 2000;128:895–902.

8. Black W, Haff R. The surgical pathology of parathyroid chief cell hyperplasia. *Am J Clin Pathol*. 1970;53:565–579.

9. DeLewis R, Dayal Y, Tischler A, et al. Multiple endocrine dysplasia MEN syndromes: cellular origins and interrelationships. *Int Rev Exp Pathol*. 1986;28:163–175.

10. Delewis R, *Tumors of the Parathyroid Gland: Atlas of Tumor Pathology*. 3rd series, fascicle 6. Washington, DC: Armed Forces Institute of Pathology; 1993:1.

11. Schantz A, Castleman B. Parathyroid carcinoma: a study of 70 cases. *Cancer*. 1973;31:600–613.

12. Shane E. Parathyroid carcinoma, clinical review 122. *J Clin Endocrinol Metab*. 2001;86(2):485–493.

13. Turner W, Pellitteri PK, Orloff LA, Baergen RN. Parathyroid lipoadenoma: case report and review of the literature. *Otolaryngology/HNS*. 1996;114(2):313–316.

14. Mather H. Hyperparathyroidism with normal serum calcium. *Br Med J*. 1953;2:424–433.

15. Forster J, Monatik J, Martin H. A comparative study of serum ultrafiltrable, ionized and total calcium in the diagnosis of primary hyperparathyroidism in patients with intermittent or no elevations in total calcium. *Surgery*. 1988;104:1137–1142.

16. Monchik J, Lamberton R, Roth U. Role of the oral calcium loading test with measurement of intact parathyroid hormone in the diagnosis of symptomatic subtle primary hyperparathyroidism. *Surgery*. 1992;112:1103–1110.

17. Heath H III. Familial benign (hypocalciuric) hypercalcemia: a troublesome mimic of mild primary hyperparathyroidism. *Endocrinol Metab Clin North Am*. 1989;18:723–740.

18. Pollack M, Brown M, Chou Y, et al. Mutations in the human Ca (2+) sensing receptor gene cause familial hypocalciuric hypercalcemia and neonatal severe hyperparathyroidism (see comments). *Cell*. 1993;75:1297–1301.

19. Budayr A, Nissenson R, Klein R, et al. Increased serum levels of a parathyroid hormone-like protein in malignancy associated hypercalcemia. *Ann Intern Med*. 1989;111:807–812.

20. Strewler G, Budayr A, Clark O, Nissenson R. Production of parathyroidal hormone by a malignant non-parathyroidal tumor in a hypercalcemic patient. *J Clin Endocrinol Metab*. 1993;76:1373–1375.

21. Kenny A, MacGillivray D, Pilbeam C, et al. Fracture incidence in postmenopausal women with primary hyperparathyroidism. *Surgery*. 1995;118:109–114.

22. Bruining H, Brikenhager J, Ong G, Lamberts S. Causes of failure in operation for hyperparathyroidism. *Surgery*. 1987;101:562–565.

23. Cristesson T. Primary hyperparathyroidism—pathogensis, incidence and natural history. In: *Progress in Surgery*, Vol 18. Basel: Karger; 1986.

24. Malmaeus J, Granberg P, Halvorsen J, et al. Parathyroid surgery in Scandinavia. *Acta Chir Scand*. 1988;154:409–420.

25. Hedback G, Ogen A, Tisell L. Parathyroid adenoma weight and the risk of death after treatment for primary hyperparathyroidism. *Surgery*. 1995;117:134–139.

26. Solomon B, Schaaf M, Smallridge R. Psychologic symptoms before and after parathyroid surgery (see comments). *Am J Med*. 1994;96:101–106.

27. Kristoffersson A, Bostrom A, Soderber T. Muscle strength is improved after parathyroidectomy in patients with primary hyperparathyroidism. *Br J Surg*. 1992;79:165–167.

28. Chou F, Sheen Chen S, Leong C. Neuromuscular recovery after parathyroidectomy in primary hyperparathyroidism. *Surgery*. 1995;117:18–25.

29. Stefanelle T, Mayr H, Bergler-Klein J, et al. Primary hyperparathyroidism: incidence of cardiac abnormalities and partial reversibility after successful parathyroidectomy. *Am J Med*. 1993; 95:197–202.

30. Sacaitudeen A, Thomas T, Sellars L, et al. Hypertension and renal dysfunction in primary hyperparathyroidism: effect of parathyroidectomy. *Clin Sci*. 1989;76:289–292.

31. Silverberg S, Gartenberg J, Jacobs T, et al. Increased bone density after parathyroidectomy in primary hyperparathyroidism (see comment). *J Clin Endocrinol Metab*. 1995;80:729–734.

32. Thorsen K, Kristoffersson A, Lorentzon R. Changes in bone mass and serum markers of bone metabolism after parathyroidectomy. *Surgery*. 1997;122:882–887.

33. Talpos G, Bone H III, Kleerekoper M, et al. Randomized trial of parathyroidectomy in mild asymptomatic primary hyperparathyroidism: patient description and effects on the SF-36 health survey. *Surgery*. 2000;128:1013–1021.

34. Ware J, Sherbourne C. The MOS 36-item, short-term health survey (SF-36): I, conceptual framework and item selection. *Med Care*. 1992;30:473–483.

35. Howe JR: Minimally invasive parathyroid surgery. *Surg Clin North Am*. 2000;80(5):1399–1426.

36. Kaplan EL, Yashiro T, Salti G. Primary hyperparathyroidism in the 1990s. Choice of surgical procedures for this disease. *Ann Surg*. 1992;215:300–316.

37. Weber CJ, Sewell CW, McGarity WC. Persistent and recurrent sporadic primary hyperparathyroidism: histopathology, complications, and results of reoperation. *Surgery*. 1994;116:991–998.

38. Proye CAG, Carnaille B, Bizard JP, et al. Single and multigland disease in seemingly sporadic primary hyperparathyroidism revisited: where are we in the 1990s? A plea against unilateral parathyroid exploration. *Surgery*. 1992;112:1118–1121.

39. Bonjer HJ, Bruining HA, Birkenhager JC, et al. Single and multigland disease in primary hyperparathyroidism: clinical follow-up, histopathology, and flow cytometric DNA analysis. *World J Surg*. 1992;16:737–744.

40. Shaha AR, Jaffe BM. Cervical exploration for primary hyperparathyroidism. *J Surg Oncol*. 1993;52:14–17.

41. Russell CF, Laird JD, Ferguson WR. Scan-directed unilateral cervical exploration for parathyroid adenoma: a legitimate approach? *World J Surg*. 1990;14:406–409.

42. Robertson CS, Johnson PR, Bolia A, et al. Long term results of unilateral neck exploration for preoperatively localized nonfamilial parathyroid adenomas. *Am J Surg*. 1996;172:311–314.

43. Lucas RJ, Welsh RJ, Glover JL. Unilateral neck exploration for primary hyperparathyroidism. *Arch Surg*. 1990;125:982–985.

44. Coakley AJ, Kettle AG, Wells CP, et al. $^{99m}$Tc sestamibi: a new agent for parathyroid imaging. *Nucl Med Comm*. 1989;10:791–794.

45. O'Doherty MJ, Kettle AG, Wells P, et al. Parathyroid imaging with technetium–99m sestamibi: preoperative localization and tissue uptake studies. *J Nucl Med*. 1992;33:313–318.

46. Borley NR, Collins RE, O'Doherty M, et al. Technetium–99m sestamibi parathyroid localization is accurate enough for scan-directed unilateral neck exploration. *Br J Surg*. 1996;83:989–991.

47. Taillefer R, Boucher Y, Potvin C, et al. Detection and localization of parathyroid adenomas in patients with hyperparathyroidism using a single radionuclide imaging procedure with technetium–99m sestamibi. *J Nucl Med*. 1992;33:1801–1807.

48. Malhotra A, Silver CE, Deshpande V, et al. Preoperative localization with sestamibi. *Amer J Surg*. 1996;172:637–640.

49. Denham DW, Norman J. Cost-effectiveness of preoperative sestamibi scan for primary hyperparathyroidism is dependent solely upon the surgeon's choice of operative procedure. *J Am Coll Surg*. 1998;186:293–304.

50. Takami H. Surgical management of hyperparathyroidism in view of a reliable parathyroid adenoma localization test. *Surgery*. 1997;122:120.

51. Gupta VK, Yeh KA, Burke GJ, et al. Technetium–99m sestamibi localized solitary parathyroid adenoma as an indication for limited unilateral surgical exploration. *Am J Surgery.* 1998;176:409–412.

52. Norman J, Chheda H, Farrell C. Minimally invasive parathyroidectomy for primary hyperparathyroidism: decreasing operative time and potential complications while improving cosmetic results. *Am Surg.* 1998;64:391–397.

53. Norman J, Chheda H. Minimally invasive parathyroidectomy facilitated by intraoperative nuclear mapping. *Surgery.* 1997;122: 998–1004.

54. Flynn MB, Bumpous JM, Scill K, et al. Minimally invasive radioguided parathyroidectomy. *J Am Coll Surg.* 2000;191:24–31.

55. Shen W, Sabanci U, Morita ET, et al. Sestamibi scanning is inadequate for directing unilateral neck exploration for first-time parathyroidectomy. *Arch Surg.* 1990;132:969–976.

56. Patel PC, Pellitteri PK, Patel NM, et al. Use of a rapid intraoperative parathyroid hormone assay in the surgical management of parathyroid disease. *Arch Otolaryngol-Head Neck Surg.* 1998;124: 559–562.

57. Nussbaum SR, Thompson AR, Hutcheson KA, et al. Intraoperative measurement of parathyroid hormone in the surgical management of hyperparathyroidism. *Surgery.* 1988;104:1121–1127.

58. Chapius Y, Icard P, Fulla Y, et al. Parathyroid adenomectomy under local anesthesia with intraoperative monitoring UcAMP and/or 1-84 PTH. *World J Surg.* 1992;16:570–575.

59. Irvin GL, Dembrow VD, Prudhomme DL. Clinical usefulness of an intraoperative "quick parathyroid hormone" assay. *Surgery.* 1993;114:1019–1023.

60. Carty SE, Worsey J, Vriji MA, et al. Concise parathyroidectomy: the impact of preoperative SPECT 99mTC sestamibi scanning and intraoperative quick parathormone assay. *Surgery.* 1997;122:1107–1116.

61. Irvin GL, Prudhomme DL, Derisio GT, et al. A new approach to parathyroidectomy. *Ann Surg.* 1994;219:574–581.

62. Kao PC, Van Heerden JA, Taylor RL. Intraoperative monitoring of parathyroid procedures by a 15-minute parathyroid hormone immunochemiluminometric assay. *Mayo Clin Proc.* 1994;69:532–537.

63. Fleetwood MK, Quinton L, Wolfe J, et al. Rapid PTH assay by simple modification of Nichols intact PTH-parathyroid hormone assay kit. *Clin Chem.* 1996;42:1498.

64. Goldstein R, Blevins L, Delbeke D, Martin W. Effect of minimally invasive radio-guided parathyroidectomy on morbidity, length of stay, and costs in the management of primary hyperparathyroidism. *Ann Surg.* 2000;231:732–742.

65. Harness JK, Rausberg SR, Nishiama R, et al. Multiple adenomas of the parathyroids: do they exist? *Arch Surg.* 1979;114:468–473.

66. Tetelman S, Shen W, Shaver J, et al. Double parathyroid adenomas: clinical and biochemical characteristics before and after parathyroidectomy. *Am Surg.* 1993;218:300–305.

# 36

# Familial Hyperparathyroidism and the Multiple Endocrine Neoplasia Syndromes

Elizabeth A. Mittendorf, M.D.
Christopher R. McHenry, M.D.

## INTRODUCTION

Familial hyperparathyroidism accounts for less than 5% of all cases of hyperparathyroidism.[1] It comprises a spectrum of autosomal dominant inherited diseases which include: multiple endocrine neoplasia (MEN) 1, MEN 2A, non-MEN, and familial neonatal hyperparathyroidism. In contrast to sporadic hyperparathyroidism, patients with familial hyperparathyroidism are younger and more likely to have multiglandular disease, as well as persistent or recurrent hyperparathyroidism following parathyroidectomy. Subtotal or total parathyroidectomy in combination with bilateral transcervical thymectomy is more frequently necessary for definitive treatment rather than simple excision of an adenoma, which is all that is required for approximately 80% of patients with sporadic primary hyperparathyroidism. Long-term follow-up of patients with familial hyperparathyroidism is imperative for early detection and treatment of other endocrine neoplasms and diagnosis of recurrent hyperparathyroidism. Screening of family members is an important aspect of the management of familial hyperparathyroidism. Identification of the causative genes in MEN 1 and MEN 2A hyperparathyroidism has been important for helping provide the basis for genetic screening of family members and allowing for better allocation of resources to those individuals identified as gene carriers. In this chapter, the clinical characteristics, genetics, and management of MEN 1, MEN 2A, non-MEN and neonatal hyperparathyroidism are reviewed.

## MULTIPLE ENDOCRINE NEOPLASIA TYPE 1 (MEN 1)

### Clinical

MEN 1 is an autosomal dominant inherited syndrome characterized by the presence of neoplastic lesions involving the parathyroid glands, the anterior pituitary, the pancreas and the duodenum. In addition, patients may have carcinoid tumors of the bronchus or thymus, tumors of ovaries, thyroid gland, adrenal glands, and multiple lipomas. It is uncommon, occurring in 2 to 20 out of every 100,000 persons.[2] The coexistence of tumors of the parathyroids, pancreatic islets, and pituitary was first noted in autopsy studies performed on patients with acromegaly in 1903.[3] In 1939, Rossier and colleagues reported two sisters with parathyroid and pancreatic islet cell tumors.[4] A paternal history of ulcers was noted but the association with the endocrine tumors of the two sisters was not made until 15 years later when, in 1954, Wermer identified the hereditary nature of this syndrome. He described a family with multiple parathyroid, pancreatic islet, and pituitary tumors, and this became known as Wermer's syndrome or multiple endocrine adenomatosis.[5] Multiple endocrine neoplasia type 1 has since become the preferred term. "Multiple" refers not only to the occurrence of tumors in multiple endocrine organs but also to the occurrence of multiple tumors in the involved organs.[6]

Not all patients with MEN 1 present with the complete syndrome. Primary hyperparathyroidism is the most common manifestation of MEN 1, occurring in greater than 95% of patients, usually before age 30 and as the initial manifestation of the syndrome.[7-9] Up to 80% of patients will develop pancreatico-duodenal neoplasms. Pancreatic endocrine tumors are most often multiple and are distributed throughout the pancreas. Nonfunctioning tumors, gastrinoma, and insulinoma are the islet cell tumors most often seen in MEN 1 (Figure 36–1). A pituitary tumor, most commonly a prolactinoma, is diagnosed in 30–40% of patients (Figure 36–2). Hyperparathyroidism can occur up to 10 years before other endocrine disorders, therefore one must consider MEN 1 in any patient diagnosed with primary hyperparathyroidism at an early age or with multiglandular disease.[8] Hyperparathyroidism in MEN 1 is most commonly due to hyperplasia of all four parathyroid glands.[8-14] O'Riordan and associates reported multiglandular disease in 90% of their patients with MEN 1.[10]

The clinical manifestations of primary hyperparathyroidism in patients with MEN 1 are similar to patients with sporadic hyperparathyroidism. Some of the more common symptoms include: fatigue, muscle weakness, depression, constipation, polyuria, polydipsia, nocturia, and bone and joint pain. Associated conditions such as nephrolithiasis, nephrocalcinosis, bone fractures, peptic ulcer disease, pancreatitis and hypertension may also be present. The symptoms of primary hyperparathyroidism in MEN 1 may be masked by Zollinger-Ellison syndrome or insulinoma.[8] Conversely, hyperparathyroidism may also aggravate the clinical manifestations of Zollinger-Ellison syndrome as a result of calcium stimulation of gastrin secretion.[8]

Calcium and PTH levels in MEN 1 patients are similar to those in patients with sporadic primary hyperparathyroidism, and the diagnosis is made by documenting hypercalcemia associated with an elevated or inappropriately high parathyroid hormone (PTH) level.[15] All patients with hyperparathyroidism should be questioned about abdominal pain, neuroglycopenic symptoms, galactorrhea, a past history of ulcer disease or other endocrinopathies and a family history of hyperparathyroidism, a pituitary tumor, hyperinsulinism or ulcer disease. If the patient has a family history of hyperparathyroidism and/or other endocrine disorders, fur-

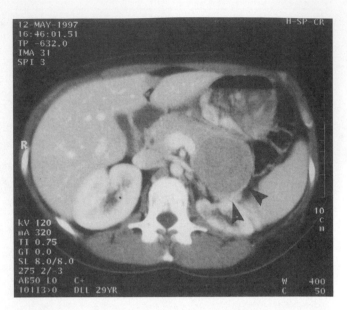

**Figure 36–1.** Large nonfunctioning islet cell tumor (arrowhead) involving the body and tail of the pancreas in a 29 year-old woman with MEN 1 who had a subtotal parathyroidectomy for hyperparathyroidism 11 years previously. (From McHenry C, Pancreatic Islet Cell Tumors, in: Baker RJ and Fischer JE eds, *Mastery of Surgery* 4th ed, Fig. 1. 2001; Boston: Little, Brown; reprinted with permission.)

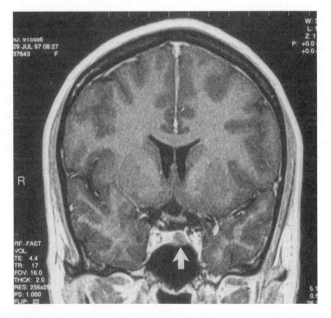

**Figure 36–2.** A prolactinoma (arrow) of the anterior pituitary gland in a patient with MEN 1.

ther screening for tumors of the pituitary gland and pancreas is warranted.[9] At minimum, this should consist of serum prolactin, glucose, basal serum gastrin and pancreatic polypeptide levels. Imaging studies should be obtained in patients with abnormal findings on history and physical examination or laboratory evaluation.

## Genetics

In 1954, Wermer observed that approximately half the offspring of an affected individual inherited the MEN 1 trait, that both sexes were affected, and that the inheritance did not skip generations.[5] This pattern of inheritance, subsequently confirmed by Johnson et al is characteristic of an autosomal dominant trait with a high degree of penetrance.[9,16]

In 1988, the MEN 1 locus was mapped to a section of chromosome 11. By comparing constitutional and tumor tissue genotypes of insulinomas from a pair of brothers who had inherited MEN 1 from their mother, Larsson et al showed that oncogenesis in these cases involved a mutation at the 11q13 locus.[17] Since that time, the gene causing MEN 1 has been identified by positional cloning. The MEN 1 gene is a tumor suppressor gene which encodes the protein menin. It is an inactivating mutation that is the cause for the various endocrine neoplasms.[6,18] One model to explain this finding is the two-hit hypothesis by Knudson et al.[19] This model for the development of hereditary cancer suggests that a mutation in the tumor suppressor gene is inherited on one parental chromosome and that a somatic event in the target organ, leading to the loss of the remaining normal copy of the gene, results in neoplasia. Greater than 90% of MEN 1 patients have germline menin gene mutations and most MEN 1 families have their own unique mutation.[20] Predisposition to MEN 1 is a heterozygotic mutation.[15] The heterogeneity in menin gene mutation may hinder the development of a rapid molecular screening test for MEN 1. Restriction fragment length polymorphism or microsatellite DNA analysis can identify the mutant gene carriers among members of a MEN 1 family; however, these techniques may not be informative for small kindreds or sporadic cases of MEN 1.[20]

## Management

The treatment of hyperparathyroidism in patients with MEN1 is extremely challenging. Multiple abnormal parathyroid glands are the rule and supernumerary parathyroid glands are common in patients with MEN 1.[8,10,11,14] Failure to recognize this may result in an inadequate operation with persistent hyperparathyroidism. Overlooking a supernumerary gland at the time of initial exploration is a well documented cause of persistent disease.[8,14,21,22]

A routine bilateral neck exploration with identification of all four parathyroid glands should be performed. We advocate a subtotal parathyroidectomy leaving a well-vascularized 30–50 mg parathyroid remnant with a bilateral transcervical thymectomy for patients with multiglandular disease Multiple authors have reported their experience with subtotal parathyroidectomy in patients with hyperparathyroidism associated with MEN1 with varying degrees of success.[8,10,11,14] Edis et al reported that 82% of their patients with chief cell hyperplasia had normal parathyroid function at least one year after subtotal parathyroidectomy.[21] However, only 6 of their 55 patients had MEN 1. Prinz et al reported that only 5 of 12 patients undergoing subtotal parathyroidectomy for MEN 1 associated hyperparathyroidism achieved normocalcemia.[14] Kraimps et al reported a 50% success rate.[8] Missed supernumerary or ectopic parathyroid glands are an important cause for persistent or recurrent hyperparathyroidism in patients with MEN 1.[8,14]

The reason that patients with MEN 1 syndrome do not do as well with subtotal parathyroidectomy as patients with isolated four gland chief cell hyperplasia may be attributable to persistent exposure to a trophic factor. In 1986, Brandi and colleagues identified a potential humoral factor contributing to hyperplasia when they demonstrated parathyroid mitogenic activity in plasma from patients with familial MEN 1. Of interest, this parathyroid mitogenic activity in the plasma persisted for up to four years after total parathyroidectomy.[23] As a result, any remnant left after subtotal parathyroidectomy will be exposed to this factor leading to recurrence of the disease. Prinz et al had one patient who had hypoparathyroidism requiring calcium supplementation for 10 years before he developed recurrence of his disease. Re-operation revealed that hyperplasia in the remnant was the cause for recurrence, a finding that supports this theory of the effects of long-lasting stimulation.[14]

Other authors advocate performing total parathyroidectomy with parathyroid autotransplantation into the brachioradialis muscle of the non-dominant forearm and routine bilateral transcervical thymectomy at the initial operation for patients with primary parathyroid hyperplasia.[24] Parathyroid tissue can be cryopreserved and successfully autotransplanted if the primary autograft does not function. However, autotransplantation of cryopreserved parathyroid autografts have been successful in only 50% of patients resulting in permanent hypoparathyroidism.[25] Wells et al pioneered this approach, and have reported that 30% of their patients have developed recurrent, graft-dependent hyperparathyroidism.[26] Malette et al reported a higher incidence of graft-dependent recurrence in MEN 1 patients treated with total parathyroidectomy with autotransplantation than in patients with sporadic hyperplasia undergoing the same operation.[12] This supports the concept that the serum from patients with MEN 1 contains a factor that stimulates parathyroid cell proliferation.[23] Persistent disease in these patients may also be caused by a supernumerary gland. Patients with persistent or recurrent disease should have localizing studies performed to identify such a gland prior to re-operation. When these localizing studies do not reveal a supernumerary gland and it is thought that the recurrent disease is caused by the autograft, a re-operation on the forearm can be performed under local anesthesia avoiding re-exploration of the neck and its potential morbidity.[14] Re-operation to excise the "right" amount of parathyroid tissue from the forearm is not a straightforward procedure. It may be difficult to determine the number, location, depth or viability of the transplanted parathyroid fragments.[27]

Although hyperplasia is the predominant pathology, up to 25% of patients may have only one or two abnormal glands. In that situation, we resect the abnormal glands. In addition, we perform a meticulous exploration for supernumerary glands and routinely perform a bilateral transcervical thymectomy. We also biopsy and mark the remaining normal glands for future identification if necessary. Clark advocates a different approach.[28] If only one abnormal parathyroid gland is identified, he advocates performing a biopsy of the two contralateral normal parathyroid glands and marking them. He then resects the abnormal and the ipsilateral normal parathyroid glands. A thymectomy on the ipsilateral side is performed. If the patient develops recurrent hyperparathyroidism, only one side of the neck will require surgical re-exploration.

Primary explorations in patients with MEN 1 can result in cure rates greater than 90%. In their series, O'Riordan and colleagues reported immediate cure in 94% of patients.[10] Persistent hypercalcemia occurred in 19% of cases in which fewer than four glands were visualized, compared with 3% of cases in which four glands or more were visualized. In addition to having persistent disease, patients may experience recurrent disease. Among the patients who underwent exploration for MEN 1 that resulted in operative cure in O'Riordan's series, recurrence rates were 2.8%, 9.5%, and 17.5% at 2, 5, and 10 years, respectively. Of interest, their results were independent of the extent of surgical resection. Other authors have reported recurrrence rates of 20% after subtotal parathyroidectomy, and higher recurrence rates following procedures where fewer then three and a half glands were resected.[9]

Long-term follow-up is important in patients with MEN 1-related hyperparathyroidism to evaluate for late recurrence of hyperparathyroidism and other endocrine tumors.[8,29] Follow-up should consist of an annual history and physical exam and serum calcium, prolactin, glucose, gastrin, and pancreatic polypeptide levels. It is also important to screen family members. As additional information accumulates regarding the genetics of MEN 1, tests that will reliably determine which family members are likely to develop the disease will be forthcoming.

## MULTIPLE ENDOCRINE NEOPLASIA TYPE 2A (MEN 2A)

### Clinical

Multiple endocrine neoplasia type 2A (MEN 2A) is a syndrome characterized by medullary thyroid cancer, pheochromocytoma, hyperparathyroidism, lichen planus amyloidosis and Hirschsprung's disease. In 1932, Eisenberg and Wallerstein first reported a pheochromocytoma and thyroid carcinoma in a patient at autopsy.[30] In 1961, Sipple et al estimated that the incidence of thyroid cancer in patients with pheochromocytoma was 14 times higher than that of the normal population.[31] In 1962, Cushman reported a family with hereditary thyroid carcinoma and pheochromocytoma in which one affected member had a parathyroid tumor.[32] The syndrome of medullary thyroid cancer, pheochromocytoma and hyperparathyroidism, once known as Sipple's syndrome, is now known as multiple endocrine neoplasia type 2A.[33]

Medullary thyroid carcinoma is seen in essentially all individuals affected with MEN 2A. The penetrance of pheochromocytoma and hyperparathyroidism, however, is variable.[34] Pheochromocytoma occurs in 70% of patients, whereas hyperparathyroidism is reported in only 20–35%.[35-38] Howe et al recently reported on 86 patients from 12 different MEN 2A kindreds who were followed for 13 years. The prevalence of hyperparathyroidism was 35%, ranging from 0% to 53% between kindreds.[36]

Hyperparathyroidism is usually diagnosed as a result of screening patients or family members with MEN 2A, or incidentally during thyroidectomy for C cell hyperplasia or medullary thyroid carcinoma.[39] In a review of 67 patients with MEN 2A and hyperparathyroidism by Raue et al, 75% were diagnosed at the time of thyroidectomy for C cell hyperplasia or medullary thyroid carcinoma. In these patients, serum calcium and PTH levels were normal and the diagnosis was based on intra-operative morphology or histology.[38] Less commonly, a diagnosis of hyperparathyroidism is made as a result of symptomatology. The clinical characteristics of MEN 2A-related hyperparathyroidism are similar to sporadic primary hyperparathyroidism.[37]

Hyperparathyroidism in MEN 2A usually develops after the third decade of life. Severe complications or hypercalcemic crises are rare and most patients have only mild hypercalcemia.[10,15,36,38] Multiple studies have shown that primary hyperparathyroidism in MEN 2A is a less aggressive condition than MEN 1 or non-MEN-related hyperparathyroidism.[10,37] In general, patients with MEN 2A have lower serum calcium levels, fewer symptoms or complications of hypercalcemia, less frequent multiple gland involvement and a lower incidence of persistent or recurrent disease following surgical treatment than patients with MEN 1 or non-MEN familial hyperparathyroidism. Supernumerary gland involvement is also much less frequent.[37]

## Genetics

MEN 2A is a genetic disease transmitted in an autosomal dominant fashion with a high degree of penetrance and variable expression. In 1987, DNA concordance studies mapped the inherited defects of the MEN 2 syndrome to the pericentromeric region of chromosome 10.[40,41] Further work identified the *ret* proto-oncogene as a segment on chromosome 10 that encodes for a specific cell surface receptor complex, the exact function of which is poorly characterized. Mutations in the segment of the *ret* proto-oncogene coding for the extracellular domain of the tyrosine kinase receptor protein are responsible for producing the MEN 2A phenotype.[42] The exact relationship to parathyroid disease is not known. The observation that the *ret* proto-oncogene is expressed in the progenitors of parathyroid cells may provide insight into the alterations found in the MEN 2A phenotype among these cells.[43]

When the MEN 2A gene was identified, it became possible to reliably determine the disease gene carrier state.[40,41] A study by Lips et al looked at the reliability of DNA analysis in identifying carriers of the MEN 2A gene. They found that such analysis for the detection of mutations in the *ret* gene was a highly reliable method for the identification of patients with MEN 2A. They encountered no false positive or false negative results and suggested that, with such a high sensitivity and specificity, clinical decisions could be based on the results of DNA analysis.[44] Among the families studied, no patient without the MEN 2A specific *ret* mutation developed medullary thyroid carcinoma or any other manifestation of MEN 2A.[44] DNA analysis looking for the presence of a *ret* point mutation on chromosome 10 should allow earlier identification of persons at risk. Identifying members of affected families who are not gene carriers will relieve anxieties they may otherwise have and eliminate the need for periodic screening with biochemical tests.[44]

## Management

Before treating the hyperparathyroidism in patients with MEN 2A, the presence of a pheochromocytoma must be excluded. Operation on a patient with an unrecognized pheochromocytoma may result in a hypertensive crisis intraoperatively. As a result, a 24-hour urine collection for catecholamines, VMA, metanephrine and non-metanephrine levels should be done prior to parathyroidectomy.

The surgical approach in patients with MEN 2A-related hyperparathyroidism is more conservative than in patients with MEN 1-related hyperparathyroidism. A routine bilateral neck exploration is performed and all 4 parathyroid glands are identified. Patients with MEN 2A-related hyperparathyroidism have a higher incidence of multiglandular disease than patients with sporadic hyperparathyroidism, although not as high as patients with MEN 1. Only the enlarged parathyroid glands are removed in patients with MEN 2A-related hyperparathyroidism. Because supernumerary gland involvement is uncommon, routine transcervical thymectomy is not necessary. Transcervical thymectomy is still performed concomitantly with subtotal parathyroidectomy in patients with four gland hyperplasia. Effort is made to protect the normal parathyroid glands during thyroidectomy for medullary thyroid carcinoma; however, if they are devascularized, autotransplantation is performed.

Surgical therapy is effective in curing MEN 2A-related hyperparathyroidism. Cance and Wells reported a 100% surgical cure rate and a 3% recurrence rate in treating patients with primary hyperparathyroidism and MEN 2A.[34] O'Riordan and colleagues reported a 100% cure rate with no recurrences whether total parathyroidectomy, subtotal parathyroidectomy or excision of enlarged glands only was performed.[10] Because MEN 2A-related hyperparathyroidism is readily cured with the excision of enlarged glands only and the recurrence rate is low, routine subtotal or total parathyroidectomy is unnecessary.

## NON-MEN FAMILIAL HYPERPARATHYROIDISM (NMFH)

### Clinical

Non-MEN familial hyperparathyroidism (NMFH), also known as familial isolated hyperparathyroidism, refers to hyperparathyroidism occurring in the absence of other endocrinopathies in a patients with at least one first degree relative with surgically proven hyperparathyroidism and no personal or family history of MEN. In 1936, Goldman and Smyth, were the first to describe familial hyperparathyroidism occurring in the absence of other endocrinopathies. They reported two siblings who had mistakenly been diagnosed with giant cell tumors. Subsequent laboratory evaluation revealed calcium levels of 18.2 and 19.2 mg/dl. Both patients were diagnosed with generalized osteitis fibrosa cystica and hyperparathyroidism and they each underwent excision of a parathyroid adenoma.[45] Since that report, a total of 97 patients with familial isolated hyperparathyroidism have been reported in the literature (Table 36–1).

**Table 36–1.** Clinical characteristics of patients with non-MEN familial hyperparathyroidism reported in the literature[27,48]

| | |
|---|---|
| Number of patients | 97 |
| Mean age (range in years) | 36.2 (11–82) |
| Gender (M/F) | 42/55 |
| Manifestations: | |
|   Kidney stones | 45 (46.4%) |
|   Bone disease | 15 (15.5%) |
|   $Ca^{2+} \geq 15$ mg/dl | 32 (33.0%) |
| Persistent or recurrent hypercalcemia | 32 (33.0%) |
| Multiple abnormal glands | 56 (57.7%) |
| Supernumerary glands | 7 (7.2%) |

It has been suggested that NMFH may be a more heterogeneous condition than previously recognized, with the majority being a variant of MEN 1 as demonstrated by novel missense mutations in the MEN 1 gene, and a subset being a variant of the hereditary hyperparathyroidism-jaw tumor syndrome. In fact, further review shows that several patients previously reported in the literature as suffering from NMFH may actually have had the hereditary hyperparathyroidism-jaw tumor syndrome.[46] This syndrome, linked to the HRPT2 gene on chromosome 1q21-q32, is characterized by solitary parathyroid adenomas/carcinomas, fibro-osseous jaw tumors, and occasionally renal lesions, namely Wilms' tumors, polycystic kidney disease, and renal hamartomas[47] (Figures 36–3, 36–4, and 36–5).

Familial hyperparathyroidism occurs in young patients with the mean age at diagnosis of 36 years. Some patients experience NMFH as children, although it is rare before 10 years of age.[48] In contrast, patients with sporadic hyperparathyroidism typically present during their fifth or sixth decades of life.[1] NMFH is more aggressive than sporadic or MEN-related hyperparathyroidism. Patients with NMFH have a high incidence of profound hypercalcemia and more frequently present with hypercalcemic crisis. Huang and co-authors reported that 44% of their patients with NMFH had $Ca^{2+} \geq 15$ mg/dl and 31% presented in hypercalcemic crisis.[49] Among a group of 51 patients previously reported in the literature, 45% presented with a $Ca^{2+}$ level $\geq 15$ mg/dl and 67% presented with a $Ca^{2+}$ level $\geq$ 13.5mg/dl.[48] Nephrolithiasis occurs in one-third to half of patients reported with NMFH, a finding consistent in all reports. It is also generally accepted that other, non-specific symptoms or signs associated with hyperparathyroidism, such as fatigue, weakness, hypertension and peptic ulcer disease, are common in patients with NMFH.[48] It has also been suggested that NMFH may be associated with an increased risk of parathyroid cancer.[48,50,51]

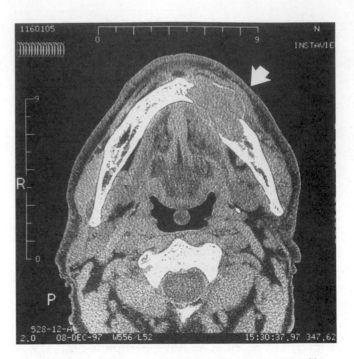

**Figure 36–3.** A computed tomogram demonstrating a fibro-osseous jaw tumor of the mandible (arrow) in a 70 year-old patient with hereditary hyperparathyroidism-jaw tumor syndrome.

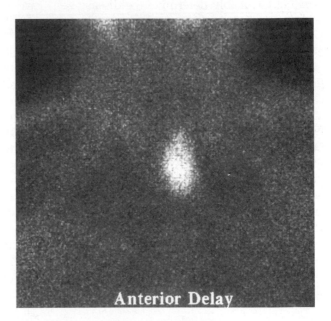

**Figure 36–4.** Parathyroid technetium-99m-sestamibi scintigraphy in a 70 year-old patient with hereditary hyperparathyroidism-jaw tumor syndrome. An anterior delayed image 2 hours after injection of 25 mCi technetium-99m-sestamibi demonstrating a single large focus of radionuclide accumulation in the left inferior position.

One impressive feature of NMFH is the high incidence of persistent or recurrent disease. The cumulative rate of persistent or recurrent disease in the 97 patients

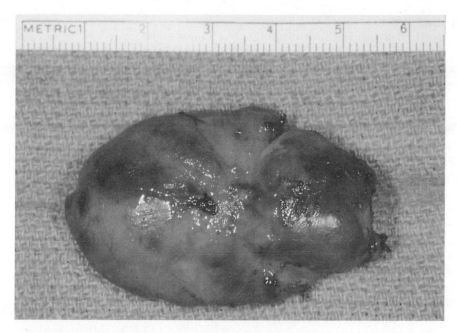

**Figure 36–5.** A giant (13.47 gram) left inferior parathyroid adenoma corresponding to the abnormal focus of sestamibi accumulation seen in Figure 36–4.

reported in the literature is 33% (Table 36–1). Barry et al reported single gland disease in 20 patients (67%) and multigland disease in 10 patients (30%) at the time of initial operation at the Mayo Clinic.[27] At the conclusion of their study, however, these numbers were reversed with single gland disease considered the final diagnosis in only 9 patients (30%) and multigland disease in 21 patients (70%). Thirteen patients (43%) required 20 repeat explorations for persistent or recurrent hyperparathyroidism. Ultimately 24 patients (80%) were cured of their disease; however, this required 50 operations in 30 patients.[27] This contrasts with cure rates of up to 99.5% in patients with sporadic hyperparathyroidism undergoing parathyroidectomy.[1] These findings have significant implications for the appropriate operative strategy in patients with NMFH.

## Genetics

NMFH is an autosomal dominant inherited disorder, although the exact mechanism of inheritance is not known. Whether NMFH is a separate clinical entity, or a variant of MEN 1, has been debated. Kassem et al were the first to implicate linkage of NMFH to MEN 1 in a Danish NMFH kindred; however, their evidence was inconclusive.[52] In subsequent studies of NMFH kindreds, some authors showed germline mutations of the MEN 1 gene, whereas others could not.[53-56]

In 1998, Teh et al reported a missense mutation in the MEN 1 gene in an NMFH family and, employing a loss of heterozygosity (LOH) study, found a loss of the wild-type allele in excised parathyroid tumors. This im-

plicated involvement of the MEN 1 tumor suppressor gene in the genesis of the parathyroid lesions in the affected family.[57] Honda et al performed a similar analysis in a Japanese kindred and identified a missense mutation in the MEN 1 gene and loss of the wild-type allele in a removed hyperplastic parathyroid gland.[58] In extending the linkage analysis in their family, Kassem et al also demonstrated that NMFH is associated with a missense mutation in the MEN 1 gene.[59] These studies showed that NMFH is a genetically heterogeneous disease with a subset linked to MEN 1, most likely representing a variant of MEN 1.[58] It is currently unclear why there are differing degrees of penetrance and why missense mutations of the MEN 1 gene located in close proximity are associated with MEN 1 in some patients and co-segregate with NMFH in others.[58] There appears to be a functionally milder missense mutation, and further MEN 1 genotyping may help define the NMFH-MEN 1 disease complex. The role of the MEN 1 gene in sporadic primary hyperparathyroidism has been investigated and no MEN 1 germ line mutations have been observed in patients with sporadic hyperparathyroidism.[60] These findings suggest that other molecular mechanisms must be involved in the tumorigenesis of adenomas in patients with sporadic hyperparathyroidism.[60]

## Diagnosis and Management

A diagnosis of NMFH is made by excluding all other possible etiologies of familial hyperparathyroidism. It should be considered in individuals presenting with hypercalcemia at a young age and patients with a family history of hyperparathyroidism without other endocrinopathies. MEN 1, MEN 2A, and benign familial hypocalciuric hypercalcemia (BFHH), should be considered in the differential diagnosis. BFHH is an autosomal dominant disorder with 100% penetrance. Linkage studies have shown that the disease locus is present on the long arm of chromosome 3 and the defect is associated with a calcium ion-sensing receptor gene. Patients with BFHH are heterozygous for the mutation.[61-63] Patients with BFHH are hypercalcemic before the age of 10 years and the calcium level is usually mildly elevated. Average calcium levels of 10.9±0.1 mg/dL were reported in a study of 21 BFHH families.[64] The capacity of renal tubular reabsorption of calcium increases in patients with BFHH and hypocalciuria is an important feature of the disease. A urinary calcium-to-creatinine clearance ratio less than 0.01 is the most reliable diagnostic criteria to distinguish BFHH from primary hyperparathyroidism.[65] Making the diagnosis of BFHH is important because no treatment is necessary.[66]

Once BFHH and other causes of familial hyperparathyroidism have been excluded, patients with NMFH should be offered surgical therapy because of the aggressive biologic behavior of this disease. Multiglandular disease occurs in 58% and supernumerary glands in 7% of patients with NMFH.[27,49] This is in contrast to patients with sporadic primary hyperparathyroidism where a single adenoma is present in 80% of patients. The high incidence of multiglandular disease and supernumerary glands is implicated in the high incidence of persistent or recurrent disease.

A bilateral neck exploration with visualization of all four parathyroid glands should be performed. If four abnormal glands are identified, a subtotal parathyroidectomy is performed leaving a 35–50 mg well-vascularized parathyroid remnant. A bilateral cervical thymectomy are also performed. Total parathyroidectomy with autotransplantation of parathyroid tissue into the brachioradialis muscle of the non-dominant forearm, bilateral cervical thymectomy and cryopreservation of parathyroid tissue is also acceptable treatment for patients with parathyroid hyperplasia. We reserve total parathyroidectomy, parathyroid autotransplantation and thymectomy for patients undergoing re-operative surgery for multiple gland disease. In patients with a single or double adenoma, these adenomas are resected and a bilateral cervical thymectomy is performed.

Surgical therapy for patients with a single or double adenoma is more controversial. Some advocate removing the adenoma as well as the normal appearing gland on the same side and performing an ipsilateral thymectomy.[48] When two adenomas are present, both are removed and one of the normal appearing glands is biopsied to evaluate for hyperplasia. The goal is to leave parathyroid tissue on only one side of the neck.[48] The authors from the Mayo Clinic have been influenced by

their need to perform 15 repeat explorations in 30 patients, eight for recurrent and seven for persistent disease. They advocate subtotal parathyroidectomy and routine transcervical thymectomy in all patients with NMFH regardless of the intra-operative findings.[27]

All authors recognize the high rate of persistent or recurrent disease. For this reason, it is advisable that these patients be treated by surgeons with a large endocrine experience. In addition, long-term follow-up is mandatory to evaluate for persistent or recurrent disease.

## FAMILIAL NEONATAL HYPERPARATHYROIDISM

### Clinical

Neonatal hyperparathyroidism is a rare condition characterized by severe hypercalcemia occurring in association with severe hypotonia, poor feeding, constipation, failure to thrive and respiratory distress. The clinical manifestations become evident during the first week of life; however, it may not become manifest until the age of 3 months or older. There have been reports of associated renal stones, limb and thoracic cage deformities and pathologic fractures.[48]

### Genetics

Hillman et al first identified the familial occurrence, and since that time, approximately half of the reported cases have been familial in origin.[48,67] The majority of cases of familial neonatal hyperparathyroidism occur in families with a known history of benign familial hypocalciuric hypercalcemia (BFHH). The disease locus for BFHH has been identified on the long arm of chromosome 3 and patients with BFHH are heterozygous for the mutation, with one affected allele.[61,62] It is thought that two defective alleles cause severe neonatal hyperparathyroidism.[63] It is uncertain if this mechanism accounts for all cases of neonatal hyperparathyroidism. It has been suggested that some patients with neonatal hyperparathyroidism may have one defective allele with an abnormal expression of the remaining allele on chromosome 3.[48] In addition, there have been reports of seven cases from three families where an autosomal recessive mode of transmission has been suggested.[67-69]

### Management

Most patients require urgent parathyroidectomy. Because there is a high recurrence rate after subtotal parathyroidectomy, total parathyroidectomy with parathyroid autotransplantation and bilateral transcervical thymectomy is recommended. At the time of exploration, diffuse enlargement of the parathyroid glands is noticed and chief cell hyperplasia is evident histologically.[70] After total parathyroidectomy with autotransplantation, some infants will have slight hypercalcemia, a normal PTH level, hypermagnesemia, and relative hypocalciuria, similar to patients with BFHH.[71]

## SUMMARY

Familial primary hyperparathyroidism is a well recognized disease which most commonly occurs in association with MEN 1 and MEN 2A, but may also occur as an isolated entity. Familial hyperparathyroidism is characteristically associated with multiple abnormal parathyroid glands and a high incidence of persistent and recurrent disease. Hyperparathyroidism occurs in greater than 95% of patients with MEN 1 and is more aggressive than sporadic hyperparathyroidism. Hyperparathyroidism occurs in approximately 35% of patients with MEN 2A and is a milder form of disease that can be cured by excision of the enlarged glands alone. NMFH is the most aggressive form of the disease with a high incidence of profound hypercalcemia and hypercalcemic crisis.

In all patients diagnosed with primary hyperparathyroidism, it is important to obtain a complete family history. If there is a family history of hypercalcemia, screening for BFHH and MEN syndromes should be performed prior to proceeding with parathyroidectomy. At operation, all four parathyroid glands are routinely identified in patients with familial hyperparathyroidism and enlarged glands are always removed. This constitutes definitive treatment for patients with MEN 2A. For patients with MEN 1 and NMFH, either a subtotal parathyroidectomy with bilateral transcervical thymectomy or total parathyroidectomy, parathyroid autotransplantation and bilateral transcervical thymectomy should be performed to optimize cure rates. Patients with familial neonatal hyperparathyroidism are preferably treated with total parathyroidectomy, parathyroid autotransplantation, and bilateral transcervical thymectomy. All patients require long-term follow-up evaluation for development of other endocrinopathies and/or recurrent hyperparathyroidism. Patients' family members should be appropriately screened for other endocrinopathies and hypercalcemia.

## References

1. vanHeerden JA, Grant CS. Surgical treatment of primary hyperparathyroidism: an institutional perspective. *World J Surg.* 1991; 15:688–692.

2. Boey JA, Cooke T JC, Gilbert JM, Sweeney EC, Taylor S. Occurrence of other endocrine tumors in primary hyperparathyroidism. *Lancet.* 1975;2:781–784.

3. Erdheim J. Zur normalen und pathologischen Histolojie der Glanula Thyreodea, Parathyroidea, and Hypophysis. *Beitr Path Anat.* 1903;33:158.

4. Rossier PH, Dressler M. Familiare Erkrankung innerskretorischer Drusen Kombiniert Mit Ulcuskrankheit. *Schweiz Med Wochenschr.* 1939;69:985–990.

5. Wermer P. Genetic aspects of adenomatosis of endocrine glands. *Am J Med.* 1954;16:363–370.

6. Spiegel AM. Endocrine neoplasias in relation to oncogenes and tumor suppressor genes at the National Institutes of Health (p 484–486). In: Marx S. Multiple endocrine neoplasia type 1: clinical and genetic topics. *Ann Intern Med.* 1998;129:484–494.

7. Brandi, ML, Marx, SJ, Aurbach, GD, Fitzpatrick LA. Familial multiple endocrine neoplasia type 1: a new look at pathophysiology. *Endocrine Rev.* 1987;8:391–405.

8. Kraimps JL, Duh, QY, Demeure M, Clark, OH. Hyperparathyroidism in multiple endocrine neoplasia syndrome. *Surgery.* 1992; 112:1080–1088.

9. Deveney CW. Multiple endocrine neoplasia type 1. In: Clark OH, Duh QY, eds. *Textbook of Endocrine Surgery.* Philadelphia: W.B. Saunders Co; 1997;70:556–561.

10. O'Riordan DS, O'Brien T, Grant CS, Weaver A, Gharib H, van Heerden JA. Surgical management of primary hyperparathyroidism in multiple endocrine neoplasia types 1 and 2. *Surgery.* 1993;114:1031–1039.

11. Van Heerden JA, Kent RB, Sizemore, GW, Grant CS, ReMine WH. Primary hyperparathyroidism in patients with multiple endocrine neoplasia syndromes. *Arch Surg.* 1983;118:533–536.

12. Mallete LE, Blevins T, Jordan PH, Noon GP. Autogenous parathyroid grafts for generalized primary hyperplasia: contrasting outcome in sporadic hyperplasia versus multiple endocrine neoplasia type 1. *Surgery.* 1987;101:738–745.

13. Hellman P, Skogseid B, Juhlin C, Akerstrom G, Rastad J. Findings and long term results of parathyroid surgery in multiple endocrine neoplasia type 1. *World J Surg.* 1992;16:718–723.

14. Prinz RA, Gamvzos OI, Sellu D, Lynn JA. Subtotal parathyroidectomy for primary chief cell hyperplasia of the multiple endocrine neoplasia type 1 syndrome. *Ann Surg.* 1981;193:26–29.

15. Kraimps JL, Barbier J. Familial hyperparathyroidism in multiple endocrine neoplasia syndromes. In: Clark OH, Duh, QY, eds. *Textbook of Endocrine Surgery.* Philadelphia: W.B. Saunders; 1997; 47:381–384.

16. Johnson GJ, Summerskill DM, Anderson VE, Keating FR. Clinical and genetic investigation of a large kindred with MEA. *N Engl J Med.* 1967;277:1379–1385.

17. Larsson C, Skogseid B, Oberg K, Nakamura, Nordenskjold M. Multiple endocrine neoplasia type 1 gene maps to chromosome 11 and is lost in insulinoma. *Nature.* 1988;332:85–87.

18. Chandrasekharappa SC, Guru SC, Manickan P, et al. Positional cloning of the gene for multiple endocrine neoplasia-type 1. *Science.* 1997;276:404–407.

19. Knudson AG Jr. Mutation and cancer: statistical study of retinoblastoma. *Proc Natl Acad Sci.* 1971;68:820–823.

20. Sato F, Duh QY. Multiple endocrine neoplasia syndrome. In: Prinz RA, Staren ED, eds. *Endocrine Surgery.* Georgetown, Texas: Landes Bioscience; 2000:263–272.

21. Edis AJ, van Heerden JA, Scholz DA. Results of subtotal parathyroidectomy for primary chief cell hyperplasia. *Surgery.* 1979;86: 462–469.

22. Cope O. Hyperparathyroidism—too little, too much surgery? (editorial) *N Engl J Med.* 1976;295:100–102.

23. Brandi ML, Aurbach GD, Fitzpatrick LA, et al. Parathyroid mitogenic activity in plasma from patients with familial multiple endocrine neoplasia type 1. *N Engl J Med.* 1986;314:1287–1293.

24. Wells SA Jr, Ellis GJ, Gunnells JC, Schneider AB, Sherwood LM. Parathyroid autotransplantation in primary parathyroid hyperplasia. *N Engl J Med.* 1976;295:57–62.

25. McHenry CR, Stenger DB, Calandro NK. The effect of cryopreservation on parathyroid cell viability and function. *Am J Surg.* 1997;174:481–484.

26. Wells SA Jr, Farndon JR, Dale, JK, Leight GS, Dilley WG. Longterm evaluation of patients with primary parathyroid hyperplasia managed by total parathyroidectomy and heterotopic autotransplantation. *Ann Surg.* 1980;192:451–456.

27. Barry MK, van Heerden JA, Grant CS, Thompson GB, Khosla S. Is familial hyperparathyroidism a unique disease? *Surgery.* 1997; 122:1028–1033.

28. Clark OH. Comment in O'Riordain DS, O'Brien T, Grant CS, Weaver A, Gharib H, van Heerden JA. Surgical management of primary hyperparathyroidism in multiple endocrine neoplasia types 1 and 2. *Surgery.* 1993;114:1031–1039.

29. Clark OH, Way LW, Hunt TW. Recurrent hyperparathyroidism. *Ann Surg.* 1976;184:391–402.

30. Eisenberg AA, Wallerstein HW. Pheochromocytoma of the suprarenal medulla (paraganglioma): a clinicopathologic study. *Arch Pathol.* 1932;14:818–36.

31. Sipple JH. The association of pheochromocytoma with carcinoma of the thyroid gland. *Am J Med.* 1961;31:163–166.

32. Cushman PJ. Familial endocrine tumors: report of two unrelated kindreds affected with pheochromocytomas, one also with multiple thyroid carcinomas. *Am J Med.* 1962;32:352–360.

33. Steiner AL, Goodman AD, Powers SR. Study of a kindred with pheochromocytoma, medullary thyroid carcinoma, hyperparathyroidism and Cushing's disease: multiple endocrine neoplasia type 2. *Medicine.* 1968;47:371–409.

34. Cance WG, Wells SA Jr. Multiple endocrine neoplasia type IIa. *Curr Probl Surg.* 1985;22:1–56.

35. Chong GC, Beahrs OH, Sizemore GW, Woolner LH. Medullary carcinoma of the thyroid gland. *Cancer.* 1975;35:695–704.

36. Howe JR, Norton JA, Wells SA Jr. Prevalence of pheochromocytoma and hyperparathyroidism in multiple endocrine neoplasia type 2a: results of long-term follow-up. *Surgery.* 1993;114:1070–1077.

37. Raue F, Kraimps JL, Dralle H, et al. Primary hyperparathyroidism in multiple endocrine neoplasia type 2A. *J Int Med.* 1995;238:369–373.

38. Raue F, Frank-Raue K, Grauer A. Multiple endocrine neoplasia type 2, clinical features and screening. *Endocrin Metab Clin North Am.* 1994;23:137–156.

39. Block MA, Jackson CE, & Tashjian AHJ. Management of parathyroid glands in surgery for medullary thyroid carcinoma. *Arch Surg.* 1975;110:617–622.

40. Matthew CGP, Chin KS, Easton DF, et al. A linked genetic marker for multiple endocrine neoplasia type 2A on chromosome 10. *Nature.* 1987;328:527–528.

41. Simpson NE, Kidd KK, Goodfellow PN, et al. Assignment of multiple endocrine neoplasia type 2A to chromosome 10 by linkage. *Nature.* 1987;328:528–530.

42. Mulligan LM, Kwok JBJ, Healey CS, et al. Germline mutation of the RET protooncogene in multiple endocrine neoplasia type 2A. *Nature.* 1993;363:458–460.

43. Miller CA, Ellison EC. Multiple endocrine neoplasia type 2B. In: Clark OH, Duh QY, eds. *Textbook of Endocrine Surgery,* Philadelphia: W.B. Saunders; 1997:619–625.

44. Lips CJM., Landvaster RM, Hoppener JWM, et al. Clinical screening as compared with DNA analysis in families with multiple endocrine neoplasia type 2A. *N Engl J Med.* 1994;331:828–835.

45. Goldman L, Smyth FS Hyperparathyroidism in siblings. *Ann Surg.* 1936;104:971–981.

46. Farnebo LO. Commentary in Huang SM, Duh QY, Shaver J, Siperstein AE, Kraimps JL, Clark OH. Familial hyperparathyroidism without Multiple Endocrine Neoplasia. *World J. Surg.* 1997;21:22–29.

47. Larsson C. Editorial: Dissecting the genetics of hyperparathyroidism—new clues from an old friend. *J Clin Endocrinol Metab.* 2000;85:1752–1754.

48. Huang SM. Familial hyperparathyroidism. In: Clark OH, Duh QY, eds. *Textbook of Endocrine Surgery.* Philadelphia: W.B. Saunders; 1997:385–393.

49. Huang SM, Duh QY, Shaver J, Siperstein AE., Kraimps JL, Clark OH. Familial hyperparathyroidism without Multiple Endocrine Neoplasia. *World J Surg.* 1997;21:22–29.

50. McHenry CR, Rosen IB, Walfish PG, Cooter N. Parathyroid crisis of unusual features in a child. *Cancer.* 1993;71:1923–1927.

51. Wassif WS, Moniz CF, Friedman E, et al. Familial isolated hyperparathyroidism: A distinct genetic entity and increased risk of parathyroid cancer. *J Clin Endocrinol Metab.* 1993;77:1485–1489.

52. Kassem M, Zhang X, Brask S, Eriksen EF, Mosekilde L, Kruse TA. Familial isolated primary hyperparathyroidism. *Clin Endocrinol.* 1994;41:415–420.

53. Shimizu, S, Tsukada T, Futami H, et al. Germline mutations of the MEN 1 gene in Japanese kindred with multiple endocrine neoplasia type 1. *Jpn J Cancer Res.* 1997;88:1029–1032.

54. Ohye H, Sato M, Matsubara S, et al. Germline mutation of the multiple endocrine neoplasia type 1 (MEN1) gene in a family with primary hyperparathyroidism. *Endocrine J.* 1998;45:719–723.

55. Tanaka C, Yoshimoto K, Yamada S, et al. Absence of germ-line mutations of the multiple endocrine neoplasia type 1 (MEN1) gene in familial pituitary adenoma in contrast to MEN1 in Japanese. *J Clin Endocrinol Metab.* 1998;83:960–965.

56. Teh BT, Kytola S, Farnebo F, et al. Mutation analysis of the MEN1 gene in multiple endocrine neoplasia type 1, familial acromegaly and familial isolated hyperparathyroidism. *J Clin Endocrinol Metab.* 1998;83:2621–2625.

57. Teh BT, Esapa CT, Houlston R, et al. A family with isolated hyperparathyroidism segregating a missense MEN1 mutation and showing loss of the wild-type alleles in the parathyroid tumors. *Am J Hum Genet.* 1998;63:1544–1549.

58. Honda M, Tsukada T, Tanaka H, et al. A novel mutation of the MEN1 gene in a Japanese kindred with familial isolated primary hyperparathyroidism. *Eur J Endocrinol.* 2000;142:138–143.

59. Kassem M, Kruse TA, Wong FK, Larsson C, Teh BT. Familial isolated hyperparathyroidism as a variant of multiple endocrine neoplasia type 1 in a large Danish pedigree. *J Clin Endocrinol Metab.* 2000;85:165–167.

60. Karges W, Jostarndt K, Maier S, et al. Multiple endocrine neoplasia type 1 (MEN1) gene mutations in a subset of patients with sporadic and familial primary hyperparathyroidism target the coding sequence but spare the promoter region. *J Endocrinol.* 2000; 166:1–9.

61. Heath H III, Jackson CE, Otterud B, Leppert MF. Genetic linkage analysis in familial benign (hypocalciuric) hypercalcemia: Evidence for locus heterogeneity. *Am J Hum Genet.* 1993;53:193–200.

62. Heath H III. Familial benign hypercalcemia—From clinical description to molecular genetics. *World J Med.* 1994;160:554–561.

63. Pollack MR, Beown EM, Wu Chou, YH, et al. Mutations in the human $Ca^{2+}$-sensing receptor gene cause familial hypocalciuric hypercalcemia and neonatal severe hyperparathyroidism. *Cell.* 1993;75:1297.

64. Law MW, Heath H III. Familial benign hypercalcemia (hypocalciuric hypercalcemia): clinical and pathogenetic studies in 21 families. *Ann Intern Med.* 1985;102:511–519.

65. Kristiansen JH. Familial hypocalciuric hypercalcemia. *Dan Med Bull.* 1992;39:321–324.

66. Marx SJ, Attie MF, Levine MA, Spiegel AM, Downs RW Jr, & Lasker RD. The hypocalciuric or benign variant of familial hypercalcemia: clinical and biochemical features in fifteen kindreds. *Medicine*. 1981;60:397–412.

67. Hillman DA, Scriver CR, Pevis S, Shragovitch I. Neonatal familial primary hyperparathyroidism. *N Engl J Med*. 1964;270:483–490.

68. Nishiyama S, Tomoeda S, Inoue F, Ohta T, Matsuda I. Self-limited neonatal familial hyperparathyroidism associated with hypercalciuria and renal tubular acidosis in three siblings. *Pediatrics*. 1990; 86:421–427.

69. Goldbloom RB, Gillis DA, Prasad M. Hereditary parathyroid hyperplasia: a surgical emergency of early infancy. *Pediatrics*. 1972;49:514–523.

70. Ross AJ III, Cooper A, Attie M, Bishop HC. Primary hyperparathyroidism in infancy. *J Pediatr Surg*. 1986;121:493–499.

71. Cooper L, Wertheimer J, Levey R, et al. Severe primary hyperparathyroidism in a neonate with two hypercalcemic parents: Management with parathyroidectomy and heterotopic autotransplantation. *Pediatrics*. 1986;78:263–268.

# 37

# Renal Failure and Secondary Hyperparathyroidism

Sanziana Roman, M.D.
Barbara Kinder, M.D.

## HISTORY

The relationship between chronic renal disease and hyperparathyroidism (HPTH ) was first suggested by Albright[1,2] in 1934. At the time he attributed the observed bone disease to the acidosis of renal failure rather than to HPTH. Castleman and Mallory[3] then described the pathologic finding of parathyroid hyperplasia of chief cells with marked gland enlargement. Over the next 25 years the theory of acidosis as the cause of bone disease in renal failure was supported by many authors thereby excluding the option of parathyroidectomy for symptomatic patients with medical failure. In 1959 Stanbury and Lumb[4] in Manchester, England, described three types of skeletal problems in renal failure: renal rickets, azotemic osteomalacia and azotemic HPTH. They also reported the first subtotal parathyroidectomy as definitive therapy for renal osteitis fibrosa.[5]

Performing surgical parathyroidectomy was not a foreign concept. The first successful parathyroidectomy had been performed in Vienna by Felix Mandl in 1925. At this time the relationship between bone diseases and the parathyroid gland changes had been demonstrated and transplantation of heterotopic parathyroid tissue had been performed as a treatment for rickets. Mandl described his patient as a healthy 38 year old man with severe osteitis who had undergone heterotopic parathyroid tissue transplant without improvement. He performed a single enlarged gland excision and the patient recovered very well.[6]

It was not until 1971 that Wilson[7] reported a retrospective 7 year experience with surgically treated patients with severe secondary HPTH and renal failure confirming the validity of subtotal parathyroidectomy as a means of preventing progression of osteitis.

This chapter encompasses the historical and current pathogeneic theories of secondary HPTH, the associated disease processes, medical and surgical treatment options as well as renal transplantation and tertiary HPTH.

## PATHOGENESIS

### Hyperphosphatemia and the "Trade-Off" Hypothesis

In 1973 Slatopolsky and Brickers[8,9] described a simple yet attractive hypothesis of development of HPTH in renal failure. They postulated that uremic hyperphosphatemia leads to hypocalcemia in turn leading to hyperparathyroidism. This then becomes a compensatory mechanism serving to maintain phosphate balance in uremia. The "trade off" was normalization of calcium and phosphate at the cost of sustained high PTH levels (Figure 37–1).

Since the 1970s advances in understanding secondary HPTH have been made. Now we know that this is a multi-factorial, complex mechanism with emerging developments (Figure 37–1).

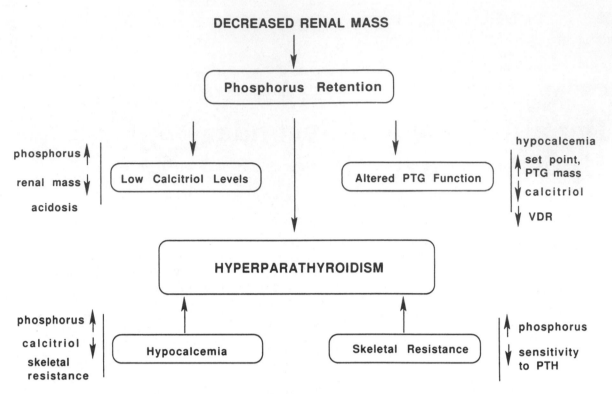

**Figure 37–1.** The "trade off " hypothesis. From Bilezikian JP, *The Parathryroids: Basic and Clinical Concepts.*[95] ©2001, 1994 by John P. Bilezikian, Robert Marcus, and Michael A. Levine, reproduced by permission of Academic Press.

## Early Renal Failure (ERF)

Studies show that phosphorus retention does not occur in early renal failure. Low serum levels are generally reported. Studies in children and adults show that ERF leads to higher urinary phosphate excretion than normal and even though these patients have no HPTH, they excrete phosphate in similar fashion to patients with primary HPTH.[10,11]

## Advanced Renal Failure (ARF)

Phosphate retention increases because of impaired renal excretion. This starts occurring once glomerular filtration rate (GFR) is less than 25–30mL/min. At this level chronic high phosphate leads to low serum calcium and the chronically high serum PTH typical of uremic patients.

## Mechanism of Phosphate Retention in Secondary HPTH

Phosphate retention induces secondary HPTH by several mechanisms:

High phosphate leads to low calcium which leads to high PTH.

High phosphate inhibits renal enzyme 1-alpha hydroxylase which converts 25-(OH)D3 to active 1,25-(OH)D3

(calcitriol). Calcitriol is the active form of vitamin D which facilitates active absorption of calcium from the gastrointestinal tract.

High phosphate decreases calcemic response to PTH, potentiating hypocalcemia.

Lucas et al[12] showed that low phosphate diets in chronic renal failure (CRF) decreased serum PTH without changing serum calcium or calcitriol. In rats Yi et al[13] showed that moderate phosphate restriction decreased levels of PTH mRNA independent of calcium and 1,25-(OH)D3. This suggests that phosphate may have direct action on the parathyroids.

## Impaired Calcemic Response to HPTH

This occurs early in renal failure. There is a skeletal resistance to PTH such that higher levels of PTH are needed to maintain normal serum calcium. It is postulated that chronically high levels of PTH in uremia desensitize the bone to the action of PTH and intiate a vicious cycle of PTH mediated bone disease.

## Altered Calcium Regulated PTH Secretion

In chronic renal failure (CRF) the calcium concentration producing half the maximal inhibition of PTH release (set point) changes; thus the normal concentration of calcium is not sufficient to suppress the PTH glands and higher levels of calcium are necessary to do so. This is potentiated by phosphate retention, lower calcitriol levels as well as an increase in PTH gland mass.[14] Whether there is a difference in increasing the set point in renal failure compared to normal patients was questioned by Ramirez et al[15] in a study of 13 patients with secondary HPTH and CRF and 20 normal volunteers. The authors induced hypercalcemia and hypocalcemia by respectively infusing intravenous calcium followed by sodium citrate and measured the resulting serum PTH levels. Calculated set points for calcium did not differ significantly between groups in this short term study. Other studies though have supported the altered set point theory.[16, 17]

## Calcitriol Effect

A calcitriol receptor has been demonstrated in the cytosol and nucleus of PTH glands. Prolonged exposure of PTH cells in vitro to calcitriol suppresses PTH secretion in a dose dependent manner, reducing PTH mRNA levels by lowering rates of gene transcription.

In ERF there is generally a reduction in serum calcitriol levels. Several studies have shown low levels of plasma calcitriol at creatinine clearance less than 70mL/min.[18-21] Calcitriol synthesis may be impaired even more in patients with tubulointerstitial disease, as 1-alpha-hydroxylase is present in the mitochondria of proximal tubular cells.

In some instances, however, investigators have noted normal, even high levels of calcitriol in ERF.[2,10,21-23] This may be caused by increasing levels of PTH, which itself is a potent stimulus of renal production of 1,25(OH) D3. Other factors such as decreased clearance of calcitriol in CRF caused by "uremic toxins" may contribute to seemingly normal calcitriol levels observed in some patients with ERF.

As renal failure progresses, the levels of circulating calcitriol decrease significantly. This major reduction may play a role in the abnormal secretion of PTH. Some researchers have noted a reduced density and binding of the calcitriol receptors in the parathyroids with advancing renal failure thus further reducing the parathyroid inhibitory effect of calcitriol.[14,24] This abnormality can be reversed by successful renal transplantation.[2]

## Parathyroid Extracellular Calcium Sensing Receptor

A cell surface calcium sensing receptor—BoPcalciumR1—has been cloned from bovine parathyroid.[25] Mutations in this receptor have been shown to cause familial hypocalciuric hypercalcemia and neonatal severe HPTH.[26] This new information opens the possibility that a BoPcalciumR1 abnormality, such as mutation or decreased expression of the receptor, may be found as early triggering mechanisms of HPTH in ERF.

## Gland Proliferation

Gland hyperplasia is a common finding in uremic patients. Enlargement histologically defined as both diffuse and nodular can be found in CRF. The term "tertiary HPTH" refers to the presence of autonomously functioning glandular elements superimposed on the diffuse hyperplasia of secondary HPTH, or to the development of persistent hypercalcemia in patients after successful renal transplantation. Hyperplastic glands that contain nodular features have a higher rate of developing recurrent HPTH after total parathyroidectomy and autotransplantation. These nodular areas appear to contain highly active secretory cells which may not suppress with hypercalcemia.[27] Areas of autonomously secreting nodular tissue have been shown to have lower levels of calcitriol receptors than those from regions of uniform hyperplasia.[28] Both calcitriol modulated specific replication associated oncogenes (*c-myc, c-fos*)[29] and allelic loss on chromosome 11 leading to inactivation of a tumor suppressor gene[30] may contribute to the proliferation of autonomously functioning monoclonal parathyroid cell population in uremic patients.

## Altered Metabolic Clearance of PTH

The kidney plays an important role in PTH degradation. Metabolic clearance of PTH is reduced in renal failure and contributes to the HPTH of uremia. Intact PTH is a 9,500 Dalton, 84 amino acid peptide chain secreted in a pulsatile fashion. It is rapidly degraded in the circulation, particularly by the liver and kidney, into a biologically active and short-lived amino-terminal portion and an inactive carboxy terminal fraction with a longer half-life. Because of the difference in fragment half-lives, older radio-immunoassays using antiserum directed to carboxy terminal regions revealed higher levels of PTH than the newer methods such as immuno-radiometric or immuno-chemiluminescent assays which detect intact PTH.[31,32]

Split PTH fragments are also produced. The 1–34 amino terminal fragment binds to cellular receptors in a manner similar to intact PTH.[33,34] The secretion of these split fragment proteins is independent of intact PTH and is influenced by extracellular calcium concentration.[35]

## Summary

The pathogenesis of secondary HPTH in CRF has multiple contributing factors including possible genetic mutations, altered vitamin D metabolism and resistance, an impaired calcemic response to PTH, phosphorus retention and altered metabolism of PTH. The pathways leading to HPTH seem to have different predominating factors depending on the severity of the renal failure. In ERF, possible mutations in calcium sensor receptors and generalized defect of calcitriol receptors could lead to incipient HPTH. Subtle changes in calcitriol levels, serum phosphate levels and the direct action of phosphate on the parathyroids may further potentiate HPTH. Altered calcitriol levels and receptor binding seem to begin altering PTH secretion.

In progressing CRF, calcitriol deficiency becomes more important and phosphate retention plays a major role in worsening HPTH. Changes in calcium set points, increasing skeletal resistance to PTH and decreased metabolic clearance of PTH contribute to the clinical syndrome of secondary hyperparathyroidism.

## PATHOPHYSIOLOGIC SEQUELAE OF CRF AND HPTH AND INDICATIONS FOR SURGICAL INTERVENTION

### Renal Osteodystrophy

Renal osteodystrophy is a term used to describe the multiple skeletal complications of end stage renal disease (ESRD). It is a disorder of bone remodeling. It is affected both positively and negatively by HPTH and the variables within.

### Normal Bone Remodeling

Normal remodeling is a coupled process of resorption of bone and its replacement by new bone along specific locations in the skeleton. Parathyroid hormone and 1,25(OH) D3, along with various cytokines such as IL-1 and TNF-$\alpha$, stimulate the production of osteoclasts at different stages of cell differentiation and allow local chemotactic matrix proteins such as osteocalcin, osteopontin and bone sialoprotein to be released under the influence of granulocyte macrophage colony stimulating factor (GM-CSF), macrophage colony stimulating factor (M-CSF), and interleukin (IL)-6 and IL-11. These matrix proteins are recognized by osteoclast integrins and act as chemotactic organizers of osteoclasts at the cortical osteon. Multi-nucleated osteoclasts are formed by fusion of precursor mononuclear pre-osteoclasts derived from bone marrow granulocyte macrophage colony forming units (GM-CFU). These matured multi-nucleated osteoclasts then adhere to the bone matrix and form the special plasma membrane resorptive domaine, the ruffled border. The products of resorption such as increased local calcium concentrations and

bone matrix factors such as TGF-beta and fibroblast growth factors lead to osteoclast separation from the surface and eventual apoptosis. These same factors act as stimulants for osteoblast precursors derived from marrow stromal osteoprogenitor cells. PTH and calcitriol potentiate osteoblastic proliferation. This results in osteoblast accumulation in the resorption lacunae with mineralization and remodeling of new bone.[36]

At the end of the normal cycle, the new bone formed is actually less than that resorbed. This resultant osteopenia becomes more evident with age and is even more pronounced in ESRD patients because of the excess PTH and excess circulating cytokines acting synergistically on resorption. Despite this, it is clear that PTH also has an anabolic effect on the osteoblasts via its direct action on differentiation and potentiation of the released insulin-like growth factor (IGF)-1 from osteoblasts (Figure 37–2).[37]

### Pathophysiology of Bone Remodeling

Renal osteodystrophy can be divided into:

1. Osteitis fibrosa
2. Osteomalacia
3. Adynamic bone disease

#### Osteitis fibrosa

This classic form of osteodystrophy is marked by marrow fibrosis with increased bone remodeling caused by the increased number and activity of osteoclasts, as well as higher rates of bone formation with non-lamellar bone deposition. High levels of PTH coupled with increased cytokines production and especially low calcitriol levels cause the above abnormality.

Osteitis fibrosa is associated with osteopenia, long bone fractures and decreased bone strength caused by dystrophic bone formation.

#### Osteomalacia

This disorder is characterized by lower bone turnover, mineralization deficiency and the accumulation of unmineralized osteoid. Deposition of aluminum and other heavy metals associated with ESRD treatment leads to defective mineralization. The incidence of osteomalacia has been decreasing since the 1970s because of increased awareness of these metals and decreased usage of aluminum salts in dialysis fluids. Despite avoidance of heavy metals, this disease entity has not disappeared completely, implying that there are other unknown factors involved.

Osteomalacia is marked by skeletal deformities, fractures and pain. Unlike non-renal osteomalacia, this form of the disease is refractory to vitamin D administration.

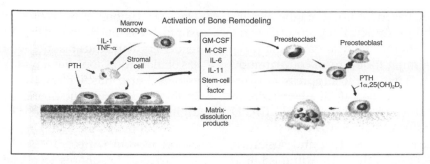

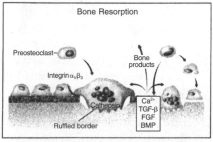

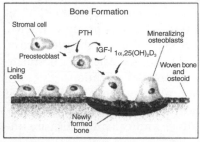

Figure 2. Bone Metabolism in Renal Osteodystrophy.

Factors such as parathyroid hormone (PTH), tumor necrosis factor α (TNF-α), and interleukin-1 (IL-1) activate the remodeling cycle (top panel) through actions on the layer of osteoblasts covering bone surfaces. Existing osteoclasts are attracted to the site and activated by matrix-dissolution products. In addition, stimulated osteoblasts and other cells in the bone microenvironment, such as marrow stromal cells, produce granulocyte–macrophage colony-stimulating factor (GM-CSF), macrophage colony-stimulating factor (M-CSF), interleukin-6 (IL-6), interleukin-11 (IL-11), and stem-cell factor, which stimulate the proliferation and differentiation of osteoclast precursor cells (preosteoclasts), leading to an enlargement of the osteoclast pool. Osteoclasts are derived from hematopoietic granulocyte–macrophage colony-forming units, and precursors fuse. The action of IL-6 depends on its circulating soluble receptor, which with IL-6 couples to the cell-membrane protein gp130, activating signal transduction.[11] In addition, cells of the osteoblast lineage (preosteoblasts), stimulated by activators of bone resorption, participate in bone resorption, participate in cell-to-cell communication. PTH and calcitriol (1α,25-dihydroxycholecalciferol [1α,25(OH)₂D₃]) are also important factors in the differentiation of committed preosteoclasts.[14] Expression of IL-1, TNF-α, IL-6, and IL-11 and their soluble receptors is increased in end-stage renal disease, suggesting that they play a part in the activation of remodeling in renal osteodystrophy.[8,11,19,20]

In the resorptive component of remodeling (bottom left panel), the multinucleated osteoclast is formed by the fusion of mononuclear precursors that differentiate from bone marrow granulocyte–macrophage colony-forming units. Recognition of bone matrix by the integrin αᵥβ₃ stimulates cellular remodeling, resulting in the adherence of osteoclasts to the bone matrix and the formation of a specialized resorbing domain of the plasma membrane, the ruffled border. The products of bone resorption, calcium and transforming growth factor β (TGF-β), inhibit osteoclast function or serve as growth factors (TGF-β, basic and acidic fibroblast growth factor [FGF], and bone morphogenetic protein [BMP]) for osteoblasts, which move into the resorption lacunae and produce new bone.

In the bone-formation component of remodeling (bottom right panel), osteoblast precursors are derived from marrow stromal osteoprogenitor cells. The precursor pool is expanded by proliferative factors, and the pool differentiates to the bone-forming cuboidal osteoblasts responsible for matrix synthesis, mineralization, and remodeling. At the completion of bone formation, the differentiated osteoblast-lining cells form a syncytial-cell layer covering endosteal and periosteal bone surfaces that are not actively involved in remodeling. PTH stimulates osteoblastic proliferation at a discrete undetermined point in osteoblast ontogeny, in part by stimulating the production of insulin-like growth factor I (IGF-I). Calcitriol (1α,25(OH)₂D₃) also regulates osteoblast ontogeny, leading to the differentiation of the osteoblast, and organizes the regulation of matrix-protein production.[21]

**Figure 37–2.** From Hruska KA, Teitelbaum SL Renal osteodystrophy. *N Engl J Med.* 1995;333:168. Used with permission of Massachusetts Medical Society.

### Adynamic bone disease

This poorly understood bone disease of ESRD is marked by hypocellular bone surfaces with little or no evidence of remodeling. This disease is common in patients with normal or low PTH or severe IDDM and aluminum intoxication. It has been associated with peritoneal dialysis (CAPD). This may be explained by the fact that during continuous peritoneal dialysis, there is greater transfer of calcium from the dialysate to the patient, which suppresses the parathyroids. Thus normal or even lower PTH levels may not be able to maintain normal rates of bone remodeling. This need for increased bone remodeling may actually be a stimulus for parathyroid oversecretion.[38,39]

There may also be suppressors and inhibitors of bone remodeling such as IL-11, IL-4[40,41] and nitrous oxide[42] and fragments of parathyroid hormone related protein.[43,44] This disease can cause fractures and microfractures leading to bone pain.

## Diagnosis and Medical Treatment of Renal Osteodystrophy

Despite the fact that a bone biopsy remains the best way to determine the type of osteodystrophy present, measurements of serum alkaline phosphatase, PTH, serum aluminum concentrations and bone scintigraphy (such as 99m Tc-pyrophosphate)[45] can help in distinguishing between the different types of bone disease.

Radiographic examination of hands, skull and long bones will show osteopenia, periosteal bone resorption and, occasionally, cysts as evidence of severe osteodystrophy.

Medical control of osteodystrophy includes a low phosphate diet, addition of phosphate binders that are calcium, not aluminum, based, limiting magnesium intake (magnesium inhibits mineralization) consistent with minimal physiologic needs. Maintaining a positive calcium balance, aiming for a serum concentration on the high end of normal in order to suppress the overactivity of the parathyroids is beneficial albeit easier to achieve with CAPD rather than hemodialysis. CAPD allows improved transfer of calcium across the peritoneal membrane in a more consistent and sustained manner than intermittent hemodialysis. Administration of vitamin D analogues has been used to treat HPTH as well as to correct the endogenous deficiency in CRF. These agents should be used carefully in the presence of hyperphosphatemia as an increased calcium phosphate ion product can lead to systemic calcifications.

New drugs, such as calcium free, aluminum free non-absorbable oral phosphate binders, non-hypercalcemic vitamin D derivatives and calcimimetics are under development.[46]

## Calciphylaxis in Secondary HPTH

Calciphylaxis, also named calcific uremic arteriolopathy, is a rare, severe complication of uremic hyperparathyroidism characterized by calcification of the media of small to medium sized arteries, resulting in ischemic damage in dermal and epidermal structures. Calcification can lead to non-healing ulcers, gangrene, sepsis and even death.

Women on hemodialysis or status post-renal transplantation are almost three times as likely to develop the disease as men. The most commonly accepted etiologic theory was described by Selye[47] in 1962, who also coined the term calciphylaxis. He studied experimentally induced calciphylaxis in rats and defined it as a condition causing calcification of various organs. Sensitization was achieved by injecting PTH, vitamin D and dihydrotachysterol and, after a latency period, a challenging factor such as eggs, metallic salts or trauma induced calcium deposits and inflammatory necrosis of the skin and subcutaneous tissues.[48-50]

Another hypothesis is that an acquired relative protein C and S deficiency leads to thrombotic occlusion of venules and skin necrosis similar to a warfarin effect.[48] Almost all patients with this disease have hyperphosphatemia and an elevated serum calcium–phosphorus product above $40mmol^2/L^2$. Serum calcium can be normal or slightly elevated and PTH can also be mildly to significantly elevated. Subperiosteal bone resorption can be seen on hand roentgenography as a sign of advanced HPTH.

The diagnosis of calciphylaxis is usually based on clinical findings of characteristic skin lesions and can be supported by microscopic examination of skin biopsy.

The skin lesions appear as mottled, violaceous and painful areas, livedo reticularis, advancing to hard, very tender erythematous plaques which develop central areas of ulceration and over days to weeks become stellate eschars. Superinfection can lead to abscesses requiring antibiotics and necrotic debridement. Dry gangrene of digits without systemic sepsis may autoamputate. Peripheral pulses may remain preserved depending on the pre-morbid status.

Serum phosphorus levels need to be lowered by binders and diet. Calcium carbonate should not be used as a phosphate binder because of the increased risk of hypercalcemia and increased calcium–phosphorus product. Dialysis may also be used to lower this product.

Parathyroidectomy seems effective in slowing progression of the disease and allowing eventual healing of the wounds with intensive local therapy. There is still controversy on the issue of altering the course of calciphylaxis with parathyroidectomy. Some studies have concluded that the prognosis depends more on the location of the disease rather than surgery.[51,52] It seems that calciphylaxis involving the trunk, shoulder, buttock or thigh have poorer prognosis than patients with distal extremity disease. Yet in patients with high PTH levels or elevated serum calcium–phosphorus product refractory to medical therapy, parathyroidectomy may prevent fatal outcomes.

Parathyroidectomy is also the only effective treatment in patients with calciphylaxis in tertiary hyperparathyroidism and renal transplantation.[53,54] Immunosuppressive therapy may worsen calciphylaxis unless there is an autoimmune vasculitic component. Cervical or lumbar sympathectomy aimed at relieving vasoconstriction in the periphery is not helpful in treating these ulcers.

Prevention is aimed at avoiding HPTH, hyperphosphatemia and elevated calcium phosphate products.

## Uremic Pruritus

Moderate to severe itching often occurs in end stage renal failure. In the majority of patients it improves, even disappears with institution of dialysis. However, there are patients who do not respond despite adequate dialysis. There have been suggestions[55,56] that this occurs because of increased calcium salts deposition in the dermis without visible skin lesions. There is no correlation between the type of bone disease present, the serum calcium level or the size of the parathyroids and the severity of pruritus. However, parathyroidectomy relieves these symptoms within a few days.[55,56] The exact etiologic mechanism of uremic pruritus has not been completely elucidated, but the metabolic electrolytic derangements of uremia along with hormonal disturbances may contribute to the intractable cases.

## General Weakness

General weakness is commonly observed in uremic patients, particularly in secondary HPTH. It is more prevalent among women and it is of particular importance in patients with diabetic and hypertensive nephropathy. Chou et al[58] describe a series of 56 patients with ESRD and HPTH who were objectively evaluated by muscle strength flexion and extension as well as level of activity. The patients subsequently underwent total parathyroidectomy and autotransplantation with resolution of the HPTH. At three months all patients showed significant increase in the muscle force measurements as well as clinical improvements in physical activity.

The symptoms of weakness are often downplayed by the patient and physician, but in the patients with secondary HPTH, they should be considered as part of the syndrome and therefore readily treatable.

## Anemia and Response to Erythropoietin

Anemia is very common in uremic patients. Its pathogenesis is multi-factorial but a deficiency in endogenous erythropoietin is likely one of the more important causes. PTH may directly inhibit renal and extra-renal production of erythropoietin.[59]

Along with the erythropoietin deficiency associated with renal dysfunction, bone marrow fibrosis potentiates uremic anemia. Excess PTH secretion in both secondary and primary HPTH can lead to marrow fibrosis. There is a significant correlation between hemoglobin concentration and serum levels of alkaline phosphatase as a marker for bone disease. A direct inhibitory effect of PTH on bone erythropoiesis has been debated.[60-62] Patients who require large doses of epogen administration may have more extensive marrow fibrosis caused by HPTH.[63]

There are more complex effects mediated by PTH which affect serum hemoglobin levels, including intracellular and extracellular calcium and phosphate levels, osteoclast resorption and the erythropoietic progenitor cell response to exogenous erythropoietin. Further study is necessary to elucidate these complex interactions.

Improvements in anemia have been reported after parathyroidectomy.

## Tertiary HPTH and Renal Transplantation

St. Goar recognized that secondary HPTH could persist even after patients underwent renal transplantation. He postulated that the parathyroids became autonomous and named this entity tertiary hyperparathyroidsm.[64]

Theoretically, reversal of parathyroid tissue hyperplasia can be expected after successful renal transplantation. Yet studies have shown that hypercalcemia can persist in ranges of 8.5% to 53% of post-transplant patients. Of these, less than 1% may require parathyroidectomy for tertiary HPTH.[65]

Pulsed calcitriol therapy can be used to decrease PTH secretion in post-transplant hypercalcemia,[66] but in some patients the high level of intact PTH may persist despite normalization of serum calcium levels.[67] This may imply independently functioning adenomatous transformation of parathyroid tissue for which surgical intervention may be necessary.

In the transplanted patient, there may be additional factors which can contribute to persistent HPTH. Steroids, cyclosporine, thiazides, GFR alterations caused by tubular injury or rejection episodes can influence parathyroid function and bone response.[68]

The best treatment option in dialysis patients with HPTH who are candidates for renal transplantation is still somewhat controversial. The duration of hemodialysis and renal disease may affect severity of HPTH. The severity of bone disease per se does not seem to be a predictor of likelihood of post-transplant normalization of parathyroid hyperplasia.

Calcium homeostasis in renal transplant patients may take different courses. First, serum calcium levels may be normal immediately post-transplant. This indicates normal physiologic response of the parathyroids to the well functioning graft and resolution of secondary HPTH. Second, hypercalcemia may persist post-transplant but gradually return to normal within the following months. This suggests that post-transplant HPTH is a transient, reversible event. Third, hypercalcemia persists post-transplant consistent with autonomously hyperfunctioning parathyroid tissue. More rarely, hypercalcemia develops months after successful renal transplantation, related to new onset HPTH or subclinical HPTH exacerbated by post-transplant factors, such as medications.[2]

It is known that severe hypercalcemia may affect graft function adversely, therefore calcium levels over 11mg/dl may need to be addressed more aggressively. Patients with symptomatic bone disease or other significant serious sequelae of uremic HPTH may benefit from surgical intervention, particularly if the timing of transplantation is unknown. Otherwise, given the observation that in most cases HPTH will resolve post-transplantation, conservative medical treatment may be indicated.

Surgical treatment of tertiary HPTH after renal transplantation is not very common and is reserved for patients without resolution of symptoms, with hormonal and chemical abnormalities, such as elevated or increasing PTH levels, and asymptomatic increase in serum calcium greater than 12.0mg/dl persisting more than one year post-transplant, and acute hypercalcemia (calcium level more than 12.5mg/dl) in the immediate post-transplant period.[65]

## SURGICAL TREATMENT OF SECONDARY HYPERPARATHYROIDISM

### Preoperative Imaging

Preoperative imaging of the parathyroids has been done quite successfully in primary HPTH where the hyperfunctioning adenoma will often have intense sestamibi uptake. Imaging techniques are also indicated in re-operative parathyroid interventions when, despite adequate first time surgical explorations, heterotopic or supernumerary glands could not be identified. Parathyroid imaging prior to initial surgery for secondary HPTH has had mixed success. The limited sensitivity and specificity of imaging modalities in end stage renal disease may be explained by variations in size and function among the different glands despite increased metabolic activity overall. Several researchers[69,70] have described improvements in these modalities by employing either subtraction techniques, such as technetium-99m-labelled sestamibi and iodine-123 or double phaseTc-99m sestamibi scintigraphy (Figure 37–3). In some of these studies, no false positive scans were documented, and among 11 patients, 42 hotspots were identified and 45 enlarged glands were found at operation.

High resolution sonography can also be used in localizing enlarged glands. This is most successful in primary HPTH, but can identify the enlarged glands seen in secondary HPTH as well.[71]

Rapid intra-operative identification of parathyroid glands with intravenously administered tetramethylthionine chloride (methylene blue) has also been described. Patients were given 5.5mg/kg of methylene blue intravenously 30–60 min prior to induction. Ninety percent of glands were observed to have identifiable staining differentiating parathyroids from surrounding tissue. One hundred percent of glands identified in patients with preoperative serum intact PTH over 700 picograms/ml had intense staining.[72]

## Subtotal Parathyroidectomy and Total Parathyroidectomy with Autotransplantation

After the first successful surgical intervention by Stanbury in 1960, subtotal parathyroidectomy became the standard operative strategy. In 1975, with the demonstration of parathyroid autograft function by PTH assay and forearm autotransplantation,[73,74] total parathyroidectomy with autotransplantation became popular. Total parathyroidectomy without autotransplantation has been described but is not widely in use.[75]

The debate over which procedure is better has been longstanding. Both approaches require a thorough neck exploration through a cervical incision. When performing the subtotal parathyroidectomy, it is well advised to choose the easiest accessible gland for the vascularized remnant. Most often this will be an inferior gland because of its more anterior location. If the remnant appears ischemic, a second gland should be chosen. The surgery consists of removal of three (or more if supernumerary glands are identified) glands in toto and 50 to 75% removal of one gland with preservation of a viable, histologically confirmed remnant. Marking the remnant with a clip will enable later identification if the need arises. Use of intra-operative PTH measurements can help assure that adequate tissue has been resected (see below).

The advantages of performing a subtotal parathyroidectomy are:

1. A well vascularized, orthotopic gland will regain function earlier and maintain it more easily than an autotransplanted gland that would need to undergo neo-vascularization post-transplantation. This contention has been supported by some studies[76] where

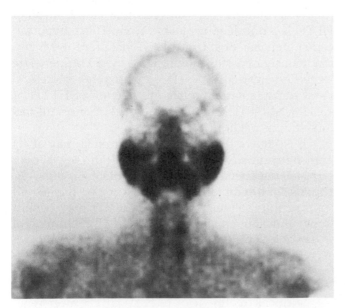

**Figure 37–3.** Te-Sestamibi scan of four gland parathyroid hyperplasia

postoperative serum calcium levels were easier to control in subtotal parathyroidectomy patients with less severe hypocalcemia.[77]

2. Choosing an accessible gland and marking it with a clip for potential later identification makes re-exploration easy without significant complication rates.

3. Avoiding an arm incision allows undisturbed hemodialysis access potential.

The disadvantages are:

1. A second neck surgery is necessary if hyperparathyroidism recurs.

2. If the remnant is not well vascularized, the patient may develop hypoparathyroidism with significant hypocalcemia.

Total parathyroidectomy with autotransplantation removes all identified glands and uses an easily accessible area, most commonly the forearm as the heterotopic site for autotransplantation. Other sites, such as the sternocleidomastoid muscle, have also been used. The gland to be transplanted is minced into 1mm pieces and appoximately 20–30 pieces are imbedded in well vascularized muscle and marked with a stich or clip. Neovascularization needs to take place to make the parathyroid tissue functional. The advantage is:

Residual parathyroid function is easily followed and recurrences can be treated by partial resection under local anesthesia without the attendant risks of a cervical reexploration.

The disadvantages are :

1. More aggressive medical treatment is necessary postoperatively to maintain adequate serum calcium levels and avoid serious hypocalcemic complications.

2. Autograft failure can lead to delayed hypoparathyroidism.[78-80]

3. Retrieval of all grafts may be difficult.

4. Invasive growth of autografts into muscle and adjacent tissue has been described requiring radical resection of the area.[81]

5. It may interfere with hemodialysis access if complications occur.

6. Supernumerary glands may still be present in the neck. Identification of the source of hyperparathyroidism may be complicated and neck exploration may still be necessary.

Subtotal parathyroidectomy seems to be the preferred surgical approach. Overall recurrence of HPTH varies in the literature from 5%–17%.[76,82,83] Nodular proliferation in glands seem to predispose to recurrence more often than homogenous gland hyperplasia.[75]

Cryopreservation of excised tissue is a good strategy if available. This will allow later transplantation of parathyroid tissue if the primary remnant or autograft is non-functional, thus avoiding hypoparathyroidism.

## Other Procedures and Intra-Operative PTH

Newer procedures aimed at minimizing potential operative complications and risks have been under evaluation.

### Percutaneous Ethanol Injection

Percutaneous ethanol injection therapy guided by color Doppler flow mapping has been described recently.[84,85] Several reports of successful percutaneous ethanol injection with pre- and post-injection MRI and MIBI scanning[86] seem hopeful in attaining controlled destruction of parathyroid tissue with minimized side effects and nerve palsy. This method has also been described as treatment for recurrent HPTH after subtotal parathyroidectomy and as an alternative to surgery in high surgical risk patients. It has several problems, such as recurrent laryngeal nerve injury by ethanol, other adnexal tissue ablation, Horner's syndrome and tissue necrosis. It should be regarded as an option in exceptional cases, not as a standard.[87]

### Endoscopic Parathyroidectomy

Endoscopic parathyroidectomy has been performed with the advent of laparoscopy and the impetus to expand the minimally invasive technology into different fields. Several animal, as well as human, endoscopic approaches have been described and both solitary adenomata and four gland hyperplasia have been approached in this fashion. A variety of techniques have been adopted for adequate visualization of the parathyroids, including balloon dissection, carbon dioxide insufflation and mechanical lifters.[88-90] This approach is still under development and its application to secondary HPTH needs further investigation.

### Intraoperative Serum PTH Measurements

Intraoperative serum PTH measurements have been possible given the short half-life of the intact PTH molecule and the development of a rapid modified immuno-chemiluminometric assay in recent years. Using portable equipment, blood samples can be collected and tested in the operating area before starting parathyroidectomy and at five minute intervals post-resection of each enlarged gland. Significant decreases in serum PTH levels after parathyroidectomy by as much as 20% to 86%[91-93] have been noted consistently. Useful in primary HPTH,[94] intra operative PTH measurements may prove to be a good tool in secondary HPTH to determine adequacy of resection as well as to identify patients with supernumerary glands.

## SUMMARY

Secondary HPTH is a complex process. Hyperplasia of the parathyroid glands and increase in the serum PTH levels appear early in the development of renal disease. The primary factors responsible for the development of HPTH in renal failure include phosphorus retention, decreased levels of calcitriol, hypocalcemia and skeletal resistance to calcemic effect of PTH. Medical treatment of HPTH is aimed at reducing serum phosphorus levels, increasing serum calcium levels, administering vitamin D analogs and maintaining an appropriate metabolic equilibrium with adequate dialysis.

The most common indications for surgical treatment of secondary HPTH are the development of renal osteodystrophy, severe pruritus associated with HPTH, calciphylaxis and tumoral calcinosis. Less clear indications for surgery are easy fatigability, proximal muscle weakness and anemia.

Patients with secondary HPTH treated surgically can expect substantial improvements in bone and joint pain and pruritus in most cases. Amelioration of fatigue and generalized well-being are often observed, albeit harder to quantify.

Surgical techniques most commonly employed include subtotal parathyroidectomy and total parathyroidectomy with autotransplantation. There may be a role for minimally invasive approaches, such as endoscopic parathyroidectomy and percutaneous ethanol ablation which are currently still investigational. Refinements in the utilization of intra-operative PTH measurements also promise improvement in the surgical technique and outcome.

## References

1. Albright F, Baird PC, Cope O, Bloomberg E. Studies on the physiology of parathyroid glands—renal complications of hyperparathyroidism. *Am J Med Sci.* 1934;187: 49–65.
2. Diethelm AG, Edwards RP, Whelchel JD. The natural history and surgical treatment of hypercalcemia before and after renal transplantation. *Surg, Gynecol & Obstet.* 1982; 154:481–490.
3. Castleman B, Mallory TB. Parathyroid hyperplasia in chronic renal insufficiency. *Am J Pathol.* 1937; 13: 553–558.
4. Stanbury WS, Lumb GA, The Association for Physicians of Great Britain and Ireland, Fifty-third Annual General Meeting. *Q J Med.*1959; 28: 583.
5. Stanbury WS, Lumb GA, Nicholson WF. Elective subtotal parathyroidectomy for renal hyperparathyroidism. *Lancet.* 1960; 1:793.
6. Organ CH. Our surgical heritage—therapeutic trial in a case of osteitis fibrosa generalizata by removal of a parathyroid tumor *Surg Rounds.* 1985;333:55–70.
7. Wilson RE, Hampers CL, Bernstein DS. Subtotal parathyroidectomy in chronic renal failure; a seven year experience in a dialysis and transplant program. *Ann Surg.* 1971; 174: 640.
8. Slatopolsky E, Bricker NS. The role of phosphorus restriction in the prevention of secondary hyperparathyroidism in renal disease. *Kidney Int.* 1973; 4: 141–148.

9. Llach F. Secondary hyperparathyroidism in renal failure: the trade-off hypothesis revisited. *Am. J. of Kid. Dis.* 1995; 5: 663–679.
10. Llach F, Massry SG. On the mechanism of the prevention of secondary hyperparathyroidism in moderate renal insufficiency. *J Clin Endocrinol Metab.* 1985; 61:601–606.
11. Portale AP, Booth BE, Halloran BP, Morris RC Jr. Effect of dietary phosphorus on circulating concentrations of 1,25 dihydroxyvitamin D and immunoreactive parathyroid hormone in children with moderate renal insufficiency. *J Clin Invest.* 1984; 73:1580–1589.
12. Lucas PA, Brown RC, Woodhead JS, Coles G. 1, 25 dihydoxycholecalciferol and parathyroid hormone in advanced renal failure: effect of simultaneous protein and phosphorus restriction. *Clin Nephrol.* 1986; 25:7–10.
13. Yi H, Fukagawa M, Kurokawa K. Mild dietary phosphorus restriction directly prevents enhanced parathyroid hormone secretion and synthesis and proliferation of parathyroid cells in chronic renal failure in rats. *J Am Soc Nephrol.* 1992; 3:703–706.
14. Delmez JA, Slatopolsky E. Recent advances in the pathogenesis and therapy of uremic secondary hyperparathyroidism. *J Clin Endocrinol. Metab.* 1991; 72:735–739.
15. Ramirez JA, Goodman WG, Gornbein J, et al. Direct in vivo comparison of calcium regulated parathyroid hormone secretion in normal volunteers and patients with secondary hyperparathyroidism. *J Clin Endocrinol Metab.* 1993; 76:1489–1494.
16. Brown EM, Wilson RE, Eastman R. Abnormal regulation of parathyroid hormone release by calcium in secondary hyperparathryoidism due to chronic renal failure. *J Clin Endocrinol Metab.*1982; 54:172–177.
17. Voigts A, Felsenfeld AJ, Andress DL, Llach F. Parathyroid hormone and bone histology: response to hypocalcemia in osteitis fibrosa. *Kidney Int.* 1984; 25:445–452.
18. Chesney RW, Hamstra AJ, Mazess RB. Circulating vitamin D metabolite concentrations in childhood renal diseases. *Kidney Int.* 1982; 21:65–69.
19. Reichel H, Deibert B, Schmidt-Gayk H, Ritz E. Calcium metabolism in early chronic renal failure: implications for the pathogenesis of hyperparathyroidism. *Nephrol Dial Transplant.* 1991; 6:162–169.
20. Portale AP, Booth BE, Tsai HC, Morris RC Jr. Reduced plasma concentration of 1,25 dihydroxyvitamin D in children with moderate renal insufficiency. *Kidney Int.* 1982; 21:627–632.
21. Martinez I, Zaracho R, Montenegro J, Llach F. The role of calcitriol in the secondary hyperparathyroidism of chronic renal failure. *J Am Soc Nephrol.* 1993; 4:725–734.
22. David DS. *Calcium Metabolism in Renal Failure and Nephrolithiasis.* New York, NY: Wiley; 1977.
23. Cheung AK, Manolagas SC, Catherwood BC, et al. Determinants of serum 1,25 dihydroxyvitamin D in renal disease. *Kidney Int.* 1983; 24:104–109.
24. Korkor AB. Reduced binding of 3(H)1,25-dihydroxyvitamin D3 in the parathyroid glands of patients with renal failure. *N Engl J Med.* 1987; 316:1573–1577.
25. Brown EM, Gamba G, Ricciardi D, et al. Cloning and characterization of an extracellular Ca-sensing receptor from bovine parathyroid. *Nature.* 1993; 366:575–579.
26. Pollak MR, Brown EM, Chou YM, et al. Mutation in the human Ca-sensing receptor gene causes familial hypocalciuric hypocalcemia and neonatal severe hyperparathyroidism. *Cell.* 1993; 75: 1297–1301.
27. Wallfelt CH, Larsson R, Gylfe E, Ljunghall S, Rastad J, Akerstrom G. Secretory disturbance in hyperplastic parathyroid nodules of uremic hyperparathyroidism. *Acta Univ Upsaliensis.* 1987; 126: v1–v18.
28. Fukuda N, Tanaka H, Sato K, et al. Decreased 1,25-dihydoxyvitamin D receptor density is associated with a more severe form of parathyroid hyperplasia in chronic uremic patients. *J Clin Invest,* 1993; 92:1436–1443 (abst).

29. Kremer R, Bolivar I, Goltzman D, Hendy GN. Influence of calcium and 1,25-dihydroxycholecalciferol on proliferation and proto-oncogene expression in primary cultures of bovine parathyroid cells. *Endocrinology.* 1989; 125:935–941.

30. Falchetti A, Bale AE, Bordi C, Cicchi P, Bandini S, Mars SJ. Progression of uremic osteodystrophy involves allelic loss on chromosome 11. *J Clin Endocronol Metab.* 1993; 76:139–144.

31. Dunlay R, Rodriguez M, Felsenfeld AJ, Llach F. Direct inhibitory effect of calcitriol on parathyroid function (sigmoidal curve) in dialysis patients. *Kidney Int.* 1989; 36:1093–1098.

32. Morita A, Tabata T, Koyama H, et al. A two-site immunochemiluminometric assay for intact parathyroid hormone and its clinical utility in hemodialysis patients. *Clin Nephrol.* 1992; 38:154–157.

33. Gardella TJ, Rubin D, Abou-Samra AB, et al. Expression of human parathyroid hormone 1-84 in *E. coli* as a factor X-cleavable fusion protein. *J Biol Chem.* 1990; 265:15854–15859.

34. Tregear GW, van Rietschoten J, Greene E, et al. Bovine parathyroid hormone: minimum chain length of synthetic peptide required for biolobical activity. *Endocrinology.* 1973; 93:1349–1353.

35. Lim SK, Gardella TJ, Baba H, Nussbaum SR, Kronenberg HM. The carboxy-terminus of parathyroid hormone is essential for hormone processing and secretion. *Endocrinology.* 1992; 131:2325–2330.

36. Hruska KA, Teitelbaum SL. Renal osteodystrophy. *N Engl J Med.* 1995; 333:166–174.

37. Aarden EM, Burger EH, Nijweide PJ. Function of osteocytes in bone. *J Cell Biochem.* 1994; 55:287–299.

38. Hamdy NAT, Kanis JA, Beneton MNC, et al. Effect of alfacalcidol on natural course of renal bone disease in mild to moderate renal failure. *Bri Med J.* 1995; 310:358–363.

39. Goodman WG, Ramirez JA, Belin T, et al. Development of adynamic bone disease in patients with secondary hyperparathyroidism after intermittent calcitriol therapy. *Kidney Int.* 1994; 38:Suppl:S62–S67.

40. Hughes FJ, Howells GL. Interleukin-11 inhibits bone formation *in vitro. Calcif Tissue Int.* 1993; 53:362–364.

41. Watanabe K, Tanaka Y, Morimoto I, et al. Interleukin-4 as a potent inhibitor of bone resorption. *Biochem Biophys Res Commun.* 1990; 172:1035–1041.

42. MacIntyre I, Zaidi M, Alam ASM, et al. Osteoclastic inhibition: an action of nitric oxide not mediated by cyclic GMP. *Proc Natl Acad Sci USA.* 1991; 88:2936–2940.

43. Orloff JJ, Soifer NE, Fodero JP, Dann P, Burtis WJ. Accumulation of carboxy-terminal fragments of parathyroid hormone-related protein in renal failure. *Kidney Int.* 1993; 43:1371–1376.

44. Fenton AJ, Kemp BE, Hammonds RG Jr, et al. A potent inhibitor of osteoclastic bone resorption within a highly conserved pentapeptide region of parathyroid hormone-related protein: PTHrP [107–111]. *Endocrinology.* 1991; 129:3424–3426.

45. Kinnaert P, Van Hooff I, Schoutens A, et al. Differential diagnosis between secondary hyperparathyroidism and aluminum intoxication in uremic patients: usefulness of 99mTc-Pyrophosphate bone scintigraphy. *World J Surg.* 1989; 13:219–224.

46. Drueke TB. Medical management of secondary hyperparathyroidism in uremia. *Am J Med Sci* 1999; 317:383–389.

47. Selye H. *Calciphylaxis.* Chicago: University of Chicago Press; 1962.

48. Duh QY, Lim R, Clark OH. Calciphylaxis in secondary hyperparathyroidism; diagnosis and parathyroidectomy. *Arch Surg.* 1991; 126:1213–1219.

49. Selye H, Gabbiani G, Tuchweber B. Calciphylaxis and the parathyroid glands. *Recent Prog Horm Res.* 1964; 20:33–58.

50. Rees JKH, Coles GA. Calciphylaxis in man. *Br Med J.* 1969; 2:670–672.

51. Chan YL, Mahony JF, Turner J, Posen S. The vascular lesions associated with skin necrosis in renal disease. *Br J Dermatol.* 1983; 109:85–95.

52. Conn J Jr, Krumlovsky FA, DelGreco F, Simon NM. Calciphylaxis: etiology of progressive vascular calcification and gangrene? *Ann Surg.* 1973; 177:206–210.

53. Fox R, Banowsky LH, Cruz AB Jr. Post renal transplant calciphylaxis: successful treatment with parathyroidectomy. *J Urol.* 1983; 129:362–363.

54. Perloff LJ, Spence RK, Grossman RA, Barker CF. Lethal post transplant calcinosis. *Transplantation.* 1979; 27:21–25.

55. Hampers CL, Katz AI, Wilson RE, Merrill JP. Disappearance of "uremic" itching after subtotal parathyroidectomy. *N Engl J Med.* 1968; 279:695–697.

56. Kleeman CR, Better O, Massry SG, Maxwell MH. Divalent ion metabolism and osteodystrophy in chronic renal failure. *Yale J Biol Med.* 1967; 40:1–45.

57. Massry SG, Popovtzer MM, Coburn JW, Makoff DL, Maxwell MH, Kleeman CR. Intractable pruritus as a manifestation of secondary hyperparathyroidism in uremia. *N Engl J Med.* 1968; 279:697–700.

58. Chou FF, Chiang HL, Chen JB. General weakness as an indication for parathyroid surgery in patients with secondary hyperparathyroidism. *Arch Surg.* 1999; 134:1108–1111.

59. Urena P, Eckhardt KU, Sarfati E. Serum erythropoietin and erythropoiesis in primary and secondary hyperparathyroidism: effect of parathyroidectomy. *Nephron.* 1991; 59:384–393.

60. Meytes D, Bogin E, Ma A, Dukes PP, Massry SG. Effect of parathyroid hormone on erythropoiesis. *J Clin Invest.* 1981; 67:1263–1269.

61. Delwiche F, Garrity MJ, Powell JS, Robertson RP, Adamson JW. High levels of the circulating form of parathyroid hormone do not inhibit in vitro erythropoiesis. *J Lab Clin Med.* 1983; 102:613–620.

62. McGonigle RJS, Wallin JD, Husserl F. Potential role of parathyroid hormone as an inhibitor of erythropoiesis in the anemia of renal failure. *J Lab Clin Med.* 1984; 104:1016–1026.

63. Rao SD, Shih MS, Mohini R. Effect of serum parathyroid hormone and bone marrow fibrosis on the response of erythropoietin in uremia. *N Engl J Med.* 1993; 328:171–175.

64. Case records of the Massachussetts General Hospital, Case 29-1963. *N Engl J Med.* 1963; 268:943–952.

65. Kerby JD, Rue LW, Blair H, Hudson S, Sellers MT, Diethelm AG. Operative treatment of tertiary hyperparathyroidism: a single center experience. *Ann Surg.* 1998; 227:878–886.

66. Hamdy NA, Brown CB, Kanis JA. Intravenous calcitriol lowers serum calcium concentrations in uremic patients with severe hyperparathyroidism and hypercalcemia. *Nephrol Dial Transplant.* 1989; 4:545–548.

67. Fang JT, Chuang CK, Chu LB, Jeng LB, Huang CC. Tertiary hyperparathyroidism after renal transplantation. *Transplant Proc.* 1996; 28:1484–1485.

68. Tominaga Y, Uchida K, Sato M, Numano Y, Tanaka Y, Takagi H. Parathyroidectomy before and after renal transplantation. *Transplant Proc.* 1992; 24:1861–1862.

69. Valli N, Leccia F, Pommereau A, Bordenave L, Laffon E, Ducassou D. Double phase Tc-99m Sestamibi scintigraphy in a patient with uremia and secondary hyperparathyroidism—an aid for subtotal parathyroidectomy. *Clin Nuc Med.* 1999; 24:189–191.

70. Hindic E, Urena P, Jeanguillaume C, et al. Preoperative imaging of parathyroid glands with Tc-99m labelled Sestamibi and iodine 123 subtraction scanning in secondary hyperparathyroidism. *Lancet.* 1999; 353:2200–2204.

71. Brabant G, Kleine P, Hesch RD, Von zur Muhlen A. Preoperative localization of parathyroid tumours by high resolution sonography. *Ultrasound Med Biol.* 1983; Suppl 2:393–396.

72. Bland KI, Tidwell S, Von Fraunhofer JA, Morris RR, McCoy MT, Wathen RL. Intraoperative localization of parathyroid glands using methylthionine chloride/tetramethylthionine chloride in secondary hyperparathyroidism. *Surg Gynecol Obstet.* 1985; 160:42–48.

73. Hickey RC, Samaan NA. Human parathyroid autotransplantation: proved function by radioimmunoassay of plasma parathyroid hormone. *Arch Surg.* 1975; 110:892–895.

74. Wells SA, Gunnells JC, Shelburne JD. Transplantation of the parathyroid glands in man: clinical indications and results. *Surgery.* 1975; 78:34–44.

75. Stracke S, Jehle PM, Sturm D, et al. Clinical course after total parathyroidectomy without autotransplantation in patients with end stage renal failure. *Am J Kid Dis.* 1999; 33:304–311.

76. Albertson DA, Poole GV, Myers RT. Subtotal parathyroidectomy versus total parathryroidectomy with autotransplantation for secondary hyperparathyroidism. *Am Surgeon.* 1985; 51:16–20.

77. Yu I, DeVita MV, Komisar A. Long term follow up after subtotal parathyroidectomy in patients with renal failure. *Laryngoscope.* 1998; 108:1824–1828.

78. Salander H, Tisell LE. Latent hypoparathyroidism in patients with autotransplanted parathyroid glands. *Am J Surg.* 1980; 139: 385–389.

79. Saxe AW, Spiegel AM, Marx SJ, Brennan MF. Deferred parathyroid autografts with cryopreserved tissue after reoperative parathyroid surgery. *Arch Surg.* 1982; 117:538–543.

80. Mozes MF, Soper WD, Jonasson O, Lang GR. Total parathyroidectomy and autotransplantation in secondary hyperparathyroidism. *Arch Surg.* 1980; 115:378–385.

81. Frei U, Klempa I, Schneider M. Tumour like growth of parathyroid autografts in uraemic patients. *Proc Eur Dial Transplant Assoc.* 1981; 18:548–555.

82. Punch JD, Thompson NW, Merion RM. Subtotal parathyroidectomy in dialysis dependent and post renal transplant patients. A 25-year single center experience. *Arch Surg.* 1995; 130:538–542.

83. Gange ER, Urena P, Leite Silva S, et al. Short and long term efficacy of total parathyroidectomy with immediate autografting compared with subtotal parathyroidectomy in hemodialysis patients. *J Am Soc Nephrol.* 1992; 3:1008–1017.

84. Kakuta T, Fukugawa M, Fujisaki T, et al. Prognosis of parathyroid function after successful percutaneous ethanol injection therapy guided by color Doppler flow mapping in chronic dialysis patients. *Am J Kidney Dis.* 1999; 33:1091–1099.

85. Fletcher S, Kanagasundaram NS, Rayner HC, et al. Assessment of ultrasound guided percutaneous ethanol injection and parathyroidectomy in patients with tertiary hyperparathyroidism. *Nephrol Dial Transplant.* 1998; 13:3111–3117.

86. Wada A, Sugihara M, Sugimura K, Kuroda H. Magnetic resonance imaging and technetium 99m methoxyisonitrile (MIBI) scintigraphy to evaluate the abnormal parathyroid gland and PEIT efficacy for secondary hyperparathyroidism. *Rad Med.* 1999; 17:275–282.

87. Khafif A, Halperin D, Marshak G. Ethanol injection to parathyroid tissue: indications and limitations. *Ear Nose Throat J.* 1998; 77:538–540.

88. Brunt LM, Jones DB, Wu JS, Quasebarth MA, Meininger T, Soper NJ. Experimental development of an endoscopic approach to neck exploration and parathyroidectomy. *Surgery.* 1997; 124:118–120.

89. Miccoli P, Bendinelli C, Vignali E, et al. Endoscopic parathyroidectomy: report of an initial experience. *Surgery.* 1998; 124: 1077–1079.

90. Gagner M. Endoscopic subtotal parathyroidectomy in patients with primary hyperparathyroidism. *Br J Surg.* 1996; 83:875.

91. Proye CA, Goropoulos A, Franz C, et al. Usefulness and limits of quick intraoperative measurements of intact (1–84) parathyroid hormone in the surgical management of hyperparathyroidism: sequential measurements in patients with multiglandular disease. *Surgery.* 1991; 110:1035–1042.

92. Martin M, de la Cruz Vigo F, Martinez JI, Larrodera ML, Ortega G. Intraoperative serum parathyroid hormone measurement in the surgical treatment of hyperparathyroidism. *Med Clin (Barc).* 1997; 109:201–206.

93. Clary BM, Garner SC, Leight GS. Intraoperative parathyroid hormone monitoring during parathyroidectomy for secondary hyperparathyroidism. *Surgery.* 1997; 122:1034–1039.

94. Nagel M, Ockert D, Zimmermann T, Saeger HD. Intraoperative determination of parathyroid hormone—an alternative to preoperative localization and diagnosis. *Langenbecks Arch Chir Suppl Kongressbd.* 1997; 114:1154–1156.

95. Bilezikian JP et al. *The Parathyroids: Basic and Clinical Concepts.* New York: Raven Press; 1994.

# 38

# Re-exploration for Hyperparathyroidism

Phillip K. Pellitteri, D.O., F.A.C.S.
Roger Levin, M.D., F.A.C.S.
Daniel W. Karakla, M.D. F.A.C.S.

## INCIDENCE

### Diagnosis

The most common etiology for primary hyperparathyroidism is a solitary parathyroid adenoma found in 85% of patients with this diagnosis.[1] Surgical excision of the parathyroid adenoma is curative and the surgical literature abounds with reports claiming this can be accomplished in 90–97% of patients with almost no morbidity.[1,2] Most believe, however, that the actual cure rate after surgery is significantly lower, often as low as 70%.[3] The reason for this disparity is that the high cure rates are described by surgeons who perform large numbers of these cases, whereas the majority of operations for this disease are performed by surgeons with less experience.[4]

Persistent and recurrent disease occurs in approximately 3.2% and 0.7% of patients, respectively.[5] Initial studies of patients with persistent or recurrent elevated calcium levels after an initial parathyroid procedure suggested that the majority of patients in this category had multiglandular disease unappreciated at the initial operation.[6-8] However, these reports originated from institutional series with considerable experience in parathyroid surgery and are not representative of the general population after failed parathyroid procedure.[9] A missed single abnormal parathyroid adenoma accounts for the majority of patients who fail initial procedures for the treatment of primary hyperparathyroidism.[2,10] The causes for failed cervical exploration include the presence of multiple abnormal, ectopic, or supernumerary glands, surgeon inexperience, inadequate exploration of the neck and/or superior mediastinum, and incomplete resection of hyperplastic glands.[5,9] Those patients not cured by the first operation pose a significant problem because of the more difficult and technically demanding nature of re-operative parathyroid surgery.

Scarring and distortion of normal tissue planes in the neck after a prior cervical exploration lead to decreased success rates and increased complications after re-operative parathyroid procedures.[9-13] The failure to identify an adenoma at an initial procedure suggests that it will not be an obvious lesion by either location or appearance. The features used to identify parathyroid adenomas such as color, shape, and tactile perception of gland may be much more difficult to appreciate because of fibrosis within the tissues from the previous surgery.[14,15] As a result, success rates at subsequent surgery for primary hyperparathyroidism are decreased and operative complications, including recurrent laryngeal nerve injury with paralysis and hypoparathyroidism can be even more daunting. The initial surgical management of this problem has already been discussed elsewhere. Importantly, the percentage of re-operation for persistent or recurrent secondary hyperparathyroidism after parathyroidectomy ranges from 6% to 25%.[16]

The first requirement for success in re-operative parathyroid surgery is proper diagnosis. By definition, hyperparathyroidism (primary or secondary) must be proven by elevation of serum calcium levels associated with high or normal parathyroid hormone levels. Elevated serum chloride and decreased serum phosphate levels are frequently noted. In addition, urinary calcium should be appropriately elevated, in order to exclude a diagnosis of familial hypocalciuric hypercalcemia. If all these parameters are not present, other causes of hypercalcemia must be considered as a repeat surgical exercise is almost guaranteed to be unsuccessful.[16] The diagnosis of hyperparathyroidism is currently more straightforward with immunoradiometric and immunochemiluminescent assays of parathyroid hormone levels. However, it has been estimated that up to 10% of surgical failures occur because of mistaken diagnosis. Diagnostic errors in hyperparathyroidism can result from: medications (calcium, vitamin D, Lasix, thiazide diuretics, calcitonin, lithium), benign familial hypocalciuria, hypercalcemia, malignancy (bone metastasis or humoral hypercalcemia), granulomatous disease, acute renal failure, bone disease (Paget's, immobilization), hyperthyroidism, or adrenal insufficiency.

The indications for surgical intervention in secondary cases must be solid, as the morbidity and technical difficulty is increased. The guidelines for surgery in primary hyperparathyroidism, as outlined in the National Institutes of Health 1991 Consensus Conference, are reviewed in the accompanying table (Table 38–1).

## CAUSES OF FAILED EXPLORATION

As mentioned earlier, the most common finding on parathyroid re-exploration by the experienced parathyroid surgeon is a missed single adenoma. Akerstrom et al reported on 84 parathyroid re-explorations in 69 patients with primary hyperparathyroidism. Thirty-seven of these patients had missed adenomas; four of these patients having double "adenomas" with only one adenoma being resected on the initial exploration.[17] The majority of the remaining patients had persistent hyperparathyroidism secondary to inadequate resection of parathyroid hyperplasia with only four patients demonstrating recurrent "single" adenomas. Rotstein and colleagues analyzed their series of 28 re-operations for primary hyperparathyroidism. They identified solitary adenomas in 24 patients, with 2 patients each having hyperplasia and carcinoma.[18] Norman and Denham utilized the technique of minimally invasive radio-guided parathyroidectomy for re-operative disease.[4] They studied 24 patients and resected 23 solitary adenomas. Jaskowiak et al reviewed their experience at the National Institutes of Health with 288 patients with persistent/recurrent hyperparathyroidism.[9] Two hundred and twenty-two (77%) of these patients were ultimately demonstrated to have solitary adenomas.

In patients with secondary hyperparathyroidism, hyperplasia is obviously expected. Cattan et al re-explored 89 patients for persistent or recurrent secondary hyperparathyroidism; 53 of these patients had undergone subtotal parathyroidectomies, while 36 had prior total parathyroidectomies with autotransplantation.[19] They identified hypertrophy of the remnant as the principal cause of recurrence in the subtotal group. In the group with total parathyroidectomy, recurrence was located in the autotransplant in half; hyperplastic disease was identified in the neck or mediastinum in the other half.

Just as important as the finding that the cause of persistent/recurrent hyperparathyroidism is a solitary adenoma in the majority of patients, is the observation that, in the majority of these cases, the adenoma is in a "standard" location. In the report by Akerstrom et al, only 8 patients required sternotomies for ectopic adenomas identified in the mediastinum despite 17 sternotomies being performed. In 5 of the 17 patients who had sternotomy, the offending lesion was ultimately identified in a normal location in the neck. Of the more unusual ectopic locations, one was ventral to the left atrium, one ventral to the aortic root, and one in the aortopulmonary window. Furthermore, only one gland was truly intra-thyroid, despite 19 thyroid lobectomies performed as part of the re-exploration. In the series by Norman and Denham, only one gland was in the mediastinum (just anterior to the right atrium), while two were intra-thyroid. Jaskowiak et al identified adenomas in the posterior superior mediastinum, specifically in the tracheoesophageal groove in 27% of their patients (59/215). This was the most common location of the adenoma in the "failed" first exploration. This site is easily explored transcervically and should be considered as an inferior extension of the normal superior gland position. Furthermore, the authors point out that these adenomas were almost always in direct apposition to the recurrent laryngeal nerve, perhaps suggest-

**TABLE 38–1.** NIH 1991 Consensus Conference—Guidelines for Surgery in Primary Hyperparathyroidism

1. Serum calcium > 12 mg/dl

2. Marked hypercalciuria (7,400 mg/dsg)

3. Any overt manifestation of primary hyperparathyroidism

4. Markedly reduced cortical bone density (Z score ≤2)

5. Reduced creatinine clearance in the absence of other cause

6. Age < 50 years

ing that inadequate dissection around the nerve initially contributed to the failure. Another 24.3% of patients had their adenomas in the normal positions adjacent to the thyroid gland.[8]

In the NIH series, the most common ectopic site was within the thymus or mediastinum, accounting for 16.7%.[8] This value is lower than other reports of 22% intra-thymic tumors at the initial operation and 38% for re-operation.[19] An intra-thyroidal lesion was noted in 10% (22 patients) of their study population. A similar percentage of patients had undescended parathyroid glands. These so-called parathymic lesions are located at the bifurcation of the carotid artery, high in the neck, and represent an inferior gland that is arrested in the descent from the third branchial pouch.[20,21] Other "typical" ectopic locations included lesions within the carotid sheath and the retroesophageal space. Unusual ectopic locations included the aortopulmonary window in two patients, the hypopharynx at the base of the tongue in one patient, the wall of the nasopharynx near the nasal septum in one patient, and within the vagus nerve high in the neck at the level of C1–C2 vertebrae. Furthermore, three patients had lesions "seeded" within the strap muscles, most likely because of the first exploration.[8]

## PREOPERATIVE ASSESSMENT

A missed single abnormal adenoma in a "standard" location accounts for the majority of patients who fail initial procedures for the treatment of hyperparathyroidism. For this reason, accessing the records from the original exploration, including the operative dictation and the pathology report are essential. Notes from the original operation may describe in detail the thoroughness of the exploration: which parathyroid glands remain in situ, whether the recurrent laryngeal nerve was identified and thoroughly skeletonized, and whether any "atypical" but regional areas were explored. These areas might include the retroesophageal compartment, the accessible carotid sheath, and the anterior mediastinum/thymus. The pathology report should document what histologic items were identified, ie, whether all normal parathyroids were biopsy proven. Ideally, all four glands should be identified before calling an initial exploration negative. Attie demonstrated that an adenoma was invariably identified in the neck in a normal location on re-exploration when the original surgeon had pathologic documentation of fewer than three normal glands. Unfortunately, the uninvolved glands can be suppressed and hypoplastic in some cases of primary hyperparathyroidism, making biopsy difficult.[20]

No matter what the original surgical and pathologic reports state, endocrine surgeons universally agree that preoperative imaging studies are an essential component of re-operative parathyroid surgery. A variety of invasive and non-invasive techniques are available to image or localize abnormal parathyroid glands. The four principal non-invasive techniques are nuclear medicine scan (Tc-99m-sestamibi), high resolution ultrasound, neck and mediastinal computed tomography scan, and neck and mediastinal magnetic resonance imaging. The principal invasive techniques include selective angiography, selective venous sampling for parathyroid hormone, or percutaneous aspiration of suspicious lesions. Furthermore, intraoperative ultrasound, radio-guidance, and parathyroid hormone assay can be helpful.

Jaskowiak et al reported their approach from the NIH. Each of their patients underwent all four modes of non-invasive testing. When the combined findings of these studies identified a non-equivocal lesion consistent with a parathyroid adenoma on two or more studies, the patients were taken to the operating room. When the data were negative, equivocal, or contradictory, the patients proceeded to invasive testing. Unfortunately, only 27% of their population met the criteria for surgical exploration based on the non-invasive studies.[9] The sensitivity and specificity of these studies were also less than optimal (see Figure 38–1). Other studies have demonstrated similar findings with regard to non-invasive localizing procedures and their sensitivities/specificities. Rodriguez et al utilized 174 localization studies on 152 patients. They recommended using ultrasonography, sestamibi scanning, and MRI for their re-operative patients. They found that multiple non-invasive studies correctly localized the site of the parathyroid tumor in 78% to 100% of patients. They further recommend reserving selective venous catheterization for equivocal or negative non-invasive studies.[22] Shen et al demonstrated equivalent sensitivities using sestamibi and MRI (77%), with ultrasound (US) and CT scanning being less effective (57% and 42%, respectively).[3] Interestingly, selective venous catheterization was no more sensitive than sestamibi or MRI. Overall, imaging studies were able to identify the lesion in 87% of cases in this study.[3] Kebebew et al evaluated imaging techniques in their cohort of patients undergoing re-operation for parathyroid carcinoma. They found the sensitivities for the non-invasive modalities sestamibi, MRI, CT scan, and ultrasound to be 79%, 93%, 67%, and 69%, respectively. Selective venous catheterization had a sensitivity of 83%.[23] Finally, Cattan et al reviewed the use of imaging studies in re-operative secondary hyperparathyroidism. They recommended high resolution ultrasound, CT scanning and MIBI scintigraphy, particularly to help differentiate between recurrence in the neck versus forearm parathyroid graft.[19] Intra-operative sestamibi scanning in re-operative parathyroid sur-

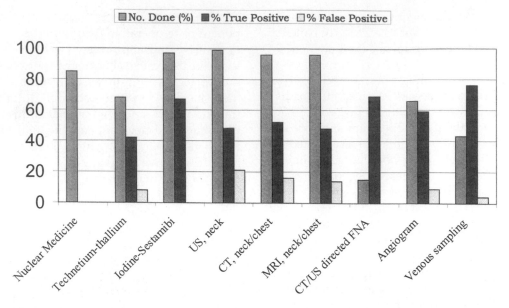

**Figure 38–1.** Sensitivity and specificity of various localization studies for abnormal parathyroid gland identification. (Adapted from Jaskowiak N, et al. *Ann Surg.* 1996;224:308–322.)

gery was investigated in eleven patients (Rossi).[24] All patients had preoperative sestamibi scintigraphy and ultrasound exams, which correctly localized 10 of 11 (91%) hyperfunctional glands. Intra-operative PTH immunochemiluminescent assay was used in all patients, and a 50% or greater drop in baseline values was used to confirm complete excision of hyper-functioning parathyroid tissue. Additionally, all patients had parathyroid tissue cryopreserved.

As mentioned above, a number of studies evaluating imaging modalities for recurrent hyperparathyroidism employ the use of selective vein catheterization with PTH analysis. Sugg et al described the experience from the NIH with this modality, and reviewed the literature. The authors evaluated a population of 86 patients with negative non-invasive studies and negative angiograms who underwent this invasive study. They determined that 88% of patients had a significant gradient. A positive gradient was defined as a step-up of at least twice the peripheral PTH determined from iliac vein samples. A true positive result in this study was defined as finding an abnormal parathyroid gland in the region of the positive PTH gradient. They reported their sensitivity with this modality to be 88% with a specificity of 86%.[25] Further reviewing the literature, they determined a success rate between 71% and 88% with selective venous catheterization. In contrast with these results are earlier reports from the Mayo clinic and University of Michigan where more than half the studies were either negative or showed false positive outcomes.[26,27]

Angiography is useful not just as a localizing technique, but in some cases as a therapeutic technique as well. Doherty et al reviewed their results using angiographic ablation of mediastinal parathyroid adenomas. They found that selective embolization was initially successful in 73%, with long-term control of hyperparathyroidism in 63%. Furthermore, unsuccessful ablations were easily salvageable by mediastinal exploration via a median sternotomy. Importantly, angiographic ablation resulted in a substantially shorter length of hospitalization, less discomfort, and easier recuperation.[28]

Cost associated with localization studies performed in preparation for re-exploration may be significant, adding to the overall expense associated with failed initial exploration. Feingold et al reviewed 62 patients, who underwent re-operation for missed adenomas. Sixty-one patients had a curative operation (98%). All patients had preoperative ultrasound, CT scan, MRI and sestamibi scan, which was estimated to cost over $7,000 in the community. If two concordant, non-invasive studies failed to localize the adenoma, then invasive studies (angiography, venous sampling, percutaneous FNA) were pursued. This group also utilized intra-operative ultrasound, and found it was useful at times in guiding the surgeon to an adenoma in a scarred operative field or unusual location. When preoperative ultrasound and sestamibi (cost $1,400) were analyzed, one or both studies actually localized the gland in 58 of 62 cases (94%).[29]

In sorting through the many choices and algorithms for preoperative localizing studies for reoperative parathyroid surgery, it would be ideal to correlate localizing physiologic and anatomic studies. It is extremely important to identify a radiologist/nuclear medicine physician, who is experienced and skillful in ultrasound and sestamibi scanning, in order to optimize localization results.

Given the need to balance cost and accuracy, preoperative sestamibi and ultrasound or MRI can be recommended as initial studies. If all non-invasive studies fail to localize, then selective venous sampling and arteriography are pursued. If the sestamibi localized to the chest, then MRI and, possibly, invasive testing may be performed. Intra-operative sestamibi, PTH assessment and ultrasound serve as additional tools to enhance the surgeon's expertise.

## SURGICAL CONSIDERATIONS

### Operative Risk: Re-exploration

Once a decision has been made to pursue re-exploration for persistent or recurrent hyperparathyroidism, the patient and surgeon must review and mutually understand the inherent risks of such surgery. Re-operation procedures conducted in any anatomic region are always associated with an increased risk to adjacent structures and potential compromise of physiologic function; this is no exception when considering cervical re-exploration. The risk of injury to the recurrent laryngeal nerve, a potentially very problematic complication, is greater in re-explored necks than that for initial exploration. In two large studies, the incidence of vocal cord paralysis exceeded 6% following parathyroid re-exploration, in sharp contrast to the exceedingly low rate (<1%) realized following initial bilateral exploration.[30] Although more limited approaches to parathyroid re-exploration (targeted exploration; minimally invasive radio-guided surgery) are likely to result in a reduced incidence of nerve injury following re-operation, it remains that surgical treatment of the operated neck will always be associated with increased risk. In addition to an increased incidence of recurrent nerve injury, re-exploration carries with it a greater likelihood for postoperative hypocalcemia, both temporary and permanent.[31] Finally, although the success rate for re-operative parathyroid surgery may exceed 90% in experienced hands, this remains substantially less than the near perfect rate of success for initial surgery. Thus, it is important that, together with re-confirmation of the diagnosis and careful patient preparation, a candid discussion of the risks associated with re-operation be held with the patient.

### Ectopic Glands

As mentioned previously, the most likely cause of an unsuccessful initial parathyroid exploration is that oc-

curring as a result of a single missed adenoma, accessible in more than 90% of instances through a cervical approach (Figure 38–2). In the majority of these situations, missed adenomas will be located in normal anatomic locations, and may be reliably found using meticulous technique and a comprehensive knowledge of the embryonic-anatomic relationship of the parathyroid glands and lower neck region. Nonetheless, parathyroid glands may be located in unusual or ectopic locations and may prove challenging to the surgeon undertaking re-exploration. The most common ectopic location encountered in re-operation for missed parathyroid adenoma is the posterior superior mediastinum.[32] Both Wang and Norton have described this entity, occurring as a result of enlargement of a superior parathyroid gland which transverses a retroesophageal course with the upper posterior mediastinal compart-

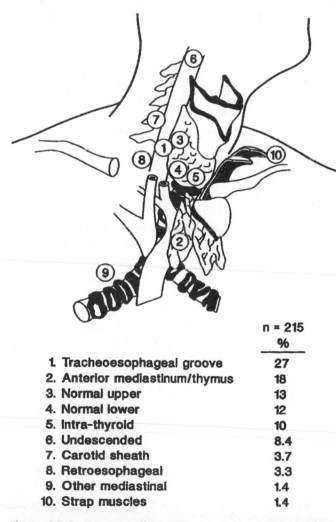

| | n = 215 |
|---|---|
| | **%** |
| 1. Tracheoesophageal groove | 27 |
| 2. Anterior mediastinum/thymus | 18 |
| 3. Normal upper | 13 |
| 4. Normal lower | 12 |
| 5. Intra-thyroid | 10 |
| 6. Undescended | 8.4 |
| 7. Carotid sheath | 3.7 |
| 8. Retroesophageal | 3.3 |
| 9. Other mediastinal | 1.4 |
| 10. Strap muscles | 1.4 |

**Figure 38–2.** Diagram illustrating anatomic regions harboring parathyroid glands missed at initial operation. (Reprinted with permission from Jaskowiak N, et al. *Ann Surg.* 1996;224:308–322.)

ment.[33,34] This entity accounts for greater than 25% of persistent hyperparathyroidism requiring re-operation. Although embryologically the superior gland is more consistent in normal location, and thus less likely to be truly ectopic, it is more difficult to identify when it does not reside in its usual location. This substantiates Norton's observation that these "ectopic" superior glands actually represent normally located glands which descend to atypical locales subsequent to enlargement.[35] Because of the more extensive course of embryonic descent involved, a missed inferior parathyroid adenoma, located within the thymus in the anterior mediastinal compartment, represents the second most common ectopic site, occurring in 18% of patients requiring re-operation in a study conducted by the NIH.[9]

The longer embryologic descent of the inferior gland may give rise to widely disparate anomalies where potential ectopic locations are widely separated. The inferior gland may not separate from the third pharyngeal anlage and thus fails to descend, ultimately remaining associated with the lateral pharyngeal musculature or carotid sheath. Although the entity has been postulated by anatomic studies to represent up to 2% of inferior gland anomalies, clinical series of primary explorations have set this incidence at a fraction of 1%. Examination of re-operative clinical series places the incidence of undescended inferior glands in a range from 1% to nearly 20%.[36] In one of these series, Edis emphasized the finding of trace amounts of thymic tissue in association with the undescended glands, so called parathymus.[37,38]

Alternatively, the inferior gland may fail to separate from the thymus during descent, thereby allowing the gland to reside within the anterior mediastinal compartment. In most series, this represents a common location for an ectopic parathyroid adenoma, discounting the so-called "ectopic" enlarged superior gland in the posterior superior mediastinum.[33,34,39]

A less commonly encountered location for ectopic parathyroid gland is within the thyroid gland. Intrathyroidal parathyroid glands have been described to occur at an incidence ranging from 3% to 10% in various clinical series.[29,40] When found in this location, they occur most likely as a result of failure of the superior gland to separate from the thyroid primordium during embryonic development. Another uncommon ectopic entity is the undescended superior parathyroid gland, noted previously and described by Simeone et al.[37] These investigators identified only five undescended superior glands in more than 3,000 patients undergoing exploration, or 0.08%. This ectopic location is defined as being at least 1.0 cm cephalad to the upper limit of the superior thyroid pole, within or in close approximation to the pharyngeal wall. As would be expected, and in

contradistinction to undescended inferior glands, thymic tissue is uncommonly associated with undescended superior parathyroid glands. Finally, distinctly uncommon ectopic locations where parathyroid glands have been described include: carotid sheath, submandibular triangle, floor of mouth and aortopulmonary window.

## Operative Strategy

Following the decision to proceed with re-exploration and having performed a review of the initial operative procedure, and localization studies, the surgeon then considers the operative approach. Ideally, the objective is to remove a single gland without extensive dissection, which may result in injury to the surrounding structures, ie, recurrent laryngeal nerve or devascularization of remaining parathyroid tissue. The likelihood of accomplishing this objective is very dependent upon two factors: the experience of the initial operating surgeon and the demonstration of an enlarged parathyroid gland on correlative localization studies.

In most cases, re-operation following initial surgery by an experienced surgeon will be difficult and tedious because the initial dissection will have been comprehensive and the surgical bed will have significant fibrosis. In contradistinction, the extensiveness of initial exploration, and resulting degree of fibrosis, may be significantly less in patients having had the original surgery performed by a relatively inexperienced surgeon. In both of these circumstances, the localizing studies will be of prime importance in targeting the putative hyperfunctional gland and limiting the re-operative dissection.

The best of all scenarios, and the most common, is unequivocal localization to a cervical site, which may also include the anterior superior mediastinum. The previous neck incision is generally used for access, in some cases by excising the old scar completely. The usual superior/inferior flaps are raised and access is gained to the side of the neck indicated by the localization studies. A lateral to medial approach to dissection is undertaken, in order to avoid the dense scarification and fibrosis in the region of the tracheoesophageal groove where the recurrent laryngeal nerve resides. In this manner, dissection proceeds medially from the sternomastoid muscle superficial to the great vessels and then directly to the region overlying the cervical spine. This approach exploits the concept of the viscerovertebral angle (VVA) as described by Tenta.[41] This potential anatomic space is defined as that area bordered laterally by the carotid sheath structures, medially by the trachea and esophagus, anteriorly by the thyroid and posteriorly by the cervical spine (Figure 30–3). In

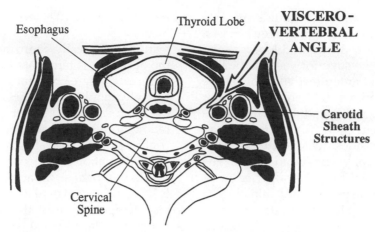

**Figure 38–3.** The viscero-vertebral angle (VVA) illustrated in coronal projections.

accessing this region, the surgeon may take advantage of a tissue plane with relatively little vascularity and fibrosis. This area will allow extension to examine the superior mediastinum inferiorly, the retroesophageal compartment medially and as far superior as the hyoid bone, all within planes of dissection that separate with relative freedom. Although not necessary in most cases, the recurrent laryngeal nerve may be identified and extensively exposed for protection by following this approach, as dense fibrosis is infrequently encountered over the prevertebral space, even following a thorough initial exploration. In the event a gland is suspected in the superior retrothyroidal area, the nerve should be identified as it may be lateral to a medially displaced superior gland. The majority of missed adenomas, which are accessible through a cervical incision, may be approached using this technique, which also allows for thyroid lobectomy, should an intra-thyroidal gland be suspected. A situation whereby localization studies indicate a mediastinal location usually mandates a thoracic approach, either by median sternotomy or lateral thoracotomy, depending on the location within the mediastinum. An enlarged gland identified within the anterior mediastinum is usually associated with the thymus, and may be accessed by median sternotomy. These glands are usually found at the level of the innominate vein within thymic tissue but may also be found adjacent to the aortic arch or between the thymus and pleura. Should the localizing studies demonstrate a posterior based mediastinal gland, a lateral or posterolateral thoracotomy should be strongly considered in order to avoid attempts at dissection through critical structures in the anterior mediastinum. These posterior glands may reside in the aorto-pulmonary window or the retroesophageal region. One should be aware that the recurrent laryngeal nerve may be injured when approaching the posterior mediastinum through a left lateral thoracotomy. Despite what may be interpreted as compelling localization results, the surgeon should be prepared to perform concurrent cervical exploration in the event that initial operative PTH levels (IOPTH) do not confirm removal of all hyperfunctional parathyroid tissue.

The most problematic preoperative scenario to confront is that in which localization fails to identify any suspicious site. It is in this situation where re-operative surgery for hyperparathyroidism is potentially the least successful and the most morbid. Failure to localize usually mandates a bilateral cervical exploration which comprehensively and methodically addresses all potential sites which may harbor a missing gland or glands. A properly constructed initial operative note which accurately documents remaining histologically identified parathyroid glands and regions explored is of utmost importance and potential value for the re-operative surgeon. An orderly systematic approach to re-exploration is necessary in these circumstances in order to locate the missing gland(s) and limit morbidity. The order in which regions are approached may vary according to the surgeon; however, it is important that all potential areas be accessed in order to increase the chance of success and avoid a failed re-exploration. Our preference is to approach each side explored through the viscero-vertebral angle via a lateral to medial orientation. We then address regions in the following manner: the anterior superior mediastinum is dissected first, with careful attention to the thyrothymic ligament and tracheoesophageal groove region adjacent to the recurrent nerve. Cervical thymectomy, if not performed during initial surgery, is completed at this time. Dissection then turns to the retropharyngeal, retroesophageal region where blunt dissection within the prevertebral space will allow for digital exploration superiorly above the cricoid larynx and inferiorly into the posterior mediastinum. Enlarged glands in this anatomic plane may often be felt before they are seen using these techniques. Next, the thyroid lobe is mobilized, possibly truncating the superior vascular pedicle in order to rotate the gland anteromedially so that the posterior thyroid capsule may be closely examined for a folded, lobulated parathyroid gland under the capsular fascia. Using this maneuver, the thyroid lobe is palpated for any nodular densities, which may be suspicious for an intra-thyroidal parathyroid gland. The carotid sheath is then opened from the superior mediastinum to the hyoid bone, inspecting and palpating for nodular structures within the sheath. Failing identification on the side explored first, the dissection proceeds contralaterally in the same manner, with orderly inspection of all regions noted above. In the event that a bilateral exploration fails to identify the offending gland, thyroid lobectomy is usually performed on the side suspected of harboring the missing gland. During these exercises it is important to document carefully all normal parathyroid tissue found, or in the instance that glands are not identified, the putative missing parathyroid gland by position.

If all maneuvers previously described are unsuccessful in identifying the missing gland, the procedure is terminated and further measures are undertaken to identify the gland's position by imaging and possibly angio-invasive studies. Mediastinal exploration should not be performed in this sitting, predominantly because of the lack of localization and the element of time involved with the unsuccessful bilateral cervical exploration just completed.

## Intra-operative Assessment of Parathyroid Hormone (IOPTH)

IOPTH represents a useful surgical adjunct in the performance of re-operative parathyroid exploration, both for single and multiple gland disease. The usefulness of biochemically confirming the removal of hyperfunctional parathyroid tissue by applying IOPTH becomes apparent when one considers the previous operative procedure(s) performed by the initial surgeon with respect to what was identified/removed and whether normal glands were identified and histo-pathologically confirmed. For example, if at initial operation a single adenoma was removed without biopsy or identification of normal parathyroid tissue, the surgeon performing re-exploration is faced with the prospect of identifying all three remaining glands in order to eliminate the existence of multigland disease—independent of what the preoperative localization study indicates. The utilization of IOPTH, however, allows the surgeon to identify the putative missing gland and determine the effect re-

moval has on the PTH level intra-operatively. If a decrement of 50–70% is achieved following removal of a histopathologically confirmed abnormal gland, then the operation is terminated without further identification or biopsy of normal parathyroid glands. Alternatively, should the IOPTH determination not achieve the minimum of 50% decrement required, the exploration proceeds until all abnormal glands are identified, confirmed pathologically and removed with biochemical confirmation provided by repeat IOPTH.

In this manner, the application of IOPTH potentially limits the extent of re-exploration required in the previously operated neck, thereby limiting the possibility of injury to the recurrent laryngeal nerve and iatrogenic hypoparathyroidism caused by manipulation/biopsy of normal glands. In addition, the utilization of IOPTH in re-operative procedures for multigland disease provides a level of confidence that a sufficient amount of hyperfunctional parathyroid tissue has been removed while leaving behind a functional remnant for achievement of normocalcemia. Ultimately the use of IOPTH in all parathyroid explorations provides a measure of biochemical confidence that will serve to limit the extent of operation and reduce re-operative morbidity.

## Mediastinal Exploration

Re-exploration for parathyroid disease may require exploration of the mediastinum. Ectopic parathyroid glands located within the mediastinum and below the level of the thymus account for a small percentage (0.2%) of all abnormally located glands.[42] In contrast, both Wang and Norton have shown that a more substantial proporation, 18 and 20% respectively, of ectopically located adenomas reside in the mediastinum accessible only through a mediastinal approach.[32,35] These inferior parathyroid glands are associated in almost all circumstances with the thymus with which they descend during embryonic development, having arisen with the thymus as a third pharyngeal pouch derivative.

Several approaches to the mediastinum are available for re-exploration. The choice of approach utilized is dependent on the location of the putative adenoma. Localization studies which, in combination, corroborate and specify the mediastinal location are required prior to undertaking exploration. In the author's experience, Tc-99m-sestamibi imaging together with magnetic resonance (MRI) represents the optimal combination of physiologic and anatomic-based imaging for localization (Figure 34–4A & B). The techniques available for approaching the mediastinum include: transcervical substernal with thymectomy using anterior retraction of the sternum for superior mediastinal glands; median sternotomy with direct approach to the anterior middle

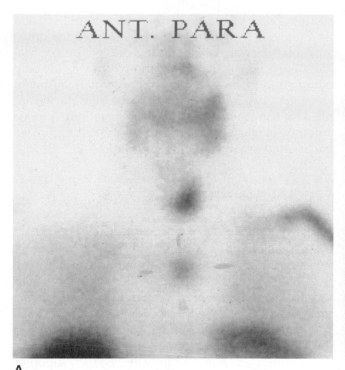

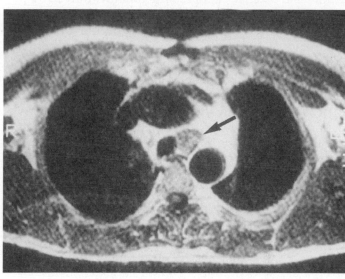

**A**                                    **B**

**Figure 38–4.** Correlative Tc-99m-sestamibi (A) and magnetic resonance (B) imaging from a patient with mediastinal parathyroid adenoma and persistent hyperparathyroidism. MRI demonstrates adenoma localized to aorto-pulmonary window (see arrow).

and caudal mediastinal compartments; posterolateral thoracotomy with selective posteriorly based glands in the lower mediastinal compartment; and endoscopic, minimally invasive mediastinal dissection for selectively focused exploration. The majority of glands will be approached via a median sternotomy, owing to this technique's capability to safely address a number of areas within the mediastinum as well as the lower cervical region immediately posterior to the clavicular heads and manubrium. This technique also allows uninterrupted visualization of both recurrent laryngeal nerves, thus preventing inadvertent injury to these structures within the mediastinum.

Surgical adjuncts which may aid in the intra-operative localization of adenomas, and which may be employed following median sternotomy, include intra-operative ultrasound (IOUS) and gamma probe following preoperative sestamibi injection.

## Gamma Probe

Minimally invasive cervical exploration utilizing a gamma radiation detection device (gamma probe) has been developed and advocated by Norman and associates in order to accurately facilitate and expedite initial surgery for parathyroid adenoma.[43] The methodology exploits both the nuclear uptake characteristics of

parathyroid adenoma with respect to Tc-99m-sestamibi, and the ability of the gamma probe to intra-operatively localize these glands in the neck following preoperative sestamibi injection.

We have found it to be most useful in identifying abnormal parathyroid tissue in the previously operated neck, whereby its application in selected instances allows for accurate, targeted dissection with minimal disturbance of surrounding structures. Norman and Denham have published their experience with minimally invasive radio-guided parathyroidectomy (MIRP) in the previously operated neck.[4] In this series of 24 previously operated patients, of whom 21 localized sufficiently to undergo MIRP, all 21 were re-operated with the gamma probe and were rendered normocalcemic postoperatively without complications.

The technique, as described by Norman, involves initial sestamibi scanning preoperatively to determine suitability for MIRP. The initial scan provides information regarding localization of putative adenomas as well as the presence of delayed uptake of nuclear material within the thyroid gland. Should excessive delayed activity be present in the thyroid, the patient is subjected to thyroid suppression for 6–8 weeks prior to re-operation in order to reduce background radiation in the thyroid bed and increase the accuracy of the probe. Correlative imaging using MRI, CT, or US may be combined with the initial sestamibi scan according to site localized and surgeon preference. The author prefers MRI in combination with sestamibi to accurately localize to either cervical or mediastinal regions. On the day of operation, patients are then injected with Tc-99m-sestamibi and taken to the operating room within 1.5 to 2.5 hours following injection and exploration performed utilizing the gamma probe. Following identification and removal of the adenoma, the gland is checked for degree of radioactivity ex vivo against background tissues in the surgical bed. Based on previous reported data, excised glandular tissue emitting radiation greater than 20% of that found in tissues in the surgical bed was confirmed as the hyperfunctional parathyroid tissue implicated in disease.[45]

The author (PKP) has applied this technique in mediastinal exploration following sternotomy with satisfactory results (Figure 38–5). Despite uptake of sestamibi by myocardial tissue, background radioactivity within the mediastinum appears to be less than that of thyroid tissue, thus facilitating a focused dissection with minimal disturbance of surrounding mediastinal structures. Re-operation for multiple gland disease in secondary and tertiary hyperparathyroidism has been aided with the use of the gamma probe, when supernumerary glands are present. In one instance, the author recovered three additional parathyroid glands (2 cervical, 1 mediastinal) in a patient with tertiary hyperparathyroidism who previously underwent document-

ed four gland parathyroidectomy during preparation for cadaveric renal transplantation. The gamma probe was instrumental in identifying one of the cervical glands and one mediastinal gland which was the only parathyroid gland that localized accurately on initial sestamibi imaging. The gamma probe may also be applied for removal of hyperfunctional parathyroid tissue autotransplanted to the forearm in the setting of secondary/tertiary hyperparathyroidism.

## SPECIAL SITUATIONS

### Secondary/Tertiary Hyperparathyroidism

Recurrent/persistent hyperparathyroidism following total or subtotal parathyroidectomy in patients with secondary/tertiary hyperparathyroidism represents a unique challenge to the surgeon. Problems with persistent disease usually result from inadequate resection following subtotal parathyroidectomy in which three or fewer glands are removed initially or when supernumerary gland(s) are not recognized during four gland parathyroidectomy. Recurrent parathyroidism usually results from delayed hyperplasia developing in cervical parathyroid remnants or within autotransplanted tissue placed during initial surgery. To a large extent, the incidence of persistent disease may be reduced by the application of IOPTH following removal of all four parathyroid glands, although the absolute trough level of serum PTH will often remain elevated above laboratory normal.

Persistent disease is more common than recurrent and is defined as a persistence or recurrence of preoperative symptoms, laboratory abnormalities and radiologic findings within six months of initial surgery.[45] Recurrence of these findings outside of six months following initial exploration is generally classified as recurrent disease and is less commonly found, especially after total parathyroidectomy.

The presence of persistent/recurrent disease is usually established by the nephrologists during dialysis therapy or as a finding during routine follow-up in patients who received a transplant and are undergoing immunosuppressive therapy. In the authors' experience, it is the nephrologist who usually recommends repeat surgical intervention, predominantly based on symptoms (bone pain, intractable pruritis, soft tissue calcification, calciphylaxis) or as a preparation for renal transplantation.

The surgical evaluation for patients recommended for re-exploration includes Tc-99m-sestamibi imaging and the determination of the serum PTH gradient in the graft-bearing arm as compared to the contralateral arm in patients who also received autotransplantation

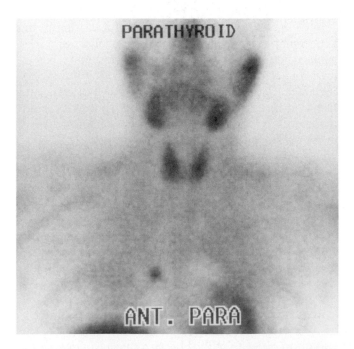

**Figure 38–5.** Tc-99m-sestamibi imaging showing mediastinal parathyroid which represented a fifth hyperplastic gland missed at initial surgery at which time four glands were removed.

initially. A gradient reflective of hyperfunctional graft tissue is defined as a 100% increase in the graft versus contralateral sample.[18] Unlike that of primary hyperparathyroidism caused by four-gland hyperplasia, it has been the author's experience that in most instances, sestamibi scanning will successfully localize remaining hyperfunctional parathyroid tissue in patients with secondary/tertiary hyperparathyroidism (Figure 38–6). This experience has been shared by others where reported accurate localization prior to re-operation for secondary hyperparathyroidism ranges from 100% to 69%.[5,22,46,47] As in all instances of re-operative surgery, the technique calls for meticulous hemostatic dissection and attention to surrounding structures, in particular, the recurrent laryngeal nerves. Gamma probe aided dissection facilitates both the cervical and mediastinal exploration in selected patients where significant postoperative fibrosis exists or where extensive dissection within the mediastinum should be avoided. The determination of PTH gradient will, in most instances, determine the need for graft removal, gradient greater than two indicating parathyroid graft hyperfunction, less than two indicating hyperfunctional gland in the neck. Uncommonly, sestamibi imaging may localize to hyperfunctional graft tissue as has been the finding in one of our patients.

Re-operation for persistent/recurrent secondary/tertiary hyperparathyroidism is associated with increased morbidity and may be minimized by initial total parathyroidectomy.[48] Re-exploration is facilitated by accurate localization using a combination of imaging studies, the utilization of IOPTH and the use of the gamma probe in selected patients.

## Parathyroid Carcinoma

The incidence of parathyroid carcinoma is quite low, occurring in less than 1% of all patients with hyperparathyroidism.[49] The ultimate prognosis of patients surgically managed for this disease depends, to a large extent, on the ability to resect all tumor at the initial operation. The recognition of parathyroid cancer at initial surgery is not always obvious, and in many cases the diagnosis is confirmed in the postoperative period precluding en bloc resection of adjacent structures. It is in this setting that local recurrence of disease is likely and re-operation may be required.

The recurrence of disease is usually heralded by recurrent hypercalcemia. Preoperative assessment should include a localization study, preferably Tc-99m-sestamibi, which may also be utilized in conjunction intraoperatively with the gamma probe (Figure 38–7).[50] Mediastinal localization indicated by nuclear imaging should be corroborated by MRI or CT so that an appropriate surgical approach may be planned. The presence

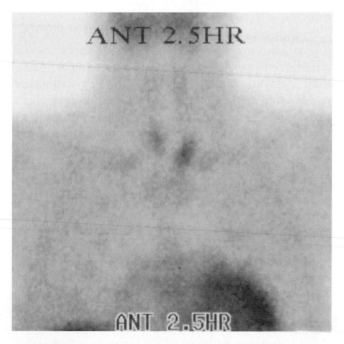

**Figure 38–6.** Tc-99m-sestamibi image demonstrating bilateral hyperplastic parathyroid glands in a patient with recurrent secondary hyperparathyroidism 10 years following initial subtotal parathyroidectomy.

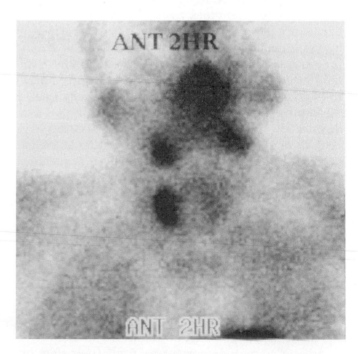

**Figure 38–7.** Tc-99m-sestamibi image demonstrating intense delayed nuclear uptake in the right paratracheal region in a patient previously operated for parathyroid carcinoma.

of regional nodal and distant (pulmonary, osseous) metastasis should be ruled out prior to contemplating re-operation. As recurrent disease occurs earliest and most often at the site of original presentation, most recurrent tumors will present low in the neck at the cervico-thoracic junction. It has been our experience that when tumor recurs in this location, a combined transcervical, trans-mediastinal approach via median sternotomy is utilized to facilitate wide en bloc resection and prevent catastrophic injury to critical vascular structures in the mediastinum. Surgery for recurrent parathyroid carcinoma is difficult and is associated with a high likelihood of recurrent laryngeal nerve injury.[51] If en bloc resection is not carried out at initial operation, every attempt should be made to do so at re-operation so as to maximize the chance of achieving normocalcemia. A central compartment and superior mediastinal lymph node dissection should be performed in conjunction with the resection. If not already accomplished at initial surgery, ipsilateral thyroid lobectomy and isthmusectomy should proceed en bloc at re-operation. Curative resection is no longer possible with the development of pulmonary or other distant metastatic foci, but may be of benefit in selected patients for palliation to control pain and hypercalcemia.[52,53]

## Autotransplantation/Cryopreservation

Parathyroid autotransplantation, or "autografting" of fresh parathyroid tissue into the forearm following removal of all parathyroid tissue, has been heavily utilized since the mid 1970s for prevention of permanent hypocalcemia following total parathyroidectomy.[54] The procedure is employed most commonly following initial surgery for secondary/tertiary hyperparathyroidism and primary hyperparathyroidism caused by the multiple endocrine neoplasia (MEN) type I syndrome. The technical aspects of the procedure have been thoroughly described in the literature as well as in Chapter 39 of this text.[55] Traditionally, the brachioradialis muscle of the non-dominant arm or that upper extremity without a hemodialysis access port represented the recipient site for the autograft. An investigation by Chou has demonstrated the potential for transplantation into the subcutaneous tissue of the arm with viability and recovery of functioning graft tissue comparable to that of muscle implantation.[56] Parathyroid autotransplantation enjoys a 90–95% success rate as defined by sustained normocalcemia without Vitamin D supplementation.[57-59]

A further application of autotransplantation is as an adjunct to re-operation for recurrent/persistent hyperparathyroidism where all functional parathyroid tissue has been removed. This may not be clearly apparent to the surgeon based upon a review of the initial procedure combined with the re-operative findings. The surgeon performing re-exploration must be prepared to autotransplant viable parathyroid tissue in the event that total removal of all glandular tissue is removed as a consequence of all operations performed. In any case, immediate autotransplantation is recommended for patients in whom a total of four glands have been removed for hyperplasia at both surgical procedures, initial and current.

The indications for autotransplantation in re-exploration for missed single gland disease are less clear, as the number of viable normal parathyroid glands remaining following initial exploration may be in question. It is in this setting that the authors have found utilization of IOPTH to be of great benefit. Following successful localization and directed removal of an adenoma during re-operation, the level of PTH determined after removal will guide the need for autotransplantation, as it will serve as an indicator of viability with respect to remaining normal glands. (*Note:* The resected adenoma should be kept in sterile iced saline until PTH level is reported.)

We generally use a post-removal PTH level of less than 10 pg/ml as an indication for autotransplantation using tissue from the resected adenoma. This methodology has proven sound in our experience but does carry with it a small chance of recurrent hyperfunction from the autograft.

Alternatively, cryopreservation of parathyroid tissue removal may be used in a delayed fashion should long-term hypocalcemia develop following re-operation. Delayed autotransplantation of cryopreserved parathyroid tissue restores hypocalcemia in approximately 50% of patients autografted and is less reliable in achieving normal parathyroid function than is immediate autografting.[60] Cryopreserved tissue may be used to supplement autotransplantation should the graft "viability" be in question following the postoperative interval necessary to achieve normocalcemia (12 weeks). We recommend autotransplantation and cryopreservation of parathyroid tissue in all patients undergoing either initial or repeat surgery for hyperparathyroidism caused by diffuse hyperplasia (MEN I, secondary/tertiary). In addition, cryopreservation may be performed in patients undergoing subtotal (3½ glands) parathyroidectomy for sporadic hyperplasia in order to supplement the remnant in delayed fashion.

During any re-operative procedure, all parathyroid tissue removed should be kept in sterile iced saline until the surgeon is satisfied that all hyperfunctional tissue has been removed and a decision has been made as to the necessity for autotransplantation/cryopreservation. The only absolute contraindication to autotransplantation of parathyroid tissue is in the surgical management of parathyroid carcinoma.

## UNSUCCESSFUL RE-EXPLORATION

The unsuccessful re-exploration for recurrent hyperparathyroidism is the most discouraging experience encountered by the endocrine surgeon. Fortunately, in experienced hands, this is an uncommon (<5%) situation resulting primarily from ectopic or supernumerary glands residing within the mediastinum which have not imaged accurately. When confronted with this situation, the entire preoperative evaluation process must be repeated, including: confirming the diagnosis of hyperparathyroidism; determining the need for surgical treatment based on biochemical criteria or symptoms; determining the optimum localization scheme and planning the surgical approach. Thorough communication between endocrinologist, surgeon and patient is necessary in order that all parties understand the indications for treatment and agree to pursue further medical or surgical therapy or conservative observation.

Consideration for medical therapy should be weighed in relation to the patient's symptom complex, age and overall medical condition/health status. If further surgical therapy is recommended, every effort should be made to confirm the location of the missing gland(s). Failing accurate localization with non-invasive imaging, invasive studies may be used to identify a side or region (cervical/mediastinal) harboring the putative gland(s). Selective arteriography may be useful in identifying an ectopic mediastinal parathyroid gland, though the sensitivity is low (60%).[22] For glands which localize accurately on arteriography, selective ablation may be carried out with potential long-term control of hyperparathyroidism.[61] Another invasive study which may prove useful is selective venous sampling of PTH concentrations. This method is costly and not without some risk but may prove valuable in patients for whom

all localization studies have failed and surgery is required. Selective venous sampling provides regional localization of abnormal parathyroid glands by establishing a PTH gradient across selected veins draining various regions of the neck and mediastinum. Large differences in PTH concentration between veins sampled establish a gradient by which a region drained by the vein at the apex of the gradient is that which is felt to harbor the missing gland. A large series of patients who underwent selective venous sampling for parathyroid localization has been reported by the NCI, and discussed previously in this chapter.[25] These investigators concluded that in the subgroup of patients who fail standard non-invasive localization studies, selective venous sampling of PTH represents the study of choice in directing re-operative procedures for ectopic hyperfunctional parathyroid glands.

Medical management for patients in whom re-operation has failed generally consists of temporary control of hypercalcemia through hydration, use of loop diuretics and a limited group of medications including bisphosphonates, calcitonin and plicamycin. The calcimimetic agent R568, currently under investigation, may offer a therapeutic alternative to re-operation in selected patients and those with parathyroid carcinoma.[62] Larger clinical trails will be required to further delineate the role of calcimimetic agents in the management of hyperparathyroidism. A full discussion on the medical management of hypercalcemia can be found in Chapter 42.

## SUMMARY

Management of recurrent hyperparathyroidism represents a unique therapeutic challenge. Opportunity for success and potential morbidity incurred as a result of re-operation differ significantly when compared with initial surgery. The utilization of surgical adjuncts such as invasive/non-invasive localization studies, IOPTH and the gamma probe offer benefit in the management of patients with recurrent hyperparathyroidism. Our management protocol is summarized in the treatment algorithm illustrated in Figure 38–8.

ALGORITHM—RE-EXPLORATION

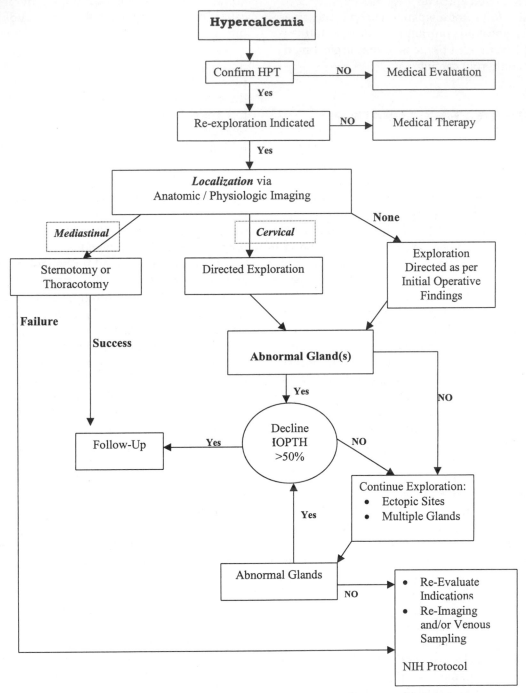

**Figure 38–8.** Management algorithm for recurrent/persistent hyperparathyroidism. IOPTH = Intra-operative Parathyroid Hormone.

# References

1. Wang C. Surgical management of primary hyperparathyroidism. *Curr Probl Surg.* 1985;22:4–50.

2. ReMine SG. Management of recurrent or persistent hyperparathyroidism. *Probl Gen Surg.* 1985;2:440–449.

3. Shen W, Duren M, Morita E, et al. Re-operation for persistent or recurrent primary hyperparathyroidism. *Arch Surg.* 1996;131:861–869.

4. Norman J, Denham D. Minimally invasive radio-guided parathyroidectomy in the re-operative neck. *Surgery.* 1998;124:1088–1093.

5. Peeler BB, Martin WH, Sandler MP, Goldstein RE. Sestamibi parathyroid scanning and preoperative localization studies for

patients with recurrent/persistent hyperparathyroidism or significant co-morbid conditions: development of an optimal localization strategy. *Am Surg.* 1997;63:37–46.

6. Haff RC, Ballinger WF. Causes of recurrent hypercalcemia after parathyroidectomy for primary hyperparathyroidism. *Ann Surg.* 1971;173:884–891.

7. Clark OH, Way LW, Hunt TK. Recurrent hyperparathyroidism. *Ann Surg.* 1976;184:391–399.

8. Martin JK, van Heerden JA, Edis AJ, et al. Persistent postoperative hyperparathyroidism. *Surg Gynecol Obstetr.* 1980;151:764–768.

9. Jaskowiak N, Norton JA, Alexander HR, et al. A prospective trial evaluating a standard approach to re-operation for missed parathyroid adenoma. *Ann Surg.* 1996;224:308–322.

10. Lang JR, Norton JA. Surgery for persistent or recurrent hyperparathyroidism. *Curr Pract Surg.* 1992;4:56–62.

11. Levin KE, Clark OH. The reasons for failure in parathyroid operations. *Arch Surg.* 1989;124:911–915.

12. Bruining HA, Birkenhager JC, Ong GL, Lamberts WJ. Causes of failure in operations for hyperparathyroidism. *Surgery.* 1987;101:562–565.

13. Katz AD, Formichella D. Fifty-three re-operations for hyperparathyroidism. *Am J Surg.* 1989;158:385–387.

14. Cohn KH, Silen W. Lessons of parathyroid operations. *Am J Surg.* 1982;144:511–517.

15. LiVolsi VA, Hamilton R. Intraoperative assessment of parathyroid gland pathology *Am J Clin Pathol.* 1993;102:365–373.

16. Thompson GB, Grant CS, Perrier ND, et al. Re-operative parathyroid surgery in the era of sestamibi scanning and intraoperative parathyroid hormone monitoring. *Arch Surg.* 199;134:699–705.

17. Akerstrom G, Rudberg C, Grimelius L, et al. Causes of failed primary exploration and technical aspects of re-operation in primary hyperparathyroidism. *World J Surg.* 1992;16:562–569.

18. Rotstein L, Irish J, Gullane P, Keller MA, Sniderman K. Re-operative parathyroidectomy in the era of localization technology. *Head Neck.* 1998;20:535–539.

19. Cattan P, Halimi B, Aidan K, et al. Re-operation for secondary uremic hyperparathyroidism: are technical difficulties influenced by initial surgical procedure? *Surgery.* 2000;127:562–565.

20. Auguste LJ, Attie JN. Initial failure of surgical exploration in patients with primary hyperparathyroidism. *Am J Surg.* 1990;160:333–336.

21. Fraker DL, Doppman JL, Shawker TH, et al. Undescended parathyroid adenoma: an important etiology for failed operations for primary hyperparathyroidism. *World J Surg.* 1990;14:342–348.

22. Rodriguez JM, Tezelman S, Siperstein AE, et al. Localization procedures in patients with persistent or recurrent hyperparathyroidism. *Arch Surg.* 1994;129:870–875.

23. Kebebew E, Arici C, Duh QY, Clark OH. Localization and re-operation results for persistent and recurrent parathyroid carcinoma. *Arch Surg.* 2001;136:878–885.

24. Rossi HL, Ali A, Prinz RA. Intraoperative sestamibi scanning in re-operative parathyroidectomy. *Surgery.* 2000;128:744–750.

25. Sugg SL, Fraker DL, Alexander R, et al. Prospective evaluation of selective venous sampling for parathyroid hormone concentration in patients undergoing re-operations for primary hyperparathyroidism. *Surgery.* 1993;114:1004–1010.

26. Edis AJ, Sheedy PF II, Beahrs OH, van Heerden JA. Results of re-operation for hyperparathyroidism with evaluation of preoperative localization studies. *Surgery.* 1978;84:384–393.

27. Cheung PSY, Borgstrom A, Thompson NW. Strategy in re-operative surgery for hyperparathyroidism. *Arch Surg.* 1989;124:676–680.

28. Doherty GM, Doppman JL, Miller DL, et al. Results of a multidisciplinary strategy for management of mediastinal parathyroid adenoma as a cause of persistent primary hyperparathyroidism. *Ann Surg.* 1992;215:101–106.

29. Feingold DL, Alexander HR, Chen CC, et al. Ultrasound and sestamibi scan as the only preoperative imaging tests in re-operation for parathyroid adenomas. *Surgery.* 2000;128:1103–1110.

30. Patow C, Norton J, Brennan M. Vocal cord paralysis and re-operative parathyroidectomy: a prospective study. *Ann Surg.* 1986;203:282–285.

31. Brennan M, Marx S, Doppman J, et al. Results of re-operation for persistent and recurrent hyperparathyroidism. *Ann Surg.* 1981;194:671–676.

32. Clark O. Mediastinal parathyroid tumors. *Arch Surg.* 1988;123:1096–1100.

33. Wang CA. Parathyroid re-exploration: a clinical and pathological study of 112 cases. *Ann Surg.* 1977;186:140–145.

34. Norton J, Schneider P, Brennan M. Median sternotomy in re-operations for primary hyperparathyroidism. *World J Surg.* 1985;9:807–813.

35. Norton J. Re-operation for missed parathyroid adenoma. *Ad Surg.* 1997;31:273–297.

36. Billingsley K, Fraker D, Doppman J, et al. Localization and operative management of undescended parathyroid adenomas in patients with persistent primary hyperparathyroidism. *Surgery.* 1994;116:982–990.

37. Simeone D, Sandelin K, Thompson N. Undescended superior parathyroid gland: a potential cause of failed cervical exploration for hyperparathyroidism. *Surgery.* 1995;118:949–956.

38. Edis A, Purnell D, Van Heerden J. The undescended "parathymus." An occasional cause of failed neck exploration for hyperparathyroidism. *Ann Surg.* 1979;190:64–68.

39. Carty S, Norton J. Management of patients with persistent or recurrent primary hyperparathyroidism. *World J Surg.* 1991;15:716–723.

40. Wang CA. Hyperfunctioning intrathyroid glands: a potential cause of failure in parathyroid surgery. *JR Soc Med.* 1981;74:49–53.

41. Tenta LT, Keyes GR. Transcervical parathyroidectomy microsurgical autotransplantation and viscerovertebral arm. *Otolaryngol Clin North Am.* 1980;13:169–179.

42. Gilmour JR. The gross anatomy of the parathyroid glands. *J Pathol.* 1938;46:133–149.

43. Norman J, Citheda H. Minimally invasive parathyroidectomy facilitated by intraoperative nuclear mapping. *Surgery.* 1997;122:998–1004.

44. Norman J. The technique of intraoperative nuclear mapping to facilitate minimally invasive parathyroidectomy. *Cancer Control.* 1997;4:500–504.

45. Brennan M, Doppman J, Marx S, et al. Re-operative parathyroid surgery for persistent hyperparathyroidism. *Surgery.* 1978;83:669–676.

46. Majors J, Burke G, Mansberger A, et al. Technetium Te-99m sestamibi scan for localization of abnormal parathyroid glands after previous neck: preliminary experience in re-operative cases. *South Med J.* 1995; 88:327–330.

47. Weber C, Vansant J, Alazrake N, et al. Value of technetium-99m sestamibi iodine–123 imaging in re-operative parathyroid surgery. *Surgery.* 1993;114:1011–1018.

48. Skinner K, Zuckerbraun L. Recurrent secondary hyperparathyroidism. An argument for total parathyroidectomy. *Arch Surg.* 1996;131:724–727.

49. Shane E. Parathyroid carcinoma. *J Clin Endo Metab.* 2001;86:485–493.

50. Martinez D, King D, Romshe C, et al. Intraoperative identification of parathyroid gland pathology: a new approach. *J Pediatr Surg.* 1995;30:1306–1309.

51. Wang C, Gaz R. Natural history of parathyroid carcinoma: diagnosis, treatment, and results. *Am J Surg.* 1985;149:522–527.

52. Dubost C, Jehanno C, Lavergne A, Carpentier Y. Successful resection of intrathoracic metastases from two patients with parathyroid carcinoma. *World J Surg.* 1984;8:547–551.

53. Koyano H, Shishiba Y, Sitimizu T, et al. Successful treatment by surgical removal of bone metastasis producing PTH: a new approach to the management of metastatic parathyroid carcinoma. *Intern Med*. 1994;33:697–702.
54. Wells S, Gunnells J, Shlebarne J, et al. Transplantation of parathyroid glands in man: clinical indications and results. *Surgery*. 1975;78:34–44.
55. Baumann D, Wells S. Parathyroid autotransplantation. *Surgery*. 1993;113:130–133.
56. Chou F, Chan H, Huang T, et al. Autotransplantation of parathyroid glands into subcutaneous forearm tissue for renal hyperparathyroidism. *Surgery*. 1998;124:1–5.
57. Shaha AR, Burnett C, Jaffe B. Parathyroid autotransplantation during thyroid surgery. *J Surg Oncol*. 1991;46:21–24.
58. Kikamori T, Imai T, Tanaka Y, et al. Parathyroid autotransplantation with total thyroidectomy for thyroid carcinoma: long term follow-up of grafted parathyroid function. *Surgery*. 1999;125:504–508.
59. Olson J, DeBenedetti M, Baumann D, Wells S. Parathyroid autotransplantation during thyroidectomy: results of long term follow-up. *Ann Surg*. 1996;223:472–480.
60. Herrara M, Grant C, Van Herden J, et al. Parathyroid autotransplantation. *Arch Surg*. 1992;127:825–830.
61. Doherty G, Doppman J, Miller D, et al. Results of a multidisciplinary strategy for management of mediastinal parathyroid adenoma as a cause for persistent primary hyperparathyroidism (see comments). *Ann Surg*. 1992;215:101–106.
62. Silverberg S, Bone H, Marriott T, et al. Short-term inhibition of parathyroid hormone secretion by a calcium-receptor agonist in patients with primary hyperparathyroidism. *N Engl J Med*. 1997;227:1506–1510.

# 39

# Cryopreservation and Autotransplantation of Parathyroid Tissue

W. Bradford Carter, M.D.

Bethany B. Tan, M.D.

## INTRODUCTION

Parathyroid autotransplantation, or the implantation of autologous parathyroid tissue into an ectopic site, has been performed routinely since 1975 when Wells et al[1] demonstrated its efficacy in preventing postoperative hypoparathyroidism in humans. Hypoparathyroidism is a dreaded complication of thyroid and parathyroid surgery. Not only may patients develop hypocalcemic tetany, but also long term consequences, include lenticular cataracts, intestinal malabsorption, electrocardiogram changes, and dry skin.[2] Additionally, over replacement of vitamin D and phosphate binders may lead to hypercalcemia, hypercalciuria and exacerbation of nephrolithiasis.[3]

The generally recognized indications for parathyroid autotransplantation include autotransplantation associated with treatment of parathyroid diseases with a total parathyroidectomy, and autotransplantation of devascularized or inadvertently removed parathyroid glands during radical head and neck surgery or total thyroidectomy.[4] Careful operative technique and a thorough understanding of the indications and application of parathyroid autotransplantation are essential to the surgeon performing endocrine surgery of the head and neck.

## ANATOMY

Understanding parathyroid anatomy is essential, not only to preserve the parathyroid blood supply during head and neck surgery, but also to locate and recognize the parathyroid glands for resection in parathyroid disease or for autotransplantation or cryopreservation. Typically, there are a total of four parathyroid glands, although supernumerary glands may be present in 6–15% of the population. Parathyroid glands are yellow to tan in color with an average size of 6 × 5 × 2 mm and an average combined weight of 120 mg.

The upper parathyroid glands are most commonly found at the level of the cricoid cartilage, approximately 1 cm above the junction of the inferior thyroid artery and the recurrent laryngeal nerve, and may be adjacent to the posterior thyroid capsule. Alternatively, upper parathyroid glands may be found within the thyroid, in the tracheo-esophageal groove or retro-esophageal space. The lower parathyroid glands are generally found lateral to the trachea at the lower pole of the thyroid. Their location is more variable and may also include the anterior mediastinum, the carotid sheath or the pharyngeal submucosa. The blood supply to the parathyroid glands is predominantly from the inferior thyroid artery, although there is most commonly a dual supply from the superior thyroid artery. The blood supply is tenuous, making parathyroid function suspect with extensive central compartment dissection or after total thyroidectomy.

## HISTORY

Following the discovery of the parathyroid glands in 1860 by a Swedish medical student, Ivan Sundstrom, the importance of the preservation of parathyroid function has been increasingly appreciated. Gley demonstrated hypocalcemia and fatal tetany in animals after total parathyroidectomy in 1891.[5] Halstead first described parathyroid autotransplantation to relieve postoperative tetany in 1907. In his landmark paper, he described a total of 130 parathyroid grafts in 60 dogs, proving successful transplantation by subsequent excision of the graft, which resulted in recurrence of symptomatic hypocalcemia.[6] Later, Lahey and associates performed the first successful parathyroid autotransplantation in humans in the 1920s.[7] Lahey performed autotransplantation of parathyroid glands inadvertently removed during subtotal thyroidectomy.

Fifty years later, interest in parathyroid autotransplantation was renewed when Wells et al[1] and Hickey and Samaan[8] demonstrated synthesis and secretion of parathyroid hormone from autotransplanted parathyroid tissue in humans. In their 1975 paper, Wells et al[1] reported a series of 29 parathyroid autotransplants and confirmed postoperative function clinically, histologically, and physiologically with a graft survival rate of 93%. These leaders in parathyroid research set the stage for the present, where the incidence of postoperative permanent hypoparathyroidism may be as low as zero to 1% through judicious use of parathyroid autotransplantation.

## INDICATIONS

There are four clinical indications for transplantation of the parathyroid: 1) total parathyroidectomy for treatment of secondary hyperparathyroidism, 2) total parathyroidectomy for treatment of primary parathyroid hyperplasia, 3) re-operative parathyroidectomy for persistent or recurrent hyperparathyroidism, and 4) autotransplantation of devascularized or inadvertently removed normal parathyroid glands during the course of radical head and neck surgery, including thyroidectomy (Table 39–1).[4]

### Secondary Hyperparathyroidism

Secondary hyperparathyroidism (or renal osteodystrophy) is the most common indication for parathyroid autotransplantation. Patients with secondary hyperparathyroidism have end stage renal disease and are on dialysis or have received a renal transplant. The

parathyroid glands develop hyperplasia as a result of abnormal calcium, phosphate and vitamin D metabolism intrinsic to renal disease. Ultimately, the parathyroid may become autonomous, causing tertiary hyperparathyroidism. Dialysis often provides adequate management of the metabolic dysfunction and maintains calcium homeostasis. However, 5–10% of patients become refractory to medical management and develop fractures, bone pain, extra-osseous soft tissue calcification or intractable pruritis, requiring surgical intervention.[4]

Surgically, secondary hyperparathyroidism may be managed with a 3½ gland (subtotal) parathyroidectomy or total parathyroidectomy and parathyroid autotransplantation. Subtotal parathyroidectomy, although more simple technically, has the disadvantage of possible hypoparathyroidism caused by hypofunction of the remaining glandular tissue or loss of remnant tissue caused by tenuous blood supply post-dissection. Persistent hyperparathyroidism may result after a subtotal resection in which a supernumerary gland is missed, or more commonly, if too much parathyroid tissue is left in situ. Although a remnant that approximates 50–75 mg of tissue should function adequately, it is an imprecise attempt to correct abnormal physiology with anatomic resection. Recurrent hyperparathyroidism has been reported to occur in 8–40 % of patients after 3½ gland parathyroidectomy,[9-11] while recurrence following total parathyroidectomy and parathyroid autotransplantation is usually much lower, 0–12%.[9,10,12-18]

## Primary Parathyroid Hyperplasia

Primary parathyroid hyperplasia may be caused by familial hyperparathyroidism, MEN1 or MEN2A, although 90% are sporadic. Essentially all patients with MEN1 have hyperplastic hyperparathyroidism, while this is only present in 25–50% of patients with MEN2A.[4] However, patients with MEN2A all develop medullary thyroid cancer, requiring total thyroidectomy and central node dissection, yet another indication for parathyroid autotransplantation. Although patients with sporadic primary hyperparathyroidism can be treated with a subtotal parathyroidectomy with an acceptable recurrence rate (0–18%),[19-21] these patients have generally an excellent result with autotransplantation. For reasons that are not well understood, recurrent hyperparathy-

**Table 39–1.** Indications for parathyroid autotransplantation

| |
|---|
| Secondary hyperparathyroidism |
| Primary parathyroid hyperplasia |
| Reoperative parathyroid surgery |
| Radical head and neck surgery including thyroidectomy |

roidism is more common after parathyroidectomy for familial hyperparathyroidism compared to sporadic hyperparathyroidism. Familial hyperparathyroidism and the MEN syndromes are therefore best treated by total parathyroidectomy and autotransplantation. All patients with MEN should also receive a cervical thymectomy at initial neck exploration. This procedure decreases the incidence of recurrence by removing the most likely location of supernumerary glands.

## Persistent or Recurrent Hyperparathyroidism

The patient with persistent or recurrent hyperparathyroidism requiring neck re-exploration also benefits from parathyroid autotransplantation. Hyperparathyroid patients who remain hypercalcemic postoperatively are designated to have persistent hyperparathyroidism, while patients who become hypercalcemic after 3–6 months of eucalcemia have recurrent hyperparathyroidism. These patients are at significant risk for morbidity following re-exploration. Postoperative hypocalcemia may be as high as 18–37%[3,19,22-26] and the risk of recurrent laryngeal nerve damage is also increased.

The surgeon given the task of re-exploration should be certain that there is no residual cervical parathyroid tissue prior to autotransplantation. If three glands were previously resected then a fourth gland should immediately be autotransplanted. If the number of prior resected glands is uncertain, parathyroid tissue found on re-exploration can be immediately autotransplanted or can be cryopreserved and subsequently autotransplanted if the patient develops symptomatic hypocalcemia.[4,27] However, restoration of calcium homeostasis is only achieved in ~50% of patients after autotransplantation of cryopreserved parathyroid tissue. Alternately, parathyroid tissue can be maintained in tissue culture with viability up to 7 days. It is yet unclear if autotransplanted tissue from tissue culture will differ from fresh autotransplanted tissue in success of restoration of calcium homeostasis.

## Radical Head and Neck Surgery

Radical neck dissections for head and neck carcinoma[28-29] or for thyroid malignancies[30-37] are an indication for parathyroid autotransplantation. The incidence of hypoparathyroidism following surgery for thyroid carcinoma may range from 3–70%,[27,30,32,36] and permanent hypoparathyroidism after total thyroidectomy has a reported incidence of 2–28%.[36-38] Thompson et al[36] achieved a low 2% incidence of permanent hypocalcemia following total thyroidectomy after a meticulous and time-consuming dissection of parathyroid glands

in situ. Many argue that this painstaking dissection to preserve blood supply to the parathyroid glands may compromise the completeness of thyroidectomy and dissection of the tracheo-esophageal groove in a cancer operation, and many surgeons perform less than a total thyroidectomy, specifically to preserve parathyroid function. An alternative is selective parathyroid autotransplantation during thyroid surgery. This will also result in a very low incidence of permanent postoperative hypocalcemia by autotransplantating every devascularized parathyroid into the ipsilateral sternocleidomastoid during any thyroid surgery. Parathyroid autotransplantation adds little operative time to radical head and neck surgery and thyroidectomy and may significantly reduce the potential morbidity of hypocalcemia.

## CONTRAINDICATIONS

There are no absolute contraindications to parathyroid autotransplantation in the eucalcemic patient except for transplantation of parathyroid carcinoma. Autotransplantation of parathyroid adenoma is a relative contraindication caused by the potential of this tissue for malignant degeneration, and a greater potential for recurrent hyperparathyroidism with adenoma.

## TECHNIQUE OF AUTOTRANSPLANTATION

The classic technique of parathyroid autotransplantation is as described by Wells et al.[1,39] Immediately following excision, the parathyroid tissue is placed in ice cold 4% saline or tissue culture medium and chilled for 30 min. Devascularized normal parathyroid glands should be placed immediately upon recognition in the cold solution. These may remain chilled until the end of the procedure.

Typically, a portion of the parathyroid gland is examined on frozen section to confirm parathyroid origin and to avoid transplantation of adenomatous glands. Lahey first demonstrated the importance of frozen section histologic confirmation in his classic 1926 paper. In an addendum to the paper, he reports that 19 of 25 transplanted specimens suspected to be parathyroid were found to be lymphoid tissue on subsequent histological examination.[7] However, as parathyroid surgery has become more common, some have questioned the necessity of routine parathyroid frozen section identification. Lo and Lam report that they were able to correctly identify parathyroid tissue in 93% of patients, leading them to conclude that routine frozen section is not necessary for experienced endocrine surgeons.[40] Alternately, "touch prep" microscopic evaluation of the putative parathyroid tissue is a fast, reliable method to confirm parathyroid tissue prior to autotransplantation, and is easily performed during the "cool-down" phase of the technique. To perform a "touch prep," the transected face of the putative parathyroid gland is placed onto a glass slide. This leaves a cellular "fingerprint" on the slide, which is air dried, and stained with hematoxylin and eosin. Parathyroid cells are easily recognized, with limited use of resources or time.

After the tissue is cooled, the glands are diced into 1-mm cubes. Ideally, 15–20 slices will provide adequate tissue for autotransplantation. For normal parathyroid tissue autotransplantation, the ultimate level of restored parathyroid hormone is proportional to the number of parathyroid glands reimplanted (Figure 39–1). This is likely caused by the normal tissue possessing limited cellular regeneration. All devascularized parathyroid glands should be reimplanted. The fascia of the ipsilateral sternocleidomastoid muscle is incised and 2–3 tissue cubes are placed within the muscle pocket, which is then closed and marked with a permanent suture (Table 39–2). Alternately, the pectoralis major muscle may be a better transplant site for patients receiving radical or extensive neck dissections, or in patients with prior head and neck irradiation, to ensure an adequate microvessel blood supply for the graft induction of neo-vascularization.

Because of the possibility of required future excision, the non-dominant brachioradialis muscle is the preferred site for autotransplantation in patients with abnormal parathyroid glands after total parathyroidectomy. This site allows monitoring of graft function by measuring parathyroid hormone levels from each antecubital vein. This manuever may prevent the considerable morbidity of a neck re-exploration, while facilitating graft re-exploration and "trimming" in cases of recurrent hyperparathyroidism caused by graft hyperfunction. Albertson et al[14] and Monchik and colleagues[41] demonstrated excellent graft function from parathyroid autotransplantation into subcutaneous tissue. This modification greatly simplifies the parathyroid graft identification and debulking in recurrent hyperparathyroidism (Table 39–3).

An alternative autograft technique for normal, devascularized parathyroid glands is to place the parathyroid tissue in saline suspension following morselation and then inject this suspension into the muscle body of choice.[42,43] Although this technique may be quicker and possibly provide better graft function, it is contraindicated in patients with abnormal parathyroid glands who are at higher risk for recurrent hypercalcemia. Re-exploration for these diffusely disseminated parathyroid cells throughout the implanted muscle would require significant muscle debridement.

A routine cervical thymectomy should be performed in all patients with secondary hyperparathyroidism or familial forms of primary hyperparathyroidism to help prevent recurrence due to supernumerary glands.

## TECHNIQUE OF CRYOPRESERVATION

Diced parathyroid tissue (1 mm³) is placed in a cytoprotective solution of 10% DMSO, 10% autologous serum, and 80% RPMI 1640, with glutamine and peni-

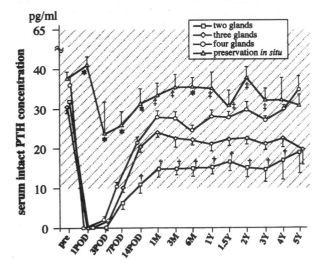

**Figure 39–1.** Profile of serum intact PTH concentrations in patients stratified by number of autotransplanted parathyroid glands. Data represent mean of each group ± SE (2 glands: *open squares*, n = 18; 3 glands: *open diamond*, n = 33; 4 glands: *open circles*, n = 33; preservation in situ: *open triangles*, n = 20). *Asterisk*, P < .01 versus 2, 3, and 4 glands; *dagger*, P < .05 versus 4 glands; *double dagger*, P < .05 versus 2, 3 glands. *Hatched area*, Normal range, POD, Postoperative day. From Kikumori et al, *Surgery.* 1999; 125:506.

**Table 39–2.** Technique of parathyroid autotransplantation

Fresh explanted tissue placed in iced saline

Tissue minced into 1 mm³

2–3 tissue slices placed in subfascial muscle compartment

Muscle pocket closed with non-absorbable suture

15–20 total slices transplanted

**Table 39–3.** Sites for parathyroid autotransplantation

Non-dominant bracioradialis muscle

Sternocleidomastoid muscle

Pectoralis major muscle

Subcutaneous tissue

cillin-streptomycin added.[39,44] Vials are then cooled to -80°C at a rate of 1°C/min and maintained in the vapor phase of liquid nitrogen. Prior to autotransplantation, the cryopreserved tissue is warmed to 37°C in a waterbath and washed three times with 4% Waymouth's medium prior to transplantation (Table 39–4).[39] The viability of dispersed parathyroid cells from cryopreserved parathyroid tissue is excellent (95–100%) as determined by trypan blue exclusion.[44] Functionally, cryopreserved tissue appears to suffer some physiologic derangement, possibly related to cellular processing or cellular expansion. Brennan and colleagues reported that maximal parathyroid hormone release was decreased 10–60%, and clinically only 50–60% of grafts achieve successful restoration of calcium homeostasis. [44]

## SUCCESS OF PARATHYROID AUTOTRANSPLANTATION

Overall, fresh parathyroid autotransplantation is successful in 94–95% of patients when performed by experienced surgeons.[45-49] Traditionally, success of parathyroid autotransplantation has been defined as maintenance of normocalcemia without calcium or vitamin D replacement, although some have monitored serum parathyroid hormone levels. Most studies show lower average values of parathyroid hormone post-autotransplantation, but calcium levels are nearly always in the normal range with few requiring calcium supplementation, and even fewer require vitamin D supplementation (< 1%).

In patients treated with total parathyroidectomy for parathyroid disease, measurement of the intact PTH concentration from bilateral antecubital veins provides the best evaluation of graft function. When comparing PTH levels between grafted and non-grafted areas, a ratio of 1.5:1 or greater is considered functional.[50] Nearly 100% of parathyroid grafts survive ex-

**Table 39–4.** Technique of parathyroid cryopreservation

| |
|---|
| Fresh explanted tissue placed in iced saline |
| Tissue minced into 1 mm³ |
| Tissue placed in cryo solution<br>   10% autologous serum<br>   10% DMSO<br>   80% RPMI 1640 culture media |
| Cooled at 1°C/min to –80°C |
| Stored in vapor phase of liquid nitrogen |

plant and autotransplantation, and ultimately produce parathyroid hormone. However, not all the autotransplants will independently regulate normocalcemia. This may be caused by too few functioning parathyroid cells or changes in the calcium/parathyroid hormone regulatory axis.

## Secondary Hyperparathyroidism

In secondary hyperparathyroidism, these changes can be complicated by the persistent physiologic stimuli of elevated serum phosphorus levels and low vitamin $D_3$. In these patients, the reported incidence of hypocalcemia after total parathyroidectomy and autotransplantation ranges broadly from 0–31%,[9-11,18,51,52] although many of these patients have evidence of parathyroid function. Malmaeus and colleagues reported their incidence of permanent postoperative hypocalcemia was initially 28%, but decreased to one of ten patients following modification of their operative technique.[10] More typically, the reported incidence is 0–8%.[9,11,18,51] The extreme ranges may be caused by technical differences in the quantity of autotransplanted parathyroid tissue or differences in the approach to control or correct the physiologic derangements seen in renal failure patients.

Recurrent secondary hyperparathyroidism is most likely caused by hyperfunction of the autograft or retained parathyroid tissue in the neck. Typically, this can be treated with partial or total excision of the autograft or neck exploration/median sternotomy following localization studies with removal of the remaining cervical parathyroid tissue. There are case reports in the literature of recurrent hyperparathyroidism refractory to these measures, prompting one author to abandon total parathyroidectomy with autotransplantation in renal patients.[17] Success in curing secondary hyperparathyroidism is dependent on complete parathyroidectomy, removing all parathyroid tissue in the neck that can potentially hyperfunction by stimulation of the abnormal physiologic conditions. With careful dissection and a thorough knowledge of parathyroid anatomy and ectopic locations, and routine cervical thymectomy to eliminate potential supernumerary glands, very low recurrence rates are achievable. Recurrence rates of 8–40% are typical for subtotal parathyroidectomy.[9-11] Recurrence following total parathyroidectomy and autotransplantation is usually much lower (0–12%)[9,10,12-18] with fewer recurrences caused by remaining parathyroid disease in the neck.

Although opinions differ, the advantages make total parathyroidectomy and autotransplantation the procedure of choice in secondary hyperparathyroidism.

These advantages include decreased incidence of recurrent hyperparathyroidism with a low incidence of permanent hypocalcemia, and decreased morbidity in the surgical management of recurrence.

## Primary Parathyroid Hyperplasia

The role of autotransplantation in sporadic primary hyperparathyroidism is debated. Recurrence rates after subtotal parathyroidectomy are generally reported to be 0–18%[19-21] with rates of hypocalcemia reported from 1–15%.[19,20,53] Surgeons with few recurrences and few patients with postoperative hypocalcemia recommend subtotal parathyroidectomy, whereas series with lesser results of subtotal parathyroidectomy recommend total parathyroidectomy and autotransplantation.[54] Recurrence after total parathyroidectomy and autotransplantation in primary hyperparathyroidism may be low (0–12%), but hypoparathyroidism has been problematic. Feldman[55] reported that only 35% of autotransplants completely restored homeostasis without any calcium supplementation, with other series ranging from 44–83%.[3,56,57] Again, most of the remaining grafts had serum parathyroid hormone detectable as evidence of graft function, but did not fully restore the calcium/parathyroid hormone axis. Nearly all these studies used 15–20 slices of parathyroid, and the quantity of viable parathyroid cells transplanted may be a significant variable in these reports.

In familial cases of primary hyperparathyroidism, there is a significantly increased rate of recurrence compared to sporadic hyperplastic disease. Malmaeus et al[58] reported that the recurrence of hyperparathyroidism in patients with MEN1 following parathyroidectomy is directly proportional to the number of glands removed. Recurrence was 86% in patients with 1–2½ glands resected, 33% in patients with 3–3½ glands resected, and 0% in patients following total parathyroidectomy and parathyroid autotransplantation.

MEN2 patients require early, total thyroidectomy with central node dissection to treat medullary thyroid carcinoma (MTC). Skinner et al demonstrated the efficacy of routine parathyroid autotransplantation with this procedure in children. Ninety-four percent of 32 patients were eucalcemic with normal parathyroid hormone levels within 3 months of surgery, with one additional child weaned from supplements at 9 months postprocedure.[49]

## Head and Neck Surgery

Normocalcemia may not be an appropriate measure of autograft function in those patients that have both in situ parathyroid and autotransplanted parathyroid tissue, as performed for devascularized normal parathyroid glands in thyroid surgery. The recommended location for these patients is the sternocleidomastoid muscle, where it is not easily monitored by parathyroid hormone gradients. However, the goal is to prevent permanent hypoparathyroidism. If in situ glands are functional postoperatively, serum calcium concentrations will not fall below 8 mg/dl. In these patients, the survival and revascularization is not essential for calcium homeostasis. In patients who have no functional in situ parathyroid glands after head and neck surgery, the risk of permanent hypoparathyroidism is high and the calcium levels will fall precipitously postoperatively. Restoration of calcium homeostasis may be achieved by the parathyroid autotransplant in 6 weeks to 6 months post-procedure. Clearly, some transiently hypofunctioning in situ glands will recover. These patients will show calcium normalization within 3 weeks, a time sequence in which revascularization and restoration of function of an autograft is unlikely. Olson and colleagues[47] reported 54% of 194 patients receiving a total thyroidectomy, with or without a node dissection, had postoperative calcium levels which fell below 8 mg/dl. Ultimately, all but one patient was weaned from vitamin D and calcium supplementation (average of 6–9 weeks). Likely, many of these patients had in situ glands which recovered function, but the overall < 1% rate of hypoparathyroidism significantly improves upon the reported 5–10 % rate of hypoparathyroidism associated with total thyroidectomy. Investigators who routinely use parathyroid autotransplantation for devascularized parathyroids during thyroid surgery report rates of hypoparathyroidism < 6 %, with more recent series near 1%. Shaha et al[45] reported a 0% incidence of permanent hypoparathyroidism after 250 thyroidectomies. Walker et al[59] reported a less than 1% incidence of permanent hypoparathyroidism following this selective autotransplantation strategy in 393 total thyroidectomies.

## RECURRENCE AFTER AUTOTRANSPLANTATION

The determination as to whether residual parathyroid tissue in the neck or hyper-functioning graft is the cause of recurrent hyperparathyroidism is of prime importance (Figure 39–2). The strategy to make this distinction first requires serum parathyroid determination from each antecubital vein. Should hyperfunction of the graft be the cause, a greater than 1.5:1 gradient of parathyroid hormone should be seen between the grafted and non-grafted arms. If the parathyroid hormone

**Recurrent hyperparathyroidism after autotransplantation**

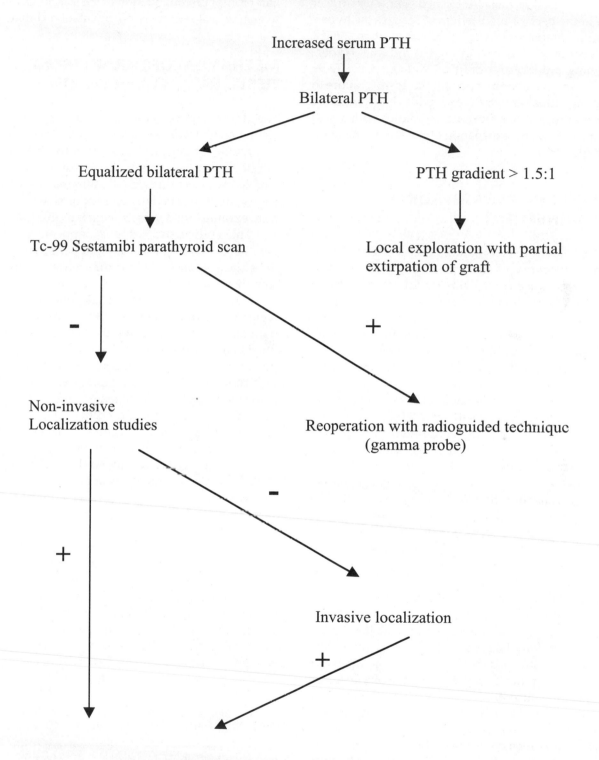

**Figure 39–2.** Decision tree for patients with recurrent hyperparathyroidism after parathyroid autotransplantation.

level is equal, the hyper-functioning tissue resides in the neck or mediastinum. A Technetium-99 Sestamibi parathyroid scan is then performed. Persistent tracer uptake in the neck or mediastinum localizes the hyper-functioning tissue, and facilitates re-exploration using a gamma probe and a radioguided technique. Hyper-functioning parathyroid graft may also uptake Tc-99 Sestamibi and be demonstrated on the scan.[50] Failure to localize the culpable parathyroid with Tc-99 Sestamibi should prompt further localization studies with a goal of re-exploration and extirpation of the remaining parathyroid glands.

## RECOVERY OF PARATHYROID AUTOTRANSPLANT

Several weeks to twelve months may be required for functional recovery of the transplanted parathyroid glands.[60-62] Because transplants do take some time to become functional, hypocalcemia will result during this transplant latency. Traditionally, some surgeons had adopted a policy of not instituting calcium and vitamin D supplementation until patients become symptomatically hypocalcemic. The belief that hypocalcemic stress would facilitate parathyroid graft recovery and enhance the return to calcium homeostasis is probably not valid. Supplementation with vitamin D has been shown not to interfere with engraftment in both nude mice[63] and humans.[64,65] Additionally, we have shown that parathyroid-induced angiogenesis and graft revascularization occurs independently of calcium concentration and parathyroid hormone levels.[66] This evidence supports a policy of routine postoperative calcium and vitamin D replacement during the graft latency period, which can then be progressively weaned over time when evidence of intrinsic parathyroid function and calcium homeostasis is seen.

For patients receiving a total parathyroidectomy and parathyroid autotransplant, our supplementation strategy is to begin oral dihydroxycholecalciferol (vitamin D$_3$) 2.0 μg/day beginning the evening of surgery for 7 days, with subsequent reduction to a maintenance dose of 0.5–1.0 μg/day. After confirmation of a fall in the serum calcium concentration to < 9.0 mg/dl, oral calcium carbonate is started at 2 g/day. Symptomatic hypocalcemic patients are begun on intravenous calcium gluconate. After a bolus of 2 g, the patients are maintained on a constant infusion of 250 mg/day. The infusion is weaned as the patient demonstrates effective oral replacement as determined by stable or rising serum ionized calcium levels, which are monitored every 12 hr. After discharge, the patients are monitored every two weeks to determine the adequacy of oral replacement. Rising calcium levels or adequate parathyroid hormone will prompt discontinuation of the vitamin D$_3$ and subsequently oral calcium supplementation (Table 39–5).

## MECHANISM OF PARATHYROID TISSUE REVASCULARIZATION

The ability of parathyroid tissue to survive autotransplantation and restore calcium homeostasis implies that this tissue revascularizes sufficiently to provide for physiologic necessity as well as restore the calcium/parathyroid hormone axis. Parathyroid tissue induces angiogenesis, or the development of new blood vessels from existing blood vessels (Figure 39–3).

The angiogenic response appears intrinsic to parathyroid tissue in that normal parathyroid cells induce the response, and no differences in angiogenic stimuli are seen between adenomatous and hyperplastic parathyroid tissue.[67] The angiogenic response is not regulated by calcium or parathyroid hormone concentrations.[66] Rather, parathyroid tissue up-regulates production of vascular endothelial growth factor (VEGF) a potent endothelial cell mitogen.[68] Although in vitro and in vivo studies have shown that VEGF can induce an angiogenic response, angiogenesis induced by parathyroid cells exceeds that induced by VEGF alone (Figure 39–4).[68] These findings suggest that other parathyroid produced factors may be involved in regulating angiogenesis with VEGF. Recently, we have shown parathyroid tissue also up-regulates angiopoietin-2, a peptide that mediates endothelial cell activity during angiogenesis. Angiopoietin-2 can augment the stimulatory effects of VEGF.[69,70]

Future studies may define the parathyroid-induced angiogenic mechanism more precisely and offer a therapeutic option to improve neo-vascularization in parathyroid autotransplantation. In turn, these processes may enhance survival and function of parathyroid autotransplanted tissue and may also shorten the latency time of graft function. More confidence in graft function post-transplant will undoubtedly drive the contro-

**Table 39–5.** Postoperative calcium and vitamin D supplementation

| | |
|---|---|
| Dihydroxycholecalciferol (vitamin D$_3$) | 2.0 μg/day (7days) |
| Maintenance vitamin D$_3$ | 0.5 – 1.0 μg/day |
| Calcium carbonate, oral | 1 – 2 g/day |
| Calcium gluconate, iv (symptomatic) | 250 mg/hr gtt |

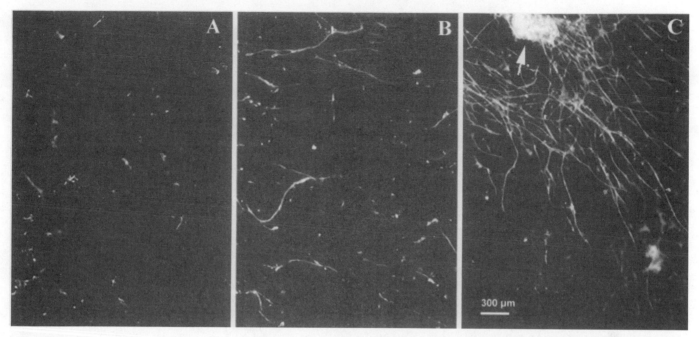

**Figure 39–3.** Induction of angiogenesis by normal parathyroid tissue. Freshly isolated rat microvessels were mixed with 1-mm³ pieces of parathyroid and cultured in a 3-D collagen gel. **A**, at day 1, isolated microvessels were uniformly distributed throughout the gel. After 11 days in culture, growing neo-microvessels show extensive arborization induced by parathyroid tissue, **C**, as compared with minimal neovessel development in control cultures, **B**. (From Carter WB, Uy K, Ward MD, Hoying JB, et al. *Surgery*. 2000;128:460.)

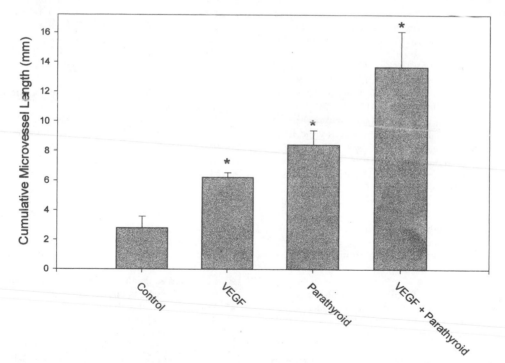

**Figure 39–4.** Comparison of neomicrovessel cumulative linear growth of control microvessel cultures to $VEGF_{165}$ treated (50 ng/ml), parathyroid tissue, and parathyroid tissue with $VEGF_{165}$ treated microvessel cultures. All experimental groups showed significant increase in cumulative length compared to control ($p < 0.01$). Parathyroid induced greater angiogenic response than $VEGF_{165}$ alone ($p < 0.05$). The addition of $VEGF_{165}$ to parathyroid tissue augmented the parathyroid-induced angiogenic response ($p < 0.05$). (From Carter WB, Uy K, Ward MD, Hoying JB, et al. *Surgery* 2000; 128:463.)

versy toward parathyroid autotransplantation as the treatment of choice in multi-gland parathyroid disease.

## References

1. Wells SA Jr, Grunnels J, Caulie S, Schneider JD, Arthur B, Sherwood L. Transplantation of the parathyroid glands in man: clinical indications and results. *Surgery.* 1975; 78: 34–44.

2. Wyngaarden JB, Smith LH. Endocrine and reproductive diseases. In: Wyngaarden JB, Smith LH, eds. *Cecil textbook of medicine.* Philadelphia: W. B. Saunders; 1985: 1423–45.

3. Herrera M, Grant C, van Heerden JA, Fitzpatrick LA. Parathyroid autotransplantation. *Arch Surg.* 1992; 127: 825–30.

4. Baumann DS, Wells SA. Parathyroid autotransplantation. *Surg.* 1993; 113: 130–3.

5. Gley E. Sur les fonctions de la glande thyroide chez le lapin et chez le chen. *CC Soc Biol (Paris).* 1891; 43: 843.

6. Halstead WS. Auto- and isotransplantation, in dogs, of parathyroid glandules. *J Exp Med.* 1909; 11: 175–98.

7. Lahey FH. The transplantation of parathyroids in partial thyroidectomy. *Surg Gynecol Obstet.* 1926; 42: 508–9.

8. Hickey RC, Samaan NA. Human parathyroid autotransplantation during thyroid surgery. *Arch Surg.* 1975; 110: 892–5.

9. Cordell LJ, Maxwell JG, Warden GD. Parathyroidectomy in chronic renal failure. *Am J Surg.* 1979; 138: 951–6.

10. Malmeus J, Akerstrom G, Johansson H, Ljunghall S, Nilsson P, Selking O. Parathyroid surgery in chronic renal insufficiency. *Acta Chir Scand.* 1982; 148: 229–38.

11. Diethelm AG, Adams Pl, Murad TM, et al. Treatment of secondary hyperthyroidism in patients with chronic renal failure by total parathyroidectomy and parathyroid autograft. *Ann Surg.* 1981; 193: 777–93.

12. Courant O, Letessier E, Moutel MG, Hamy A, Paineau J, Visset J. Surgical treatment of secondary hyperparathyroidism in chronic kidney failure. Results of total parathyroidectomy with parathyroid autotransplantation. *J Chir Paris.* 1993; 130: 327–34.

13. Kinnaert P, Salmon I, Decoster GC, et al. Total parathyroidectomy and presternal subcutaneous implantation of parathyroid tissue for renal hyperparathyroidism. *Surg Gynecol Obstet.* 1993; 176: 135–8.

14. Albertson DA, Poole GV, Myers RT. Subtotal parathyroidectomy versus total parathyroidectomy with autotransplantation for secondary hyperparathyroidism. *Am Surg.* 1985; 51: 16–20.

15. Rothmund M, Wagner PK. Total parathyroidectomy and autotransplantation of parathyroid tissue for renal hyperparathyroidism. A one to six year follow-up. *Ann Surg.* 1983; 197: 7–16.

16. Max MH, Flint LM, Richardson JD, Ferris FZ, Nagar D. Total parathyroidectomy and parathyroid autotransplantation in patients with chronic renal failure. *Surg Gynecol Obstet.* 1981; 153: 177–80.

17. Korzets Z, Magen H, Kraus L, Bernheim J, Bernheim J. Total parathyroidectomy with autotransplantation in haemodialysed patients with secondary hyperparathyroidism—should it be abandoned ? *Nephrol Dial Transplant.* 1987; 2: 341–6.

18. Block MA, Frame B, Jackson CE. The efficacy of subtotal parathyroidectomy for primary hyperparathyroidism due to multiple gland involvement. *Surg Gynecol Obstet.* 1978; 147: 1–5.

19. Edis AJ, van Heerden JA, Scholz DA. Results of subtotal parathyroidectomy for primary chief cell hyperplasia. *Surgery.* 1979; 86: 462–9.

20. Geis WP, Popovtzer MM, Corman JL, Halgrimson CG, Groth CG, Starzl TE. The diagnosis and treatment of hyperparathyroidism after renal homotransplantation. *Surg Gynecol Obstet.* 1973; 137: 997–1010.

21. Niederle B, Roka R, Brennan MF. The transplantation of parathyroid tissue in man: development, indications, technique and results. *Endocr Rev.* 1982; 3: 245–79.

22. Saxe AW, Brennan MF. Reoperative parathyroid surgery for primary hyperparathyroidism caused by multiple-gland disease: total parathyroidectomy and autotransplantation with cryo-preserved tissue. *Surgery.* 1982; 91: 616–21.

23. Beazley RM, Costa J, Ketcham AS. Reoperative parathyroid surgery. *Am J Surg.* 1975; 130: 427–9.

24. Brennan MF, Doppman JL, Marx SJ, et al. Reoperative parathyroid surgery for persistant parathyroidism. *Surgery.* 1978; 83: 669–76.

25. Edis AJ, Sheedy PF, Beahrs OH, van Heerden JA. Results of reoperation for hyperparathyroidism, with evaluation of preoperative localization studies. *Surgery.* 1978; 84: 384–93.

26. Wang C. Parathyroid re-exploration. A clinical and pathological study of 112 cases. *Ann Surg.* 1977; 186: 140–5.

27. Wells SA, Ross AJ, Dale JK, Gray RS. Transplantation of the parathyroid glands: current status. *Surg Clin North Am.* 1979; 59: 167–77.

28. Matsuura H, Sako K, Marchetta FC. Successful reimplantation of autogenous parathyroid tissue. *Am J Surg.* 1969; 118: 779–82.

29. Paloyan E, Lawrence AM, Brooks MH, Pickleman JR. Total thyroidectomy and parathyroid autotransplantation for radiation associated thyroid cancer. *Surgery.* 1976; 80: 70–6.

30. Paloyan E, Lawrence AM, Paloyan D. Successful autotransplantation of the parathyroid glands during total thyroidectomy for carcinoma. *Surg Gynecol Obstet.* 1977; 145: 364–8.

31. Katz AD, Bronson D. Total thyroidectomy. The indications and results of 630 cases. *Am J Surg.* 1978; 136: 450–4.

32. Beahrs OH, Ryan RF, White RA. Complications of thyroid surgery. *J Clin Endocrinol Metab.* 1956; 16: 1456–69.

33. Thompson NW, Harness JK. Complications of total thyroidectomy for carcinoma. *Surg Gynecol Obstet.* 1970; 131: 861–8.

34. Ohman U, Granberg PO, Lindell B. Function of parathyroid glands after total thyroidectomy. *Surg Gynecol Obstet.* 1978; 146: 773–8.

35. Harrold CC. Wright J. Management of surgical hyperparathyroidism. *Am J Surg.* 1966; 112: 482.

36. Thompson NW, Olsen WR, Hoffman GL. The continuing development of the technique of thyroidectomy. *Surgery.* 1973; 73: 913–27.

37. Wingert DJ, Friesen SR, Iliopoulos JI, Pierce GE, Thomas JH, Hermreck AS. Post-thyroidectomy hypocalcemia. *Am J Surg.* 1986; 152: 606–10.

38. Burnett HF, Mabry CD, Westbrook KC. Hypocalcemia after thyroidectomy: mechanisms and management. *South Med J.* 1977; 70: 1045–8.

39. Wells SA, Gunnels JC, Gutman RA, Shelburne JD, Schneider AB, Sherwood LM. The successful transplantation of frozen parathyroid tissue in man. *Surgery.* 1977; 81: 86–90.

40. Lo C, Lam K. Parathyroid autotransplantation during thyroidectomy: is frozen section necessary? *Arch Surg.* 1999; 134: 258–60

41. Monchik JM, Bendinelli C, Passero MA Jr, Roggin KK. Subcutaneous forearm transplantation of autologous parathyroid tissue. *Surgery.* 1999; 126: 1152–8.

42. Tenta LT, Keyes GR. Transcervical parathyroidectomy microsurgical autotransplantation and viscerovertebral arm. *Otolaryngol Clin North Am.* 1980; 13: 169–79.

43. Billings PJ, Milroy E. Autotransplantation of human parathyroid glands. *Ann R Coll Surg Engl.* 1986; 68: 11–13.

44. Brennan MF, Brown EM, Sears HF, Aurbach GD. Human parathyroid cryopreservation: in vitro testing of function by parathyroid hormone release. *Ann Surg.* 1978; 187: 87–90.

45. Shaha AR, Burnett C, Jaffe BM. Parathyroid autotransplantation during thyroid surgery. *J Surg Oncol.* 1991; 46: 21–24.

46. Kikumori T, Imai T, Tanaka Y, Oiwa M, Mase T, Funahashi H. Parathyroid autotransplantation with total thyroidectomy for thyroid carcinoma: long-term follow-up of grafted parathyroid function. *Surgery.* 1999; 125: 504–8.

47. Salander H, Tisell LE. Incidence of hypoparathyroidism after radical surgery for thyroid carcinoma and autotransplantation of parathyroid glands. *Am J Surg.* 1977; 134: 358–62.

48. Olson JA Jr, DeBenedetti MK, Baumann DS, Wells SA Jr. Parathyroid autotransplantation during thyroidectomy: results of long-term follow-up. *Ann Surg.* 1996; 223: 472–80.

49. Skinner MA, Norton JA, Moley, DeBenedetti MK, Wells SJ. Heterotopic autotransplantation of parathyroid tissue in children undergoing total thyroidectomy. *J Ped Surg.* 1997; 32: 510–3.

50. Sierra M, Herrera MF, Herrero B, et al. Prospective biochemical and scintigraphic evaluation of autografted normal parathyroid glands in patients undergoing thyroid operations. *Surgery.* 1998; 124: 1005–10.

51. Rothmund M, Wagner PK. Assessment of parathyroid graft function after autotransplantation of fresh and cryopreserved tissue. *World J Surg.* 1984; 8: 527–33.

52. Mozes MF, Soper WD, Jonasson O, Lang GR. Total parathyroidectomy and autotransplantation in secondary hyperparathyroidism. *Arch Surg.* 1980; 115:378–385.

53. Castleman B, Schantz A, Roth IS. Parathyroid hyperplasia in primary hyperparathyroidism. *Cancer.* 1976; 38: 1668–78.

54. Senapati A, Young AE. Parathyroid autotransplantation. *Br J Surg.* 1990; 77: 1171–4.

55. Feldman LA, Sharaf RN, Skarulis MC, et al. Results of heterotopic parathyroid autotransplantation: a 13-year experience. *Surgery.* 1999; 126: 1042–1048.

56. Saxe AW, Speigel AM, Marx SJ, Brennan MF. Deferred parathyroid autografts with cryopreserved tissue after reoperative parathyroid surgery. *Arch Surg.* 1982; 117: 538–43.

57. Wells SA Jr, Farndon JR, Dale JK, et al. Long-term evaluation of patients with primary parathyroid hyperplasia managed by total parathyroidectomy and heterotopic autotransplantation. *Ann Surg.* 1980; 192:451–8.

58. Malmeus J, Benson L, Johansson H, et al. Parathyroid surgery in the multiple endocrine neoplasia type I syndrome: choice of surgical procedure. *World J Surg.* 1986; 10: 668–72.

59. Walker RP, Paloyan E, Kelley TF, Gopalsami C, Jarosz H. Parathyroid autotransplantation in patients undergoing a total thyroidectomy: a review of 261 patients. *Otolaryngol Head Neck Surg.* 1994; 111: 258–64.

60. Wells SA, Stirman JA, Bolman RM. Parathyroid transplantation. *World J Surg.* 1977; 1: 747–56.

61. Malette LE, Eisenberg K, Wilson H, Noon GP. General primary parathyroid hyperplasia: studies of the evolution of autogenous parathyroid graft function. *Surgery.* 1983; 93: 254.

62. Barnett HF, Thompson BW, Barbour GL. Parathyroid autotransplantation. *Arch Surg.* 1977; 112: 373–9.

63. Funahashi H, Tanaka Y, Imai T, et al. Parathyroid hormone suppression by 22-oxacalcitrol in the severe parathyroid hyperplasia. *J Endocrinol Invest.* 1998; 21: 43–7.

64. Ueda M, Funahashi H, Satoh Y, Kato M, Takagi H. Evaluation on our procedure for autotransplantation of parathyroid glands by the intact-PTH. *Nippon Geka Gakkai Zasshi.* 1993; 94: 840–6.

65. Imai T, Tanaka Y, Kikumori T, Ohiwa M, Matsuura N, Funahashi H. Surgical management of preclinical medullary thyroid carcinoma in MEN2A. *Thyroidol Clin Exp.* 1998; 10: 143–7.

66. Carter WB, Crowell SL, Boswell CA, Williams SK. Stimulation of angiogenesis by canine parathyroid tissue. *Surgery.* 1996; 120: 1089–1094.

67. Saxe AW. Angiogenesis of human parathyroid tissue. *Surgery.* 1984; 66:1138–43.

68. Carter WB, Uy K, Ward MD, Hoying JB. Parathyroid-induced angiogenesis is VEGF-dependent. *Surgery.* 2000; 127: 1–7.

69. Holash J, Maisonpierre PC, Compton D, et al. Vessel cooption, regression, and growth in tumors mediated by angiopoietins and VEGF. *Science.* 1999; 284:1994–8.

70. Asahara T, Chen D, Takahashi T, et al. Tie2 receptor ligands, angiopoietin-1 and angiopoietin-2, modulate VEGF-induced postnatal neovascularization. *Circ Res.* 1998; 83:233–40.

# 40

# Carcinoma of the Parathyroid Glands

Ana M. Grau, M.D., Douglas B. Evans, M.D., Ana O. Hoff, M.D., and Jeffrey E. Lee, M.D.

## EPIDEMIOLOGY

Primary hyperparathyroidism (HPT) can be caused by parathyroid adenoma, hyperplasia and carcinoma. The incidence of primary HPT is reported to be 1 per 2,000,[1,2] and parathyroid carcinoma is reported to be the cause of primary HPT in only 0.1% to 4% of cases. [3–6] Parathyroid carcinoma is thus a rare entity, even more so when one considers that this incidence probably represents an overestimate caused by the frequent referral of these patients to tertiary care centers that will in turn report their series in the literature. The National Cancer Data Base (NCDB), a national electronic registry system currently capturing more than 60% of incident cancers in the United States, recently reported that 286 cases of parathyroid carcinoma were treated in the United States between 1985 and 1995.[7] Parathyroid carcinoma occurred with equal frequency in male and female patients; in contrast, parathyroid adenomas occur more frequently in female patients. The mean and median ages for the cohort were 54.5 years and 55.1 years, respectively (range, 14 to 88 years), similar to those previously reported in the literature.[2] There was no significant clustering within ethnic or income groups or unusual geographic clustering.

## ETIOLOGY

The epidemiology of parathyroid carcinoma offers few clues about its etiology and pathogenesis. Parathyroid carcinoma has been described in association with chronic renal failure and dialysis, with a total of 12 such reported cases.[8–10] It has been proposed that a malignant transformation of benign parathyroid hyperplastic tissue occurred in these cases. Previous reports of parathyroid carcinomas arising in patients with well-documented four-gland parathyroid hyperplasia support this theory.[11] Parathyroid carcinomas have been documented in association with both familial and sporadic parathyroid hyperplasia.[12] Associations of parathyroid carcinoma with familial HPT in patients with multiple endocrine neoplasia types 1 and 2A have been described. Two other forms of familial HPT, hereditary HPT-jaw tumor and familial isolated primary HPT have been associated with parathyroid carcinoma.[13] HPT-jaw tumor is characterized by recurrent parathyroid adenomas, fibro-osseous tumors of the mandible, and Wilms' tumors. Familial isolated primary HPT is characterized by parathyroid tumors with no evidence of other neoplasms. The synchronous occurrence of both an adenoma and carcinoma in a single patient has been reported.[13,14]

External irradiation has been associated with parathyroid neoplasms; however, these neoplasms are more frequently adenomas than carcinomas.[15,16]

## PATHOLOGY

The diagnosis of parathyroid cancer on the basis of histopathologic examination alone remains a challenge. Not infrequently, the diagnosis is made after the appearance of metastatic disease.[17,18] Nonetheless, criteria associated with malignancy have been identified[19] and include the presence of a fibrous capsule or trabeculae, a trabecular or rosette-like cellular architecture, mitotic figures, and capsular or vascular invasion.[18,20] However, none of these criteria is specific to parathyroid cancer, and some of them have been described in parathyroid adenomas as well.

Smith and Coombs analyzed the pathologic features of 20 parathyroid carcinomas. Nearly all carcinomas were greyish white in color and firm or hard to the touch. They found that a fibrous capsule and/or fibrous trabeculae were present in 18 of 20 specimens, a trabecular or rosette-like cellular architecture was present in 19, and mitotic figures were found in 19. The authors then stratified their 20 patients according to the patients' clinical course: development of metastasis; local invasion present; or no initial invasion and no development of metastasis. The presence of a fibrous capsule and/or trabeculae, a trabecular or rosette-like cellular architecture, and mitotic figures was common in all groups, including those patients without advanced disease. The findings in this study support the use of these three pathologic criteria for the diagnosis of parathyroid carcinoma, even in the absence of intra-operative evidence of adjacent organ or soft tissue invasion, or radiographic evidence of metastasis.[21]

## PRESENTATION

Parathyroid carcinoma occurs with equal frequency in male and female patients. The age at diagnosis reported in the literature typically ranges from 30 to 78 years,[22] although parathyroid carcinoma has also been reported in children.[23,24]

In general, patients with parathyroid cancer have higher serum calcium levels, higher levels of intact parathyroid hormone (iPTH), and more profound metabolic abnormalities than do patients with parathyroid adenomas or hyperplasia. Approximately 70% of patients with parathyroid carcinoma have serum calcium levels over 14 mg/dl and iPTH levels at least 5 times the upper limit of normal.[2,17,18,20,25] Metabolic abnormalities associated with parathyroid cancer include renal disorders (eg, nephrolithiasis, renal dysfunction, or pyelonephritis), in 30% to 60% of patients; skeletal abnormalities (eg, osteitis fibrosa cystica) in 40% to 90%; and pancreatitis in up to 15%. Polyuria, polydipsia, or nocturia is observed in 40% of patients and fatigue in 30%. 20% of patients are asymptomatic and approximately 40% were found to have a palpable neck mass.[2,18] This contrasts with the presentation in patients with benign causes of HPT: up to 50% of that group are asymptomatic at diagnosis, and the presence of a neck mass is rare.

Levin et al[26] analyzed differences between patients with parathyroid carcinomas and patients with adenomas with similar degrees of hypercalcemia.

Although patients with carcinomas had a higher frequency of combined bone and renal disease, no differences were observed in the frequencies of other metabolic abnormalities. The authors concluded that the metabolic abnormalities in patients with carcinoma are comparable to those in patients with adenomas and profound hypercalcemia.[26]

A definitive preoperative diagnosis of parathyroid carcinoma is impossible to make; metabolic manifestations of parathyroid cancer overlap with those of patients with adenomas. A high index of suspicion of parathyroid carcinoma should be maintained especially in patients with serum calcium levels over 14 mg/dl and a palpable neck mass.[2,18,25] Palsy of the recurrent laryngeal nerve in a patient with HPT is also suggestive of parathyroid cancer.[27]

Preoperative fine needle aspiration biopsy is contraindicated in patients with suspected parathyroid cancer because of the risk of local dissemination.[20] Furthermore, it is still difficult to distinguish parathyroid carcinoma from adenoma even on histologic examination, much less cytologic examination.[20]

Intra-operative recognition of parathyroid carcinoma is essential. Parathyroid cancer should be suspected in the presence of a gray, firm, adherent parathyroid gland; fibrosis is not seen in normal or adenomatous glands.[3,28] Local invasion of adjacent tissues and cervical lymph node metastasis, when present, further support the intra-operative diagnosis of parathyroid carcinoma.

## NATURAL HISTORY AND PATTERNS OF DISEASE RECURRENCE

Parathyroid carcinoma will recur in 37% to 80% of patients after successful initial resection.[2,4,18,22,29–31] Obara and Fujimoto[2] published the largest review of the natural history of parathyroid cancer in 1991. Their review included 163 cases reported in the English language medical literature between 1981 and 1989. Local invasion was present at the initial operation in 23% of the patients; 63% of the cases of invasion involved the thyroid gland and 16% the recurrent nerve, with the remaining cases involving the strap muscles, esophagus, and/or trachea. Cervical lymph nodes dissected during the initial operation were involved in only 4% of patients; 17% of patients ultimately developed lymph node metastasis, mostly in the neck and mediastinum. Distant metastases were present at the time of the initial operation in 2% of the patients; 25% of the patients developed distant disease. Sites of distant metastasis included the lung, bone, liver, and pancreas; the lung was the most frequent site of distant disease.

Metastatic parathyroid carcinomas were clinically non-functioning in only 2 patients, making it possible to use iPTH levels for surveillance for recurrence.

Among the 107 patients for whom follow-up information was available in Obara and Fujimoto's study, the recurrence rate was 37%, and the mean interval between the initial operation and the first recurrence was 2.6 years, with 4 patients having an interval of 7 to 19 years. Approximately 35% of patients died of recurrent or persistent hypercalcemia, with a mean survival after the initial operation of 6.6 years (range, 1 month to 17 years). 43% of patients were alive without disease with a mean follow-up of 4.6 years, and 22% were alive with disease for a mean of 7 years. Recurrence rates and patterns in this and other series are summarized in Table 40–1.[2,4,19,22,29,32] This Table demonstrates the wide range in the interval between the initial operation and the manifestation of recurrence, which likely reflects diversity in the biologic behavior of these tumors.

Similarly, recurrence after re-operation for parathyroid cancer presents at variable intervals. Favia et al[32] reported 6 patients with recurrent parathyroid cancer requiring a total of 12 re-operations. The mean disease-free interval was 15 months (range, 2 to 74 months). Sandelin et al[33] reported 36 patients with parathyroid carcinoma requiring 1 to 9 re-operative procedures for recurrent disease. Twenty-two patients had local disease with a median survival time from the first recurrence to death of 39 months (range, 1 to 204 months). Nine patients underwent resection of lung metastases; 4 were alive with disease for 74, 72, 48, and 34 months, respectively. The prognosis of patients with distant disease was not different from those with local spread only.

A more recent review comes from the NCDB report on 286 cases of parathyroid carcinoma treated in the United States between 1985 and 1995. Overall survival rates in the 134 cases followed for more than 5 years were 85% and 49% at 5 and 10 years, respectively. Survival results for this and other series are summarized in Table 40–2. [4,6,7,18,19,22,25,30,33] The 5-year survival rate for the 297 patients in other series was inferior to

that in the NCDB report; this difference could be caused, at least in part, by the inclusion of older series with lower survival rates[4,19] and series of patients with metastatic disease.[33]

No clear evidence of a plateau in the 10-year survival curve was noted in the NCDB report. This is consistent with previous reports of deaths from parathyroid carcinoma up to 30 years after initial diagnosis,[31] and with the high variability in the time to appearance of recurrence in these patients.

The available data on tumor size and lymph node involvement support neither of these factors as important prognostic markers. A multi-variate analysis of prognostic factors in 95 patients with parathyroid carcinoma reported by Sandelin et al[22] found that the extent of surgery when consisting of tumor resection and en bloc unilateral or bilateral thyroidectomy correlated most strongly with a longer survival and longer relapse-free period. They emphasize the importance of maintaining a high level of suspicion for parathyroid cancer based upon the gross findings intra-operatively.

## TREATMENT

Parathyroid cancer frequently recurs in the central neck and typically exhibits a natural history marked by recurrent hypercalcemia. Most patients who have recurrences after initial surgery will ultimately die of cancer related causes,[25] usually of the metabolic complications of hypercalcemia. Therefore, performance of the appropriate surgical procedure during the initial operation is critical and is one of the most important prognostic factors in parathyroid cancer.[22]

En bloc resection of the tumor and areas of potential invasion is indicated. The integrity of the parathyroid capsule should be maintained during dissection by performance of an en bloc resection of the ipsilateral central neck contents including the thyroid lobe and

**Table 40–1.** Rates and patterns of recurrence for parathyroid cancer

| First Author and Year | No. Patients | DFI (mo) | Local Recurrence % | †Distant Metastases % |
|---|---|---|---|---|
| Favia 1998[32] | 16 | 24* (7–72) | 50 | 80 |
| Cordeiro 1998[29] | 10 | 22 (6–48) | 55 | 44 |
| Sandelin 1992[22] | 95 | 33 (1–228) | 32 | 12 |
| Obara 1991[2] | 107 | 30 (0–19) | 36 | 25 |
| Wang 1985[4] | 28 | NA (6–36) | 32 | 36 |
| Schantz 1973[19] | 70 | NA | 30 | 30 |

Abbreviations: DFI, disease-free interval; NA, not available

*DFI for 10 patients with no persistent hypercalcemia

†The majority were lung metastases (30–100%)

**Table 40–2.** Survival rates for parathyroid cancer

| First Author and Year | No. Patients | Follow-up (yrs) | 5-Year Survival % | 10-Year Survival % |
|---|---|---|---|---|
| Sandelin 1994[33] | 40 | NA | 50 | 35 |
| Hakaim 1993[6] | 7 | NA | 85 | 57 |
| Sandelin 1992[22] | 95 | 6 | 85 | 70 |
| Wynne 1992[18] | 43 | 6.9 | 69 | 50 |
| Vetto 1993[30] | 14 | 6 | 55 | 55 |
| Wang 1985[4] | 28 | 7 | 57 | NA |
| Schantz 1973[19] | 70 | NA | 37 | NA |
| **Total** | **297** | | **63** | **58** |
| Hundahl 1999[7] | 134* | >5 | 85 | 49 |

*Collective review (includes patients from the other series)
Abbreviations: NA, not available

tracheo-esophageal soft tissues and lymphatics.[3] Structures, such as the recurrent laryngeal nerve, esophageal wall, or strap muscles should be sacrificed if the tumor adheres to them; this will reduce the risk of tumor spillage and local recurrence. The increased local control achieved with resection of the recurrent laryngeal nerve outweighs the complication of vocal cord paralysis, which can be managed if clinically necessary, with Teflon injection of the paralyzed cord, or phonosurgical rehabilitation procedures.

Lymph node metastases lateral to the jugular vein are rare during the initial presentation of parathyroid cancer[2]; therefore, prophylactic neck dissection (modified radical or selective neck dissection) is not recommended. Neck dissection is reserved for patients with lymph node metastasis detected radiographically or by clinical examination in the jugular distribution, or for patients with extensive soft tissue invasion.

Although cure after resection of recurrent parathyroid carcinoma is rare, aggressive re-resection of local recurrences is recommended. Selected patients will achieve prolonged disease-free intervals after one or more surgical procedures for recurrence in the neck.[32]

An aggressive surgical approach to metastatic parathyroid cancer has been advocated to control marked hypercalcemia. Obara et al[34] analyzed 22 patients who underwent lung resection for metastases from parathyroid cancer. 32% achieved a significant decrease in serum calcium levels and 14% achieved long-term survival (9 to 30 years). Patients who are good candidates for resection of metastases include those with local control of disease; no untreated metastasis at other sites; and an indolent tumor characterized by a long disease free interval.

Surgery for locally recurrent or metastatic disease should be guided by preoperative localization studies to better define the extent and location of recurrent disease.[35] However, tests performed during the early phase of calcium and iPTH elevation may fail to localize the recurrence. Thallium-201 scintigraphy and technetium[99m] Tc-Sestamibi scintigraphy are useful in locating cervical or upper mediastinal recurrences and regional lymph node metastases, but frequently fail to localize lung metastases.[36] A potential pitfall of these studies is that in patients with elevated iPTH, focal uptake of the radionuclide can be observed in brown tumors, mimicking metastases.[37,38] Computed tomographic scans are effective for identification and localization of pulmonary metastases. Venous catheterization and selective venous sampling, although more invasive, are useful when noninvasive studies fail to show recurrent tumors.[35] More recently, intra-operative use of hand-held gamma detectors after preoperative sestamibi injection has been used to aid in the intraoperative localization of recurrent parathyroid cancer.[39]

The low incidence of parathyroid cancer has made it difficult to study the roles of radiation and chemotherapy. The NCDB report described the use of radiation therapy in combination with surgery in less than 7% of the 286 cases included.[7] In Chow et al's[40] review of 10 patients treated for parathyroid cancer, 6 received adjuvant radiation therapy for microscopic residual disease. No evidence of recurrence was observed in these 6 patients with a mean follow-up of 62 months (range, 12 to 156 months).[40] Based on these results, the authors recommended adjuvant radiation with 40 to 50 Gy in patients at high risk of local relapse. Earlier reports point to the importance of complete en bloc resection followed by radiation therapy in order to increase local control. Lillemoe and Dudley[41] reported 3 patients who received postoperative radiation therapy for a high risk of microscopic residual disease. The 3 patients had no evidence of disease at 46, 22, and 16 months of follow-up, respectively. The results of these two series contrast with the common idea that radiation therapy is not effective in the treatment of parathyroid carcinoma. This belief has been based on anecdotal reports of failure of treatment involving radiation therapy; however, most patients in these reports had advanced, unresectable disease.[42,43] Wynne et al[18] reviewed their experience with 43 parathyroid cancer patients. Of the 5 patients treated with radiation therapy who had adequate follow-up, 4 had no response. The fifth patient who had surgically documented, invasive, residual parathyroid carcinoma in the neck, had no evidence of disease 11 years after radiation therapy.

Chemotherapy has a very limited role in the management of parathyroid cancer. Several agents, alone or in combination, have been tried. Anecdotal response to therapy has been seen with combination of 5-fluorouracil, cyclophosphamide, and *dacarbazine*[44] and the combination of methotrexate, doxorubicin, cyclophosphamide, and lomustine.[45]

## ILLUSTRATIVE CASES

The following three patients are currently being managed by the authors and all patients have undergone surgery within the past year. They illustrate the natural history of parathyroid carcinoma and the unique therapeutic challenges which parathyroid carcinoma presents for physicians and patients.

## Case 1

A 53-year-old man was recently referred to us by the orthopedic surgery service at our institution with cytologic confirmation of a presumed parathyroid adenoma in the left neck. He had undergone left shoulder disarticulation for a recurrent chondrosarcoma of the left upper extremity in 1998. On recent magnetic resonance imaging done as part of his routine follow-up evaluation, he was noted to have a hyperintense mass approximately 2 cm in size in the region of the left thyroid lobe (Figure 40–1). Under the assumption that the mass represented a thyroid nodule, he underwent ultrasound-guided fine needle aspiration. The cytologic findings were consistent with parathyroid tissue, and immunohistochem-

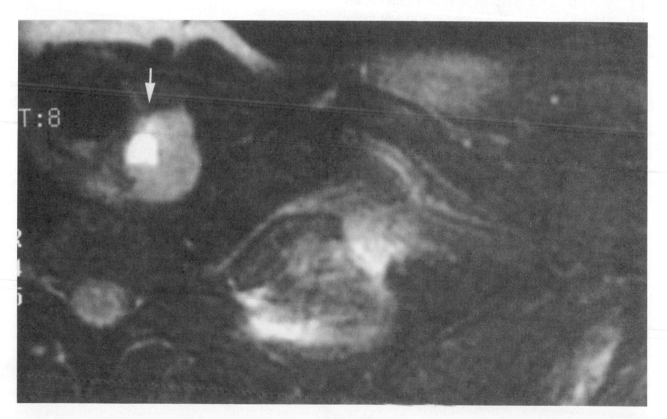

**Figure 40–1.** Axial T2 weighted MRI image of the upper chest demonstrating a well-circumscribed lesion (arrow) seen in relation to the left thyroid lobe. This was interpreted as a thyroid nodule and subjected to fine needle aspiration biopsy. At surgery this proved to be a parathyroid carcinoma.

ical staining was positive for parathyroid hormone. Interestingly, the patient had recently experienced an episode of ureterolithiasis and passed a stone, which was retrieved; analysis demonstrated that the stone was composed of calcium oxalate. This was his second episode of ureterolithiasis; his first episode occurred 5 years prior to his referral for management of hypercalcemia. The patient also gave a history of some form of external-beam radiation therapy as a young child for what he thought was an enlarged thymus. Laboratory data are described in Table 40–3.

The patient was scheduled to undergo minimally invasive parathyroidectomy under local anesthesia. He therefore received a sestamibi scan the morning of surgery; it confirmed the presence of a presumed parathyroid adenoma in the location of the mass identified on magnetic resonance imaging. At the time of surgery, the patient was found to have a greyish white, sclerotic, hard 3-cm mass posterolateral to the recurrent nerve and inseparable from the outer layer of the esophageal wall. Because of a concern about the possibility of parathyroid carcinoma based on the gross intra-operative findings, the patient was electively intubated and the anesthetic converted to general anesthesia. We then performed an en bloc resection of the left central neck compartment involving the parathyroid neoplasm, left thyroid lobe, and associated lymphatic and soft tissue contents. Final pathologic analysis demonstrated parathyroid carcinoma based upon the presence of necrosis and soft tissue invasion. Nine paratracheal lymph nodes demonstrated no evidence of metastatic carcinoma.

Because of a microscopically positive margin along the wall of the esophagus, the patient received postoperative adjuvant external-beam radiation therapy in 30 fractions to a total dose of 60 Gy utilizing an AP/PA technique with 6 MV photons. The patient tolerated this therapy well, with the only complications being sore throat, mild hoarseness, and moderate xerostomia. There was no delay in therapy caused by treatment-related complications. Approximately 3 months following completion of external-beam radiation therapy, his total and ionized calcium levels were normal.

This case demonstrates that parathyroid carcinoma can be associated with modest elevations in the levels of calcium and parathyroid hormone; dramatic elevations are not present in all patients. In addition, this case highlights two important management concepts. First, fine needle aspiration of a parathyroid neoplasm is unnecessary and can lead to parathyroid implantation of surrounding soft tissues. This can theoretically occur with both benign and malignant parathyroid neoplasms. In this case, the needle biopsy was performed under the assumption that the patient had a thyroid mass. Second, when performing minimally invasive parathyoidectomy under local or regional anesthesia, surgeons should not be afraid of conversion to general anesthesia when intra-operative findings suggest that a more extensive dissection is required. Although parathyroid carcinoma is rare, the surgeon must be aware of the gross characteristics of parathyroid carcinoma to allow appropriate intra-operative management.

## Case 2

A 25-year-old man presented to his physicians with complaints of fatigue and myalgias. Evaluation disclosed a total serum calcium level of 15.3 mg/dl and an elevated iPTH level. He underwent neck exploration, which demonstrated a 3-cm parathyroid neoplasm in the location of the left inferior parathyroid adjacent to the esophagus and the lower pole of the thyroid. Final pathologic analysis revealed parathyroid carcinoma based upon the presence of vascular and soft tissue invasion. Postoperatively, his calcium level normalized;

**Table 40–3.** Laboratory values for case 1

| Laboratory Values | Preop | Postop | Immediate Post EBRT | 3 Months Post EBRT |
|---|---|---|---|---|
| Total calcium (mg/dl) | 10.4 | 8.6 | 9.6 | 9.3 |
| Ionized calcium (mmol/l) | 1.38 | 1.11 | 1.26 | 1.18 |
| Phosphorus (mg/dl) | 2.9 | 2.5 | 3.3 | 2.8 |
| Intact PTH (pg/mL) | 61 | 81 | 39 | 55 |
| Urinary calcium (mg/24 hr) | 88 | | | |
| Creatinine (mg/dl) | 1.7 | 1.5 | 1.4 | 1.1 |

however, in approximately one year, he developed recurrent hypercalcemia. He underwent a second operation approximately 18 months after his first operation. This consisted of left thyroid lobectomy and resection of recurrent parathyroid carcinoma within the central neck compartment.

Following this operation, the patient was referred to our institution, at which time his total calcium level was 15.9 mg/dl with an ionized calcium level of 2.0 mmol/l, and his iPTH level was 350 pg/mL. Physical examination and radiographic images demonstrated a healing esophageal fistula as a complication of the most recent cervical operation. There was no evidence of measurable disease within the neck, although there were indeterminate pulmonary nodules suspicious for metastatic disease. There was no evidence of liver or bone metastasis. It was felt that the patient likely had diffuse soft tissue seeding in the left aspect of the central neck region and, probably, pulmonary metastasis. His calcium level was controlled with pamidronate, and he received doxorubicin-based systemic therapy.

Approximately one year later, cervical ultrasonography demonstrated two subcutaneous nodules in the central neck and a fairly large lymph node metastasis posterior to the base of the left internal jugular vein. These were treated surgically at our institution. His calcium level normalized for only a few months, following which he again required intravenous hydration and pamidronate. Approximately one year later, cervical ultrasonography demonstrated a recurrent mass just medial to the left carotid artery in the bed of the previously resected thyroid. The patient underwent re-operation with the aid of an intraoperative gamma detector, which required injection of 10 mCi of sestamibi 2 hours prior to surgery; the tumor mass was successfully localized and resected. To achieve complete resection, partial resection of the lateral wall of the cervical esophagus was necessary. The recurrent tumor measured approximately 3 x 2 cm and was completely re-sected. Following recovery the patient then received 60 Gy of external-beam radiation therapy (EBRT). There has been no evidence of progressive extracervical disease. The patient has not required pamidronate therapy post EBRT. Laboratory data are illustrated in Table 40–4.

This case demonstrates the problem of local-regional disease control even in the setting of probable distant metastases. The use of the hand-held gamma detector for intra-operative localization of recurrent parathyroid carcinoma was first reported by Mitchell and colleagues at Yale University in 1995. Success in re-operative parathyroid surgery (for malignant and benign disease) is greatly facilitated by the use of intra-operative ultrasonography, gamma probe localization, and the quick intra-operative parathyroid hormone assay, techniques used by the authors routinely in re-operative cases.

## Case 3

A 53-year-old man underwent subtotal thyroidectomy for a $T_1N_0$ follicular carcinoma of the thyroid. He had undergone low-dose irradiation for enlarged tonsils at the age of 5 years. Nine years after the thyroidectomy, he was found to be hypercalcemic, with biochemical evidence of primary HPT. Surgical exploration of the neck revealed an enlarged left-sided parathyroid gland, which was removed. Approximately 7 years later, he was noted to have recurrent hypercalcemia and underwent re-operation. At this procedure, thyroid tissue was removed and showed no evidence of carcinoma; there was no parathyroid tissue within the operative specimen. Postoperatively, his calcium level remained elevated (11 to 12 mg/dl). Approximately 2 years following his third cervical operation (and 18 years following his subtotal thyroidectomy), he underwent a fourth operation because of persistent hypercalcemia;

**Table 40–4.** Laboratory values for case 2

| Laboratory Values | *Preop #1 | †Preop #2 | Immediate Pre EBRT | Immediate Post EBRT | 7 Months Post EBRT |
|---|---|---|---|---|---|
| Total Calcium (mg/dl) | 11.9 | 14.6 | 13.1 | 12.6 | 9.1 |
| Ionized Calcium (mmol/l) | 1.56 | 1.88 | 1.81 | NA | 1.32 |
| Phosphorus (mg/dl) | 2.8 | 2.5 | 2.2 | 2.2 | 3.7 |
| Intact PTH (pg/ml) | 367 | 987 | 513 | NA | 66 |

* Prior to first operation at our institution; calcium level reflects extensive medical therapy
† Prior to second operation at our institution

during surgery multiple implants were noted throughout the left tracheo-esophageal groove. These were resected, and the pathologic findings were consistent with hypercellular parathyroid tissue. His calcium level normalized for a few months, only to increase once again to approximately 14 mg/dl. Approximately 2 years later (20 years following his initial subtotal thyroidectomy and 11 years following his initial parathyroidectomy), he underwent re-operation at which time multiple implants consistent with hypercellular parathyroid were again removed from the tracheo-esophageal groove and the lateral wall of the esophagus. Normocalcemia lasted only a few months, and the patient again became hypercalcemic. He was then referred to our institution 2 years after his fourth cervical operation and 17 years after his initial parathyroidectomy.

At the time of referral, the patient complained of mild depression, severe fatigue, arthralgias in the knees, elbows, and shoulders, and continuing symptoms from recurrent ureterolithiasis. His hypercalcemia was profound, with a total calcium level of 16 mg/dl. He was treated with intravenous hydration and pamidronate. Radiographic imaging demonstrated recurrent disease in the neck manifested by a lobulated,

approximately 4 cm mass in the left central neck compartment anterior to the vertebral artery and posterior to the jugular vein and carotid artery (Figure 40–2). Sestamibi imaging (Figure 40–3) demonstrated no other evidence of focally increased activity suggesting extracervical metastasis. Computed tomography of the chest and bone scintigraphy demonstrated no clear evidence of pulmonary or osseous metastasis. Following medical management of his hypercalcemia, he was brought to the operating room for surgical exploration, which revealed the recurrence in the left side of the neck to be most consistent with a nodal metastasis; it appeared as a relatively soft, encapsulated mass. There was no evidence of esophageal invasion. The mass was dissected sharply off the posterior surface of the carotid artery, the medial aspect of the jugular vein, and the anterior surface of the vertebral artery (Figure 40–4). The sympathetic ganglion and the vagus nerve were removed en bloc with the tumor; the phrenic nerve was preserved. Postoperatively, the patient recovered without complication and had a significant decline in the serum levels of both calcium and parathyroid hormone. He received 60 Gy of adjuvant external-beam radiation therapy. Laboratory data are described in Table 40–5.

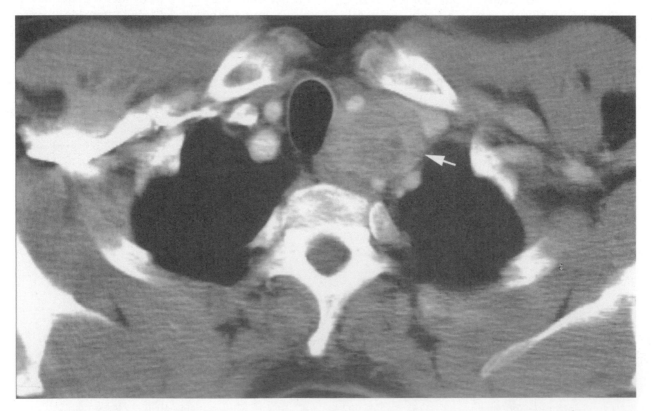

**Figure 40–2.** Axial post-contrast CT image of the chest demonstrating a 4.5 cm recurrent parathyroid carcinoma (arrow) in the lower left neck. Note the relationship of this mass to the vertebral artery posteriorly and the trachea medially. The large mass displaces the jugular vein laterally and the carotid artery anteriorly.

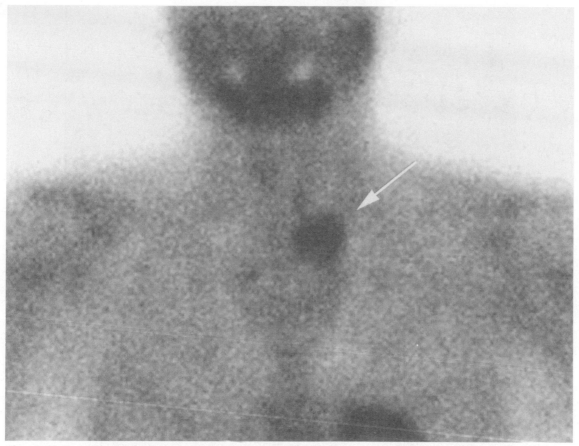

**Figure 40–3.** Whole body Sestamibi scan performed with 25 mCi of 199m Tc-Sestamibi given intravenously. There is focal increased activity seen in the left thoracic inlet within the anterior-superior mediastinum corresponding to the mass seen on CT.

The biologic behavior of this tumor appeared to become more aggressive over time, a phenomenon seen in many other solid tumors. Because of the demonstrated propensity for local-regional recurrence, we recommended external-beam irradiation following complete gross resection of recurrent disease.

## SUMMARY

Parathyroid carcinoma is a rare cause of HPT that affects men and women equally, predominantly during the 4th to 6th decades of life. The etiology of parathyroid carcinoma is unknown, although associations with chronic renal failure and dialysis, familial and sporadic HPT, and external irradiation have been described in a limited number of patients.

The preoperative diagnosis of parathyroid cancer remains a challenge. The importance of maintaining a high index of suspicion during the preoperative and intra-operative evaluation of patients with HPT cannot be overemphasized since the performance of an adequate surgical procedure during the initial exploration is critical in terms of prognosis. Preoperative findings associated with parathyroid carcinoma in patients with HPT include serum calcium levels over 14 mg/dl, high levels of iPTH elevation, profound metabolic abnormalities, a palpable neck mass, and recurrent laryngeal nerve palsy. Intra-operatively, the diagnosis should be suspected in the presence of a gray, firm, adherent parathyroid gland, evidence of local invasion, and cervical lymph node metastasis. Preoperative fine needle aspiration biopsy is contraindicated.

Adequate treatment of the primary lesion involves en bloc resection of the tumor and areas of potential invasion, with care taken to maintain the integrity of the parathyroid capsule. En bloc resection of the ipsilateral central neck contents including the thyroid lobe and tracheo-esophageal soft tissues and lymphatics as well as adherent structures should be performed.

Recurrence from parathyroid carcinoma will occur in 37% to 80% of patients after initial surgery, with a wide range in the interval between the initial operation and the manifestation of recurrence. In general, recur-

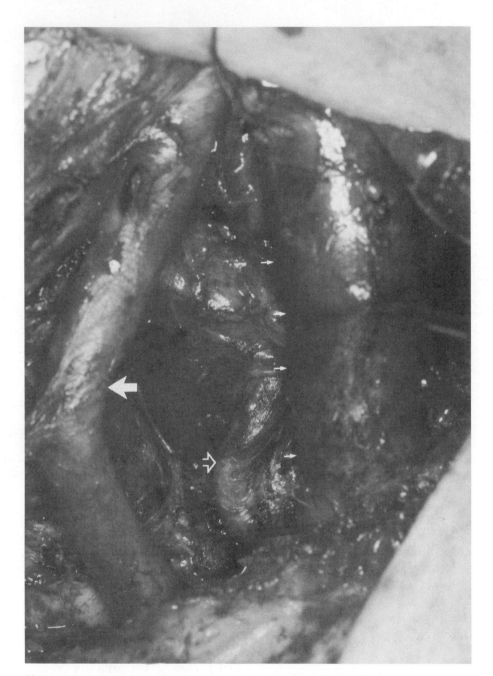

**Figure 40–4.** Intraoperative photograph following resection of recurrent parathyroid carcinoma from the left lower neck and upper mediastinum. The tumor mass did not invade the wall of the esophagus and most likely represented an enlarged nodal metastasis. The mass was sharply dissected off the posterior surface of the carotid artery (large arrow), the medial aspect of the jugular vein (small arrows), and the anterior surface of the vertebral artery (open arrow). En bloc resection did require removal of the sympathetic ganglion and the vagus nerve; the phrenic nerve was preserved.

rent disease should be treated with surgical resection; although cure after recurrence is rare, some patients will achieve prolonged disease-free intervals by facilitating the control of hypercalcemia.

Radiation therapy may play a role as an adjuvant treatment in patients at high risk for local relapse. Chemotherapy has a very limited role in the management of parathyroid cancer.

**Table 40–5.** Laboratory values for case 3

| Laboratory Values | Preop | Postop | Pre EBRT | Immediate Post EBRT | 3 Months Post EBRT |
|---|---|---|---|---|---|
| Total calcium (mg/dl) | 16.0 | 9.3 | 8.4 | 8.3 | 8.9 |
| Ionized calcium (mmol/l) | 2.05 | 1.27 | 1.11 | NA | NA |
| Phosphorus (mg/dl) | 2.3 | 2.4 | 3.3 | 3.2 | NA |
| Intact PTH (pg/ml) | 1,085 | 279 | 352 | 233 | NA |
| Creatinine (mg/dl) | 1.7 | 1.7 | NA | 1.7 | 1.6 |

# References

1. Heath HD, Hodgson SF, Kennedy MA. Primary hyperparathyroidism. Incidence, morbidity, and potential economic impact in a community. *N Engl J Med*. 1980;302:189–93.
2. Obara T, Fujimoto Y. Diagnosis and treatment of patients with parathyroid carcinoma: an update and review. *World J Surg*. 1991;15:738–44.
3. Cohn K, Silverman M, Corrado J, Sedgewick C. Parathyroid carcinoma: the Lahey Clinic experience. *Surgery*. 1985;98:1095–100.
4. Wang CA, Gaz RD. Natural history of parathyroid carcinoma. Diagnosis, treatment, and results. *Am J Surg*. 1985;149:522–7.
5. van Heerden JA, Weiland LH, ReMine WH, Walls JT, Purnell DC. Cancer of the parathyroid glands. *Arch Surg*. 1979;114:475–80.
6. Hakaim AG, Esselstyn CB, Jr. Parathyroid carcinoma: 50-year experience at The Cleveland Clinic Foundation. *Cleve Clin J Med*. 1993;60:331–5.
7. Hundahl SA, Fleming ID, Fremgen AM, Menck HR. Two hundred eighty-six cases of parathyroid carcinoma treated in the U.S. between 1985–1995: a National Cancer Data Base Report. The American College of Surgeons Commission on Cancer and the American Cancer Society. *Cancer*. 1999;86:538–44.
8. Miki H, Sumitomo M, Inoue H, Kita S, Monden Y. Parathyroid carcinoma in patients with chronic renal failure on maintenance hemodialysis. *Surgery*. 1996;120:897–901.
9. Takami H, Kameyama K, Nagakubo I. Parathyroid carcinoma in a patient receiving long-term hemodialysis. *Surgery*. 1999;125:239–40.
10. Boyle NH, Ogg CS, Hartley RB, Owen WJ. Parathyroid carcinoma secondary to prolonged hyperplasia in chronic renal failure and in coeliac disease. *Eur J Surg Oncol*. 1999;25:100–3.
11. de Papp AE, Kinder B, LiVolsi V, Gupta SM, Stewart AF. Parathyroid carcinoma arising from parathyroid hyperplasia: autoinfarction following intravenous treatment with pamidronate. *Am J Med*. 1994;97:399–400.
12. Jenkins PJ, Satta MA, Simmgen M, et al. Metastatic parathyroid carcinoma in the MEN2A syndrome. *Clin Endocrinol (Oxf)*. 1997;47:747–51.
13. Yoshimoto K, Endo H, Tsuyuguchi M, et al. Familial isolated primary hyperparathyroidism with parathyroid carcinomas: clinical and molecular features. *Clin Endocrinol (Oxf)*. 1998;48:67–72.
14. Shapiro DM, Recant W, Hemmati M, Mazzone T, Evans RH. Synchronous occurrence of parathyroid carcinoma and adenoma in an elderly woman. *Surgery*. 1989;106:929–33.
15. Takeichi N, Dohi K, Ito H, et al. Parathyroid tumors in atomic bomb survivors in Hiroshima: a review. *J Radiat Res (Tokyo)*. 1991;32 Suppl:189–92.
16. Hickey RC, Jung PJ, Merrell R, Ordonez N, Samaan NA. Parathyroid adenoma in a cancer center patient population. *Am J Surg*. 1991;161:439–42.
17. Anderson BJ, Samaan NA, Vassilopoulou-Sellin R, Ordonez NG, Hickey RC. Parathyroid carcinoma: features and difficulties in diagnosis and management. *Surgery*. 1983;94:906–15.
18. Wynne AG, van Heerden J, Carney JA, Fitzpatrick LA. Parathyroid carcinoma: clinical and pathologic features in 43 patients. *Medicine (Baltimore)*. 1992;71:197–205.
19. Schantz A, Castleman B. Parathyroid carcinoma. A study of 70 cases. *Cancer*. 1973;31:600–5.
20. Obara T, Okamoto T, Kanbe M, Iihara M. Functioning parathyroid carcinoma: clinicopathologic features and rational treatment. *Semin Surg Oncol*. 1997;13:134–41.
21. Smith JF, Coombs RR. Histological diagnosis of carcinoma of the parathyroid gland. *J Clin Pathol*. 1984;37:1370–8.
22. Sandelin K, Auer G, Bondeson L, Grimelius L, Farnebo LO. Prognostic factors in parathyroid cancer: a review of 95 cases. *World J Surg*. 1992;16:724–31.
23. McHenry CR, Rosen IB, Walfish PG, Cooter N. Parathyroid crisis of unusual features in a child. *Cancer*. 1993;71:1923–7.
24. Meier DE, Snyder WH, 3rd, Dickson BA, Margraf LR, Guzzetta PC, Jr. Parathyroid carcinoma in a child. *J Pediatr Surg*. 1999;34:606–8.
25. Shane E, Bilezikian JP. Parathyroid carcinoma: a review of 62 patients. *Endocr Rev*. 1982;3:218–26.
26. Levin KE, Galante M, Clark OH. Parathyroid carcinoma versus parathyroid adenoma in patients with profound hypercalcemia. *Surgery*. 1987;101:649–60.
27. Shane E. Parathyroid carcinoma. *Curr Ther Endocrinol Metab*. 1997;6:565–8.
28. Holmes EC, Morton DL, Ketcham AS. Parathyroid carcinoma: a collective review. *Ann Surg*. 1969;169:631–40.
29. Cordeiro AC, Montenegro FL, Kulcsar MA, et al. Parathyroid carcinoma. *Am J Surg*. 1998;175:52–5.
30. Vetto JT, Brennan MF, Woodruf J, Burt M. Parathyroid carcinoma: diagnosis and clinical history. *Surgery*. 1993;114:882–92.
31. Shortell CK, Andrus CH, Phillips CE, Jr., Schwartz SI. Carcinoma of the parathyroid gland: a 30-year experience. *Surgery*. 1991;110:704–8.
32. Favia G, Lumachi F, Polistina F, D'Amico DF. Parathyroid carcinoma: sixteen new cases and suggestions for correct management. *World J Surg*. 1998;22:1225–30.
33. Sandelin K, Tullgren O, Farnebo LO. Clinical course of metastatic parathyroid cancer. *World J Surg*. 1994;18:594–8; discussion 599.
34. Obara T, Okamoto T, Ito Y, et al. Surgical and medical management of patients with pulmonary metastasis from parathyroid carcinoma. *Surgery*. 1993;114:1040–8; discussion 1048–9.
35. Sandelin K, Thompson NW, Bondeson L. Metastatic parathyroid carcinoma: dilemmas in management. *Surgery*. 1991;110:978–86; discussion 986–8.
36. Fujimoto Y, Obara T, Ito Y, Kodama T, Nobori M, Ebihara S. Localization and surgical resection of metastatic parathyroid carcinoma. *World J Surg*. 1986;10:539–47.

37. Lu G, Shih WJ, Xiu JY. Technetium-99m MIBI uptake in recurrent parathyroid carcinoma and brown tumors. *J Nucl Med*. 1995;36: 811–3.

38. Stokkel MP, van Eck-Smit BL. Tc-99m MIBI in a patient with parathyroid carcinoma. What to expect from it. *Clin Nucl Med*. 1996;21:142–3.

39. Mitchell BK, Merrell RC, Kinder BK. Localization studies in patients with hyperparathyroidism. *Surg Clin North Am*. 1995;75: 483–98.

40. Chow E, Tsang RW, Brierley JD, Filice S. Parathyroid carcinoma—the Princess Margaret Hospital experience. *Int J Radiat Oncol Biol Phys*. 1998;41:569–72.

41. Lillemoe KD, Dudley NE. Parathyroid carcinoma: pointers to successful management. *Ann R Coll Surg Engl*. 1985;67:222–4.

42. Palnaes Hansen C, Lau Pedersen M, Christensen L. Diagnosis, treatment and outcome of parathyroid cancer. A report of eight patients. *Eur J Surg*. 1991;157:517–20.

43. Flye MW, Brennan MF. Surgical resection of metastatic parathyroid carcinoma. *Ann Surg*. 1981;193:425–35.

44. Bukowski RM, Sheeler L, Cunningham J, Esselstyn C. Successful combination chemotherapy for metastatic parathyroid carcinoma. *Arch Intern Med*. 1984;144:399–400.

45. Chahinian AP, Holland JF, Nieburgs HE, Marinescu A, Geller SA, Kirschner PA. Metastatic nonfunctioning parathyroid carcinoma: ultrastructural evidence of secretory granules and response to chemotherapy. *Am J Med Sci*. 1981;282:80–4.

# 41

# Management of Thyroid and Parathyroid Disease During Pregnancy

Michael Friedman, M.D., Jessica Landsberg, M.D., and Roee Landsberg M.D.

## INTRODUCTION

Since thyroid disorders are very common in women at their fertile age, not infrequently physicians have to deal with their occurrence in pregnant women. As is true for other disorders that occur during pregnancy, the desire to maintain the well-being of the mother and fetus and to minimize the risks of abortion or preterm labor dictate management guidelines. Thyroid disorders are especially challenging because the changes in thyroid function tests associated with pregnancy are among the most profound seen as a result of a normal physiologic condition. Similarly, findings associated with the hypermetabolic state of normal pregnancy can overlap with the clinical signs and symptoms of thyroid disease. In addition, some irreplaceable antithyroid drugs readily cross the placenta and affect the fetal thyroid at any time throughout gestation.

Pregnant patients sometimes seem "enigmatic" to physicians who do not take care of them on a daily basis. The goal of this chapter is to provide an insight into the effects of pregnancy on thyroid gland function and to elucidate specific aspects in the natural course and management of common thyroid disorders in pregnant patients. Although not commonly encountered in pregnancy, hyperparathyroidism may occur, and concepts directed at management of this disorder will also be addressed.

## THYROID GLAND ADAPTATION TO PREGNANCY

### Functional Changes

The production, circulation and disposal of thyroid hormones are all altered in pregnancy. To add to the complexity, some changes are specific to the stage of pregnancy, which should be taken into account when one attempts to interpret the results of thyroid function studies.

Pregnancy is characterized by an increasing maternal demand for iodine caused by the transfer of iodine and iodothyronines through the placenta to the fetus.[1] Fetal production of thyroid hormone, and thus its consumption of iodine, increase with the progression of pregnancy, reaching their peak at term.[2] In addition, the increase in maternal glomerular filtration rate (GFR) further contributes to a reduction in serum inorganic iodine levels. Both of these factors can lead to iodine deficiency and goiter where iodine intake is inadequate.[3]

The earliest and most marked change in thyroid function tests is an increase in serum thyroxine-binding-globulin (TBG).[4] Estrogen stimulates an increase in the synthesis of TBG and inhibits its hepatic clearance, thereby leading to an increase in serum concentrations of TBG with the subsequent increase in serum total $T_4$ and total $T_3$ levels. These levels plateau after 12 to 14 weeks of gestation. Thyroid gland enlargement in some women may also contribute to the increase in serum TBG (see Table 41–1).

Except for a transient increase in the first trimester, serum free $T_4$ ($FT_4$) level shows only minimal, if any, changes and usually remains within the normal range for non-pregnant women.[3,4] However, there is an increase in $T_4$ requirements during pregnancy, which is most evident in women with hypothyroidism who were treated with thyroxine before conceptions. In these groups of patients the thyroxine dose should be increased during pregnancy by 25–50% in order to maintain normal serum free $T_4$ concentrations.[5]

Human chorionic gonadotropin (hCG), initially produced during the first week after fertilization has a thyrotropin-like bioactivity.[6] The levels of this hormone rise steadily through the first trimester of pregnancy leading to the transient increase in serum $FT_4$ previously mentioned. During this period the thyroid gland shows histologic features of stimulation with increased iodine uptake. These phenomena become very profound in conditions associated with very high hCG levels, such as multifetal pregnancy.[6,7] After the first trimester, hCG concentration declines with a concomitant return of $FT_4$ levels to their normal values. Since the normal feedback mechanism in the hypothalamus-pituitary-thyroid axis is maintained during pregnancy, thyrotropin (TSH) levels reflect the trends in $FT_4$ levels with a slight decrease during the first trimester and normalization thereafter.[8]

Anti-thyroid antibodies (anti-thyroglobulin and/or anti-thyroperoxidase) are detected in as many as 20% of pregnant women (as compared to approximately 3% in non-pregnant women). A large fraction of these women will develop postpartum thyroiditis, although in some cases these antibodies disappear after delivery.[9]

## PLACENTAL–FETAL THYROID PHYSIOLOGY

Although an in-depth review of placental-fetal thyroid physiology is beyond the scope of this chapter, some facts should be mentioned. Thyroid hormones have important roles in embryogenesis and fetal maturation from the earliest days of gestation.[4] Fetal rat tissues, including the brain, contain $T_4$ and $T_3$ even before fetal thyroid hormones are produced.[11] The most ominous effects of fetal hypothyroidism are defects in IQ and neurologic function as seen with congenital cretinism.[12]

The fetal thyroid gland and pituitary-thyroid axis become functional late in the first trimester. Before that time the maternal circulation is the sole source for fetal thyroid hormones.[4] As will be discussed later, this is one reason to postpone maternal thyroid surgery to the second trimester. With progression of pregnancy, fetal thyroid gland, pituitary-thyroid axis and liver gradually mature as reflected by a consistent increase in the production of thyroid hormones and TBG. Fetal serum TSH levels also show a gradual increase starting at the first trimester caused by increased stimulation of the fetal thyroid by thyrotropin-releasing hormone (TRH). Although it is not clear whether maternal $T_4$ and $T_3$ play any important role in fetal development during the second and third trimesters, placental transfer of these hormones can occur late in pregnancy.[13] Because iodine is actively transported across the placenta throughout gestation, the fetus is susceptible to iodine-induced goiter and hypothyroidism when iodine is administered to

**Table 41–1.** Change in common thyroid function tests during pregnancy

| Parameter | TBG | Total $T_4$ | Total $T_3$ | Free $T_4$ | Free $T_3$ | TSH | Antithyroid Antibodies |
|---|---|---|---|---|---|---|---|
| Change observed during pregnancy | Increase First change to be observed | Increase As a consequence of increased TBG | Increase As a consequence of increase TBG | No change A transient increase in first trimester | No change A transient increase in first trimester | No change A slight decrease in first trimester concomitant with the increase in hCG | Increase in as many as 20% of pregnant women Usually reflect a predisposition to postpartum thyroiditis. Occasionally without any consequences |

Adapted from data in Brent GA, Maternal thyroid function: interpretation of thyroid function tests in pregnancy. *Clin Obstet Gynecol.* 1997; 40:3–15.[10]

the mother.[14] This is true not only for intravenous or oral routes but also for topical percutaneous applications, for example during the preparation of a surgical field or treatment of surgical wounds.

## Structural Changes

In ancient Egypt and ancient Rome, pregnancy was sometimes diagnosed by measuring the swelling in the neck of married young women.[15] As previously mentioned, women who live in areas in which iodine intake is insufficient or marginal may have an absolute or relative iodine deficiency during pregnancy resulting in an enlargement of the thyroid gland.[3]

When iodine intake is sufficient, some degree of thyroid enlargement may be evident because of glandular hyperplasia and increased vascularity. A study performed in the United States demonstrated a 10–20% increase in the volume of the thyroid gland in pregnant women.[16] Studies of thyroid volume measured by ultrasonography detected a 13% reduction in thyroid size in healthy women after delivery.[17] Frank goiter, however, should by no means be interpreted as a normal finding during pregnancy and warrants immediate further investigation. Another aspect of the enhanced thyroid vascularity during pregnancy is a possibility of an increased amount of bleeding during thyroid surgery, which should be taken into account.

## USE OF ANTITHYROID DRUGS IN PREGNANCY

### Thioamides

Propylthiouracil and methimazole are both utilized for the treatment of hyperthyroidism in pregnancy. Since both drugs cross the placenta and may induce fetal goiter and hypothyroidism, they should be used in the lowest possible doses. This usually means up to 300 mg/day of PTU or up to 20 mg/day of methimazole—doses that keep the mother's $FT_4$ concentrations at the upper normal limit. After thyrotoxicosis is controlled, doses can be reduced to 50–100 mg PTU or 5–10 mg of methimazole daily.[18] Maternal complications of these drugs do not differ between pregnant and nonpregnant patients.

### Radioiodine

The use of radioiodine is absolutely contraindicated during pregnancy and lactation. Lethal effects on the embryo are seen with exposure around the time of im-plantation with doses as low as 10cGy. Malformations can be induced during organogenesis and the threshold for these is believed to be as low as 5cGy. Exposure between 8–15 weeks is a special hazard for mental retardation since this is the time for development of the frontal brain. The fetal thyroid begins to accumulate radioiodine around week 12 of pregnancy. This carries an additional unique risk for fetal hypothyroidism with its serious implications, including attention deficit disorder and figurative memory impairment. Women exposed to radioiodine (mean dose of 109 mCi) in the year before pregnancy suffered a 40% rate of abortions.[19]

## Inorganic Iodine

Iodine is actively transported across the placenta; thus the fetus is susceptible to iodine-induced goiter and hypothyroidism when the mother is given pharmacological doses of iodine. This may occur with intravenous, oral, mucosal or even topical iodine administration.

## Thyroxine

Thyroxine can be safely administered as a replacement therapy for hypothyroidism or as a suppressive therapy for thyroid tumors without any adverse effects on the fetus. The dose of thyroxine needed to achieve a therapeutic effect may be higher in pregnant women, and titration with TSH levels is usually advocated.

## HYPERTHYROIDISM IN PREGNANCY

Hyperthyroidism occurs in about 0.2% of pregnant women in the United States. In addition to the classic complications of heart failure and thyroid storm, unique to pregnancy are the possible occurrence of pre-eclampsia and premature labor.[14] Fetal complications include minor malformations, intrauterine growth restriction and stillbirth.[18] Although some pregnancy manifestations, such as heat intolerance, fatigue and tachycardia, may mimic hyperthyroidism, pregnant thyrotoxic women ususally present with more severe symptoms and signs such as weight loss, noticeable goiter and tremor.

The most common cause of hyperthyroidism in pregnant women is Graves' disease, which, in most cases, pre-existed before pregnancy.[18,20] It is important to mention that the course of this autoimmune disorder is usually ameliorated in the second and third trimesters of pregnancy because of suppression of the maternal immune response that promotes tolerance of the fetus. The disease may worsen during the first trimester because of the thyrotropic effects of hCG and tends to relapse in the postpartum period.[20] Other causes of hyperthyroidism during pregnancy include nodular goiter, gestational trophoblastic disease and hyperemesis gravidarum.[18]

Diagnosis of hyperthyroidism during pregnancy is based on the findings of elevated serum $FT_3$ and $FT_4$ as well as undetectably low levels of TSH. Unique to Graves' disease may be the ophthalmopathy and the existence of thyroid-stimulating immunoglobulins.

## Management

The best time to initiate therapy for hyperthyroidism is prior to conception in order to prevent potential adverse effects on the fetus.[20] Except for mild cases, hyperthyroidism during pregnancy should be treated. The value of early and aggressive treatment of hyperthyroidism cannot be underscored in view of a study showing increased risk of perinatal mortality, preterm labor and maternal heart failure in pregnant women who did not receive adequate treatment for hyperthyroidism.[21]

The first line of treatment for hyperthyroidism is medical in most cases (except for hydatidiform mole, where evacuation of the uterus is mandatory). The goal of therapy is to gain control of the hyperthyroidism while minimizing fetal side effects and chances for intrauterine hypothyroidism.[22] As previously mentioned, the use of radioiodine is absolutely contraindicated in pregnant women. PTU is the drug of choice in the United States and methimazole is more common in Europe. The doses are adjusted until the maternal $FT_4$ level can be kept in the high normal range or only slightly elevated.[18] For rapid control of hyperthyroid symptoms, beta-blockers such as propranolol are very effective.[22]

In severe cases unresponsive to medical management or when patient's compliance to therapy is poor, thyroidectomy is indicated. If diagnosed at first trimester, efforts should be made to postpone surgery to the second trimester.[18] In the meantime, some authors recommend a brief preparatory course of iodine (usually two weeks) in order to decrease the vascularity of the gland.[23] Beta-blockers are utilized for perioperative control of cardiovascular manifestations. In the most severe cases, thyroid surgery should be promptly performed because of maternal indications regardless of gestational age. Esmalol, an ultra-short-acting cardioselective beta-blocker can be a substitute for propranolol should an emergency surgery be performed.[23]

Complications of total thyroidectomy during pregnancy do not differ from those of thyroidectomy performed in non-pregnant patients; these include hypoparathyroidism and vocal cord paralysis caused by recurrent laryngeal nerve injury as the most common.[23] Meticulous surgical technique and the preoperative administration of iodine will minimize intra-operative blood loss.

## THYROID NODULAR DISEASE IN PREGNANCY

### Epidemiology

Thyroid tumors, the most common endocrine neoplasms, are three to four times more common in women than in men.[24] Some tumors occur predominantly in younger women of a childbearing age. Thus, it is not uncommon to encounter a thyroid tumor in a pregnant patient. In fact, it is believed that around 2% of pregnant women have thyroid nodules[18] (whereas Hay[25] quotes a much higher number—10%). About 10% of thyroid cancers occurring during the reproductive years are diagnosed during pregnancy or in the first year after birth.[24]

Because of the strong association between thyroid nodules and female gender, reproductive factors have been implicated in the development of such tumors. Some studies have demonstrated a positive correlation between the number of pregnancies (either miscarriages or live birth) and the occurrence of thyroid neoplasms.[26,27] However, estrogen and progesterone receptors were not found to be relevant in the development of such tumors.[28] In addition, there is no evidence for adverse effects of pregnancy on the behavior or prognosis of thyroid cancers.[29,30] Altogether, if indeed parity is a causal factor in thyroid neoplasia, the precise hormonal and molecular mechanisms as well as the magnitude of its influence are yet to be defined.

### Histopathology

The histopathology of thyroid nodules diagnosed during pregnancy has been evaluated in a number of studies; a study from the Mayo Clinic evaluated 40 patients with thyroid nodules by fine needle aspiration biopsy (FNAB). Sixty-four percent of the nodules were benign, 7% positive for papillary carcinoma and 23% suspicious for malignancy. This distribution was comparable with figures obtained for 910 women aged 15–40 treated over a period of 4 years at the same institution.[31] In a Washington University Medical Center series evaluating 57 pregnant women with thyroid nodules using FNAB, 67% were found to have benign nodules, 21% had a papillary carcinoma, 3% had follicular carcinoma and 9% of the aspirates were suspicious of malignancy.[32] The largest series describing the histopathology of thyroid nodules in pregnant patients came from Mount Sinai Hospital in Toronto. Over 15 years, 61 patients underwent fine needle biopsy followed by surgical exploration. Fifty of the 61 patients had a solitary nodule. Overall, 82 % of the samples were positive for neoplasia and 50 % for cancer. All but one of the cancer cases was papillary carcinoma.[33] The apparent high frequency of malignancy in thyroid nodules diagnosed during pregnancy is not necessarily evidence for biologic effects of pregnancy on thyroid nodules. It may merely reflect the more complete and frequent physical examination provided to pregnant women and the fact that pregnant women with firm thyroid nodules are more likely to undergo FNAB.

## DIAGNOSIS AND MANAGEMENT OF THYROID NODULAR DISEASE DURING PREGNANCY

The most significant difference between management of thyroid nodules in pregnant and non-pregnant patients is the absolute banning of the use of radioactive iodine. Its utilization, either for thyroid scans or treatment of thyroid cancer, is absolutely contraindicated during all trimesters of pregnancy and during breast-feeding.[24]

Other than that, the diagnostic, management and follow-up schemes for thyroid nodules in non-pregnant patients are applicable for pregnancy, although timing considerations should be taken into account.

Serum TSH measurement is considered by many a basic test for patients with thyroid diseases.[33] The vast majority of patients with thyroid tumors in pregnancy are, however, euthyroid.[24] TSH level can definitely serve as an indicator for thyroid suppression in pregnant patients receiving thyroxine. The gold standard in the evaluation of thyroid nodules is FNAB.[24,32,33] Most thyroid cancers in pregnancy present as palpable, non-tender solitary nodules. FNAB can be performed at any time during pregnancy even if treatment is postponed for a later stage. The safety as well as the yield of FNAB are comparable for pregnant and non-pregnant patients.[24]

Ultrasound of the neck is considered a valuable tool in the evaluation of both intra-thyroidal and regional disease. It can be safely used during pregnancy either for initial assessment or for follow-up. Although the thyroid undergoes physiologic changes during pregnancy, these do not appear to affect the features or the accuracy of sonographic evaluation.[24]

The use of CT scans during pregnancy is not desirable. MRI, on the other hand is both safe and reliable and can be used for both baseline evaluation and follow-up.

When a thyroid nodule is diagnosed in a pregnant patient before 20 weeks of gestation, FNAB is unanimously advocated.[24] There is some controversy regarding the management of such a nodule discovered after 20 weeks; while some authors advocate immediate FNAB,[34] others will perform this procedure in pregnancy only for rapidly growing nodules[35] or nodules which grow under suppressive therapy.[18] These authors believe that FNAB should be performed only "when the outcome will directly alter immediate management." Since most nodules found after 20 weeks will be operated on after delivery, through the rest of the pregnancy the patient will have to deal with an anxiety derived from "a diagnosis for which no therapy is going to be immediately instituted."[35]

If FNAB is performed and cytology is benign (as occurs in the majority of pregnant patients), the patient should be reassured and real time ultrasound can serve for monitoring of nodule growth during pregnancy. Thyroxine suppressive therapy is not a common practice for such nodules. If a follicular adenoma or Hürthle cell adenoma are suspected, neck exploration is recommended postpartum.[33]

If FNAB yields cellular cytology, even without atypia a careful monitoring of the growth of the nodule is advocated. For very anxious patients diagnosed before 20 weeks, surgery can be offered in the second trimester.[33]

For papillary or follicular carcinomas, neck exploration is usually recommended at the "soonest safe date."[25] This refers to the 22nd through 26th week for tumors diagnosed in the first and early second trimester or the immediate postpartum period for tumors diagnosed later in gestation. The patient should be reassured that thyroidectomy and even neck dissection at midtrimester do not carry significant risks for the fetus and that maternal complications are comparable to non-pregnant patients. If cancer is diagnosed early in pregnancy but the patient declines surgery, deferment of intervention until after labor is an option, supported by a recent study by Moosa and Mazzaferri.[36] These authors compared 61 pregnant patients with differentiated thyroid cancer with 598 age-matched controls and found no differences in the natural history and prognostic parameters between the two groups. The conclusion from this study was that "there are no compelling reasons to perform thyroidectomy during pregnancy even for more bulky or advanced tumors." Still, most patients would find it stressful to bear the thought of an untreated cancer throughout gestation. Also, intervention performed immediately postpartum may be perceived by the parents-to-be as an interference with the initial bonding between the mother and her offspring.

The criteria used to determine the extent of surgical intervention and the need for thyroxine suppressive therapy in non-pregnant patients apply to pregnant patients as well. Monitoring the degree of thyroid suppression is based upon serum TSH levels. The therapeutic doses of thyroxine in pregnant patients may be higher than in non-pregnant patients, although in rare cases the dose should be reduced because of tachycardia.[37]

Luckily, reports of medullary or undifferentiated cancers in pregnant patients are very scarce, since these tumors predominantly affect an older age group. Because of the aggressive nature of these tumors, the "luxury" of deferring surgery to a safe date for the fetus does not exist. When medullary carcinoma is diagnosed, surgery should immediately follow at any gestational age. For cases of undifferentiated carcinoma prognosis is almost invariably grave. If surgery is indicated for palliation, it should be immediately performed. Prior to the commencement of chemotherapy and radiotherapy, pregnancy should be terminated regardless of gestational age.

## Prognosis

The behavior and prognosis of thyroid cancer diagnosed in pregnant women do not appear to differ from that of comparable non-pregnant controls (matched for age, histologic type and stage at diagnosis). In the Toronto series, during a follow up period of 1 to 15 years, there was no evidence of recurrent malignancy or mortality for papillary thyroid cancer diagnosed during pregnancy.[33]

## PRECONCEPTIONAL COUNSELING FOR PATIENTS WITH THYROID TUMORS

Ideally, a woman should plan a pregnancy when her health is at its optimal status. This means that diagnostic procedures for uninvestigated lesions are performed and appropriate therapy for coexisting illnesses implemented prior to conception. Thyroid tumors are no exception to the rule and ought to be fully investigated and treated before pregnancy. However, if a woman with thyroid cancer conceives before therapy is completed, pregnancy may be allowed to continue unless other indications for abortion, (such as an exposure to radioiodine or a need for adjuvant radiotherapy or chemotherapy) exist. This is based on evidence for the lack of adverse effects of pregnancy on the course of thyroid cancer in patients who conceived before completing therapy.[24]

There are no clear guidelines in the literature regarding the desired length of a disease-free interval between thyroid cancer and a subsequent pregnancy. However, patients with a history of thyroid cancer can

be reassured that a future pregnancy is not considered a promoting factor for cancer recurrence.

## PRIMARY HYPERPARATHYROIDISM DURING PREGNANCY

### The Parathyroid Gland and Calcium Metabolism During Pregnancy

Typical to pregnancy is a decrease in serum calcium, which can be attributed to several factors; the most significant one is the increasing transport of calcium to the fetus which is most prominent during the third trimester. Maternal serum albumin also decreases, resulting in a decrease in total calcium. The expansion of maternal extracellular volume and an increase in urinary calcium loss are two additional contributing factors. Protein-bound serum calcium is predominantly affected while ionic calcium usually demonstrates only a minimal decrease.

As a consequence of the decrease in serum calcium, maternal parathyroid hormone (PTH) increases. This increase brings about an increase in $1,25(OH)_2D$ and a decrease in serum phosphorous.[38]

All these pregnancy-induced changes are prominent enough to obscure the classic presentation of hyperparathyroidism in non-pregnant patients—asymptomatic hypercalcemia.[38]

### Histopathology

Hyperparathyroidism during pregnancy is rare, and pregnant women usually represent a very small fraction of the total number of patients treated for this disease.[39] As in non-pregnant patients, a single parathyroid is most likely to be found as the cause of hyperparathyroidism,[38] although hyperplasia and carcinoma have been reported.[40,41]

### Clinical Presentation

During pregnancy, there is a degree of protection in the mother against hypercalcemia provided by calcium transport across the placenta.[38] The large amounts of calcium depress the fetal parathyroid function and result in fetal hypoparathyroidism. After delivery, when maternal calcium is no longer available, neonatal tentany develops as a consequent of hypercalcemia and this, in fact, is the most common presenting sign for maternal hyperparathyroidism in pregnancy.[11] Additional fetal complications described in mothers with hyperparathyroidism include abortion, prematurity, intrauterine growth restriction and stillbirth.[39]

While many pregnant women are asymtomatic, presenting symptoms of hyperparathyroidism can include muscle weakness, abdominal symptoms, disorientation and even coma and death.[40] Pre-eclampsia, osteoporosis, peptic ulcer and pancreatitis have all been described in conjunction with hyperparathyroidism during pregnancy.[40] It is important to remember that even in a previously asymptomatic pregnant patient a hypercalcemic crisis can occur. The immediate postpartum period is especially vulnerable for such a crisis to occur, when calcium is no longer transferred to the fetus.

## Diagnosis

As previously mentioned, the diagnosis of primary hyperparathyroidism in pregnancy is often made postpartum, as the neonate develops tetany. Occasionally, high serum calcium levels are picked up during a routine perinatal screening. While total serum calcium levels above 10.5 mg/dl confirm the diagnosis of primary hyperparathyroidism, it cannot be ruled out in a pregnant patient when the levels are normal or only slightly elevated. In such cases ionized serum calcium should be measured. The diagnosis is then confirmed by finding inappropriately elevated PTH concentrations as well as an increase in urinary nephrogenic cyclic AMP (camp) levels.[38]

Because of the potential for severe consequences of hyperparathyroidism to the mother and the fetus, a physician should maintain a high index of suspicion and refrain from automatically considering lethargy, nausea and vomiting normal manifestations of pregnancy.

Imaging techniques that can be safely applied for further evaluation include ultrasonography of the neck and MRI.

## Treatment

The risk of obstetrical complications has been shown to be significantly greater in women who do not undergo surgery for hyperparathyroidism while pregnant.[40] Even so, some controversy exists regarding the true necessity of surgical therapy in milder cases. Gelister et al, as well as others,[41,42] believe that neonatal hypocalcemia is transient and treatable while maternal disease can be successfully controlled medically when the diagnosis is already known. The opposite opinion is that regardless of the severity of symptoms, all pregnant patients with hyperparathyroidism should undergo neck exploration in order to prevent the array of maternal and fetal complications.[43]

All authors agree that in severely symptomatic patients surgery should not be postponed until after delivery. The ideal time for parathyroidectomy is the second trimester, when chances of pregnancy loss or premature labor as a consequence of surgical interventions are minimal.[43] If the diagnosis is made during the third trimester, surgery can usually be postponed until after labor. Preoperative hypercalcemia can be successfully controlled with fluids, diuretics and orally administered phosphate. Mithramycin, an antineoplastic agent, should be avoided during pregnancy as it is highly toxic to the fetal bone marrow, liver and kidney. In the most severe cases hemodialysis may be necessary.[38] The consideration employed to determine the extent of the surgical procedure in nonpregnant patients apply to pregnancy as well. In more than 80% of cases a single parathyroid adenoma should be anticipated. In 18–19% of cases hyperplasia will be found although carcinoma is very rare, occurring only in 1–2%, which limits its reports in the literature to a very few cases.[39]

Parathyoidectomy complications in pregnant women are infrequent and resemble those in non-pregnant patiets. Postoperative hypocalcemia is easily managed with calcium supplementation. Vocal cord paralysis secondary to recurrent laryngeal nerve injury may also occur.

## References

1. Burrow GN. Thyroid status in normal pregnancy. *J Clin Endocrin Metab*. 1990;71:274–275.
2. Ballabio M, Nicolini U, Jowett T, et al. Maturation of thyroid function in normal human foetuses. *Clin Endocrinol (Oxf)*. 1989;31: 565–571.
3. Glinoer D, Lemone M. Goiter in pregnnancy: a new insight into an old problem. *Thyroid*. 1992;2:65–70.
4. Burrow GN, Fisher DA, Larsen PR. Mechanism of disease: maternal and fetal thyroid function. *N Engl J Med*. 1994; 331(15): 1072–1078.
5. Mandel SJ, Larsen PR, Seely EW, et al. Increased need for thyroxine during pregnancy in women with primary hypothyroidism. *N Engl J Med*. 1990;323:91–96.
6. Yoshimura M, Hershman JM. Thyrotropic action of human chorionic gonadotropin. *Thyroid*. 1995; 5:425–429.
7. Rajatanavin R, Chailurkit L, Srisupandit S, et al. Trophoblastic hyperthyroidism: clinical and biochemical features of five cases. *Am J Med*. 1988; 85:237–241.
8. Ballabio M, Poshyachinda M, Ekins RP. Pregnancy-induced changes in thyroid function: role of human chorionic gonadotropin as putative regulator of maternal thyroid. *J Clin Endocrinol Metab*. 1991;73:824–831.
9. Loaroyd DL, Fung HYM, McCregor AM. Postpartum thyroid dysfuction. *Thyroid*. 1992;2:73–80.
10. Brent GA. Maternal thyroid function: interpretation of thyroid function tests in pregnancy. *Clin Obstet Gynecol*. 1997; 40(1): 3–15.
11. Obergon MJ, Mallol J, Pastor R, et al. l-Thyroxine and 3,5,3'-triiodo-l-thyronine in rat embryos before onset of fetal thyroid function. *Endocrinol*. 1984;114:305–307.
12. Liu H, Momotani N, Yoshimura NJ, et al. Maternal hypothyroidism during early pregnancy and intellectual development in the progeny. *Arch Intern Med*. 1994;154:785–787.

13. Fisher DA, Polk DH. Development of the thyroid. *Baillieres Clin Endocrinol Metab.* 1989;3:627–657.

14. Becks GP, Burrow GN. Diagnosis and treatment of thyroid disease during pregnancy. In: Degroot LJ, *Endocrinology.* 3rd ed. Philadelphia: Saunders; 1995. 799–820.

15. Medvei VC. *A history of endocrinology.* Boston: MTP Press; 1982:57.

16. Glinoer D, de Nayer P, Bourdoux P. Regulation of maternal thyroid during pregnancy. *J Clin Endocrinol Metab.* 1990; 71:276–287.

17. Emerson CH. Thyroid disease during and after pregnancy. In: Braverman L, Utiger R, eds. *The Thyroid.* 6th ed. Philadelphia: J.B. Lippincott; 1991: 1263–1280.

18. Mazzaferri EL. Evaluation and management of common thyroid disorders in women. *Am J Obstet Gynecol.* 1997;176(3):507–514.

19. Gorman CA. Radioiodine and pregnancy. *Thyroid.* 1999;9(7):721–728.

20. Salvi M, How J. Pregnancy and autoimmune thyroid disease. *Endocrinol Metab Clin North Am.* 1987;16:431–444.

21. Davis CE, Lucas MJ, Hankins GVD, et al. Thyrotoxicosis complicating pregnancy. *Am J Obstet Gynecol.* 1989; 160:63–70.

22. Cunnigham FG, McDonald PC, Gant NF, et al. Endocrine disorders. In: *Williams Obstetrics.* 20th ed. Stanford, CT: Appleton & Lange: 1993:1223–1227.

23. Seely BL, Burrow GN. Thyroid disease and pregnancy. In: Creasy RB, Resnik R, eds. *Maternal Fetal Medicine—Principles and Practice.* 3rd ed. Philadelphia: Saunders; 1994:979–996.

24. Morris PC. Thyroid cancer complicating pregnancy. *Obstet Gynecol Clin No Am.* 1998;25(2):401–408.

25. Hay ID. Nodular thyroid disease diagnosed during pregnancy: how and when to treat. *Thyroid.* 1999;9(7):667–675.

26. Paoff B, Preston MS, Mack WJ. Case control study of maternal risk factors for thyroid cancer in young women. *Cancer Causes Control.* 1995; 6:389–397.

27. Galanti M, Lam M, Eckbaum A. Risk of thyroid cancer. *Cancer. Causes Control.* 1995;6:37–44.

28. Jacklic B, Rushin J, Ghosh B. Estrogen and progesterone receptors in thyroid lesions. *Am J Surg Oncol.* 1995; 2:429–434.

29. Hill C, Clark R, Wolf M. The effects of subsequent pregnancy on patients with thyroid carcinoma. *Surg Gynecol Obstet.* 1966;122: 1219–1224.

30. Rosvoll R, Winship T. Thyroid Carcinoma and Pregnancy. *Surg Gynecol Obstet.* 1965;121:1038–1045.

31. Tan GH, Gharib H, Goellner JR, et al. Management of thyroid nodules in pregnancy. *Arch Intern Med.* 1996; 156:2317–2320.

32. Marley EF, Oertel YC. Fine-needle aspiration of thyroid lesions in 57 pregnant and postpartum women. *Diag Cytopathol.* 1997;16: 122–128.

33. Rosen IB, Korman M, Walfish PG. Thyroid nodular disease in pregnancy: Current diagnosis and management. *Clin Obstet Gynecol.* 1997; 40(1): 81–89.

34. Walfish PG. Single thyroid nodule. In: Krieger DJ, Bardin E, ed. In: *Current Therapy In Endocrinology and Metabolism 1985-1986.* Philadelphia: BC Decker; 1985:79–86.

35. Doherty C. Shindo M, Rice D, et al. Management of thyroid nodules during pregnancy. *Laryngoscope.* 1995;105:251–255.

36. Moosa M, Mazzaferri EL. Outcome of differentiated thyroid cancer diagnosed in pregnant women. *J Clin Endocrinol Metab.* 1997; 82:2862–2866.

37. Wonsick C, McDougall R. Thyroid cancer in pregnant patients: diagnosis and therapeutic management. *Thyroid.* 1994;4(4):433–440.

38. Nader S. Other endocrine disorders. Creasy RB, Resnik R, eds. In: *Maternal Fetal Medicine—Principals and Practice.* 3rd ed. Philadelphia: Saunders; 1994:1004–1026.

39. Kort KC, Schiller HJ, Numann PJ. Hyperparathyroidism and pregnancy. *Am J Surg.* 1999;177(1):66–68.

40. Kristofferson A, Dhalgren S, Lithner F, et al. Primary hyperparathyroidism and pregnancy. *Surgery.* 1985;97:326–330.

41. Gelister JSK, Sanderson JB, Chapple CR, et al. Management of hyperparathyroidism in pregnancy. *Br J Surg.* 1989;76:1207–1208.

42. Lowe DK, Orwoll ES, McClung MR, et al. Hyperparathyroidism and pregnancy. *Am J Surg.* 1983; 145:611–614.

43. Nudelman J, Deutsch A, Sternberg A, et al. The treatment of hyperparathyroidism during pregnancy. *Br J Surg.* 1984;71:217–218.

# Medical Management of Hypercalcemia Caused by Hyperparathyroidism

Ronald P. Monsaert, M.D., F.A.C.P.
Phillip K. Pellitteri, D.O., F.A.C.S.

## GENERAL CONSIDERATIONS

Parathyroid surgery is generally not recommended in patients who do not meet any acknowledged surgical indications, as discussed in Chapter 35. In patients who do not receive surgical intervention, serum calcium measurements should be performed every 6 months, whereas bone densitometry and urinary calcium excretion should be evaluated annually. Prolonged immobilization should be avoided and these patients should be encouraged to maintain good hydration and avoid thiazide diuretics. This discussion offers a perspective on medical therapy for patients with asymptomatic and symptomatic hyperparathyroidism. Other etiologies of elevated serum calcium less commonly encountered by the surgeon are discussed in the context of the differential diagnosis of hypercalcemia, as presented in Chapter 31.

## SYMPTOM COMPLEX

Oftentimes the onset of hypercalcemia is insidious and thus may not be recognized by the patient or family. The symptoms of hypercalcemia are similar in all patients whatever the etiology of the hypercalcemia. The severity of symptoms is usually proportionate to the degree of hypercalcemia, although older patients may have more prominent symptoms compared to a younger cohort with equal degrees of hypercalcemia. In general, all patients have some symptoms once the serum calcium reaches 12.5 mg/dl or greater.

Symptoms may vary from patient to patient but often fatigue is the earliest and most frequent symptom noted. Because hypercalcemia aggravates neuromuscular function, myopathic symptoms (usually proximal muscle weakness) can be prominent. Hypercalcemia decreases intravascular volume by not only causing an osmotic diuresis but may also cause nephrogenic diabetes insipidus. Thus patients may have polydipsia, polyuria and orthostatic symptoms. Azotemia may occur as a result of dehydration and nephrotoxic effects of the hypercalcemia. Gastrointestinal symptoms are common and include nausea, vomiting, constipation and abdominal pain. Pancreatitis may occur also. Mental status changes range from depression to coma depending on the severity of the hypercalcemia.

## TREATMENT CONSIDERATIONS

A limited number of general management schemes may be used to treat hypercalcemia. Expansion of intravascular volume by hydration together with the administration of loop diuretics should enhance urinary calcium excretion. Pharmaceuticals which reduce osteoclastic bone resorption such as the bisphosphonates calcitonin and plicamycin may be employed for various clinical settings.

The type of treatment employed generally depends upon the severity of the hypercalcemia and resultant clinical setting. In patients not fulfilling any criteria for surgery and in the absence of any circumstances that would make the patient no longer suitable for medical monitoring as described above, no treatment is recommended except adequate hydration and avoidance of thiazide diuretics and immobilization. Estrogens have a theoretical advantage of potentially lowering serum calcium while providing known beneficial effects on bone in the prevention of osteoporosis in postmenopausal women. The potential for development of malignancies of the uterus and breast with estrogen use limits the practicality of this approach to reduce calcium levels. In addition, estrogen use may raise levels of parathyroid hormone (PTH). Considering these variables, estrogen should be used cautiously in these patients and if needed to control calcium levels, surgical exploration should be advocated.

For patients in whom calcium levels are 12 mg/dl or less, enhancement of urinary calcium excretion should be the initial approach. Most patients in this category are volume depleted as a result of the loss of water resulting from hypercalciuria. Volume correction with appropriate oral intake of salt and fluids will most often correct the serum calcium level. Diuresis should be implemented carefully in these patients as the use of diuretics may worsen volume depletion and exacerbate hypercalcemia. If diuresis is warranted to enhance calciuria, loop diuretics such as furosemide may be used. Thiazide compounds, which may worsen hypercalcemia, are to be avoided.

The use of oral phosphate salts has been advocated in the treatment of mild hypercalcemia in controlled situations.[1] This approach may lower the serum calcium by up to 1 mg/dl through a series of complex mechanisms involving decreased calcium absorption from the gut, decrease in circulating 1,25 dihydroxyvitamin D and the reciprocal lowering of serum calcium by increasing serum levels of phosphorus. Chronic usage has the disadvantage of poor gastrointestinal tolerance, increasing PTH levels and the development of soft tissue calcifications, all of which limit the use of oral phosphates in primary hyperparathyroidism. Bisphosphonates conceptually offered an alternative in treatment for mild hypercalcemia caused by primary hyperparathyroidism but thus far have not provided for a substantial reduction in serum calcium levels. They appear to transiently lower serum calcium concentrations while effecting a rise in PTH levels.[2]

Long-term medical management of hypercalcemia in patients with mild hyperparathyroidism or those in whom surgery may carry unacceptable risk remains problematic. Direct reduction of parathyroid hormone levels by manipulating the calcium sensing receptors on parathyroid cells has ushered in a new class of pharmaceuticals called calcimimetic agents.[3,4] These agents act at the level of the parathyroid cell calcium receptor as a G-protein, such that when coupled with the receptor, the receptor G-protein complex recognizes calcium as its ligand.[5] In the presence of increased extracellular calcium, the receptor complex is activated, which results in a signal to the cell via a G-protein transducing pathway to raise intracellular calcium, thus inhibiting PTH secretion. One such calcimimetic agent is R-568, which was found to increase cytoplasmic calcium and reduce PTH secretion in vitro.[4] Further investigational experience was noted in postmenopausal women with primary hyperparathyroidism where administration of R-568 resulted in decreased PTH secretion and reduced serum calcium concentrations.[3] Larger clinical trials will further clarify the therapeutic potential of these calcimimetic compounds but it appears that they may offer a therapeutic alternative to parathyroidectomy in the long-term management of hypercalcemia, especially in patients with mild hyperparathyroidism or those in whom surgery is contraindicated or not possible, ie, parathyroid carcinoma.

Management of the hypercalcemia from primary hyperparathyroidism utilizing dietary manipulations is controversial. It has been customary to advise limiting intake of calcium through the diet so as not to exacerbate the hypercalcemia. This recommendation is complicated by the finding that restriction of dietary intake of calcium may result in rises in PTH levels in normal subjects.[6] Patients with primary hyperparathyroidism may demonstrate a rise in PTH levels with strict restriction of dietary calcium, whereas dietary increases in calcium have been shown to depress levels of PTH in these patients.[7] Levels of 1,25 dihydroxyvitamin D will also influence the response in PTH levels to dietary intake of calcium. Whereas patients in whom 1,25 dihydroxyvitamin D levels are normal will not exhibit a change in urinary calcium excretion with elevated dietary intake of calcium, those with elevated levels of vitamin D will demonstrate hypercalciuria. Thus, patients with hyperparathyroidism and elevated levels of 1,25 dihydroxyvitamin D should be controlled as to the intake of calcium, and those on vitamin D or analogues (ie, calcitriol) should be discontinued for a period until hypercalcemia is reduced. The administration of corticosteroids (ie, prednisone) will shorten the hypercalcemic episode if vitamin D is the etiology of the hypercalcemia.

In contrast to patients with mild to moderate hypercalcemia (< 12.0 mg/dl) who are asymptomatic, those in whom serum calcium levels are 12.5 mg/dl or greater are said to have "parathyroid storm" or "crisis" and require more urgent aggressive therapy to lower the calcium concentration. Although these patients and those who are symptomatic require surgery, they should initially be admitted to the hospital in order to decrease serum calcium concentration to a safe level in preparation for surgical exploration. Saline hydration is the first order of therapy with up to 4 liters of fluid administered intravenously over 2–6 hours of treatment provided the patient's cardiovascular system can tolerate the volume expansion. Following adequate rehydration, loop diuretics may be administered to induce diuresis together with calciuria and sodium excretion. This treatment can be expected to reduce serum calcium levels up to 2 mg/dl. Patients in whom the serum calcium levels exceed 14 mg/dl should also receive agents that inhibit osteoclast function, provided intravascular volume is restored following initial diuresis. Pamidronate (60–90 mg), a bisphosphonate, may be infused over 24 hours and salmon calcitonin (4 IU/Kg) may be administered subcutaneously or intramuscularly every 12 hours. One may expect to encounter tachyphylaxis to calcitonin within several days. Responsiveness during prolonged acute therapy may be boosted by the concomitant administration of corticosteroids. Plicamycin (25 mcg/kg), a tumoricidal antibiotic originally used to treat embryonal cell carcinoma of the testes, may also be administered by infusion over 4–6 hours to acutely decrease calcium levels. Administration of these additional agents may be expected to lower the serum calcium to normal levels within 24–48 hours. Once normocalciuria has been restored, parathyroidectomy should proceed without delay before hypercalcemia returns.

## PARATHYROID CARCINOMA

Inoperable patients with parathyroid carcinoma require a maintenance regimen in order to palliate disease and prevent serious metabolic disturbances secondary to hypercalcemia. In contrast to the treatment of acute hypercalcemia of benign parathyroid etiology, these patients should be placed on the therapeutic agents described above earlier in the course of treatment as there is generally a lag period before optimum activity is achieved. Calcitonin, with or without corticosteroids, pamidronate and plicamycin (as described above) are all potential agents for use in patients with parathyroid carcinoma and intractable hypercalcemia. Plicamycin should be used with caution as it has significant serious hepato- and nephrotoxicity in addition to local irritative and thrombocytopenic effects.

## CONCLUSION

The endocrine surgeon may encounter hypercalcemia not only in patients with hyperparathyroidism awaiting surgery, but also in postsurgical patients who are iatrogenically hypoparathyroid and who become hypercalcemic on their medications. Hypercalcemia can be a life-threatening condition and thus recognition of its symptoms and prompt appropriate treatment are essential.

Medical therapy of hypercalcemia is dependent upon the surgical status of the patient, the symptom complex and the degree of hypercalcemia. Volume expansion with accompanying loop diuretic-induced diuresis is the initial modality of therapy employed for a mild condition, whereas more significant or symptomatic hypercalcemia demands urgent therapy with additional agents followed by surgery. Patients with parathyroid carcinoma deserve special attention because of the serious metabolic disturbances which occur consequent to the degree of hypercalcemia associated with this disorder. Calcimimetic agents hold promise as a potential long-term medical alternative to surgery.

## References

1. Broadus AE, Mogel JS, Mallete AE, et al. A detailed evaluation of oral phosphate therapy in selected patients with primary hyperparathyroidism. *J Clin Endo Metab.* 1983;56:953–961.
2. Reasner CA, Stone MD, Hoskin DJ, et al. Acute changes in calcium homeostasis during treatment of primary hyperparathyroidism with risedronate. *J Clin Endocrinol Metab.* 1993;77:1067–1071.
3. Silverberg SJ, Bone HG, Marriott TB, et al. Short-term inhibition of parathyroid hormone secretion by a calcium-receptor agonist in patients with primary hyperparathyroidism. *N Engl J Med.* 1997;337:1506–1510.
4. Collins MT, Skarulis MC, Bilezikian JP, Silverberg SJ. Treatment of hypercalcemia secondary to parathyroid carcinoma with a novel calcimimetic agent. *J Clin Endocrinol Metab.* 1998;93:1083–1088.
5. Brown EM, Pollak M, Seidman CE. Calcium ion sensing cell surface receptors. *N Engl J Med.* 1995;333:234–240.
6. Barger-Lux MJ, Heaney RP. Effects of calcium restriction on metabolic characteristics of pre-menopausal women. *J Clin Endocrinol Metab.* 1993;76:103–107.
7 Insogna KL, Mitnick ME, Stewart AF, et al. Sensitivity of the parathyroid hormone 1,25-dihydroxyvitamin-D axis to variations in calcium intake in patients with primary hyperparathyroidism. *N Engl J Med.* 1985;313:1126–1130.

# Index